TEXTBOOK OF DIAGNOSTIC RADIOLOGY

VOLUME 1: IMAGING PRINCIPLES AND CLINICAL PERSPECTIVES

Farid Ezat

ALLIED HEALTH PRESS

Textbook of Diagnostic Radiology

Volume 1: Imaging Principles and Clinical Perspectives

Author: **Farid Ezat**

Allied Health Press
4164 Lakeshore Road
Burlington ON L7L 1A4
Canada
www.alliedhealthpress.com
Email: orders@arclereducation.com

ISBN: 978-1-77956-783-3

ABOUT THE AUTHOR

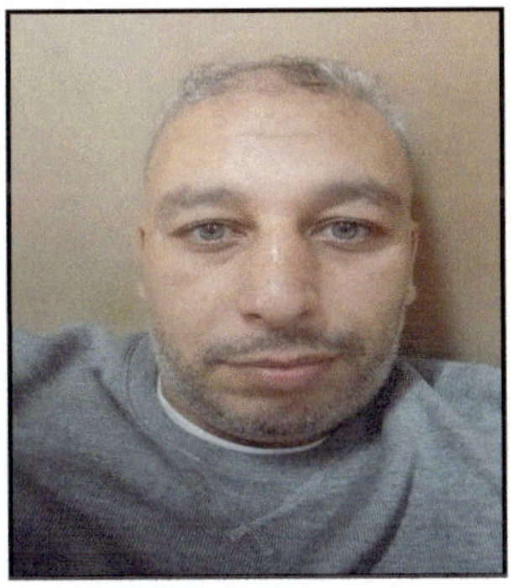

Farid ezat is a dedicated medical doctor with a diverse background in radiology, general practice, and research. Currently serving as a consultant teleradiologist for teleradiology solution , Bangaluru , India , He meticulously analyzes radiological images and engages in research. Previously, Farid honed his clinical skills as a General Practitioner in Alexandria main university hospitals. Farid's academic journey includes earning his Master degree from the Alexandria university ", Faculty of Medicine in Egypt. Committed to continuous learning, Farud actively participates in extracurricular activities and preparing for final FRCR exam.

Brief Table of Contents

Chapter Openers

A list of Chapter Outline is presented providing a brief Introduction to what will be covered in the chapter.

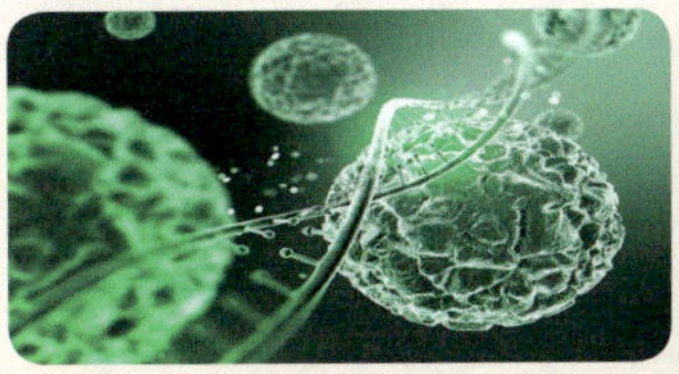

LEARNING OBJECTIVES

After studying this chapter, you will be able to:

1. Discuss the scientific method in biology;
2. Explain the cell theory;
3. Discuss the genetics and heredity;
4. Evolution and natural selection;
5. Focus on ecology and ecosystems;
6. Learn about human biology;
7. Evaluate the plant biology;
8. Explain the microbiology;
9. Focus on current trends in biology.

Introduction

Often referred to as the science of life, biology is a broad field of study aimed at comprehending the several kinds of life on Earth, from tiny creatures to sophisticated multicellular entities. Comprising several subfields, including molecular biology, ecology, and evolutionary biology, each of which advances our knowledge of living systems, this field clarifies the mechanisms controlling life events, including development, reproduction, and interaction with the surroundings, which is the central goal of biology. Moreover, biology fills in the void between the natural sciences and medicine by offering a necessary understanding of health, illness, and the interactions between organisms and their environments. Dealing with urgent global issues such as climate change, biodiversity loss, and new diseases depends on an awareness of these complex biological interactions, therefore highlighting the critical part biology plays in modern civilization. Fundamentally, biology explores and tests ideas about the living world using the scientific method. Through methodical observation and experimentation,

1.1. The Scientific Method in Biology

Learning Outcome

1. Describe the steps of the scientific method;
2. Focus on hypothesis formation;
3. Learn about experimental design.

Learning Outcomes

The beginning of each section of every chapter contains a set of Learning Outcomes that inform students of concepts they should understand. These outcomes help students understand what they should be able to do if they have mastered the material in that section.

Test Your Knowledge

Throughout each chapter, Test Your Knowledge cues you to note which topics have been covered and to self-test your understanding of the material presented.

Test Your Knowledge

1. Explain why correlation does not imply causation in scientific experiments.
2. How does the scientific method help reduce the influence of personal opinions in research?

Chapter Summary

The Summary Section appear at the end of each chapter and summarize main concepts covered throughout the chapter. These points provide key concepts in an engaging and meaningful way.

Summary

The investigation of biological principles highlights the importance of a comprehensive view of life by reflecting the intricate interactions that occur within living systems. The complexity of biology goes beyond individual species or systems, as this essay highlights; it also includes the interactions that mold ecosystems and affect biodiversity. Researchers can conduct in-depth analyses of metabolomic data using sophisticated technologies like MetaboAnalyst, which offer insights into the molecular mechanisms underlying these interactions. As demonstrated by the developments in MetaboAnalyst, for example, the integration of diverse omics data promotes a thorough understanding of metabolic pathways and helps identify important biological markers necessary for research on development and disease (Chong et al., 2018). Additionally, the phenomenon of ecological invasions is a key component of biological research and a vital field of study. The introduction of non-native species into unfamiliar habitats has significant ramifications and calls for multidisciplinary management strategies. Examining the origins and effects of these biological incursions, invasion science has become a crucial field that highlights the need to comprehend ecological dynamics and community interactions. As interest in biological invasions increases, new findings are emerging that put conventional ecological theories and practices to the test. The importance of incorporating various scientific viewpoints is shown by this developing discipline, which also highlights how invasive species shape ecosystems and advances our knowledge of ecological resilience (David et al., 2013). When taken as a whole, these discoveries from invasion science and metabolomics highlight the value of multidisciplinary biology research. Fostering cross-disciplinary collaboration and utilizing technological breakthroughs to improve our comprehension of intricate biological interactions are crucial as we look to the future of biological research. In addition to deepening our understanding of the complexities of life, this method lays the groundwork for tackling urgent environmental issues. Future studies can ensure the continued relevance of biology in a world that is constantly changing by acknowledging the interconnection of biological systems and opening the door to creative solutions that support sustainability and biodiversity conservation. We might imagine a thorough comprehension of life that serves both academia and society at large through ongoing investigation and integration of scientific knowledge.

Knowledge Assessment

The chapter includes material designed to review and reinforce each content. It includes Critical Thinking Questions to help test of your understanding of information presented in the chapter and Short answer Questions to review your understanding of the key concepts presented in the chapter.

Critical Thinking Questions

1. **Who is known as the "Father of Modern Biology"?**
   a. Aristotle
   b. Charles Darwin
   c. Gregor Mendel
   d. Louis Pasteur
2. **What is the basic unit of life?**
   a. Atom
   b. Molecule
   c. Cell
   d. Organism
3. **Which branch of biology studies the interaction of organisms with their environment?**
   a. Genetics
   b. Ecology
   c. Physiology
   d. Botany
4. **Which macromolecule is the main source of energy for living organisms?**
   a. Proteins
   b. Lipids
   c. Carbohydrates
   d. Nucleic acids
5. **DNA is primarily responsible for which function in living organisms?**
   a. Energy production
   b. Protein synthesis
   c. Storing genetic information
   d. Regulating body temperature

Short Answer Questions

1. What is biology, and why is it important to study biology?
2. What are the three main domains of life, and how are they different from one another?
3. Define homeostasis and give an example of how it works in living organisms.
4. What is the cell theory, and why is it fundamental to biology?
5. How do autotrophs and heterotrophs differ in the way they obtain energy?
6. What is the scientific method, and how is it applied in biological research?
7. Discuss how biology helps address global challenges such as climate change, disease, and food security.
8. Explain the levels of biological organization from the smallest unit to the largest. Provide examples at each level.
9. Describe the relationship between structure and function in biology, giving specific examples from cells or organs.
10. How has the discovery of genetics shaped our understanding of inheritance and variation among organisms?

Supplementary Materials

Key Terms: A list of key terms is given for quick reference

KEY TERMS FROM THIS CHAPTER

Annotation enrichment analysis	Biological structure	Cell
Cell theory	Cellular structure	Ecology
Ecosystems	Genetics	Human biology
Microbiology	Natural selection	Organism
Plant biology		

Further Resources: Recommendations for additional readings, websites, and multimedia resources.

References

1. Argelaguet, R., Velten, B., Arnol, D., Dietrich, S., Zenz, T., Marioni, J. C., Buettner, F., et al. (2018). Multi-omics factor analysis—A framework for unsupervised integration of multi-omics data sets. *Molecular Systems Biology, 14*. https://doi.org/10.15252/msb.20178124.
2. Bacher, S., Blackburn, T. M., Essl, F., & Genovesi, P. (2017). *Socio-Economic Impact Classification of Alien Taxa (SEICAT).* https://core.ac.uk/download/286567949.pdf (accessed on 8th March 2025).
3. Barnett, R., Brace, S., Cucchi, T., & Dobney, K. (2013). *Divergent Evolutionary Processes Associated with Colonization of Offshore Islands.* https://core.ac.uk/download/20664364.pdf (accessed on 8th March 2025).

Detailed Table of Contents

CHAPTER 2

Radiation Physics 33

CHAPTER 3

Radiation Protection and Safety 65

CHAPTER 6

Chest Radiology 143

CHAPTER 7

Cardiovascular Imaging 175

LIST OF FIGURES

PREFACE

Diagnostic radiology is right at the heart of modern medicine, giving doctors information that is essential for them to know about the inner workings and anatomy of the human body without invasive techniques. Since the discovery of X-rays in 1895, imaging technology has moved significantly, from plain films to advanced modalities such as computed tomography (CT) and ultrasound. This imaging equipment has changed patient care by enabling early detection of disease, guiding treatment, and monitoring the results of treatment. Volume 1 of this book lays the foundation for understanding the blending of radiology with clinical practice, achieving a balance between image acquisition, interpretation, and safety measures. It addresses the physical principles of imaging, the biology of the action of ionizing radiation, and the anatomical knowledge required in making effective diagnoses.

Textbook of Diagnostic Radiology Volume 1 aims to present a comprehensive and unified summary of the science and practice of radiology. Constructed on building blocks, volume 1 presents clear explanations of the science of imaging, the technique employed to minimize risk to patients and professionals, and the anatomical landmarks that define normal and disease appearances. Through the integration of theory and case illustration, it prepares students to read studies confidently, understand the limitations of each modality, and appreciate the imaging contribution to multidisciplinary care.

The following chapters are described in detail to guide the reader through a tour of what needs to be done in radiology.

Chapter 1 presents an introduction to a focus on the history and organizational principles of radiology, illustrating how imaging is integrated into clinical decision-making, the organizational structure of a radiology department, and the mechanisms by which consistency and quality are maintained in study acquisition and reporting.

Chapter 2 describes the physics of diagnostic image formation in the context of X-ray tube design, photon–matter interactions such as photoelectric absorption and Compton scattering, and the physics of image contrast, spatial resolution, and noise behavior.

Chapter 3 explores strategies and regulations for the protection of staff and patients from unnecessary radiation exposure, including dose measurements, shielding requirements, personnel monitoring strategy, and national and international safety standards, and considers in particular dose reduction in children and pregnant women.

Chapter 4 covers the effect of ionizing radiation on living tissue, from the molecular level damage to DNA and cellular repair mechanisms through to clinical manifestations of stochastic and deterministic action of radiation, and how these principles direct diagnostic intervention as well as therapeutic application.

Chapter 5 is a thorough systematic review of normal anatomy as presented in cross-sectional and radiographic imaging, correlating appearance on plain film, CT, and ultrasound, and landmarks, variant anatomy, and the use of anatomical information in the differentiation between typical structures and pathology.

Chapter 6 deals with thoracic radiology with a description of the evaluation of lung parenchyma, airways, pleura, and mediastinum; it says patterns of pulmonary disease—e.g., consolidation, interstitial processes, nodular lesions—and describes how positioning, technique, and adjunct imaging may clarify nonspecific findings.

Chapter 7 discusses cardiovascular imaging techniques, providing protocols for CT angiography, MR angiography, and Doppler ultrasound; it explains how each of the methods is used to assess coronary artery disease, aortic disease, and peripheral vascular disease, and discusses stenosis quantification and aneurysm evaluation criteria.

Chapter 8 outlines abdominal imaging techniques, including contrast-enhanced CT and ultrasound methods for the gastrointestinal tract and abdominal organs; it addresses the selection of imaging phases, contrast media, and multiplanar reconstructions to delineate inflammatory, neoplastic, and vascular disease.

Chapter 9 addresses hepatobiliary and pancreatic imaging, such as MR cholangiopancreatography techniques, hepatobiliary scintigraphy basics, and contrast-enhanced ultrasound techniques; it draws attention to the imaging features of common pathologies such as cholangiocarcinoma, gallstones, and pancreatic tumors.

Chapter 10 shows genitourinary imaging, presenting CT urography techniques, intravenous urography basics, and pelvic ultrasound protocols; it depicts imaging criteria for renal masses, urinary tract obstruction, bladder disease, and prostatic enlargement or malignancy.

Chapter 11 illustrates practice in obstetric ultrasound, from first-trimester viability scans to full anatomic surveys in the second and third trimesters; it covers fetal biometry norms, assessment of amniotic fluid volume, placental localization, and Doppler evaluation of uteroplacental and fetal circulation.

Chapter 12 covers gynecologic imaging methods, reviewing transvaginal and transabdominal sonography, pelvic MRI protocols, and CT applications; it illustrates the imaging appearance of fibroids, endometriosis, ovarian cysts, and gynecologic cancers, and elucidates how imaging guides intervention procedures.

Chapter 13 discusses breast imaging methodologies, outlining screening and diagnostic mammography techniques, ultrasound examination of palpable and nonpalpable lesions, and breast MRI protocols; outlines lesion characterization criteria, BI RADS evaluation categories, and image-guided biopsy methods.

This text is intended for radiology residents, medical students, and allied health professionals who must have a solid background in imaging science and anatomy. Physicians desiring greater insight into radiologic reports and technologists wishing to improve practice will find the material easy to comprehend and clinically applicable immediately. Upon finishing this book, readers will have the information to interpret radiologic studies with accuracy and confidence.

FUNDAMENTALS OF RADIOLOGY

1

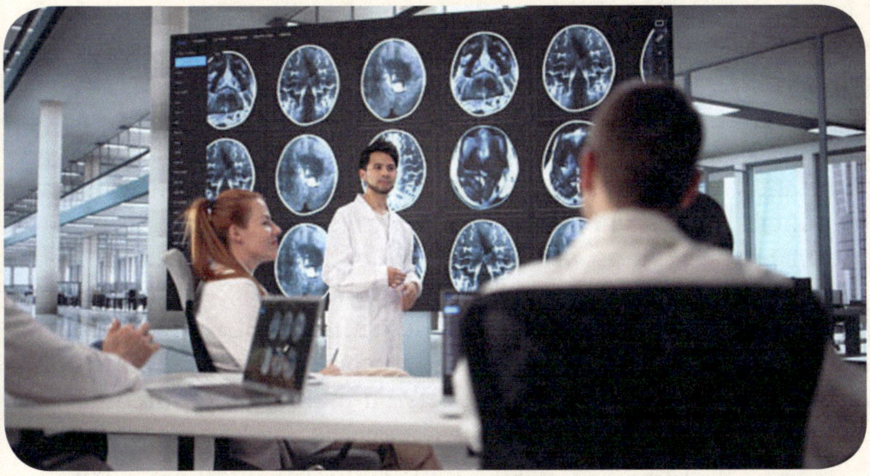

LEARNING OBJECTIVES

After studying this chapter, you will be able to:

1. Identify types of radiological imaging
2. Learn principles of radiological techniques
3. Discuss clinical applications of radiology
4. Focus on radiology and patient care

Introduction

The development of medical imaging has had a profound effect on the methods of diagnosis, permitting clinicians to obtain crucial information regarding human anatomy and disease. Radiology, an integrating discipline, employs a variety of imaging modalities to visualize internal structures without invasion, permitting accurate diagnosis and best treatment planning. Understanding the principles of radiology requires knowledge of both its technical advances and clinical uses, which span across a diversity of medical specialties. This chapter begins with investigating the fundamental principles of radiological techniques, emphasizing their use in detecting pathological conditions such as tumors and other lesions. Adding radiology to pathology and clinical data enhances diagnostic sensitivity, particularly in heavily structured anatomical regions such as the sellar region, where high-resolution imaging becomes essential in differentiating benign from malignant masses (Ugga et. al., 2023). In addition, the multidisciplinary nature of radiologic assessment mirrors broader medical complexity in the atypical conditions where combination with clinical judgement is paramount to effective management (Fêde et. al., 2021).

Definition of Radiology

Advances in medical imaging have significantly enhanced the ability to diagnose and treat a wide range of conditions, marking the ever-growing field of radiology. Radiology is basically the medical field employing various imaging techniques to visualize the body's internal structures and functions for diagnosis and therapy. These include X-rays, computed tomography (CT), magnetic resonance imaging (MRI), ultrasound, and nuclear medicine, which all provide detailed information that is vital for accurate diagnosis and treatment planning. Radiology has transitioned from traditional imaging to the integration of sophisticated computational methods, including deep learning algorithms, which improve the detection and analysis of conditions like diabetic retinopathy with excellent precision and accuracy (Gulshan *et. al.*, 2016).

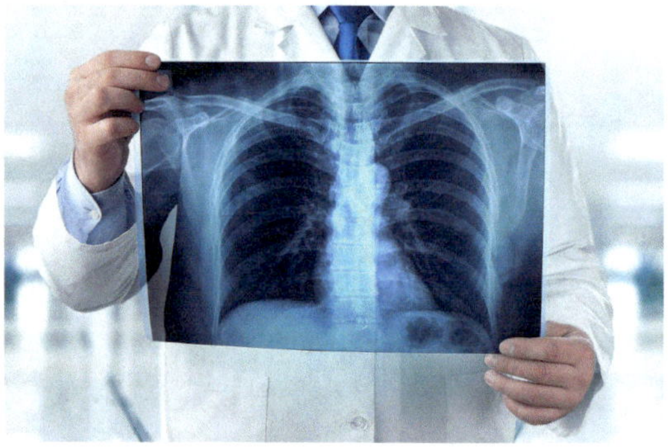

Figure 1.1. Radiology is fundamentally the branch of medicine that employs various imaging techniques to visualize the internal structures and functions of the body for diagnostic and therapeutic purposes.

Source: https://static.wixstatic.com/media/87a6fb_0fa46bf46d444d0c89bdc10aa73aa8e1~mv2.jpg/v1/fill/w_1000,h_667,al_c,q_85,usm_0.66_1.00_0.01/87a6fb_0fa46bf46d444d0c89bdc10aa73aa8e1~mv2.jpg.

Besides, radiology takes a central position in modern oncology, with advanced imaging protocols and staging systems, such as those adopted in the American Joint Committee on Cancer, taking a central place in individualized patient care and particular treatment regimens (Figure 1.1).

Importance of Radiology in Medicine

Technological advancements in medical education and assessment have further emphasized the role of competence in diagnostic technology, with radiology being an important component of patient management. Integration of imaging modalities enables accurate diagnosis, guides therapeutic interventions, and enhances perioperative care in specialties. Models of medical education, such as those developed by accrediting entities, emphasize competency-based learning (CBL) involving radiologic skills, underscoring their significant input to clinical decision-making and outcome improvement. Moreover, the evolving uses of radiology, such as ultrasound techniques, have transcended traditional boundaries, becoming critical tools for both anesthesiologists and critical care professionals alike (Mahmood *et. al.*, 2016). These developments herald a broader recognition of the value of radiology not only for diagnosis but also for real-time procedural guidance, risk assessment, and monitoring. Therefore, mastery of radiologic principles and practices is imperative for today's physicians to deliver high-quality, evidence-based healthcare.

Historical Development of Radiology

The use of technology in medical imaging has been a defining point in radiology, transforming the profession from being predominantly mechanistic to a high-tech science of diagnosis. This process gained unimaginable speed once artificial intelligence (AI) came along, with machine learning (ML) and deep learning algorithms entirely redefining image analysis, enabling greater precision in segmentation and diagnosis of medical images. The transition from traditional X-rays to AI modalities illustrates the increased functionality and increasing sophistication of radiological techniques, paralleling more universal technological trends like the handling of big data and cloud computing that have enhanced access to and interpretation of data. The history of evolutionary radiology thus involves not only technological advances but also overcoming challenges concerned with data quality, ethics, and infrastructural demands. The development of digital twins and other AI tools in medicine further underscores ongoing development in radiology towards a future in which ongoing synergy between technologists and clinicians will be crucial (Barricelli *et. al.*, 2019; Najjar, 2023).

Overview of Radiological Techniques

Advances in medical imaging have dramatically transformed diagnostic capability to enable better detection and characterization of pathological conditions. Of the many radiological modalities, contrast-enhanced ultrasonography (CEUS) with agents like Sonazoid has emerged as a key modality, particularly in hepatocellular carcinoma diagnosis, by highlighting specific imaging features such as arterial phase hyperenhancement and Kupffer phase washout to improve diagnostic performance (Jeong, 2023). Simultaneously, the introduction of ML, especially deep learning methods, to image analysis has introduced new facets to interpretation and prognosis and has found applications from image acquisition to disease prediction in imaging modalities like MRI (Selvikv *et. al.*, 2018). These innovations illustrate the dynamic nature of radiological methods, the premise that contemporary radiology is not only based on traditional imaging technology but increasingly engages computational advances to enhance image quality, automate detection, and support clinical decision-making. Overall, these advances reflect a general introduction to evolving radiological practices vital to present-day medical care.

Role of Radiologists in Healthcare

Advances in technology have profoundly impacted many areas of healthcare, with radiology setting a shining example. Radiologists serve as vital interpreters between advanced imaging technology and clinical decision-making, translating information that directly impacts patient diagnosis and treatment. In addition to interpreting images, their function is to collaborate with multidisciplinary teams to validate appropriate and timely provision of care to patients. Current implementation of AI in radiology has further enhanced the role of the radiologist by automating image segmentation, computer-aided diagnosis, and workflow efficiency, improving diagnostic accuracy and personalized medicine approaches (Najjar, 2023).

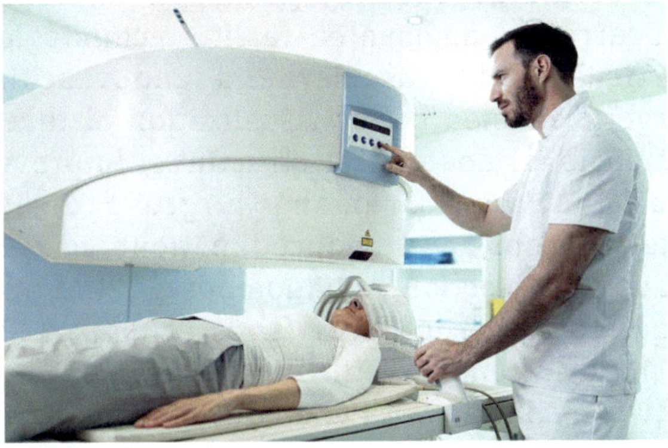

Figure 1.2. Radiologists serve as crucial intermediaries between complex imaging technologies and clinical decision-making, interpreting data that directly influences patient diagnosis and treatment.

Source: https://orthomiami.com/wp-content/uploads/2023/11/Can-Diagnostic-Imaging-Help-in-Monitoring-Treatment-Progress.jpg.

Nevertheless, this technological transformation requires radiologists to keep evolving, embracing new digital technology while following the ethical guidelines embedded in medicine. Evolution in radiology follows broader organizational trends within healthcare, with digital innovation structuring professional professions and value propositions to focus on the shifting role of the radiologist from image interpreter to engaged participant in digitally evolving healthcare systems (Wessel *et. al.*, 2021) (Figure 1.2).

Advances in Radiology Technology

The integration of state-of-the-art technologies has greatly influenced the radiology environment, enhancing both procedure effectiveness and diagnostic accuracy. Technologies such as AI and augmented reality have introduced new facets to radiology practice. AI-assisted software, like ChatGPT, provides personalized, interactive learning experiences, enabling radiologists to better understand intricate imaging information and work independently (İsmail *et. al.*, 2023). Concurrently, augmented reality technologies, particularly in vascular and endovascular surgery, enabled better visualization of three-dimensional anatomical structures, improved spatial awareness among surgeons during interventions, and reduced patient risk by reducing dissection, radiation dosage, and time required for procedures (Eves *et. al.*, 2022). Such advancements affirm an interconnection between clinical work and education, ushering in new paradigms that enhance the precision and safety of radiological procedures and facilitate continuous professional development. As processing speed and real-time imaging integration evolve, the industry stands to see even more revolutionary expansion, ultimately for the betterment of healthcare professionals and patients alike.

Ethical Considerations in Radiology

Advances in radiology, particularly with the implementation of AI, have revolutionized diagnostic capability but concurrently created urgent ethical challenges that must be carefully confronted. The promise of AI-enhanced radiology is accompanied by increased accuracy and productivity. However, it presents accompanying issues such as data confidentiality, transparency of algorithms, and accountability that are far-reaching in nature. Ethical frameworks must address the "black box" of AI systems, where it becomes challenging for clinicians to understand and account for diagnostic outputs, thus undermining patient trust and informed consent. Equitable distribution of technology and fair representation of data are also necessary to prevent unequal access to health care and differential diagnostic performance. Radiologists and teachers are increasingly being asked to provide ethical training that is focused on these topics alongside technological proficiency, thereby facilitating appropriate deployment of AI technologies in the clinical setting (Najjar, 2023; Paranjape *et. al.*, 2019). In the end, creating a culture for ongoing ethical discussion is essential to maintain patient safety and maintain the integrity of radiological practice (Figure 1.3).

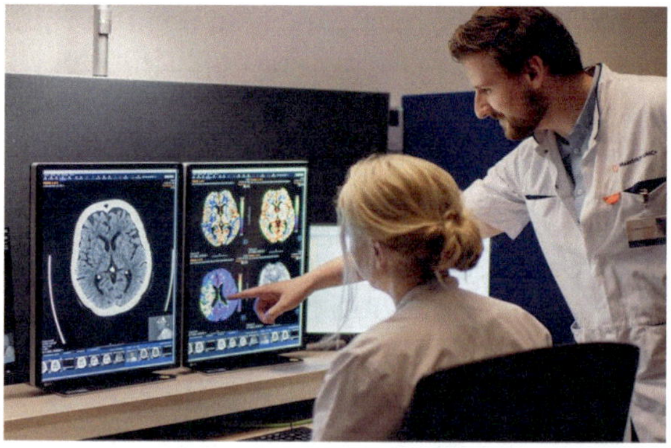

Figure 1.3. Ethical considerations in radiology.

Source: https://media.licdn.com/dms/image/v2/D4D12AQHunULH80Qkng/article-cover_image-shrink_720_1280/article-cover_image-shrink_720_1280/0/1681886001795?e=2147483647&v=beta&t=rf1mVFhZGEHbMzDz6xN0rYr5-5sNsJvwL3t3ISuu-0U.

Future Trends in Radiology

Trends in technology and growing focus on patient safety are set to define the radiology environment of the future. Emerging imaging technology aims to enhance diagnostic accuracy with reduced doses of radiation, in response to long-standing issues related to intraoperative imaging. For instance, access to more sophisticated fluoroscopy, CT, and MRI imaging offers new opportunities for limiting unnecessary radiation, thereby making interventions safer for both patients and physicians (Nathaniel *et. al.*, 2021). Paralleling the above, personalized medicine must affect radiological planning, especially through the integration of molecular and genetic information in order to tailor imaging protocols and therapy. Although these advancements are already underway in oncology, for example, novel diagnostic and therapeutic strategies for tumors like cholangiocarcinoma (Jesús *et. al.*, 2020), their translation to other aspects of radiology is full of promise. Overall, the future of radiology will hinge on the balance between technological innovation and risk reduction, ultimately improving clinical outcomes and standards of patient care.

1.1. Types of Radiological Imaging

Learning Outcome

1. Compare imaging modalities
2. Describe fluoroscopy and mammography
3. Discuss nuclear medicine
4. Explain magnetic resonance imaging (MRI)
5. Focus on X-ray imaging
6. Know interventional radiology
7. Learn ultrasound imaging
8. Understand computed tomography (CT)

An understanding of the different modalities of radiologic imaging is essential for accurate diagnosis and the best management of patients. Radiology encompasses a multitude of modalities, each with unique mechanisms, advantages, and limitations. Plain X-rays use ionizing radiation to produce images primarily of bones and dense structures, while computed tomography (CT) scans produce cross-sectional images optimized for visualization of soft tissue. Magnetic resonance imaging (MRI) employs magnetic fields and radio waves instead of ionizing radiation. It is better suited to high-resolution soft tissue contrast, making it very useful in neurological and musculoskeletal imaging. Ultrasound imaging employs high-frequency sound waves and generates real-time images with no radiation exposure and is commonly used in obstetrics and abdominal scanning. While some modalities, such as CT and PET, subject patients to high ionizing radiation, others, such as MRI and ultrasound, do not, and therefore, one needs to be cautious about the risks and benefits of radiation when applying different methods (Hoveidaei *et. al.*, 2025). Proficiency in interpreting various imaging modalities demands statistical knowledge to critically evaluate diagnostic efficacy and accuracy (Kumar *et. al.*, 2025).

1.1.1. X-Ray Imaging

Advances in radiological technology have significantly enhanced the precision and efficiency of diagnostic examinations, particularly through improved imaging methods. A prime example is X-ray imaging, still a mainstay, that provides vital information regarding the internal anatomy of the body at amazingly high speed and resolution. New technologies in free-electron laser (FEL) technology, such as the Soft X-ray Laser (SXL) at MAX IV Laboratory, will produce ultrashort and high-intensity soft X-ray pulses to enhance the capabilities of traditional X-ray techniques for scientific and medical applications (Werin *et. al.*, 2017). The new technologies have the potential to achieve improved spatial and temporal resolution that will enable improved visualization of molecular structures and soft tissues. In parallel, the inclusion of advanced information processing methods in radiology facilitates the improved interpretation of X-ray images by mitigating noise, artefacts, and physiological dynamic changes, thus facilitating more accurate diagnosis and intervention guidance (Barratt *et. al.*, 2014). Such integrated developments demonstrate the evolving role of X-ray imaging in the overall landscape of radiology, improving the accuracy of diagnosis and patient care (Figure 1.4).

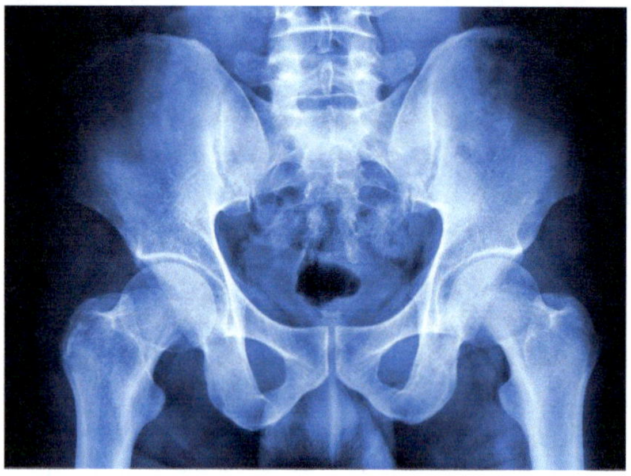

Figure 1.4. X-ray imaging.

Source: https://media.post.rvohealth.io/wp-content/uploads/2020/08/pelvis-x-ray_thumb-1-732x549.jpg.

1.1.2. Computed Tomography (CT)

Advances in imaging technology have profoundly changed diagnostic capability, with CT as a necessary modality because it can provide high-resolution cross-sectional images of the body. With X-ray beams that rotate around the patient, CT can generate volumetric data reconstructed to visualize complex anatomical structures at high resolution. The technology is founded mainly upon the interaction of X-rays with tissue and upon differential absorption and attenuation principles, which are required for differential image contrast and visibility (Vrdoljak *et. al.*, 2024). Though diagnostic benefits, the ionizing radiation typical of CTneeds to be optimized in order not to cause likely damage to patients, and this needs to be taken into serious consideration. Recent breakthroughs with the incorporation of artificial intelligence (AI) have enhanced low-dose CT scans by reducing noise and image noise degradation while preserving diagnostic performance, thus addressing safety concerns (David-Olawade *et. al.*, 2025). These breakthroughs validate the interface between physics, technology, and patient care, reiterating CT's pivotal role in contemporary radiology (Figure 1.5).

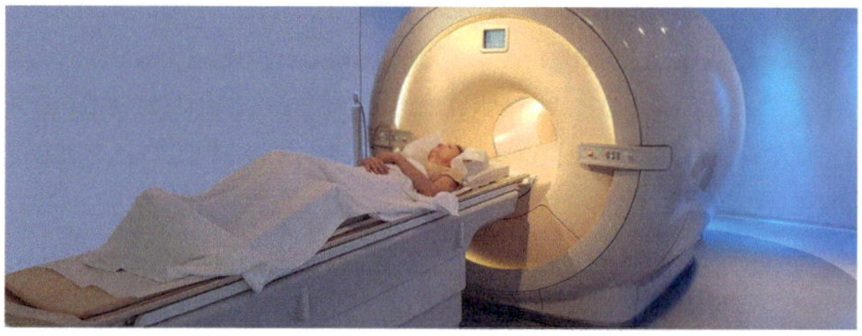

Figure 1.5. Computed tomography (CT).

Source: https://www.hopkinsmedicine.org/-/media/images/health/2_-treatment/neurology/ct-scan-of-brain-hero.jpg?h=500&iar=0&mh=500&mw=1300&w=1297&hash=F94B8AFCB5E27E8776892990B9A84FA7

1.1.3. Magnetic Resonance Imaging (MRI)

Medical imaging advances have revolutionized the potential for diagnosis, particularly by integrating MRI, which offers the best soft tissue contrast without ionizing radiation. Unlike X-rays and CT scans, MRI makes use of strong magnetic forces and radiofrequency pulses to create excellent images, and it is invaluable for assessing neurological, musculoskeletal, and cardiovascular diseases. Recent developments in AI have also further optimized MRI use through reduced image quality and acquisition times, improving patient safety and diagnostic quality without increased radiation exposure (David-Olawade *et. al.*, 2025). In neurosciences investigation as well, contrast-enhanced MRI is critical in understanding brain clearance mechanisms, with gadolinium-based contrast agents tracking cerebrospinal fluid dynamics and solute exchange between blood, brain, and CSF spaces. These observations, based on differential pharmacokinetics across routes of injection, have significant ramifications for the understanding of brain pathologies and the study of neurodegenerative disorders (Van *et. al.*, 2024). Therefore, MRI remains a cornerstone of radiology, uniting technological advancement with clinical utility in modern medicine (Figure 1.6).

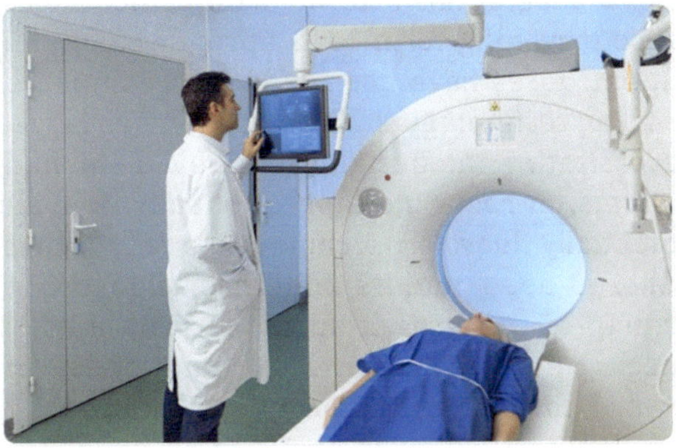

Figure 1.6. Magnetic resonance imaging (MRI).

Source: https://d2jx2rerrg6sh3.cloudfront.net/image-handler/picture/2016/11/MRI_shutterstock_509318605.jpg.

1.1.4. Ultrasound Imaging

Medical imaging technology has further revolutionized diagnostic radiology, with ultrasound imaging also playing an irreplaceable role due to its non-invasive nature and real-time capabilities. Microbubble contrast agents have further enhanced the diagnostic function of ultrasound significantly by providing improved blood flow echoes and enabling better measurement of microvascular circulation, further increasing their clinical applications, particularly in cardiology and radiology (Yusefi *et. al.*, 2022). Moreover, the novel 3-D ultrasound imaging technology surpasses established 2-D approaches through volumetric visualization, which is required in complex clinical scenarios as prenatal imaging and interventional therapy. Innovative technologies, like fast acoustic steering by tilting electromechanical reflectors (FASTER), have been incorporated to achieve low imaging volume rates with increased spatial precision, without incurring higher costs (Dong *et. al.*, 2020). These developments underscore the increasing complexity of ultrasound imaging, reaffirming its importance in radiology's fundamental procedures and its contribution to more sophisticated and faster diagnostic testing (Figure 1.7).

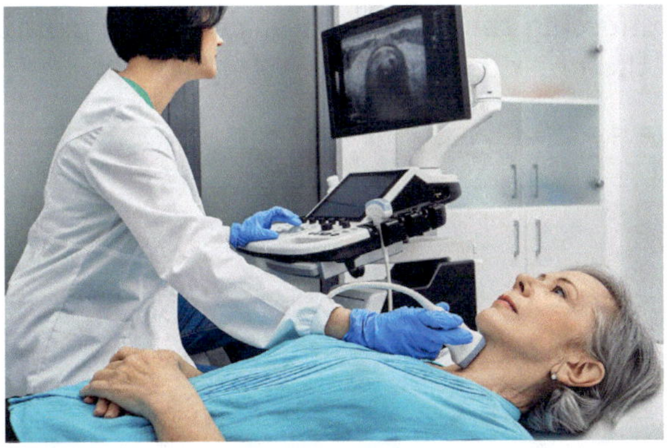

Figure 1.7. Ultrasound imaging.

Source: https://www.health.com/thmb/vh8ENHy0WGOvbZvK75-slUV2dP4=/1500x0/filters:no_upscale():max_bytes(150000):strip_icc()/Health-GettyImages-1400264257-96cad1815ad34f4794c716414fbf5efc.jpg.

1.1.5. Nuclear Medicine

Medical advancements now rely more and more upon precise diagnostic and therapeutic techniques that include the application of medicine and physics. Nuclear medicine is a subspecialty of radiology that utilizes radiopharmaceuticals to image organ function at the molecular level, making possible the early diagnosis and targeted treatment of disease. Advanced nuclear medicine practice, with safe and effective use, underscores the pivotal role of health physics professionals in providing radiation protection and adherence to regulations within medical settings (Michael *et. al.*, 2022). Enhanced demand for diagnostic precision is also underpinned by the necessity for available and reliable nuclear medicine services within multiservice delivery systems (Fleming *et. al.*, 2021). Technological advancements, workforce education, and quality control join forces to optimize nuclear medicine's potential, justifying its value within the radiologic environment. With changing diagnostic challenges, nuclear medicine serves as the prime model for blending specialized knowledge with state-of-the-art technology, thereby enhancing patient care and reinforcing the fundamental principles central to the practice of radiology (Figure 1.8).

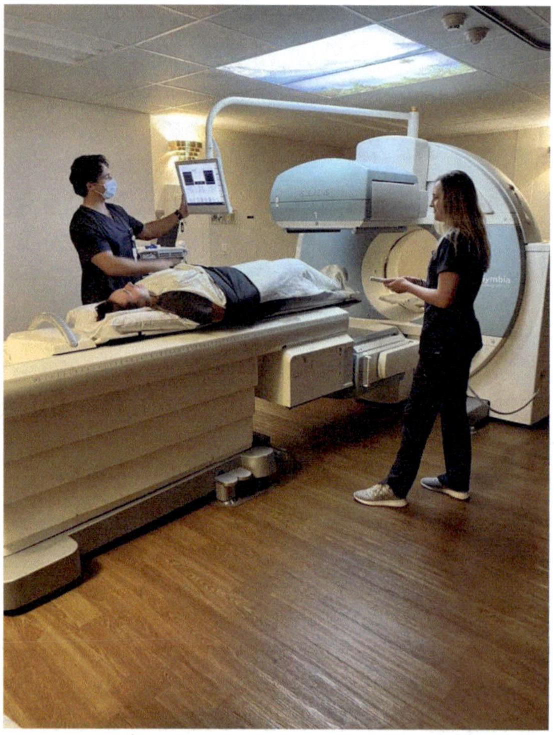

Figure 1.8. Nuclear medicine technology.

Source: https://www.uwlax.edu/globalassets/academics/programs/nuclear-medicine-technology/siemenscamera.jpg/Xlarge.

1.1.6. Fluoroscopy

The evolution of medical imaging has revolutionized interventional and diagnostic procedures, and fluoroscopy is a mainstay as it permits real-time visualization. Fluoroscopy enables physicians to image dynamic processes within the body, such as gastrointestinal motility or catheter guidance, by producing continuous X-ray images. However, the technology inherently demands the use of ionizing radiation, which is of great concern to both healthcare workers and patients. Occupational hazards include not just the risk of cataracts, cancers, and other chronic diseases due to radiation, but also a substantial rate of orthopedic disease caused by long-term lead apron wear. While patient doses have been reduced by improved imaging technology, staff protection has lagged, necessitating the design of improved shielding systems, in-room monitoring of radiation, and potentially fluoroless techniques to reduce these risks. A deep understanding of fluoroscopy principles, as presented in current medical imaging physics, underlies ongoing endeavors toward the reconciliation of maximum safety and diagnostic efficiency (Lloyd *et. al.*, 2020).

1.1.7. Mammography

Breast cancer diagnosis and detection have been significantly enhanced by improvements in imaging modalities, with early detection through mammography playing a central role. Using low-dose X-rays to create accurate images of breast tissue, mammography offers *in vivo* high-resolution visualization that is capable of identifying microcalcifications and narrow masses that would otherwise go undetected through physical exam. The technological advancement of mammographic equipment, including improvement of focal spot size and image receptor sensitivity , has enabled improved images and reduced radiation dosage, with an increased focus on optimizing image quality while maintaining patient safety. These improvements, as evidenced by advances in focal spot technology, directly affect diagnostic accuracy by reducing image distortion and increasing spatial resolution. Hence, mammography remains an essential component among the radiological fundamentals, marrying precision and earlier detection to optimize patients' outcomes in breast cancer management (Figure 1.9).

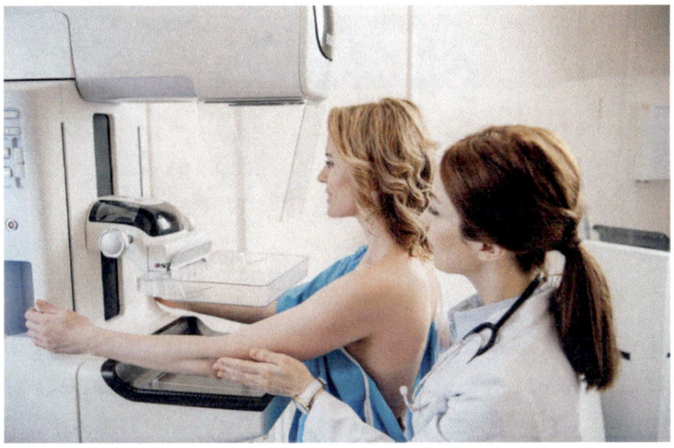

Figure 1.9. Mammography.

Source: https://empliving.com/wp-content/uploads/2023/07/How-to-Make-Mammography-Exams-Easier-.jpeg.

1.1.8. Interventional Radiology

Medical technology innovations have turned traditional diagnostic radiology into an actively therapeutic discipline in the guise of interventional radiology. It is a minimally invasive, image-guided subspecialty that diagnoses and treats disease, with special emphasis on lymphatic pathology induced by trauma or surgery. New techniques such as intranodal Lipiodol lymphangiography and dynamic magnetic resonance lymphangiography provide better visualization and control of post-operative lymphatic leaks with greater accuracy and reduced invasiveness than the previous techniques. Furthermore, lymphatic embolization with liquid embolic agents, such as N-BCA glue, is an excellent example of how interventional radiology surpasses imaging to deliver final interventions with the assurance of a significant reduction in morbidity for patients with intractable lymphatic leakage (Hur *et. al.*, 2021). In addition, the integration of deep learning techniques in imaging analysis fosters improvements in anatomical boundary markers and procedural guidance, thereby enhancing the accuracy and efficacy of interventional procedures (Shen *et. al.*, 2017). Such improvements underscore the central role of interventional radiology in the new paradigm of modern-day radiology (Figure 1.10).

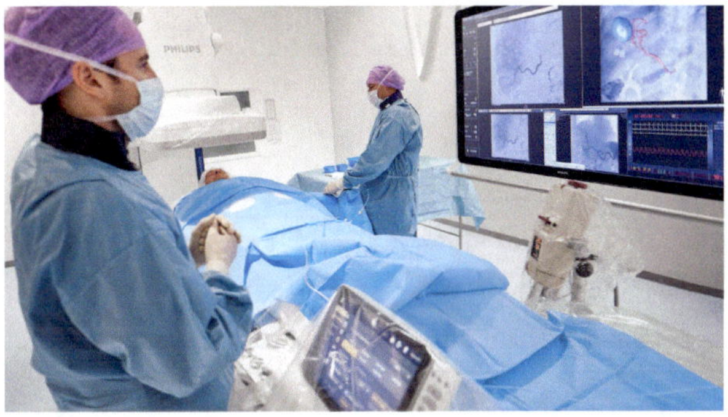

Figure 1.10. Interventional radiology.

Source: https://www.itnonline.com/sites/default/files/field/image/Screen%20Shot%202019-02-27%20at%202.47.30%20PM.png.

1.1.9. Comparison of Imaging Modalities

The evolution of imaging modalities has transformed diagnostic capabilities for all medical specialties, prompting judicious modalities comparison to provide the best clinical decision-making. Technologies such as optical coherence tomography (OCT) offer unparalleled micrometer-scale detail, enabling the accurate visualization of vascular microanatomy and device interactions in real-time, surpassing traditional modalities like intravascular ultrasound, based on resolution and specificity (Matthew *et. al.*, 2018). Conversely, modalities like traditional angiography provide more anatomical context but lack the high resolution necessary for assessment of plaque morphology or thrombosis formation, which are critical for precise interventional planning. Although OCT's limited tissue penetration constricts its capability to examine deeper structures, it optimally defines superficial lesions and device apposition, which significantly contribute to procedural success. By comparison, other imaging modalities may offer greater penetration, but at the expense of spatial resolution, as they suggest an unavoidable trade-off on clinical grounds. In proper diagnosis and effective therapeutic intervention of advanced diseases, such as cholangiocarcinoma, when non-invasive methods are unsuccessful without histological confirmation (Jesús *et. al.*, 2020).

Test Your Knowledge

1. What is ultrasound?
2. Explain the key differences between MRI and CT scans in terms of imaging technique, radiation exposure, and clinical use.

1.2. Principles of Radiological Techniques

Learning Outcome

1. Describe quality assurance in radiology
2. Discuss image acquisition techniques
3. Explain contrast agents in imaging
4. Focus on radiation safety and protection
5. Identify challenges in radiological techniques
6. Identify digital imaging technologies
7. Know the role of artificial intelligence in radiology
8. Learn image processing and interpretation
9. Understand basic physics of radiology

The specificity and accuracy of radiological diagnostic images depend significantly on the basic principles that govern radiological techniques. The principles involve optimizing exposure parameters, such as kilovoltage, milliamperage, and exposure time, to achieve the appropriate image quality with the minimum amount of patient exposure. It is essential to understand the interaction between X-rays and tissue, including attenuation and scatter, to produce high-resolution and contrast images. Furthermore, tube design and operation, particularly focal spot size, play an important role in image resolution and detail fidelity, since smaller focal spots offer greater spatial resolution. Advances in tube technology and detectors also further enhance these techniques, maximizing diagnostic performance over safety issues. Control of these fundamental elements ensures that radiological procedures not only provide accurate diagnostic information but also adhere to the principles of radiation protection and patient care, which are at the core of modern radiology.

1.2.1. Basic Physics of Radiology

The origin of radiology lies in the comprehension of fundamental physical principles underlying the creation of radiation and its interaction with matter. Fundamental physics principles enable practitioners to comprehend how X-rays and other ionizing radiation are generated, move through tissues, and deposit energy in order to form images for diagnosis or produce therapy. Mastery of atomic and nuclear structure, beam production of radiation, and processes of radiation interaction is important not merely for accurate diagnosis and effective therapy but for patient safety as well. As technology improves, influencing radiological practice, the physics rules remain the same, serving as the intellectual conveyance that supports innovation and clinical practice. Thus, a thorough comprehension of basic radiological physics is crucial for future development of critical thinking as well as safe practice in both diagnostic and therapeutic contexts (Beriwal *et. al.*, 2023). With continuously advancing modern developments, ongoing education in physics is crucial to the multidisciplinary spirit of radiology (Chang *et. al.*, 2024) (Figure 1.11).

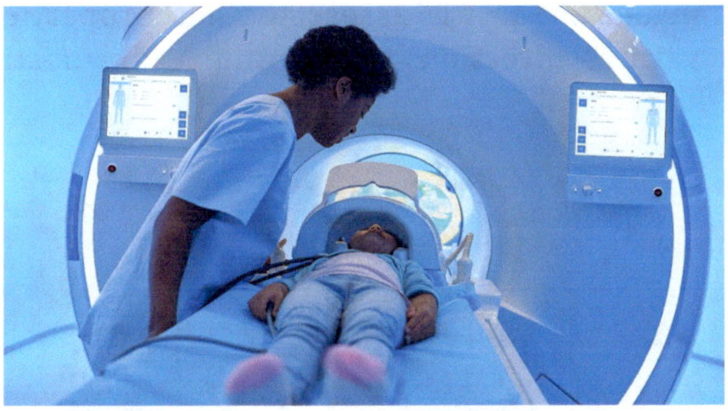

Figure 1.11. The foundation of radiology lies in understanding the fundamental physical principles governing radiation production and interaction with matter.

Source: https://www.philips.com/c-dam/corporate/innovation-and-you/global/nov-2020/hero-radiology-workflow.jpg.

1.2.2. Radiation Safety and Protection

The convergence of the latest imaging modalities has immensely contributed to diagnostic capability, but at the same time, underlines the sheer importance of embracing stringent radiation safety principles. Ionizing radiation, such as X-rays and CT scanning, possesses intrinsic risks due to its ability to damage biological tissues and to induce mutations with implications for carcinogenesis. Therefore, adherence to ordered radiation protection principles—justification, optimization, and limitation of dose—is essential in balancing the benefits of diagnostics with the risks. The ALARA approach (as low as reasonably achievable) is used to guide practice in a way that minimizes exposure without impairing image quality. Further, measures of quality assurance and equipment evaluation by diagnostic medical physicists are necessary to ensure uniformity in safety levels and protection of patients, medical staff, and the general public from excessive doses of radiation. Industry, regulation, and medical professionals need to collaborate to ensure that radiological procedures are safe while enhancing medical treatment (Gambo *et. al.*, 2024; Kim, 2016).

1.2.3. Image Acquisition Techniques

Technology has significantly contributed to how medical images are acquired, enhancing diagnostic and clinical usefulness. Traditional radiographic procedures rely on differential X-ray absorption by various tissues, resulting in contrast that demarcates anatomical features. Modern procedures entail advanced modalities such as CT, MRI, and ultrasound that use unique physical principles to acquire high-resolution images of the internal structures. Besides, recent developments in AI have enabled optimization of image acquisition parameters and interpretative imaging automatically, hence optimizing workflow effectiveness and diagnostic precision in radiology (Esteva *et. al.*, 2021). Nevertheless, despite these developments, problems with controlling image quality, patient comfort, and radiation dose remain to be addressed through ongoing optimization of acquisition protocols. Efficient imaging acquisition techniques therefore remain at the base of radiology, balancing technological potential with clinical demands to enable accurate diagnosis and treatment planning (Jesús *et. al.*, 2020) (Figure 1.12).

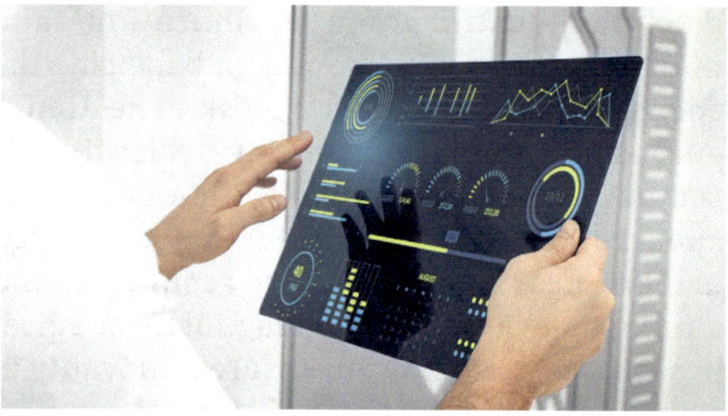

Figure 1.12. Image acquisition techniques.

Source: https://miro.medium.com/v2/resize:fit:1400/1*1OxjLRasKYjuL-aH-TBsDA.jpeg.

1.2.4. Contrast Agents in Imaging

Technological advancements in imaging technologies have significantly enhanced diagnostic specificity via enhanced tissue differentiation and lesion characterization. One such pivotal advance has been the use of contrast agents, whereby the visual contrast within imaging modalities is increased, thereby providing vital functional and anatomical information. Such contrast agents could be endogenous, such as hemoglobin in photoacoustic imaging, or drugs that can be exogenously administered to delineate structures more vividly. Photoacoustic imaging, for instance, takes advantage of both contrast modalities to deliver rich details of vascular and soft tissue content, which finds utility in a myriad of clinical applications, including breast and vascular imaging (Attia *et. al.*, 2019). Similarly, for rectal cancer, contrast-enhanced MRI optimizes tumor staging through the excellent outlining of anatomical boundaries as well as tumor infiltration, enabling precision treatment planning and monitoring of therapy response (Horvat *et. al.*, 2019). Accordingly, contrast agents continue to be the cornerstone of radiology, improving image quality and supporting clinical decision-making.

1.2.5. Image Processing and Interpretation

Advances in medical imaging have revolutionized the power of diagnostics to an extent that visualization and examination of anatomical structures are possible with greater accuracy. Image processing translates raw medical data into clinically useful information, which helps in improving accurate interpretation by radiologists. Techniques such as three-dimensional reconstruction make it possible to have global views of difficult-to-visualize structures such as pulmonary nodules, where clinicians are able to assess nodules' properties in various directions and optimize diagnostic efficacy.

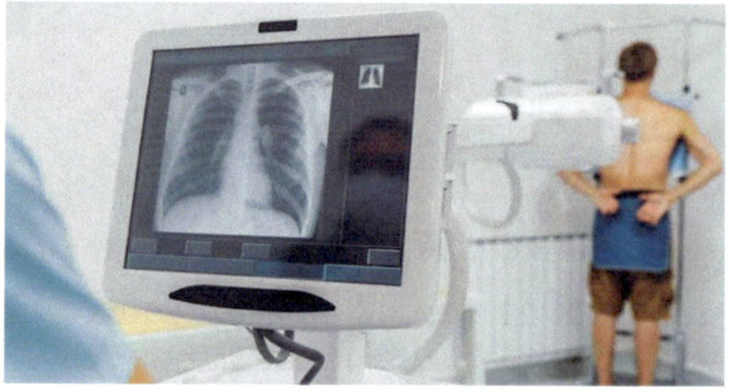

Figure 1.13. Advancements in medical imaging have revolutionized diagnostic capabilities by enabling more precise visualization and analysis of anatomical structures.

Source: https://medicalbuyer.co.in/wp-content/uploads/2024/01/Pioneering-the-future-%E2%80%93-Medical-imaging-solutions-unleashed-through-digital-radiography-systems.jpg.

Despite this, difficulties persist in achieving models that can be universally used due to variations in imaging machines, acquisition time, and lesion features, posing a challenge in standardizing interpretation (Xue *et. al.*, 2023). Integrating heterogeneous imaging modalities, including CT, MRI, and X-rays, with ML and deep learning algorithms enhances class separation of lung diseases by detecting sophisticated features and enhancing diagnostic processes. Despite progress, shortcomings such as unavailability of annotated datasets and interpretability challenge clinical adoption, necessitating explainable AI architectures and multi-modal data fusion to facilitate effective image interpretation and decision-making in radiology (Kumari *et. al.*, 2023) (Figure 1.13).

1.2.6. Quality Assurance in Radiology

Maximum patient results in radiology need careful quality assurance processes, incorporating not only technical competency but also patient care. Effective quality assurance ensures imaging techniques provide accurate diagnoses with minimal discomfort and anxiety, which can significantly influence patient compliance and satisfaction. For example, in mammography screening care, client satisfaction has a direct association with service accessibility, as well as how radiographers communicate and provide care. Women who experienced high discomfort underwent mammography reported lower satisfaction based on perceived inadequacies in radiographers' confidence and empathetic care, which underscores the importance of technical expertise with patient-empathetic interaction. Further, the anxiety levels prior to and during screening highlight the significance of quality assurance to satisfy psychological as well as physical aspects of the patient experience. Overall program satisfaction, as defined by these factors, has a vital role in ensuring sustained participation and compliance with follow-up care, thereby enhancing early detection and treatment outcome (Curtis *et. al.*, 2015). Standard imaging protocols and visual documentation further serve as intrinsic components in ensuring quality via radiological practices.

1.2.7. Digital Imaging Technologies

Medical imaging technologies have contributed extensively to diagnostic capability, particularly by incorporating digital imaging technology. These technologies provide high-resolution imaging of internal body organs with increased detail and function compared to traditional modalities. Among these, OCT has been an important device, as it provides cross-sectional images at the micrometer scale through measurement of backscattered light and thus gives a precise assessment of vascular and tissue diseases. The OCT translation to intravascular application allows doctors to evaluate plaques in coronary arteries and deploy stents with unprecedented accuracy, significantly influencing interventional choices (Matthew et al., 2018). Simultaneously, computer vision strategies based on AI take the interpretive value of digital images to an unprecedented level, optimizing complicated diagnosis workloads and delivering tailored therapeutic strategies across various medical fields (Esteva *et. al.*, 2021). Collectively, digital imaging technologies form the backbone of modern radiology, synergizing advanced optics, computational algorithms, and clinical insights to improve patient care through precise, minimally invasive imaging and intervention (Figure 1.14).

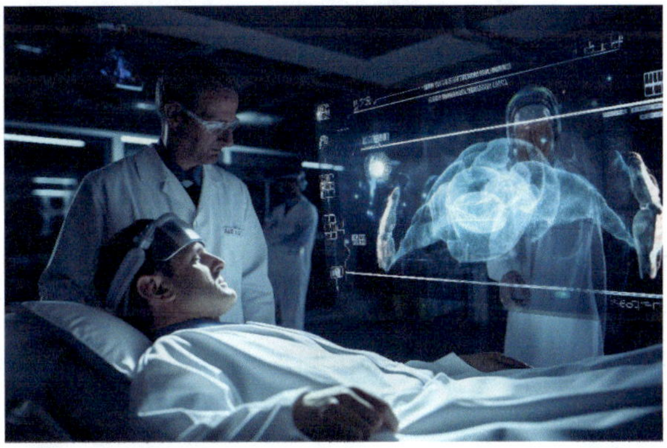

Figure 1.14. Advancements in medical imaging have profoundly transformed diagnostic capabilities, particularly through the integration of digital imaging technologies.

Source: https://miro.medium.com/v2/resize:fit:10752/1*El2D7cGxDk1D5KbQeotLGg.jpeg.

1.2.8. Role of Artificial Intelligence in Radiology

Advances in technology have consistently revolutionized radiology practice, and AI has been a game-changer in the process. AI enhances diagnostic accuracy through computerized analysis of images, allowing the faster and more accurate identification of abnormalities that human error would otherwise miss. Moreover, AI algorithms also contribute to minimizing cognitive biases inherent in manual readings, which improves consistency and effectiveness in clinical processes. However, the adoption of AI is not without problems; such machines tend to learn biases from training data, which can appear as errors in diagnosis or differential patient outcomes. Avoidance of such biases, detection of them, and ethical decision-making are necessary for achieving the best benefits of AI in radiology. This equilibrium guarantees AI not only complements the radiologists but also maintains patient safety and justice, and represents a significant step in medical image evolution (Bluethgen *et. al.*, 2025) (Figure 1.15).

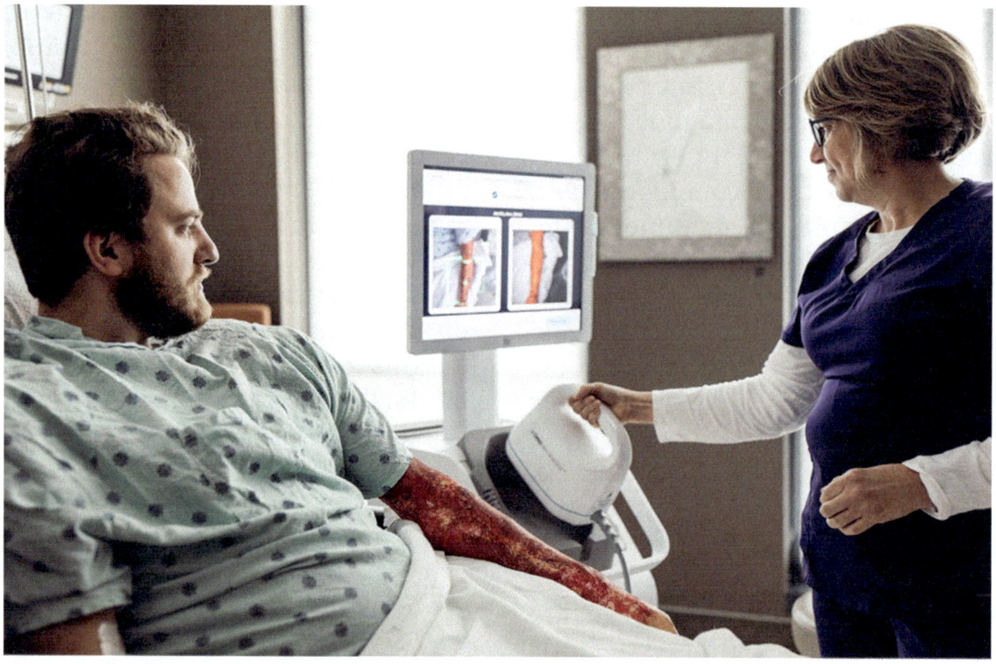

Figure 1.15. AI enhances diagnostic accuracy by automating image analysis, allowing for faster and more precise identification of abnormalities that may be overlooked by human interpretation.

Source: https://www.spectral-ai.com/wp-content/uploads/2024/08/artificial-intelligence-medical-imaging.jpg.

1.2.9. Challenges in Radiological Techniques

Radiological imaging has come a long way in the diagnostic accuracy field, but much remains to be overcome in terms of its clinical utility. Part of the largest obstacle to this is the segmentation of medical images accurately, which is required for detecting abnormalities such as tumors, but is always clouded by tissue heterogeneity and image quality. Recent breakthroughs, like the Segment Anything Model (SAM), make positive contributions through enhanced segmentation dependability across a broad spectrum of modalities, though fine-tuning and testing these models in complex clinical environments remain in progress (Ranem *et. al.*, 2023). In addition, integration of imaging techniques like CT, MRI, and X-rays using multimodal approaches in comprehensive disease description poses challenges related to data preprocessing, feature extraction, and algorithmic interpretation. The growing reliance on ML and deep learning strategies amplifies these challenges, particularly when faced with small annotated datasets and the need for transparent, clinically interpretable models (Kumari *et. al.*, 2023). Addressing these challenges is necessary to advance radiological practice and optimize patient outcomes.

Test Your Knowledge

1. Describe the basic physics behind X-ray generation.
2. How does contrast media work, and when is it used?

1.3. Clinical Applications of Radiology

Learning Outcome

1. Discuss emergency radiology
2. Explain the application of radiology in oncology, orthopedics, cardiology, and neurology
3. Focus on pediatric radiology
4. Know the importance of radiology in women's health
5. Learn case studies in clinical radiology
6. Understand the role of radiology in surgical planning

The developments in technology have significantly transformed the landscape of medical diagnosis and treatment, enabling more precise and efficient clinical decision-making. Radiology, as a critical aspect of the revolution, has expanded beyond traditional imaging to accommodate sophisticated AI algorithms. These technologies augment, improve, and enhance the detection, characterization, and tracking of many diseases, enhancing both diagnostic performance and patient outcomes. For instance, deep learning techniques have been integrated into medical imaging modalities such as cardiology and pathology, with capabilities of automatic interpretation and assisting physicians under challenging cases (Esteva *et. al.*, 2021). Moreover, radiology plays a crucial role in radiation oncology by providing functionalities such as auto-contouring and treatment planning, maximizing therapeutic maneuvers, and limiting human errors (Naqaa *et. al.*, 2020). Despite holding out some promise, their validation and application in regular clinical practices are complex and will need continued research and cross-disciplinary collaborations in order to unlock their full potential for personalized medicine.

1.3.1. Radiology in Oncology

Quick advances in radiological techniques have immensely enhanced the precision and efficacy of oncology treatment planning and assessment. New imaging technologies not only facilitate the identification and staging of tumors but also permit intense scrutiny of anatomical features even under challenging circumstances, such as the presence of metal artifacts due to implantable devices. For instance, sophisticated deep learning models have been developed to automatically detect and inpaint metal artifacts in cardiac CT scans, thereby improving the visualization and segmentation of cardiac structures critical for stereotactic arrhythmia radiotherapy patients (McKeown *et. al.*, 2024). Besides, radiology plays a key role in making therapy decisions, and one such example is the use of preoperative radiotherapy in the treatment of resectable rectal carcinoma, wherein imaging helps fine-tune therapy in a bid to reduce local recurrence and improve patient' results (Figueredo *et. al.*, 2003). Collectively, these advances bear witness to the extensive contribution of radiology to oncology in diagnostic accuracy and best therapeutic maneuvers (Figure 1.16).

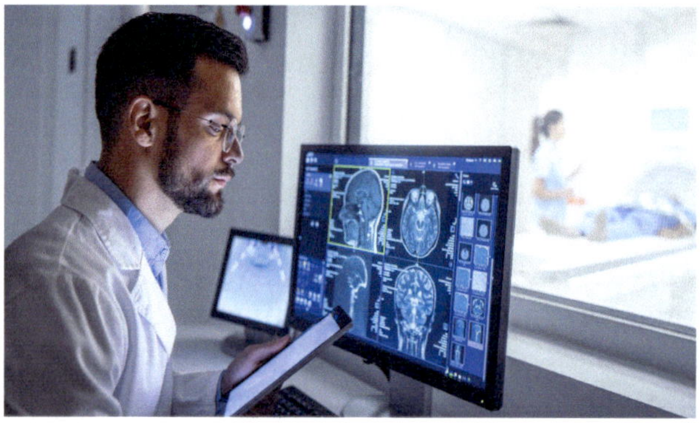

Figure 1.16. Radiology in oncology.

Source: https://www.stillwater-medical.org/wp-content/uploads/2024/03/Radiation-Oncology-scaled.jpg.

1.3.2. Radiology in Orthopedics

Pedagogic innovations have had a significant influence on how challenging fields in medicine are addressed, perticularly in specialties such as orthopedics. The union of Three-Dimensional Multimodality Imaging (3DMMI) and Case-Based Learning (CBL) is a good example of how technologies in radiology enhance insight into nuances of pelvic anatomy and tumor dynamics to promote enhanced diagnostic performance and theoretical competence among postgraduate students (Hu *et. al.*, 2023). This imaginative use of imaging not only enhances student engagement and clinical thinking but also improves teaching efficiency in orthopedic education. Additionally, the inclusion of near-peer teachers who are experienced in ultrasonography (EUS) and clinical anatomy further improves the learning experience, providing pragmatic, clinically focused perspectives that bridge the gap between theoretical knowledge and application (Quiroga *et. al.*, 2020). Cumulatively, these approaches underline the inseparable role of radiology in orthopedics by promoting improved anatomical understanding, effective diagnosis, and improved surgical planning, reinforcing radiology's core role in modern orthopedic education and practice.

1.3.3. Radiology in Cardiology

Imaging technology has made dramatic advances in cardiology's diagnostic and treatment functions, particularly through radiology. Cardiac CT plays a central role in visualizing the anatomical structures of the heart as well as cardiac movement, although metal artifacts from implanted devices can reduce the quality of images. New developments using deep learning models have addressed these limitations by automatically identifying metal artifacts and inpainting the areas of damage with anatomically conforming information, thereby improving the accuracy of heart chamber segmentation and cardiac motion analysis (McKeown *et. al.*, 2024). Moreover, the integration of radiological data must be followed by proper clinical judgment, because over-reliance on imaging can lead to overconfidence in diagnosis and therapy. Precautions for such risks include exercising professional humility and regularly renewing interpretative skills, reminding the need to blend radiological knowledge with clinical wholism (Yagil *et. al.*, 2020). Radiology in cardiology is thus a sophisticated union of technology and clinical judgment integral to modern medical practice (Figure 1.17).

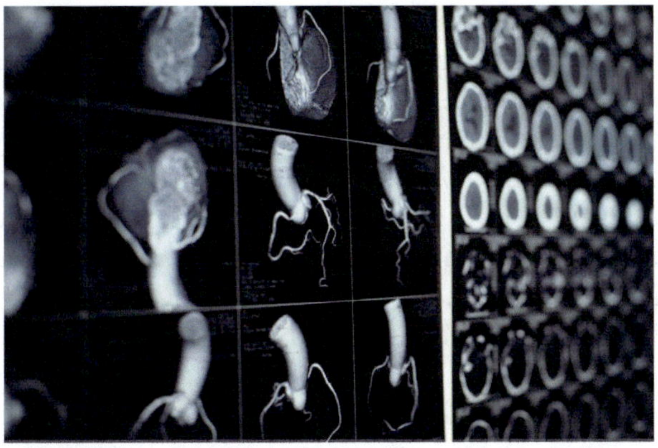

Figure 1.17. Cardiac computed tomography (CT).

Source: https://my.clevelandclinic.org/-/scassets/images/org/health/articles/16834-heart-ct-scan.

1.3.4. Radiology in Neurology

Advances in imaging technology have significantly impacted the diagnostic approach to neurological disorders and enabled earlier and more specific intervention. Modern radiological techniques, including multi-parametric MRI, provide valuable information beyond that of conventional anatomical imaging by assessing the histology, biology, and physiology of brain tissue, thus enabling radiophenotyping of complex neurologic disorders. This enhanced information is likely to be utilized to inform individualized treatment strategies, especially in combination with emerging AI algorithms that combine extensive imaging and clinical data further to develop prognostic models and decision-making in neurological care (Pringle *et. al.*, 2022). In addition, radiology is also essential in the acute identification of potentially fatal pathologies like cerebral herniation, where the rapid imaging on CT or MRI can expedite diagnosis and guide emergent therapeutic interventions. Recognition of the various subtypes of herniations' imaging appearance is important for localizing, assessing complications, and correlating clinical symptoms in neurologic patients (Gilardi *et. al.*, 2019). These together emphasize the central role of radiology in enhancing neurological diagnosis and patient outcomes.

1.3.5. Pediatric Radiology

Radiologic imaging technology advances have made a very significant contribution to the diagnostic resources in all patient groups, yet disproportionately so for children. Children's unique physiological characteristics and higher susceptibility to ionizing radiation make them uniquely in need of special approaches to radiologic imaging. The most recent technological advancements, for example, in photon-counting CT, have had remarkable benefits, including decreased radiation dose and better image quality, which are highly valuable for reducing the risks of several imaging examinations in children.

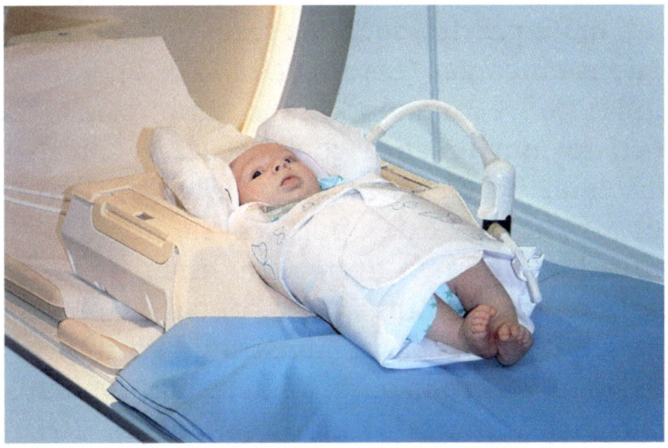

Figure 1.18. Pediatric radiology.

Source: https://www.pearl-technology.ch/hubfs/BBFC_Spule_Baby_1.png.

Also, the ability to obtain high-resolution images with reduced noise levels enables proper diagnosis without unnecessary dose limitation, a concern in pediatric radiology. Also, the widespread use of thoracic support lines and tubes among hospitalized children highlights the importance of radiologists' expertise to interpret these devices toward ensuring treatment monitoring as well as prevention of complications. Monitoring for the position and orientation of devices through radiographic inspection is an essential practice in pediatric imaging (Liszewski *et. al.*, 2019). All these technologies work in concert to enhance diagnostic accuracy and patient safety in pediatric radiology (Figure 1.18).

1.3.6. Emergency Radiology

Early and accurate diagnosis is essential in critical care situations, particularly in trauma and severe injury scenarios where prompt intervention may be a matter of life and death. Emergency radiology plays a vital part in enabling quick imaging exams that guide clinical action, particularly in the management of severe bleeding and coagulopathy following traumatic injury. Advances in imaging technologies and the use of artificial intelligence have significantly enhanced diagnosis in emergency settings, with more precise, complex cases and improved patient outcomes (Esteva *et. al.*, 2021). Clinical guideline recommendations emphasize the need to individualize goal-directed treatment strategies based on imaging findings, thereby personalizing care pathways. Besides, a multidisciplinary approach incorporating radiological findings into decision-making pathways has been demonstrated to improve the standardization of care and reduce avoidable trauma deaths worldwide (Donat *et. al.*, 2019). Therefore, emergency radiology is a very essential component of contemporary trauma care, emphasizing its underpinning position within the realm of radiology.

1.3.7. Radiology in Women's Health

Technological innovation in medical imaging has had profound effects on the diagnosis and treatment of diseases uniquely occurring in women, demonstrating the crucial function of radiology in women's health. Interventional radiology, more than any other discipline, has expanded enormously, being an important tool in the management of complex gynecologic disorders, such as pelvic venous disease, uterine fibroids, and adenomyosis. This specialty enables minimally invasive treatments, like uterine artery embolization, which have transformed patient care by providing efficacious alternatives to surgery, reducing recovery times and associated risks (Tanaka *et. al.*, 2023). In addition, radiology supports more widespread public health activities by providing information on the trends in the oral health of women, as seen through the study of extreme partial edentulism, which shows the crosstalk between systemic health and imaging diagnosis (Go *et. al.*, 2024). These developmentsreflect the ongoing improvements in imaging technologies and treatment regimens, highlighting the central role played by radiology in improving women's health outcomes and creating individually personalized therapeutic plans (Figure 1.19).

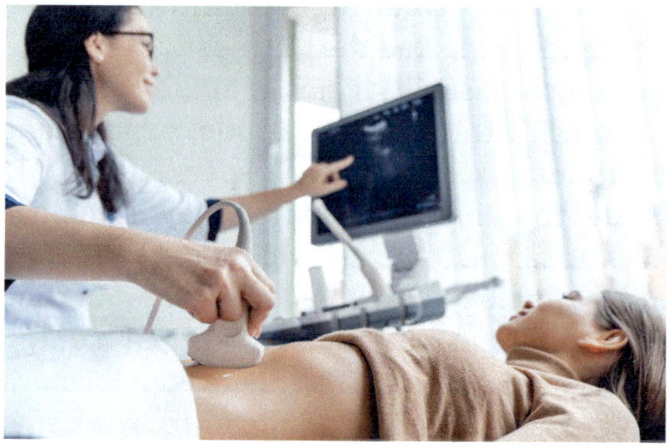

Figure 1.19. Importance of radiology in women's health.

Source: https://www.healthimages.com/content/uploads/sites/2/2021/03/women-ultrasound.jpg.

1.3.8. Role of Radiology in Surgical Planning

Accurate diagnosis and complete anatomical awareness are indispensable prerequisites for efficacious surgical interventions, and radiology is inevitably engaged in fulfilling these requisites.

Advanced imaging modalities enable surgeons to possess accurate visualization of complex regions, such as the sellar and suprasellar compartments, where diverse pathologies, including neoplastic and vascular lesions, may be located. Distinguishing between these "chameleon" lesions on radiological evaluation enables proper preoperative planning, guiding surgical approach, and informs intraoperative decision-making, exemplified by cases with glioblastomas, neuroendocrine tumors, and cavernous malformations (Bove *et. al.*, 2023). Moreover, incorporating newer technologies, such as AI and deep learning, enhances image interpretation and workflow effectiveness, with the potential to transform surgical planning by predicting the outcome and better outlining crucial structures (Esteva *et. al.*, 2021). This synergistic multi-disciplinary union of radiology and surgery not only optimizes patient safety but also strengthens surgical efficacy, emphasizing the central role of radiology in modern operative methods within the broader framework of medical practice.

1.3.9. Case Studies in Clinical Radiology

Effective diagnosis and management of complex clinical cases often rely on thorough examination of individual cases, illustrating the essential role of case studies in clinical radiology. Case studies not only reinforce practical radiological understanding but also enable a better understanding of atypical or challenging presentations. For example, radiological imaging of giant recurrent colloid cysts of the third ventricle highlights the need for urgent radiological assessment to prevent complications that could be life-threatening, emphasizing the role of imaging in guiding minimally invasive interventions and patient prognosis (Nadia *et. al.*, 2024). Additionally, the development of advanced medical natural language processing models on a limited but annotated set of radiology reports illustrates how clinical data can be applied in maximizing diagnostic performance and automating clinical workflow under privacy constraints and limited resources (Yada *et. al.*, 2024). As a whole, these illustrations illustrate how clinical radiology employs both imaging and data-driven methods to inform efficient patient care in an interdisciplined medical model.

Test Your Knowledge

1. What role does ultrasound play in obstetrics and gynecology?
2. Which imaging modality is most commonly used in the evaluation of head trauma?

1.4. Radiology and Patient Care

Learning Outcome

1. Discuss informed consent in radiology
2. Explain patient education on radiological procedures
3. Focus on communication between radiologists and patients
4. Know the impact of radiology on patient outcomes
5. Know radiology reports and their importance
6. Learn a multidisciplinary approach to patient management
7. Manage patient anxiety and comfort
8. Perform follow-up care and imaging
9. Understand patient preparation for radiological procedures

Effective patient care in radiology extends beyond proper imaging to encompass the overall experience of patients undergoing diagnostic testing. Research highlights that patient satisfaction is not solely dependent on the technical quality of radiological care but also on accessibility, communication, and the demonstration of empathy by radiology staff. For instance, the Maltese Breast Screening Program reported that, despite high levels of reported satisfaction with care and a willingness to recommend the program, issues like difficulty in attending the unit and discomfort during mammography negatively impacted patient experience (Curtis *et. al.*, 2015). These results highlight the importance for radiology departments to embrace patient-focused care approaches, such as clear communication , anxiety reduction, and comfort support. Moreover, simplifying routine operations like appointment scheduling and training personnel can significantly enhance overall care quality . Thus, balancing technical proficiency with empathetic patient relations is key to pushing radiology's role in integrated healthcare (Figure 1.20).

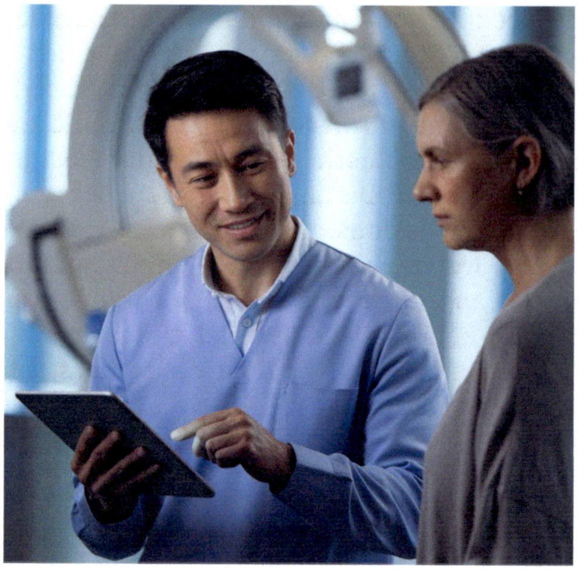

Figure 1.20. Effective patient care within radiology extends beyond accurate imaging to encompass the holistic experience of individuals undergoing diagnostic procedures.

Source: https://www.cidrad.com/wp-content/uploads/36.jpg.

1.4.1. Patient Preparation for Radiological Procedures

Success in imaging diagnosis depends in large part on adequate patient preparation in order to obtain both high-quality images and the safety of the patients. Adequate preparation involves compliance with standardized protocols for specific contrasted examinations as recommended by established radiology literature and clinical guidelines. For instance, some radiology examinations adhere to preparations developed by experienced authors, such as Bontrager and Lampignano, such as fasting, hydration, and allergenic risk stratification prior to contrast injection. These planning steps minimize side effects and artifacts, thereby increasing diagnostic accuracy. Advances in imaging technology, including ML tools, also highlight precise patient positioning and preparation to optimize image segmentation and anomaly detection algorithms in modalities like MRI (Ghorbel *et. al.*, 2022). Thus, gaining knowledge and implementing total patient preparation protocols is crucial for radiology professionals to produce accurate diagnostic images and enable sound clinical decision-making in modern medical practice.

1.4.2. Communication Between Radiologists and Patients

Successful radiological communication transcends technical interpretation of the image and plays a key role in patient care and outcomes. Radiologists must balance explaining results clearly and empathetically while condensing complex information so that patients understand what the implications are without undue distress.

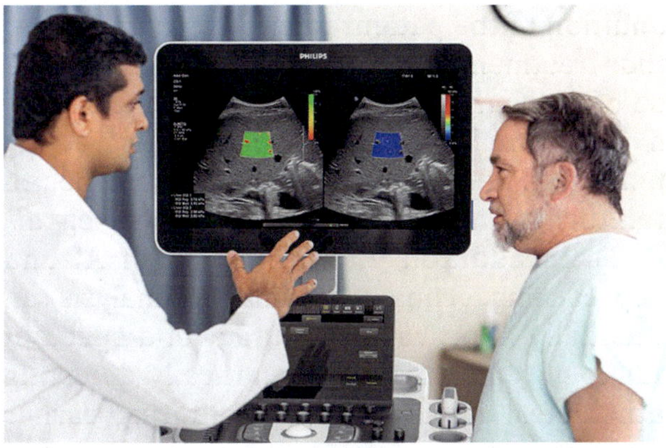

Figure 1.21. Effective communication in radiology extends beyond technical image interpretation, playing a crucial role in patient care and clinical outcomes.

Source: https://www.philips.com/c-dam/corporate/innovation-and-you/global/dec-2021/02-image-blog-ultrasound-lfq.jpg.

This interaction is especially important as radiology increasingly employs advanced technologies like AI, which, while enhancing diagnostic accuracy and workflow, has the potential to complicate communication through issues like the "black box" phenomenon inherent to AI solutions (Najjar, 2023). Moreover, organizational changes brought about by digital transformation require radiologists to redefine themselves not just as diagnosticians but also as communicators who actively engage patients in their healthcare journey (Wessel *et. al.*, 2021). Improvement in radiologist-patient communication develops confidence and facilitates joint decision-making and, finally, enhances the healing process under the new environment of radiology's expanding technological and ethical foundation (Figure 1.21).

1.4.3. Informed Consent in Radiology

Patient autonomy and patient safety are hallmark of ethical clinical practice, particularly in radiology, with its associated risks of exposure to ionizing radiation. Educating patients about the benefits, risks, and alternatives of radiologic exams is most important in ensuring informed consent. Not only does it provide transparency, but it also allows patients to make choices in consultation with their healthcare providers. Because of the potential for injury associated with radiation exposure, including cellular and genetic damage, clinicians are required to explain these risks clearly and emphasize dose optimization methods following the ALARA principle to minimize risks without compromising diagnostic accuracy (Dudhe *et. al.*, 2024). Besides, patient education is more than a verbal description but includes authoritative documentation and answers to specific questions relevant to specific conditions, as radiologic findings are prone to influence future clinical management (Chandel *et. al.*, 2023). Lastly, radiologic informed consent reestablishes trust, encourages patient-centered care, and satisfies legal and ethical expectations as part of the larger matrix of fundamental radiology practice.

1.4.4. Managing Patient Anxiety and Comfort

Patient anxiety and comfort management are necessary in radiology to ensure quality imaging and an overall satisfactory healthcare experience. Radiologic studies provoke stress through unknown environments, confinement, and fear of diagnosis, which tends to erode patient cooperation and image quality. Technologies such as AI-supported patient monitoring and tailored interventions offer possible answers to alleviate anxiety by pre-empting patient stress responses and scaling communication (Varnosfaderani *et. al.*, 2024).

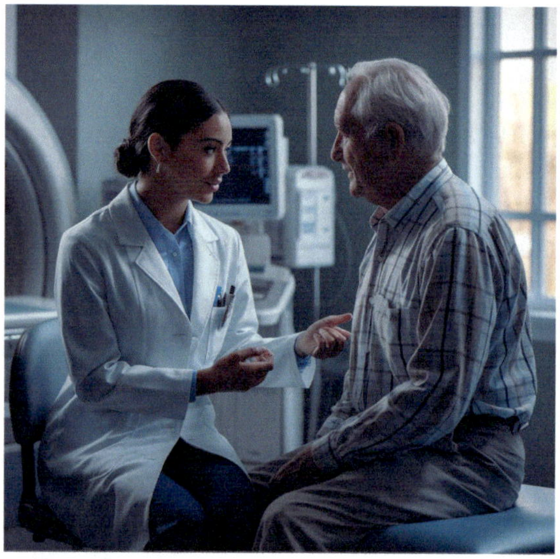

Figure 1.22. Effective management of patient anxiety and comfort is crucial in radiology to ensure accurate imaging and a positive overall healthcare experience.

Source: https://www.cidrad.com/wp-content/uploads/45.jpg.

New technologies on the Metaverse platform integrate virtual and augmented reality to provide immersive, calming settings that distract and reassure patients during imaging (Chengoden *et. al.*, 2023). These innovations enhance not only patient compliance but also provide more empathetic care by addressing both psychological and physical needs. Incorporating such measures into routine radiologic practice underscores the importance of a patient-centered model, with technological progress used to maximize emotional health as well as diagnostic outcomes, and improve overall patient satisfaction (Figure 1.22).

1.4.5. Radiology Reports and Their Importance

Timely and precise data transmission of diagnostic information is crucial in medical practice, especially when managing advanced imaging data. Radiology reports serve as the essential interface between imaging technology and clinical decision-making, relaying accurate interpretation information to inform patient care. They not only report imaging findings but also position them in context with the entire condition of the patient to enable physicians to tailor treatments properly. Advances, such as the use of unmanned aerial vehicles for measuring environmental radiation, highlight the growing application of radiological data in public health monitoring and regulations (Borbinha *et. al.*, 2020). In addition, the utilization of AI and deep learning techniques in imaging analysis can potentially improve the accuracy and speed of radiology reporting by automatically detecting pathological features, thus facilitating earlier diagnoses and improved outcomes (Gulshan *et. al.*, 2016). Hence, radiology reports are integral aids that connect technology and clinical understanding, which augments their supreme significance in medical delivery.

1.4.6. Follow-Up Care and Imaging

Effective patient care in radiology often extends beyond the initial diagnosis, emphasizing the critical value of follow-up imaging and care to monitor disease course or response to treatment. Ongoing evaluation allows clinicians to recognize subtle changes that may influence therapeutic decisions or foreshadow complications in an early phase. Advancing imaging modalities offer high-resolution visualization, enabling accurate measurement of clinical status over time. Moreover, standardized follow-up protocols improve the reproducibility and consistency of imaging studies, facilitating comparisons at multiple time points and among multiple clinical teams.

Radiologists must balance the benefits of repeated imaging against concerns for radiation exposure,expense, and ensure that follow-up plans are clinically justified and best timed. The incorporation of systematic follow-up into radiological practice not only optimizes patient outcomes but also highlights imaging's cooperative role in multidisciplinary care, emphasizing its critical position within radiology's building blocks (Figure 1.23).

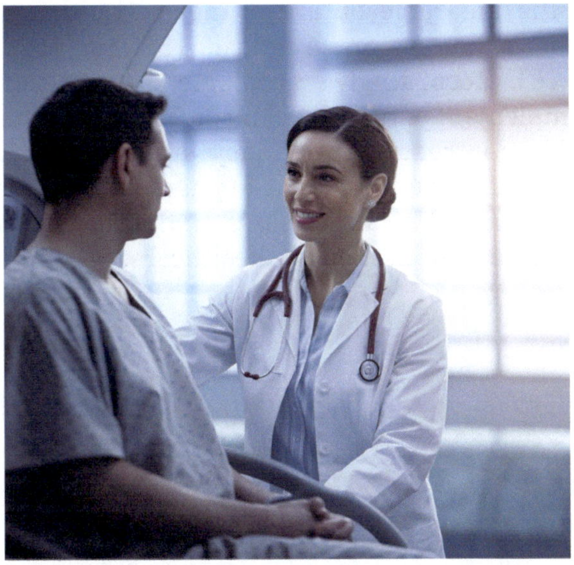

Figure 1.23. Effective management of patients in radiology often extends beyond initial diagnosis, emphasizing the critical role of follow-up care and imaging to monitor disease progression or treatment response.

Source: https://www.cidrad.com/wp-content/uploads/20.jpg.

1.4.7. Multidisciplinary Approach in Patient Management

Effective patient care in radiology is more and more dependent on interdepartmental collaboration, allowing for holistic care to assemble many different types of expertise. Radiologists must be closely in touch with clinicians, surgeons, pathologists, and, increasingly, data scientists to achieve diagnostic precision and optimal treatment outcomes. Multidisciplinary working enhances decision-making by combining the expertise of imaging with clinical information and new technologies, such as AI, which can further improve diagnosis and therapeutic regimens. The inclusion of an AI curriculum in radiologist training is a quintessential demonstration of this transformation, equipping radiologists with the skills to communicate and collaborate with AI experts , ultimately providing better quality and safety in patient care (Hofmeijer *et. al.*, 2024). Illustrations of such blended models demonstrate how teamwork harmony is required, illustrating how teamwork expertise across specialties can be enhanced to reduce errors. Adopting this collaborative paradigm is vital to moving radiology's position forward in today's healthcare networks and maximizing patient-focused results.

1.4.8. Patient Education on Radiological Procedures

Effective communication between patients and medical professionals is crucial to ensure safe and proper use of radiological tests. Educating patients on the purpose, benefit, and potential risks, most importantly the radiation exposure, promotes informed choice and reduces fear related to imaging tests. This procedure conforms to the essential principles of justification and optimization, which seek to minimize radiation doses while maximizing diagnostic quality and ensuring that every procedure's benefits are greater than its risks. Evidence-based clinical imaging guidelines play a crucial role in standardizing the education of patients and achieving consistency in care delivery (Jang *et. al.*, 2024). Besides, clear procedural guidance tailored to individual procedures, such as pre-third molar removal assessments, , is also seen to increase patient understanding and promote shared decision-making. In conclusion, patient education maximizes safety and compliance while also improving overall healthcare outcomes by promoting transparency and patient-centered medicine within radiology (Figure 1.24).

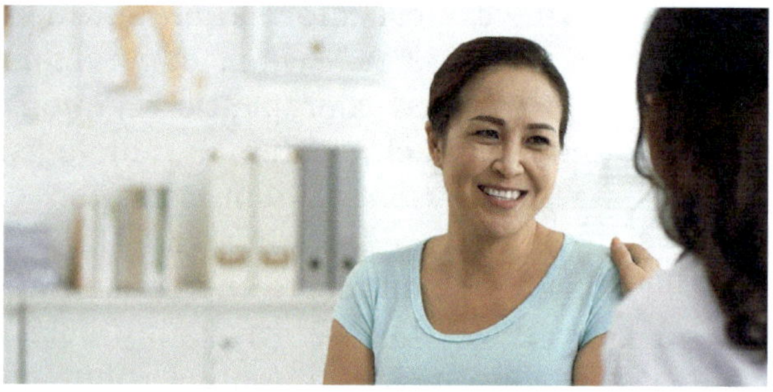

Figure 1.24. Educating patients about the purpose, benefits, and potential risks, particularly regarding radiation exposure, fosters informed decision-making and reduces anxiety related to imaging tests.

Source: https://f.hubspotusercontent00.net/hubfs/5834805/patient-care-in-radiology.jpg.

1.4.9. Impact of Radiology on Patient Outcomes

The evolution of diagnostic and imaging modalities has significantly transformed patient care practices in oncology and chronic disease management. Radiology plays an integral role in early detection, accurate staging, and continuous monitoring of disease, which in turn has a direct impact on management and prognostic prediction. For instance, advancements in staging melanoma, as reflected in updated AJCC criteria, are greatly based on precise radiologic evaluation to quantify tumor thickness and nodal involvement, thereby enhancing patient stratification and treatment planning (Jeffrey *et. al.*, 2017). Similarly, in diseases like metastatic breast cancer, imaging facilitates an early diagnosis of metastatic disease, which is significant in the context of the incurable nature of metastatic disease and its impact on prognosis (Fátima *et. al.*, 2016). Accordingly, radiologic interventions complement personalized medicine approaches, enhance treatment efficacy, and ultimately optimize patient outcomes by facilitating more discerning clinical decisions, underlining their inherent role in modern healthcare.

Test Your Knowledge

1. A child is brought in with abdominal pain. Which imaging technique would be most suitable and least harmful?
2. A patient presents with sudden chest pain and shortness of breath. What imaging modalities would be appropriate, and why?

SUMMARY

In total, radiology is an excellent combination of technical data and clinical expertise, and both of which are required to provide accurate diagnosis as well as patient treatment. Disease information and disease diagnosis have been greatly enhanced with technological developments, but within constraints whereby multifactorial causes of death necessitate radiological data to be interpreted against pathological and clinical data to develop a conclusive diagnosis, e.g., in complex forensic cases (Vedashree *et. al.*, 2025). Moreover, the performance of radiology experts also relies on psychological factors such as work stress and resilience, which directly affect diagnostic quality and overall performance. Advanced care in radiologic practice needs to be assured by addressing such human factors through stress management and resilience training (Shen *et. al.*, 2024). Lastly, a fair mix of technical expertise, clinical acumen, and psychological health is the basis for good radiology, with its highest significance to modern medicine.

Follow-up of good radiological practice is built on an intimate understanding of clinical and technological factors, the cornerstone of accurate patient protection and diagnosis. The most significant items are concerned with the significance of awareness of weather, environmental factors influencing image interpretation, such as climatic factors, weather changes that might influence patient status and radiological findings, as discussed in studies on extreme weather impacts on health information (Luiz *et. al.*, 2025). Also, the credibility and accuracy of radiologic data depend heavily on proper data handling methods. Proper quality, normalized, and anonymized data sets must be maintained, particularly with increased use of AI in imaging to enable effectiveness and accuracy (Galbusera *et. al.*, 2024). Specifically designed image annotation and processing software tools also accomplish this goal, supporting regulatory compliance and improved diagnostic precision. These are all the fundamental elements to further the roots of radiology and enhance patient care.

KEY TERMS FROM THIS CHAPTER

Anatomy	Clinical applications	Clinical judgement
Clinicians	Computed tomography	Diagnosis
Fluoroscopy	Lesions	Magnetic resonance imaging MRI)
Mammography	Nuclear medicine	Pathology
Radiologic assessment	Technological advancements	Treatment
Tumors	Ultrasound imaging	X-ray imaging

CRITICAL THINKING QUESTIONS

1. **Which imaging technique uses sound waves to create images of internal organs?**
   a. X-ray
   b. CT Scan
   c. Ultrasound
   d. MRI
2. **What is the main advantage of MRI over CT scans?**
   a. Faster scan time
   b. Better bone imaging
   c. No radiation exposure
   d. Lower cost
3. **Which imaging method provides real-time moving images of the internal body?**
   a. MRI
   b. PET Scan
   c. X-ray
   d. Fluoroscopy
4. **What is commonly used for breast cancer screening?**
   a. CT
   b. Ultrasound
   c. Mammography
   d. PET Scan
5. **Which modality is best for imaging soft tissues like the brain or spinal cord?**
   a. X-ray
   b. MRI
   c. CT Scan
   d. Mammography

Short Answer Questions

1. What is radiology and what are its primary clinical applications?
2. Differentiate between diagnostic and interventional radiology.
3. Name the main types of radiological imaging techniques.
4. What is ionizing radiation, and which radiological techniques use it?
5. Why is patient positioning important in radiological imaging?

Answers to Critical Thinking Questions

1.(c); 2.(c); 3.(d); 4.(c); 5.(b)

REFERENCES

1. Attia, A. B. E., Balasundaram, G., Moothanchery, M., Dinish, U. S., Bi, R., Ntziachristos, V., & Olivo, M. (2019). A review of clinical photoacoustic imaging: Current and future trends. *Photoacoustic, 16*, 100144. https://doi.org/10.1016/j.pacs.2019.100144.

2. Bañales, J. M., Marín, J. J. G., Lamarca, Á., Rodrigues, P. M., Khan, S. A., Roberts, L. R., Cardinale, V., *et. al.* (2020). Cholangiocarcinoma 2020: The next horizon in mechanisms and management. *Nature Reviews Gastroenterology & Hepatology, 17*(557–588). https://doi.org/10.1038/s41575-020-0310-z.

3. Barratt, D., Jannin, P., Fichtinger, G., & Cotin, S. (2014). Information processing in computer-assisted interventions: 4th international conference, 2013. *International Journal of Computer Assisted Radiology and Surgery, 9*(6), 755–757. https://www.semanticscholar.org/paper/04a31adde96205906b9c23deddb7120d246e5c4d (accessed on 30 May 2025).

4. Barricelli, B. R., Casiraghi, E., & Fogli, D. (2019). A survey on digital twin: Definitions, characteristics, applications, and design implications. *IEEE Access, 7*, 167653–167671. https://doi.org/10.1109/access.2019.2953499.

5. Beriwal, S., Corrigan, K. L., McDermott, P. N., Ryckman, J. M., Tsao, M., Zheng, D., Joiner, M. C., *et. al.* (2023). Three discipline collaborative radiation therapy (3DCRT) special debate: Radiation oncology has become so technologically complex that basic fundamental physics should no longer be included in the modern curriculum for radiation oncology residents. *Journal of Applied Clinical Medical Physics, 24*. https://doi.org/10.1002/acm2.14128.

6. Koçak B, Ponsiglione A, Stanzione A, Bluethgen C, Santinha J, Ugga L, Huisman M, Klontzas ME, Cannella R, Cuocolo R. Bias in artificial intelligence for medical imaging: fundamentals, detection, avoidance, mitigation, challenges, ethics, and prospects. Diagn Interv Radiol . 2025 Mar;31(2):75-88. doi:10.4274/dir.2024.242854.

7. Borbinha, J., Romanets, Y., Teles, P., Corisco, J., Vaz, P., Carvalho, D. D., Brouwer, Y., *et. al.* (2020). Performance analysis of Geiger–Müller and cadmium zinc telluride sensors envisaging airborne radiological monitoring in NORM sites. *Sensors, 20*(1538). https://doi.org/10.3390/s20051538.

8. Boujida, N., Messaoud, O., Lahfidi, A., Kettani Ech-Chrif, N., Fikri, M., & Touarsa, F. (2024). A giant colloid cyst of the third ventricle: A case report. *Erodium Journal of Radiology*. https://www.semanticscholar.org/paper/e8417212c179cade725d955c5dbaf3403abd760d (accessed on 30 May 2025).

9. Bove, I., Franca, R. A., Ugga, L., Solari, D., Elefante, A., Del Basso De, M., & Cavallo, L. M. (2023). The "chameleon" sellar lesions: A case report of unexpected seller lesions. *Frontiers in Neurology, 14*. https://doi.org/10.3389/fneur.2023.1149858.

10. Cardoso, F., Costa, A., Senkus, E., Aapro, M., André, F., Barrios, C. H., Bergh, J., *et. al.* (2016). 3rd ESO–ESMO International consensus guidelines for advanced breast cancer (ABC 3). *Annals of Oncology, 28*(1), 16–33. https://doi.org/10.1093/annonc/mdw544.

11. Chandel, D., Sanghavi, P., & Verma, R. (2023). Clinical profile and cytogenetic correlations in females with primary amenorrhea. *Clinical and Experimental Reproductive Medicine, 50*(3), 192–199. https://www.semanticscholar.org/paper/64c341e50142a2b35c3f727200271f2357d049f1 (accessed on 30 May 2025).

12. Chang, Y., Wang, X., Wang, J., Wu, Y., Yang, L., Zhu, K., Chen, H., *et. al.* (2024). A survey on evaluation of large language models. *ACM Transactions on Intelligent Systems and Technology, 15*, 1–45. https://doi.org/10.1145/3641289.

13. Chengoden, R., Victor, N., Huynh-The, T., Yenduri, G., Jhaveri, R. H., Alazab, M., Bhattacharya, S., *et. al.* (2023). Metaverse for healthcare: A survey on potential applications, challenges and future directions. *IEEE Access, 11*, 12765–12795. https://doi.org/10.1109/access.2023.3241628.

14. Curtis, J., Marmara, D., & Marmarà, V. A. (2015). Women's satisfaction of the Maltese breast screening programmed: A cross-sectional survey. https://core.ac.uk/download/46603757.pdf (accessed on 30 May 2025).

15. David-Olawade, A. C., Olawade, D., Vanderbloemen, L., Rotifa, O. B., Fidelis, S. C., Egbon, E., Akpan, A. O., *et. al.* (2025). AI-driven advances in low-dose imaging and enhancement—A review. *Diagnostics, 15.* https://www.semanticscholar.org/paper/44051b152f1c9fdf0599bfc6f3bf4a45b07ac104 (accessed on 30 May 2025).

16. Dong, Z., Li, S., Lowerison, M. R., Pan, J., Zou, J., & Song, P. (2020). Fast acoustic steering via tilting electromechanical reflectors (FASTER): A novel method for high volume rate 3-D ultrasound imaging. *IEEE Transactions on Ultrasonics, Ferroelectrics, and Frequency Control, 68*(2), 675–687. https://www.semanticscholar.org/paper/af03c6d561cf9fd8862b3bc223faa373c7d7fb7c (accessed on 30 May 2025).

17. Dudhe, S., Mishra, G., Parihar, P., Nimodia, D., & Kumari, A. (2024). Radiation dose optimization in radiology: A comprehensive review of safeguarding patients and preserving image fidelity. *Cureus, 16.* https://www.semanticscholar.org/paper/d9b72b4ebe65054d721bbd828f1508b37c495c6f (accessed on 30 May 2025).

18. El Naqa, I., & Das, S. K. (2020). The role of machine and deep learning in modern medical physics. *Medical Physics, 47.* https://doi.org/10.1002/mp.14088.

19. Esteva, A., Chou, K., Yeung, S., Naik, N., Madani, A., Mottaghi, A., Liu, Y., *et. al.* (2021). Deep learning-enabled medical computer vision. *npj Digital Medicine, 4.* https://doi.org/10.1038/s41746-020-00376-2.

20. Eves, J., Sudarsanam, A., Shalhoub, J., & Amiras, D. (2022). Augmented reality in vascular and endovascular surgery: Scoping review. *JMIR Serious Games, 10*, e34501. https://doi.org/10.2196/34501.

21. Fêde, Â., Souza, R. P., Doi, M., De Brot, M., Osório, C. A. B. de T., Gondim, G. R. M., Rocha, J. C. C. da, *et. al.* (2021). Malignant phyllodes tumor of the breast: A practice review. *Clinics and Practice, 11*(2), 205–215. https://doi.org/10.3390/clinpract11020030.

22. Figueredo, A., Zuraw, L., Wong, R., Agboola, O., Rumble, R., Tandan, V., *et. al.* (2003). The use of preoperative radiotherapy in the management of patients with clinically respectable rectal cancer: A practice guideline. *BMC Medicine, 1*(1), 1. https://www.semanticscholar.org/paper/3cadf9da24aed9336d80594cf4867d3538ec5e54 (accessed on 30 May 2025).

23. Fleming, K. A., Horton, S., Wilson, M. L., Atun, R., DeStigter, K., Flanigan, J., Sayed, S., *et. al.* (2021). The Lancet Commission on diagnostics: Transforming access to diagnostics. *The Lancet, 398*(1997–2050). https://doi.org/10.1016/s0140-6736(21)00673-5.

24. Galbusera, F., & Cina, A. (2024). Image annotation and curation in radiology: An overview for machine learning practitioners. *European Radiology Experimental, 8*, Article 1. https://

www.semanticscholar.org/paper/d921426c19b3e56c37ac1179a6d3142d3e42ac26 (accessed on 30 May 2025).

25. Gambo, N., & Shehu, M. (2024). The role of diagnostic medical physics in medicine: An overview. *Sahel Journal of Life Sciences FUDMA*. https://www.semanticscholar.org/paper/372a33a3ed2cd5bb3d645657730b8c7801785d41 (accessed on 30 May 2025).

26. Gershenwald, J. E., Scolyer, R. A., Hess, K. R., Sondak, V. K., Long, G. V., Ross, M. I., Lazar, A. J., *et. al.* (2017). Melanoma staging: Evidence-based changes in the American Joint Committee on Cancer eighth edition cancer staging manual. *CA: A Cancer Journal for Clinicians, 67*(472–492). https://doi.org/10.3322/caac.21409.

27. Ghorbel, A., Aldahdooh, A., Albarqouni, S., Hamidouche, W., Univ. Rennes, I., *et. al.* (2022). Transformer-based models for unsupervised anomaly segmentation in brain MR images. *arXiv*. https://www.semanticscholar.org/paper/46ea50841fee9b43331e40ff45753ae160b4f1dd (accessed on 30 May 2025).

28. Gilardi, B. R., Muñoz López, J. I., Hernández Villegas, A. C., Garay Mora, J. A., Rico Rodríguez, O. C., Chávez Appendini, R., De la Mora Malváez, M., *et. al.* (2019). Types of cerebral herniation and their imaging features. *Radiographic, 39*(6), 1598–1610. https://doi.org/10.1148/rg.2019190018.

29. Go, H., Jung, H., Ahn, S. V., Ahn, J., Shin, H., Amano, A., & Choi, Y. H. (2024). Trend in the incidence of severe partial edentulism among adults using the Korean National Health Insurance Service claim data, 2014–2018. *Yonsei Medical Journal, 65*(234–240). https://www.semanticscholar.org/paper/5a69ba45d6d661a1b0866483f67a7dd595dabc0f (accessed on 30 May 2025).

30. Gounis, M. J., Ughi, G. J., Marosföi, M., Lopes, D. K., Fiorella, D., Bezerra, H. G., Liang, C. W., *et. al.* (2018). Intravascular optical coherence tomography for neurointerventional surgery. *Stroke, 50*(2), 218–223. https://doi.org/10.1161/strokeaha.118.022315.

31. Gulshan, V., Peng, L., Coram, M., Stumpe, M. C., Wu, D., Narayanaswamy, A., Venugopalan, S., *et. al.* (2016). Development and validation of a deep learning algorithm for detection of diabetic retinopathy in retinal fundus photographs. *JAMA, 316*(22), 2402–2410. https://doi.org/10.1001/jama.2016.17216.

32. Hofmeijer, E. I. S., Kwee, T., Lamers, M., *et. al.* (2024). A framework to integrate artificial intelligence training into radiology residency programs: Preparing the future radiologist. https://core.ac.uk/download/620143327.pdf (accessed on 30 May 2025).

33. Holmboe, E. S., Yamazaki, K., Edgar, L., Conforti, L. N., Yaghmour, N. A., Miller, R. S., & Hamstra, S. J. (2015). Reflections on the first 2 years of milestone implementation. *Journal of Graduate Medical Education, 7*(3), 506–511. https://doi.org/10.4300/jgme-07-03-43.

34. Horvat, N., Rocha, C. C. T., Oliveira, B. C., Petkovska, I., & Gollub, M. J. (2019). MRI of rectal cancer: Tumor staging, imaging techniques, and management. *Radiographic, 39*(2), 367–387. https://doi.org/10.1148/rg.2019180114.

35. Hoveidaei, A., Some'eh, S. H., Goradel, R. R., Didar, H., Khonji, M. S., Khadembashiri, M. M., Fazeli, P., *et. al.* (2025). Medical radiation knowledge among medical doctors and students in Iran: A nationwide cross-sectional study. *Journal of Medical Imaging and Interventional Radiology*. https://www.semanticscholar.org/paper/897c82be65c81d6f6de38c67008853962472e204 (accessed on 30 May 2025).

36. Hu, X., Wang, Y., Li, J., Qing, P., Yang, X., Zeng, J., Min, L., *et. al.* (2023). Three-dimensional multimodality image reconstruction as teaching tool for case-based learning among medical postgraduates: A focus on primary pelvic bone tumor education. *BMC Medical Education, 23*. https://doi.org/10.1186/s12909-023-04916-8.

37. Hur, S., Jun, H., & Jeong, Y. S. (2021). Novel interventional radiological management for lymphatic leakages after gynecologic surgery: lymphangiography and embolization. *Gland Surgery, 10*(4), 1260–1267. https://doi.org/10.21037/gs-2019-ursoc-10.

38. Jang, H. Y., & Choi, C. H. (2024). Clinical imaging guidelines: Current status and challenges. *Journal of the Korean Medical Association*. https://www.semanticscholar.org/paper/42374a1ce44497e726b2e8ea5878317973208da8 (accessed on 30 May 2025).

39. Jenkins, N. W., Parrish, J. M., Sheha, E., & Singh, K. (2021). Intraoperative risks of radiation exposure for the surgeon and patient. *Annals of Translational Medicine, 9*, 84. https://doi.org/10.21037/atm-20-1052.

40. Jeong, W. K. (2023). Diagnosis of hepatocellular carcinoma using Sonazoid: A comprehensive review. *Journal of Liver Cancer, 23*(4), 272–283. https://doi.org/10.17998/jlc.2023.08.25.

41. Kim, D. I. (2016). PREFACE: How dangerous are X-ray studies that we undertake every day? *Journal of Korean Medical Science, 31*(Suppl 2), S2–S3. https://www.semanticscholar.org/paper/bbd1d226b331f27b7ccd45c60e9f895280596c35 (accessed on 30 May 2025).

42. Klein, L. W., Goldstein, J. A., Haines, D. E., Chambers, C. E., Mehran, R., Kort, S., Valentine, C. M., *et. al.* (2020). SCAI multi-society position statement on occupational health hazards of the catheterization laboratory: Shifting the paradigm for healthcare workers' protection. *Catheterization and Cardiovascular Interventions, 95*, 1327–1333. https://doi.org/10.1002/ccd.28579.

43. Kumar, A. A., Valakkada, J., Ayyappan, A., & Kannath, S. (2025). Basic statistics for radiologists: Part 1—Basic data interpretation and inferential statistics. *The Indian Journal of Radiology & Imaging, 35*, S58–S73. https://www.semanticscholar.org/paper/58e914931fb0e5a6c62c591bd6dec5a46d402f3e (accessed on 30 May 2025).

44. Kumari, C. S., & Seethalakshmi, K. (2023). Synthesizing radiological insights: Enhancing lung disease classification through multimodal imaging. *International Journal of Pharmaceutical Quality Assurance*. https://www.semanticscholar.org/paper/72338b8d5ae6054edf037405ba5663a016b47f85 (accessed on 30 May 2025).

45. Liszewski, M., Daltro, P., & Lee, E. Y. (2019). Back to fundamentals: Radiographic evaluation of thoracic lines and tubes in children. *AJR. American Journal of Roentgenology*. https://www.semanticscholar.org/paper/c97162c546387e56e9579e9badb3d9ffb44e6761 (accessed on 30 May 2025).

46. Luiz-Silva, W., Bazzanela, A. C., Dereczynski, C., Oscar-Júnior, A. C., & Raupp, I. (2025). Temperature and precipitation extremes in the Brazilian Legal Amazon: A summary of climatological patterns and detected trends. *Atmosphere*. https://www.semanticscholar.org/paper/71dad33260a22e8afc417a910c619af14e40b1b2 (accessed on 30 May 2025).

47. Lundervold, A. S., & Lundervold, A. (2018). An overview of deep learning in medical imaging focusing on MRI. *Zeitschrift für Medizinische Physik, 29*(2), 102–127. https://doi.org/10.1016/j.zemedi.2018.11.002.

48. Lydiatt, W. M., Patel, S. G., O'Sullivan, B., Brandwein, M., Ridge, J. A., Migliacci, J., Loomis, A., *et. al.* (2017). Head and neck cancers—Major changes in the American Joint Committee on Cancer eighth edition cancer staging manual. *CA: A Cancer Journal for Clinicians, 67*(2), 122–137. https://doi.org/10.3322/caac.21389.

49. Mahmood, F., Matyal, R., Skubas, N. J., Montealegre-Gallegos, M., Swaminathan, M., Denault, A., Sniecinski, R. M., *et. al.* (2016). Perioperative ultrasound training in anesthesiology: A call to action. *Anesthesia & Analgesia, 122*(6), 1794–1804. https://doi.org/10.1213/ane.0000000000001134.

50. McKeown, T., Gach, H., Hao, Y., An, H., Robinson, C. G., Cuculich, P., Yang, D., *et. al.* (2024). Small metal artifact detection and inpainting in cardiac CT images. *ArXiv*. https://www.semanticscholar.org/paper/38f9934ae70ba5fd4df41aba9134d85b39d75b3c (accessed on 30 May 2025).

51. Meher, V. R., Huntsman, R. J., Green, F. H. Y., Wooff, J. C., & Auer, R. (2025). Cause of death analysis in a 9½-year-old with COVID-19 and Dravet syndrome. *Pathophysiology, 32*. https://www.semanticscholar.org/paper/5b9f3194cf2b1329bff7bdcde88ca79743605bee (accessed on 30 May 2025).

52. Meşe, İ., Taşlıçay, C. A., Kuzan, B. N., Kuzan, T. Y., & Sivrioğlu, A. K. (2023). Educating the next generation of radiologists: A comparative report of ChatGPT and e-learning resources. *Diagnostic and Interventional Radiology, 30*(163–174). https://doi.org/10.4274/dir.2023.232496.

53. Najjar, R. (2023). Redefining radiology: A review of artificial intelligence integration in medical imaging. *Diagnostics, 13*, 2760. https://doi.org/10.3390/diagnostics13172760.

54. Noska, M. A., Borrás, C., Holahan, E. V., Dewji, S., Johnson, T. E., Hiatt, J. W., Newhauser, W., *et. al.* (2022). Health physics workforce in the United States. *Journal of Applied Clinical Medical Physics, 23*. https://doi.org/10.1002/acm2.13757.

55. Paranjape, K., Schinkel, M., Panday, R., Car, J., & Nanayakkara, P. W. B. (2019). Introducing artificial intelligence training in medical education. *JMIR Medical Education, 5*, e16048. https://doi.org/10.2196/16048.

56. Pringle, C., Kilday, J. P., Kamaly-Asl, I., & Stivaros, S. (2022). The role of artificial intelligence in paediatric neuroradiology. *Pediatric Radiology, 52*(12), 2159–2172. https://doi.org/10.1007/s00247-022-05322-w.

57. Quiroga-Garza, A., Elizondo-Omaña, R. E., Salinas-Alvarez, Y., & Guzman-Lopez, S. E. (2020). Effective near-peers in anatomy. *The FASEB Journal, 34*(S1), 1. https://doi.org/10.1096/fasebj.2020.34.s1.00413.

58. Ranem, A., Babendererde, N., Fuchs, M., & Mukhopadhyay, A. (2023). Exploring SAM ablations for enhancing medical segmentation in radiology and pathology. *arXiv, abs/2310.00504*. https://www.semanticscholar.org/paper/d5e46d745bcd746d65fe5b7f7dce22815afe212b (accessed on 30 May 2025).

59. Shen, D., Wu, G., & Suk, H. I. (2017). Deep learning in medical image analysis. *Annual Review of Biomedical Engineering, 19*, 221–248. https://doi.org/10.1146/annurev-bioeng-071516-044442.

60. Shen, L., Lu, Y., He, Y., Wang, P., Chen, Y., Li, H., Yang, Z., *et. al.* (2024). Work stress and competency among radiology residents: The mediating effect of resilience. *Frontiers in Public Health, 12*. https://www.semanticscholar.org/paper/cb1c6950f780ea9872ef5a79eec568d2b5c9d502 (accessed on 30 May 2025).

61. Spahn, D. R., Bouillon, B., Černý, V., Duranteau, J., Filipescu, D., Hunt, B. J., Komadina, R., *et. al.* (2019). The European guideline on management of major bleeding and coagulopathy following trauma: Fifth edition. *Critical Care, 23*, Article 98. https://doi.org/10.1186/s13054-019-2347-3.

62. Tanaka, M., Keefe, N. A., Caridi, T., Kohi, M., & Salazar, G. (2023). Interventional radiology in obstetrics and gynecology: Updates in women's health. *Radiographic: A Review Publication of the Radiological Society of North America, Inc., 43*(3), e220039. https://www.semanticscholar.org/paper/fc8e6cfd3985a6210c693e69cb5158498872b5ea (accessed on 30 May 2025).

63. Ugga, L., Franca, R. A., Scaravilli, A., Solari, D., Cocozza, S., Tortora, F., Cavallo, L. M., *et. al.* (2023). Neoplasms and tumor-like lesions of the seller region: Imaging findings with correlation to pathology and 2021 WHO classification. *Neuroradiology, 65*(675–699). https://doi.org/10.1007/s00234-023-03120-1.

64. Van Osch, M. V., Wåhlin, A., Scheyhing, P., Mossige, I., Hirschler, L., Eklund, A., Mogensen, K., *et. al.* (2024). Human brain clearance imaging: Pathways taken by magnetic resonance imaging contrast agents after administration in cerebrospinal fluid and blood. *NMR in Biomedicine*. https://www.semanticscholar.org/paper/9f30da6234a545704eace368644b26b082bc4d7d (accessed on 30 May 2025).

65. Varnosfaderani, S. M., & Forouzanfar, M. (2024). The role of AI in hospitals and clinics: Transforming healthcare in the 21st century. *Bioengineering, 11*(4), 337. https://doi.org/10.3390/bioengineering11040337.

66. Vrdoljak, I., & Bradarić, A. (2024). Medical physics in radiological practice. *Journal of Applied Health Sciences*. https://www.semanticscholar.org/paper/3062f5c5bf3e4222cd2d8fb11e0d706966920462 (accessed on 30 May 2025).

67. Werin, S., Andersen, J., Bonetti, S., Curbis, F., Goryashko, V., Isaksson, L., Johnsson, P., *et. al.* (2017). The soft X-ray laser project at MAX IV. https://www.semanticscholar.org/paper/6c3befaa0ed3d74eac470a2fe16f547f629c032b (accessed on 30 May 2025).

68. Wessel, L., Baiyere, A., Ologeanu-Taddeï, R., Cha, J., & Jensen, T. B. (2021). Unpacking the difference between digital transformation and IT-enabled organizational transformation. *Journal of the Association for Information Systems, 22*, 102–129. https://doi.org/10.17705/1jais.00655.

69. Xue, J., Xing, F., Liu, Y., & Liang, T. (2023). A 3D digital model for the diagnosis and treatment of pulmonary nodules. *Journal of Visualized Experiments (JoVE), 195*. https://www.semanticscholar.org/paper/ef7b97453d5bd0d1dfda0a746c950c47fcffc4ee (accessed on 30 May 2025).

70. Yada, S., Nakamura, Y., Wakamiya, S., & Aramaki, E. (2024). Cross-lingual natural language processing on limited annotated case/radiology reports in English and Japanese: Insights from the Real-MedNLP Workshop. *Methods of Information in Medicine*. https://www.semanticscholar.org/paper/851ddb06e25d3fe2286eb492735e943ae59c3b8e (accessed on 30 May 2025).

71. Yagil, D., Reuveni, Y., & Segal-Karpas, D. (2020). Physicians' cognitive strategies for avoiding overconfidence. *Journal of Evaluation in Clinical Practice*. https://www.semanticscholar.org/paper/d5e4c5921643a2ee876ad83823de90c3fea2efc2 (accessed on 30 May 2025).

RADIATION PHYSICS

2

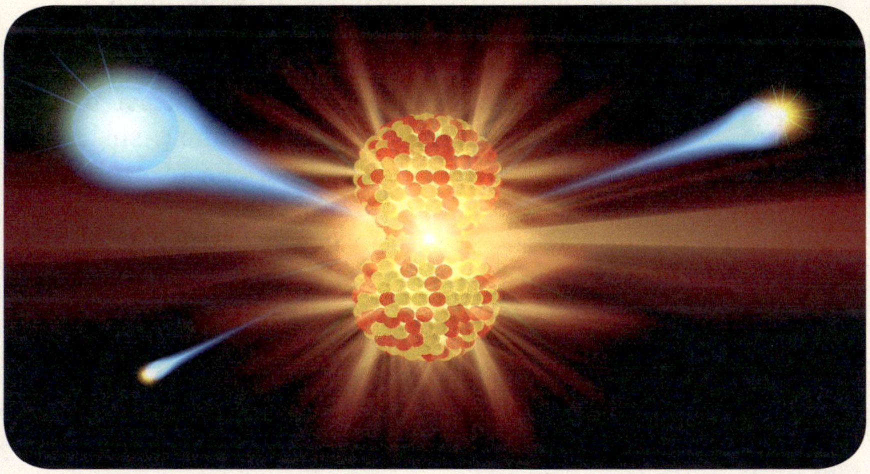

LEARNING OBJECTIVES

After studying this chapter, you will be able to:

1. Understand fundamental concepts of radiation
2. Know sources of radiation
3. Explain the biological effects of radiation
4. Discuss applications of radiation physics

Introduction

The two-way relationship between energy and matter has fascinated researchers for centuries, driving progress across the entire spectrum of physics and engineering. Radiation physics, a science that focuses on the emission, transmission, and absorption of energy in the form of particles or waves, encompasses fundamental principles that are equally applicable in theoretical studies as in practical applications. Radiation physics examines a range of phenomena, including electromagnetic radiation, particle emissions, and their atomic and subatomic interactions. Progress in this area not only deepens our knowledge of physical principles but also promotes technological advancements, such as semiconductor material, which is the foundation of modern electronics and facilitates information processing (Tolasa, 2025). Quantum information theory concepts also explain microscopic radiation behavior, relating fundamental physics to advanced technological challenges like quantum information processing and information transmission (Grazioso, 2015). As such, radiation physics is at the intersection of classical theory and state-of-the-art research, providing essential information on natural phenomena and applied sciences.

Definition of Radiation Physics

The science behind the study of matter and energy is the foundation for most advanced medical technology, particularly that involving radiation. Radiation physics is a branch of applied physics that examines the nature, behavior, and effects of ionizing and non-ionizing radiation when they collide with material, including biological ones like the human body. The field applies principles borrowed from classical mechanics and electromagnetism to interpret how radiation can be used effectively and safely, particularly in therapeutic and diagnostic medicine. Over time, applications of radiation physics have evolved to keep pace with heightened requirements for precision and customized treatment, illustrating a region of intersection between physics and medical practice beyond traditional boundaries (Samei *et. al.*, 2018). Moreover, through the integration of knowledge of physical hazards associated with energy and electromagnetic radiation, radiation physics aids in setting safety standards that protect workers as well as patients (Wald, 2016). Thus, radiation physics is an essential branch that combines fundamental physics with beneficial, life-saving medical technology (Figure 2.1).

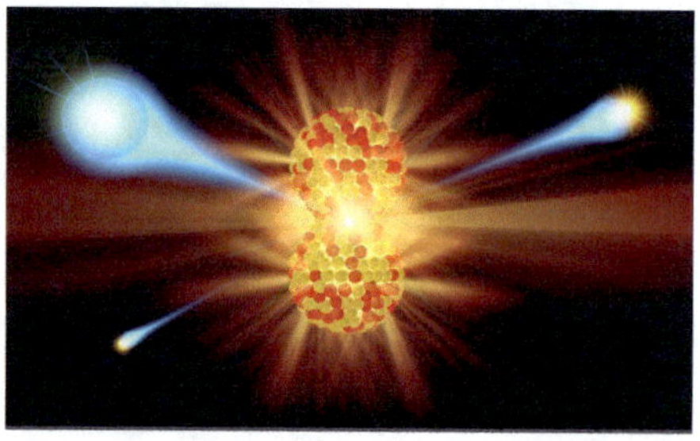

Figure 2.1. Radiation physics.

Source: https://www.thoughtco.com/thmb/fhok5Y1gFTXL5Cm7u7_eNXfBTHY=/1500x0/filters:no_upscale():max_bytes(150000):strip_icc()/atom-splitting-in-nuclear-fission-587169643-5792680a3df78c1734990723.jpg.

Historical Background

The course of radiation physics is forever intertwined with advances in particle physics and computer technology, which have increasingly enabled us to extend our understanding of things at the atomic and subatomic level. Early discoveries, such as X-rays and radioactivity, laid the basis upon which phenomena concerning the interaction between matter and radiation could be investigated. However, it is the latest breakthroughs in experimental and theoretical models, including large-scale collider experiments like those planned in the Future Circular Collider study, that attest to the dynamic evolution of the discipline (Asmâa *et. al.*, 2019). These researchers aim to probe fundamental particles to unprecedented levels of energy, refining accuracy and discovering new physics. Coincidentally, the use of digital twins—virtual models that replicate real systems—is revolutionizing simulation and predictive ability in radiation physics to allow for closer monitoring and control of complex experiments (Rasheed *et. al.*, 2020). Together, these technological and temporal developments highlight how radiation physics has matured into a field essential to both basic research and applications.

Importance of Radiation Physics in Modern Science

Diagnostic medical and renewable energy technologies exemplify the vital role played by radiation physics in current science. In medicine, radiation physics enables imaging techniques such as X-rays and MRI for accurate disease diagnosis, monitoring, and treatment planning. Every imaging technique has its advantages and limitations, necessitating a comprehensive understanding of radiation-matter interaction to streamline their applications in hospitals (Kamel *et. al.*, 2024). Outside of medicine, principles of radiation physics are at the core of solar photovoltaic system design, where the knowledge of semiconductor-photon interactions enables efficient light-to-electricity energy conversion (Shahid *et. al.*, 2023). This fusion of theory and practice emphasizes radiation physics as a basis for innovation, enabling advancements that promote human health and accelerate sustainable energy technology. Thus, the impact of the discipline extends across various scientific and engineering disciplines, advancing technologies, and addressing fundamental societal problems (Figure 2.2).

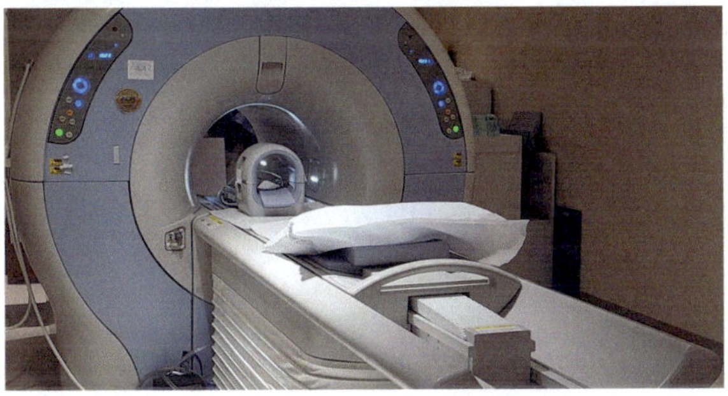

Figure 2.2. In healthcare, radiation physics underpins imaging techniques such as X-rays and MRI, which are essential for accurate disease diagnosis, monitoring, and treatment planning.

Source: https://medicalbuyer.co.in/wp-content/uploads/2022/02/MRI-Equipment_870x470.jpg.

Overview of Types of Radiation

Radiation encompasses a broad range of energy emissions, which are usually categorized as ionizing and non-ionizing depending on the ability to ionize atoms. Ionizing radiation includes alpha particles, beta particles, gamma rays, and neutrons, and each of which differs in mass, charge, and penetration capacity. Alpha particles, for example, have low penetration but high ionization capacity, while gamma rays comprise highly penetrating electromagnetic radiation. Non-ionizing radiation, such as radio waves and visible light, lacks sufficient energy to displace tightly held electrons but is still capable of inducing heat effects. Recognizing these distinctions is not only critical in the realm of nuclear accidents but also in cutting-edge technological applications, such as high-energy physics experiments, where radiation-hardened equipment, like the Low-Power Gigabit Transceiver, is rigorously tested for functional resilience under radiation exposure (Montesinos *et. al.*, 2024). In addition, careful monitoring and assessment in nuclear accidents underscore the importance of radiation type differentiation for effective risk communication and health physics responses (Yokoyama *et. al.*, 2024).

Applications of Radiation Physics

Manipulation and control of particle and electromagnetic radiation beams have significantly advanced scientific exploration and applications across a broad spectrum of science. They are focused bundles of energy and information, enabling specific interactions with matter of significant value in medicine, therapeutic applications, and material science. Major breakthroughs in beam dynamics, superconducting magnets, and accelerator design have enabled the conception of new devices, like the Gamma-Gamma and Muon Colliders, which expand particle physics discovery and medical imaging techniques (Chattopadhyay *et. al.*, 1994). Concurrently, the development of laser technology founded on a comprehensive understanding of radiation-matter interaction has revolutionized industrial applications and scientific inquiry. Laser beams provide unrivaled precision and efficiency in manufacturing, communication, and surgery, attesting to the extensive application of radiation physics principles in modern technology (Deneva *et. al.*, 2017). These advancements together underscore the pivotal role of radiation physics in determining both cutting-edge research and transformational industrial applications.

Key Concepts in Radiation Physics

Fundamental concepts of radiation physics include ionizing radiation-matter interactions, energy transfer mechanisms, and dose effect measurements, which together form the foundation for theoretical understanding as well as for practical use. Important concepts are particles and electromagnetic waves, linear energy transfer (LET), and stochastic versus deterministic effects, all of which are determinants of the effects radiation produces on biological systems and materials. The evolving research emphasizes the use of immersive learning tools, such as virtual and augmented reality, that are being brought more and more into the realm of pedagogy for radiation physics to make the abstract concepts easier to learn and to improve hands-on ability (Tene *et. al.*, 2024). Furthermore, earlier and ongoing conflicts over dose thresholds and model reliability for assessing radiation risk demonstrate the necessity of rigorous scientific scrutiny, revealing the nuances of interpreting epidemiological data and experimental findings in the field of radiation physics (Beyea, 2024). Taken together, these elements present an advanced appreciation of radiation's behavior and its significance to scientific and regulatory forums (Figure 2.3).

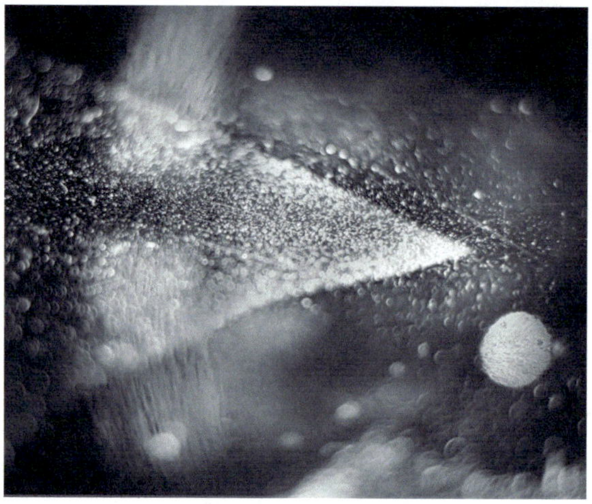

Figure 2.3. Nature of particles.

Source: https://howardlewisphotographs.com/wp-content/uploads/2020/04/The-Nature-of-Particles-47.jpg.

Significance of Understanding Radiation

The complications of radiation-matter interaction point towards the importance of recognizing how radiation behaves in various contexts, from astrophysics phenomena to biological systems. For instance, in high-energy astrophysics, the detection of quasi-periodic variation trends in gamma-ray activity from blazars enhances our understanding of the involved underlying radiation mechanisms and their variability, which suggests non-linear and multiplicative processes rather than simple Gaussian noise trends, with significant consequences for modeling these cosmic sources (Benkhali *et. al.*, 2019). Similarly, in the field of crystallography, accurate comprehension of radiation damage at different resolution spaces reveals damage evolution to be an exponentially dose-dependent phenomenon regulated by energy deposition and electron density smearing, necessitating resolution-dependent dose restrictions to ensure structure integrity during experiments (Atakisi *et. al.*, 2019). These perceptions are not only important for making experimental procedures more precise but also in advancing the technological and medical utilization of radiation, where use must be scrupulously controlled and intuited in order to avoid inadvertent effects.

2.1. Fundamental Concepts of Radiation

Learning Outcome

1. Describe measurement units in radiation physics
2. Discuss the interaction of radiation with matter
3. Explain the electromagnetic spectrum
4. Explain types of radiation
5. Focus on properties of radiation
6. Know particle vs. wave theory
7. Know the role of photons in radiation
8. Understand the nature of electromagnetic radiation
9. Understand quantum theory and radiation

The interaction between matter and electromagnetic waves gives rise to advanced phenomena that are now vital for advancing today's technologies. Central to such progress is the ability to control radiation beyond natural limits , such as employing concepts like topology to control light behavior, especially in optoelectronic technology. Unlike conventional Hermitian systems with energy conservation, non-Hermitian systems allow for radiation leakage, leading to new phenomena like bound states in the continuum that support perfect light trapping by topological invariants known as topological charges. The topological nature makes it possible to control the radiation channels with high precision, giving rise to applications such as vortex beam generation with custom-designed far-field patterns and ultrafast beam switching. Furthermore, reconfigurable intelligent surfaces demonstrate how controlling radiation's wavefront—phase, amplitude, frequency, and polarization—can revolutionize wireless communications by transcending natural propagation limits. All such advancements emphasize paradigmatic influence that principles of radiation impose in selecting cutting-edge technology solutions (Ertuğrul *et. al.*, 2019; Yin *et. al.*, 2020).

2.1.1. Nature of Electromagnetic Radiation

The effect of electromagnetic radiation on matter reveals subtle processes outside the range of common thermal phenomena that lead to a more complicated intrinsic nature of such waves. Microwave frequencies, for instance, induce rotation of dipolar molecules in a dielectric material, resulting in polarization and reorientation of hydrogen bonds that influence viscosity and enhance diffusion regardless of thermal energy. This effect highlights the significance of the collective action of coherent electromagnetic fields, which have measurable effects despite their relatively low energy compared to molecular binding energies (Hinrikus *et. al.*, 2018). Furthermore, enhanced quantum-mechanical descriptions of exciton-plasmon coupled systems illustrate how electromagnetic radiation influences material responses at the nanoscale, displaying nonlinear and dephasing effects not adequately captured by classical dielectric models (Sukharev *et. al.*, 2017). These points underscore that electromagnetic radiation inherently involves both quantum and wave characteristics, which necessitate sophisticated theoretical and computational approaches to fully characterize its nature in various physical contexts (Figure 2.4).

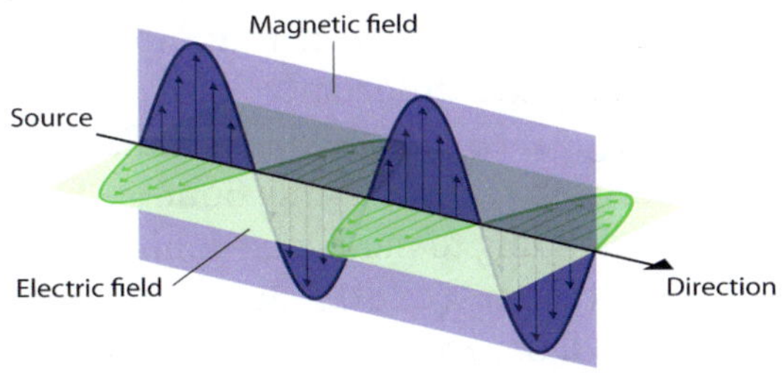

Figure 2.4. Electromagnetic radiation.

Source: https://chem.libretexts.org/@api/deki/files/32367/40e36bb375b3849544da98d03a00f649.jpg?revision=1&size=bestfit&width=588&height=305

2.1.2. Particle vs. Wave Theory

The nature of radiation has been debated over decades through the lens of particle and wave theory, each with different but complementary accounts for electromagnetic phenomena. Wave theory held sway in describing diffraction and interference, but with the advent of quantum mechanics, the concept of the photon, localized, quantized packets of light with both particulate and wavelike qualities-emerged. This duality unseats classical conceptions, showing radiation to be neither wholly particulate nor wholly wave-like but as quantum entities exhibiting the properties of both, depending on the conditions. Contemporary theoretical frameworks transcend straightforward dichotomies by incorporating the complex interplay of quantum fields and entanglement wherein particles emerge from concealed wave functions and higher-dimensional abstractions. Such hypotheses, derived from advanced string and multi-fold theories, suggest that gravity and quantum interactions are a unification phenomenon due to entangled particle states, thus combining wave and particle accounts in a single coherent microscopic framework in radiation physics (Cicoli *et. al.*, 2024; Stéphane, 2023).

2.1.3. Types of Radiation: Ionizing and Non-Ionizing

Knowledge of how ionizing and non-ionizing radiation differ is crucial in radiation physics since they interact differently with matter as well as biological tissues. Ionizing radiation has enough energy to remove tightly bound electrons from atoms, leading to molecular ionization that can cause extreme cellular damage; thus, its application is a hazard in medical diagnosis and therapies. Alternatively, non-ionizing radiation lacks sufficient energy to ionize atoms but rather primarily induces excitation or heating effects. Despite its widespread application for therapeutic purposes, such as dermatology and imaging, non-ionizing radiation is less defined and demands strict dosage control to prevent harmful effects (Omer, 2021). Technological developments like free-electron lasers demonstrate the potential of employing strong, short-wavelength ionizing radiation to perform high-resolution imaging and probing of atomic-scale phenomena and reflect the frontier research of ionizing radiation's potential in physics and medicine (Roßbach *et. al.*, 2019). This dualism reflects the importance of systemic knowledge for safe and efficient use of both forms of radiation (Figure 2.5).

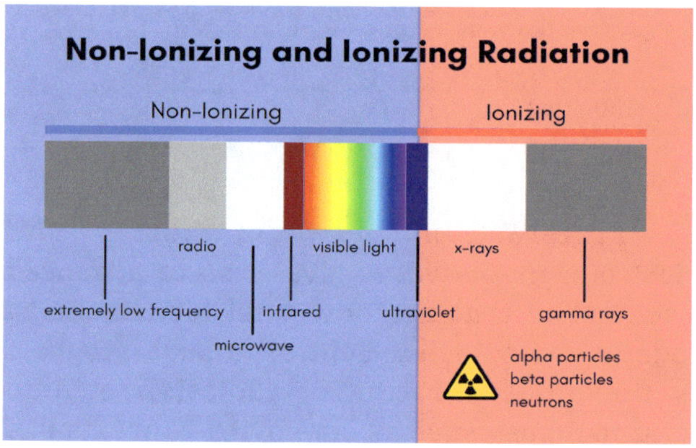

Figure 2.5. Ionizing and non-ionizing radiation.

Source: https://sciencenotes.org/wp-content/uploads/2021/04/Ionizing-and-Non-Ionizing-Radiation.png.

2.1.4. Properties of Radiation

Understanding the inherent properties of radiation entails learning how it has different properties, including wavelength, frequency, and energy, which are closely related by the electromagnetic spectrum. Radiation can come in the form of particles or waves, with different interaction characteristics with matter, influencing absorption, reflection, and transmission effects. Significantly, the stochastic gravitational wave background generated by cosmic string networks is an example of a class of radiation for which the cumulative emission contains detailed information about cosmic evolution and fundamental physics, as illustrated by proposed observations from probes like LISA (Auclair *et. al.*, 2020). Also among phenomena related to radiation are neutrino emissions, where precise information regarding neutrino mass ordering improves knowledge of particle properties and the underlying physics governing flavor and mass correlations (de Salas *et. al.*, 2018).

The above illustrations demonstrate the diversity of properties of radiation, which is not only vital to traditional physics but also to contemporary cosmology and particle physics, thereby improving the overall knowledge of the environment of radiation physics.

2.1.5. Interaction of Radiation with Matter

Understanding the fundamental processes by which radiation acts on matter is necessary to advance physics and technology. Historical milestones, such as the Saha ionization formula, Bose statistics, and Raman effect, uncovered the complex processes in matter-radiation interactions and paved the way for quantum mechanics and atomic physics. These findings stemmed from trailblazing studies in early 20th-century India, which identified how radiation can ionize atoms, determine statistical particle behaviors, and scatter light to expose material properties, respectively (Choudhuri, 2024).

The complex interactions involved include processes such as absorption, scattering, and emission, all affecting how energy transfer happens at the atomic and molecular levels. These principles not only underpin theoretical understanding but also form the foundation of applied uses,, ranging from spectroscopy to nuclear medicine and radiation detection (Choudhuri, 2024). The study of the interaction of radiation with matter thus remains fundamental to radiation physics, both underpinning scientific investigation and technological innovation (Figure 2.6).

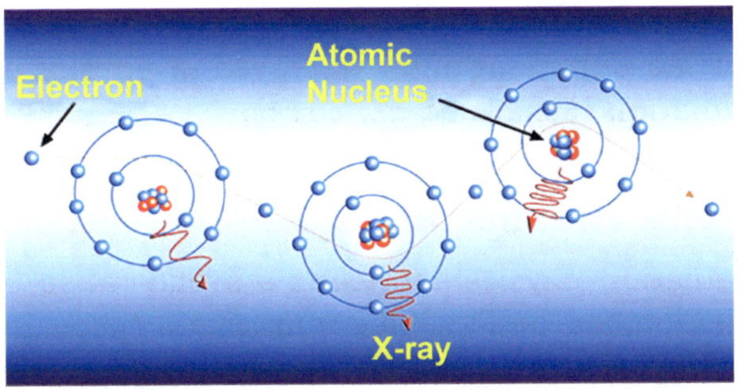

Figure 2.6. Understanding the fundamental ways in which radiation interacts with matter is essential for advancements in various fields of physics and technology.

Source: https://www.nde-ed.org/NDEEngineering/RadiationSafety/Graphics/ISU034.jpg.

2.1.6. Measurement Units in Radiation Physics

Understanding the effects and behavior of ionizing radiation necessitates precise quantification, which is provided by measurement units inherent to the physics of radiation. They allow correct and reliable communication and comparison across various applications, ranging from medical imaging to radiotherapy and monitoring the environment. The base units are the becquerel (Bq), which expresses activity of radioactive decay, and the gray (Gy), which expresses absorbed dose—that is, energy deposited per unit of tissue mass. With them are units such as the sievert (Sv), scaling absorbed dose for biological effect and for different tissue sensitivities to radiation. Such measurements depend on advanced comprehension of electromagnetic interactions, which is commensurate with advancement in related fields studying wave propagation and energy transfer, such as the development of reconfigurable intelligent surfaces in wireless communication systems (Renzo *et. al.*, 2020). In addition, computational modeling techniques in astrophysics and hydrodynamic simulations inform the calibration and validation of estimates of radiation dose, forming the basis for measurement units employed in physics of radiation (Schaye *et. al.*, 2014).

2.1.7. The Electromagnetic Spectrum

Radiation physics addresses a broad range of phenomena, and the electromagnetic spectrum is employed as a point of departure that sorts radiation by wavelength and frequency. It extends from low-energy radio waves to high-energy gamma rays, which respond differently when interacting with matter and dictate different technological uses. For instance, the knowledge of coupling of surface and volume electromagnetic fields in complicated structures leads to innovations in radiation sources and absorbers, illustrating how fundamental spectrum knowledge gets translated into functional devices such as free-electron lasers and solar cells (MacLachlan *et. al.*, 2019).

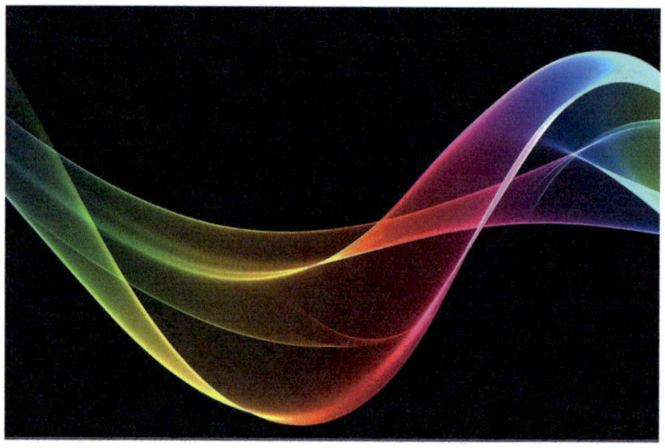

Figure 2.7. The electromagnetic spectrum.

Source: https://images.newscientist.com/wp-content/uploads/2020/02/26151654/electromagnetic-spectrum-shutterstock_1236662800_web.jpg.

Additionally, precise modeling of electromagnetic phenomena, for example, neutrino-electron scattering, necessitates the inclusion of radiative corrections in the spectrum to improve theoretical predictions and experimental interpretation (Tomalak *et. al.*, 2020). Together, these notes point towards the electromagnetic spectrum's function not only in describing the physical nature of radiation but also its optimization for application in all forms of scientific and engineering work, and consequently its importance in the grand scheme of radiation physics (Figure 2.7).

2.1.8. Quantum Theory and Radiation

It is the quantum-level interaction between matter and electromagnetic radiation that lies at the heart of radiation physics. The quantum theory, which forms the basis of this interaction, describes how particles such as electrons emit and absorb energy in quanta form. This process of quantization accounts for phenomena such as the photoelectric effect and blackbody radiation, which classical physics could not explain. Furthermore, quantum field theory also expands these concepts by putting special relativity and quantum mechanics into a framework in which particles and fields actively transform and switch back into one another, like in high-energy particle collisions studied at facilities like the Large Hadron Collider (Cohen *et. al.*, 2016). In periodic media, the behavior of the wave function is characterized by topological invariants, allowing photonic systems to exhibit robust quantum Hall effects and thus opening new regimes for manipulating radiation (Ozawa *et. al.*, 2019). These advances demonstrate that not only quantum theory describe microscopic interactions, but also it stimulates technological advances in manipulating radiation through novel quantum and topological effects.

2.1.9. The Role of Photons in Radiation

Advances in knowledge of the fundamental character of radiation have increasingly emphasized the complex photon behaviors beyond those described by classical theory. Photons, as quantum bearers of electromagnetic energy, play a significant role not only in light propagation but also in high-energy processes that extend their influence to particle physics and cosmology. Recent research indicates that photons can acquire orbital angular momentum during emission under specific conditions, such as in helical undulators or with intense laser interactions, and thus be able to create twisted states, making them suitable for a range from X-rays through to gamma rays. This adds another contribution to the arsenal of diagnostics for exploring hadronic structures and spin dynamics, demonstrating the enormous versatility of photons in radiation processes (Karlovets *et. al.*, 2023). Further, astrophysically, Lyman-Werner band photons are central in regulating molecular dissociation within early cosmos environments, impacting star formation and evolution of initial structures by regulating chemo-thermal conditions during the infancy of the Universe (Incatasciato *et. al.*, 2023). Such observations place photons as key dynamic drivers of terrestrial and cosmic radiation physics (Figure 2.8).

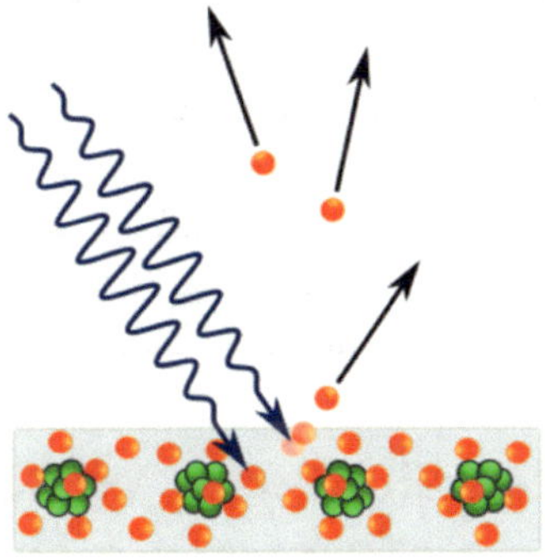

Figure 2.8. Photons play a crucial role not only in light propagation but also in high-energy phenomena that extend their influence into particle physics and cosmology.

Source: https://encyclopedia.pub/media/common/202210/mceclip0-635536464903e.png.

Test Your Knowledge

1. What are the main types of ionizing radiation?
2. What is the difference between ionizing and non-ionizing radiation?

2.2. Sources of Radiation

Learning Outcome

1. Describe nuclear power and radiation
2. Discuss terrestrial radiation
3. Explain industrial uses of radiation
4. Focus on cosmic radiation
5. Identify natural and artificial sources of radiation
6. Identify radiation from consumer products
7. Know the environmental impact of radiation sources
8. Know medical applications of radiation

It is significant to understand the sources of radiation in order to comprehend its effects and behavior under various environments. Sources of radiation can be broadly classified as natural and artificial origins, which individually contribute to the local field of radiation. The natural sources include cosmic rays, terrestrial radionuclides, and radon gas, which permeate everywhere and are location and environmental condition-dependent. Man-made sources are largely a product of human action, such as medical diagnosis, industrial consumption, and nuclear study centers. For example, sophisticated nuclear-physical methods have been employed to analyze the content of elements in soil samples surrounding research centers to establish impurities linked with anthropogenic activities, indicating the relevance of the protection of the environment in radiation physics (Maryna *et. al.*, 2024). In addition, characterization of radiation sources is extended to acoustic phenomena, such that spatial distribution and directivity of the sound source can be modeled for greater accuracy using computational methods, and there are parallels between sound and methods of radiation source analysis (Lemke *et. al.*, 2025).

2.2.1. Natural Sources of Radiation

The widespread availability of radiation in our environment does not only stem from human-made sources but also from natural sources. These natural sources, which have been present since the Earth's formation, contribute a significant share of the radiation dose received by humans annually. Cosmic radiation from outer space constantly bombards the Earth's atmosphere, creating secondary radiation that finds its way to the Earth's surface, varying by altitude and geomagnetic latitude.

In addition, soil, rocks, and building materials inherently contain terrestrial sources such as uranium, thorium, and decay products in the forms of alpha, beta, and gamma radiation. Radon gas, one of the decay products of uranium, is a significant indoor airborne radioactive hazard since it tends to concentrate within enclosed areas. Radiological outcomes and biological relevance of such exposures are explored in detail in the area of radiation physics, necessitating precise dosimetric assessment in order to understand their contribution to total dose and risk estimation. Such an understanding forms a foundation for principles in radiation protection that can be used in both environmental and medical applications (Modarai *et. al.*, 2022; Shultis *et. al.*, 2016) (Figure 2.9).

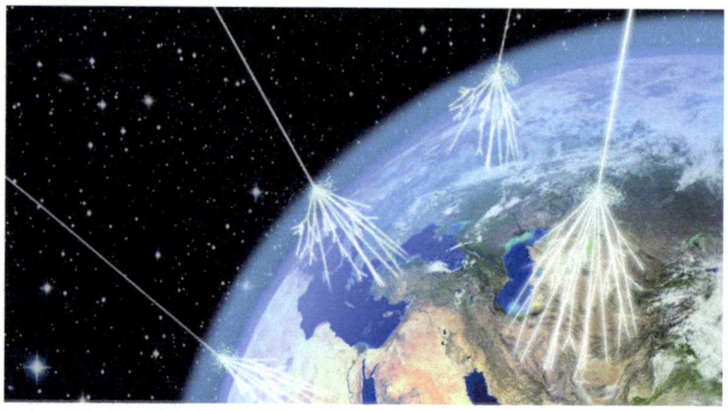

Figure 2.9. Cosmic rays from outer space continuously bombard the Earth's atmosphere, generating secondary radiation that reaches the surface, varying with altitude and geomagnetic latitude.

Source: https://news.uchicago.edu/sites/default/files/images/2023-12/cosmic-rays-illustration-explainer-hero.jpg.

2.2.2. Artificial Sources of Radiation

The technological advancement has enormously enhanced the range of sources of artificial radiation present in modern society largely because of their usage in medical, industrial, and research purposes. Of these, medical imaging techniques such as X-ray radiography, computed tomography (CT), and fluoroscopy constitute the bulk of artificial exposure, employing ionizing radiation to generate diagnostic images with significant clinical benefits but necessitating strict dose management to minimize patient and operator hazards (Modarai *et. al.*, 2022). Industry employs controlled radiation sources in determining structural quality and integrity and in quality assurance. Moreover, artificial radiation includes nascent fields like photonic systems in topological photonics, demonstrating how engineered periodic media can manipulate electromagnetic waves, opening new horizons for radiation-based technology (Ozawa *et. al.*, 2019). Despite being useful, these artificial sources must be managed by strict safety standards and regulatory regimes to minimize stochastic and deterministic health effects, underlining the central significance of radiation physics for advancing innovation and safeguarding.

2.2.3. Cosmic Radiation

Knowledge of the nature and influence of cosmic radiation is necessary to move forward in the field of radiation physics, especially since this type of radiation comes from external locations beyond Earth's atmosphere and has special challenges. Cosmic radiation is composed primarily of high-energy particles that interact with the atmosphere of the Earth, creating secondary particles that affect terrestrial and space environments.

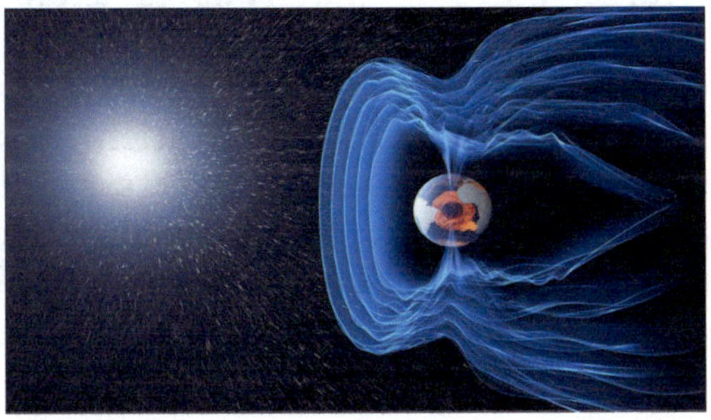

Figure 2.10. Cosmic radiation.

Source: https://www.esa.int/var/esa/storage/images/esa_multimedia/images/2014/02/earth_s_protective_shield/14265082-1-eng-GB/Earth_s_protective_shield_pillars.jpg.

Instruments on-board spacecraft are especially vulnerable to such high-energy particles, inducing damage in the form of displacement damage affecting operational integrity. Interacting processes are multi-nuclear scattering and energy loss mechanisms associated with screened nucleus-nucleus collisions within a wide energy spectrum spanning tens of keV to relativistic speeds (Boschini *et. al.*, 2010). In addition to charged particles, there exists a ubiquitous cosmic neutrino background which, though weakly interacting and hence difficult to detect directly, holds crucial cosmological importance. The neutrinos affect primordial nucleosynthesis and cosmological analysis of the cosmic microwave background as well as offer indirect signatures for dark radiation and lepton asymmetry in the cosmos (Steigman *et. al.*, 2012). Detailed study of cosmic radiation consequently merges astrophysical observations and particle physics of interactions to deepen our understanding of the nature of radiation and its influence (Figure 2.10).

2.2.4. Terrestrial Radiation

It is crucial to recognize the impact of cosmic phenomena on planetary climates in order to better appreciate the nature of radiation exposure on Earth. Terrestrial radiation primarily originates from natural radio content in the Earth, cosmic rays, and their interactions with the atmosphere, and secondary particles generated by these interactions. The Earth's magnetic field and atmospheric depth both have important roles in modulating this radiation and effectively shielding the surface from more harmful cosmic particles. Alterations in these barriers impact the radiation dose absorbed on the planet's surface, influencing biological and technological assets. Research from exoplanets reveals that an atmosphere that is thinner or a magnetic field that is weaker results in higher radiation levels, indicating the importance of such shields on planets in protecting life (Atri *et. al.*, 2013). Moreover, radiation effects considerations extend beyond the ground to problems with space travel, with radiation exposure impacting not just human health but also pharmaceutical stability on long-duration missions (Antonsen *et. al.*, 2019). Terrestrial radiation thus encompasses the complex interplay between cosmic, ground, and biological effects intrinsic to radiation physics.

2.2.5. Medical Applications of Radiation

Radiation physics innovations have deeply influenced medical diagnostics and treatment, transforming patient care through targeted therapy and precise imaging. Diagnostic radiology using ionizing radiation, such as X-rays and CT, allows physicians to image internal tissues without surgical intrusion, which aids in early detection and precise diagnosis of a variety of conditions. Therapeutically, radiation finds its most essential application in oncology, where specified quantities are given to kill cancer cells with minimal damage to the surrounding healthy tissue, demonstrating the attainability of precision through in-depth knowledge of radiation-matter interactions. Improvements in radiation sources and beam modulation have improved treatment effectiveness and reduced side effects, testifying to the intervention of physics principles in ensuring maximum clinical effectiveness. Detailed studies of radiation emission and absorption procedures have also enhanced safety regulations, minimizing hazards to patients and healthcare professionals (Figure 2.11).

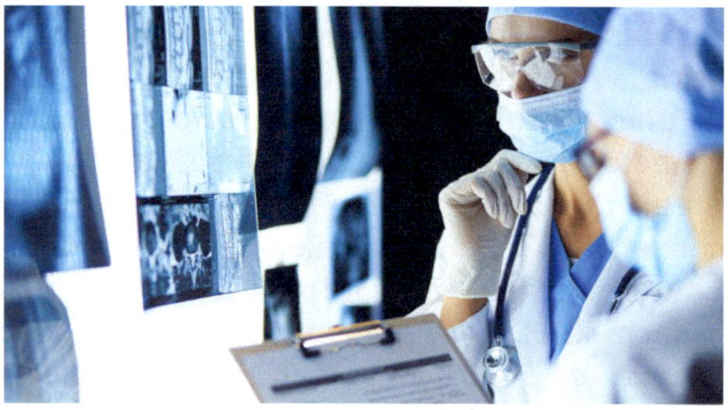

Figure 2.11. Medical uses of radiation.

Source: https://energy.ec.europa.eu/sites/default/files/styles/oe_theme_medium_no_crop/public/2024-04/MicrosoftTeams-image%20%287%29.png?itok=gDlboDqC.

2.2.6. Industrial Uses of Radiation

Advancements in the areas of materials science and energy technology have significantly expanded the industrial applications of radiation, particularly with the application of rare earth oxides (REOs). The material enhances the efficiency and lifespan of devices based on radiation in the use of energy conversion, protection against radiation, and sensor technology. For instance, REOs possess excellent chemical stability and neutron absorptivity, making them the optimum materials for gamma and neutron radiation protection in industrial processes, thereby improving the level of safety while promoting increased use of radiation (Hossain *et. al.*, 2022). In addition, gamma radiation is of great importance in various industrial processes, including sterilization, treatment of materials, and inspection. Its ability to induce controlled chemical and physical changes in materials is exploited for enhancing mechanical properties and decontaminating products efficiently (Basim, 2019). The employment of radiation in such industrial processes highlights its strength and importance in the discipline of radiation physics, connecting basic science with applied technology across industries.

2.2.7. Nuclear Power and Radiation

Enhanced computational modeling has significantly contributed to the understanding of nuclear power system safety analysis, particularly with the use of multiphysics simulations. A case in point is DireWolf software, which integrates various physical phenomena such as nuclear reactor physics, radiation transport, and heat pipe thermal hydraulics to simulate the performance of heat pipe–cooled nuclear microreactors under steady-state and transient conditions. This combined strategy is capable of capturing the complex nonlinear interactions typical of nuclear systems and providing invaluable inputs towards design optimization and failure scenario analysis (Matthews *et. al.*, 2021). Combined with such reactor-scale calculations, particle transport codes like PHITS have seen significant advancements in nuclear reaction and atomic interaction models, which enable enhanced simulation of electron and positron transport for radiation shielding and protection studies. The wider applicability of the software to medical physics, cosmic-ray research, and accelerator design shows the broad applicability of radiation transport physics for dealing with radiation safety and improving nuclear power technologies (Sato *et. al.*, 2018) (Figure 2.12).

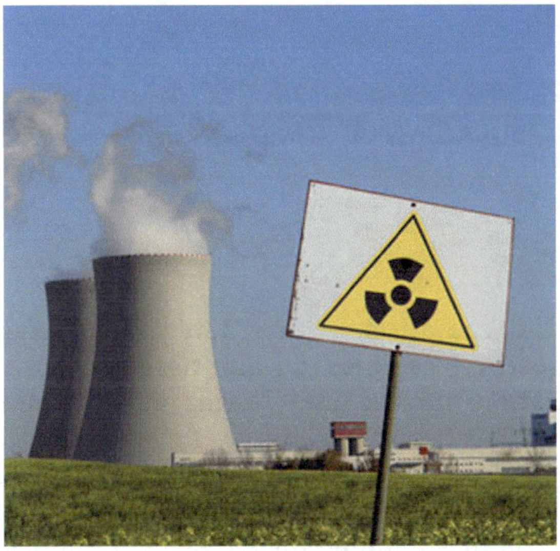

Figure 2.12. Nuclear power and radiation.

Source: https://static.scientificamerican.com/sciam/cache/file/D5B975F6-5EF8-4999-9B8C88368D25328E_*source*.jpg?w=1200

2.2.8. Radiation from Consumer Products

The application of radiation technology in food and consumer goods has provoked widespread controversy on the basis of varying perceptions regarding its safety and advantages. Ionizing radiation is applied to store certain foods like seafood and agricultural products to extend shelf life as well as inhibit microbial contamination, which can yield handsome economic returns, particularly for regions like Alaska, where product longevity matters most (Das *et. al.*, 1988). In spite of this, consumer acceptance remains a serious challenge. Studies show that distrust of regulatory bodies and insufficient knowledge about irradiation procedures are leading reasons for global skepticism of irradiated foods (Fletcher *et. al.*, 2025).

The above points highlight the importance of transparent communication and education to help build public confidence. Through the eradication of myths and re-establishing the effectiveness of control, the health risks of radiation from consumer products can be minimized so that the benefits of radiation technology for preservation and safety in food can be better enjoyed by society.

2.2.9. Environmental Impact of Radiation Sources

Advances in sources of radiation, particularly those utilizing accelerated charged particles, have enabled massive scientific achievement but raised concerns about their environmental implications. Synchrotrons and Free Electron Lasers (FELs) are such centers that emit intense electromagnetic radiation, essential for research in the fields of material and biological sciences; however, their operation necessitates radical control measures to prevent uncontrolled radiation exposure and environmental contamination (Mitri *et. al.*, 2011).

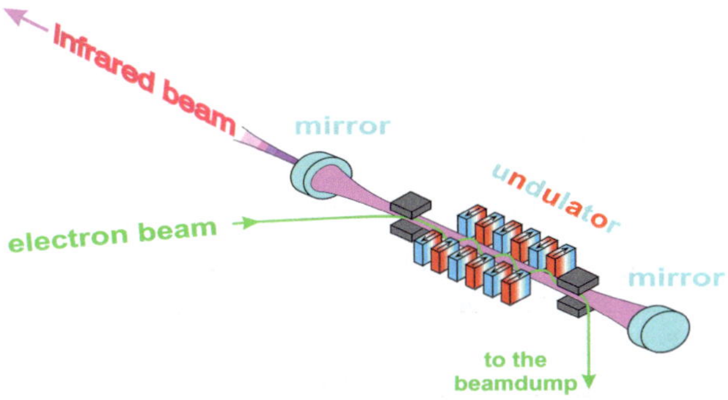

Figure 2.13. Free electron lasers (FELs).

Source: https://www.hzdr.de/db/Pic?pOId=11699

In addition, radiation from man-made sources, i.e., materials used in building construction and infrastructure, also contributes considerably to background radiation levels and has effects on human and environmental health (George *et. al.*, 2015). Mapping and tracking these radioactive discharges are critical for determining cumulative impacts and for establishing safeguarding limits of exposure. Thus, environmental stewardship in radiation physics does not just require technological progress but also integrated assessment approaches to balance scientific progress against ecological preservation. This approach ensures safe use of sources of radiation while attempting to minimize their ecological footprint (George *et. al.*, 2015) (Figure 2.13).

Test Your Knowledge

1. Name three natural sources of ionizing radiation.
2. What is cosmic radiation, and where does it come from?

2.3. Biological Effects of Radiation

Learning Outcome

1. Describe radiation-induced cancer
2. Discuss radiation dose and biological response
3. Explain acute vs. chronic radiation exposure
4. Focus on the genetic effects of radiation
5. Identify psychological effects of radiation exposure
6. Know cellular damage and repair mechanisms
7. Learn regulatory standards for radiation exposure
8. Understand mechanisms of radiation interaction with biological systems
9. Understand radiation safety and protection

A comprehension of how ionizing radiation interacts with biological systems is fundamental in ascertaining both its damaging and potentially therapeutic impacts. Radiation has the ability to damage at the molecular, cellular, and systemic levels, influencing survival, fertility, and organismal health. Surprisingly, the nature and severity of the biological effects depend extensively on the linear energy transfer (LET) of the radiation, which determines energy deposition regimes within tissue. High-LET radiation, for instance, yields more compact ionization tracks, leading to higher-order DNA damage that is more difficult for cellular repair mechanisms to rectify. Simulation tool research, such as that founded on TOPAS, has confirmed that all cells of irradiated animals, including bdelloid rotifers, are affected by ionizing particles, and that observed biological effects are due to direct radiation-induced damage, and not the probability of misses by particle impacts (Hespeels *et. al.*, 2023). Research encompassing these dynamics is of great value in understanding somatic effects, medical uses, and radiological safety protocols.

2.3.1. Mechanisms of Radiation Interaction with Biological Systems

Understanding of the intricate processes through which radiation interacts with the biosphere is facilitated by advanced modeling of particle tracks at microscopic scales. Advanced computer codes, such as the Particle and Heavy-Ion Transport code System (PHITS), enable the in-depth simulation of the radiation tracks within aquatic systems that replicate the atomic-level collisions that result in DNA damage and ensuing biological effects. By explicitly showing every atomic interaction, such simulations provide valuable information regarding microdosimetric distributions relevant to cellular response, including survival fraction and initial DNA lesion formation. These high-resolution track structure simulations are vital to both basic radiobiology and applied fields, such as radiation therapy, where therapeutic outcome depends on accurately modeling radiation-induced damage (Matsuya *et. al.*, 2021). Complementing PHITS, the Geant4 toolkit adds to this capability by simulating particle transport in matter in a range of fields with advanced models of physics and multithreading techniques to reconcile computational speed and accuracy. Together, these two tools explain the physical mechanism of radiation interaction with biological tissue to yield more insight and improved application in medical physics (John *et. al.*, 2016) (Figure 2.14).

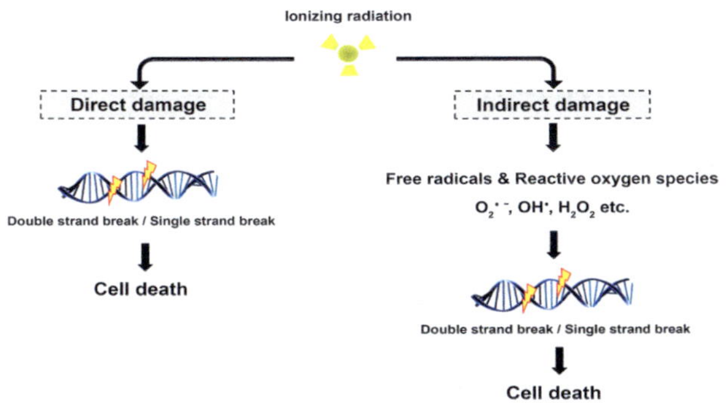

Figure 2.14. Mechanisms of radiation interaction with biological systems.

Source: https://www.mdpi.com/ijms/ijms-18-02749/article_deploy/html/images/ijms-18-02749-g001.png.

2.3.2. Acute vs. Chronic Radiation Exposure

The biological effects of ionizing radiation vary substantially based on acute or chronic exposure, and both the nature and severity of the damage. Acute radiation exposure, in which the administration of high doses over a short time, typically results in deterministic consequences such as erythema, sterility, and acute radiation syndromes (ARS), whose threshold exists below which no symptoms manifest and above which the severity will correspond directly to the magnitude of the dose (Kathren *et. al.*, 2002). In contrast, chronic exposure involves lower doses over a longer duration, with the majority of effects being stochastic, for example, cancer and genetic mutation, where risk increases linearly with dose without the existence of any measurable threshold (Kathren *et. al.*, 2002). This dichotomy complicates the assessment of risk, particularly in an environment like space, because of the difficulty presented by chronic low-dose radiation not adequately modeled by terrestrial models, diminishing predictive capability for astronaut health. Understanding the nuances between acute and chronic radiation exposure is therefore pivotal in radiation physics to get an accurate dose of the biological effect and to construct a correct protection regime.

2.3.3. Cellular Damage and Repair Mechanisms

It is significant to recognize the fine balance between repair and injury processes of cells in establishing the biological consequences of ionizing radiation. Ionizing radiation induces a variety of DNA damage, and double-strand breaks (DSBs) are the most radiosensitive type as they can result in genomic instability or cell death. Organisms have complex repair pathways like homologous recombination and non-homologous end-joining that are very efficient for the detection and repair of these breaks. Mutations within these repair proteins, in addition to enhancing radiosensitivity, are linked to inherited diseases that include immunodeficiency and cancer predisposition, a testament to the significance of DNA repair to maintain cellular integrity after exposure to ionizing radiation (Agrawal *et. al.*, 2009). Moreover, the low-dose radiation effects controversy emphasizes the complexities of the biological response, as the degree of damage and concomitant repair profoundly influence outcomes ranging from harmful mutations to adaptive resistance (Gonzalez *et. al.*, 2002). Thus, the interactive equilibrium between radiation-induced damage and cellular repair mechanisms fundamentally dictates organismal health and susceptibility to disease (Figure 2.15).

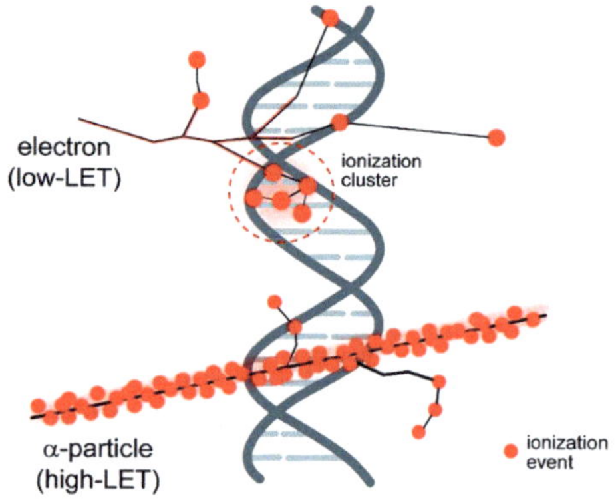

Figure 2.15. Radiation induces a spectrum of DNA lesions, with double strand breaks (DSBs) representing the most lethal form due to their potential to cause genomic instability or cell death.

Source: https://www.mdpi.com/cancers/cancers-11-01671/article_deploy/html/images/cancers-11-01671-g001.png.

2.3.4. Radiation Dose and Biological Response

The interaction of ionizing radiation with biological tissue is complex, influencing immediate and delayed health effects. Medical imaging examinations, primarily X-rays and CT scans, expose patients to different doses of radiation that are capable of causing stochastic and deterministic biological effects. Stochastic effects, such as cancers and genetic mutations caused by radiation, are chance in character and are believed to adhere to the linear non-threshold (LNT) model which states that, all incremental doses of radiation proportionally raise risk and is disputed by scientists (Kathren *et. al.*, 2002). Deterministic effects, such as erythema and sterility, only occur above a threshold dose and become progressively worsen with dose. Understanding these dose-response relationships is crucial to optimizing imaging protocols to minimize harm and optimize diagnostic yield. This balance is both for clinical practice and the derivation of radiation protection standards for patient protection (Thubab *et. al.*, 2024).

2.3.5. Radiation-Induced Cancer

The action of ionizing radiation on tissues in the body induces a cascade of damage in molecules, specifically DNA, that consequently leads to cancer development. Radiation-induced cancer is a consequence of mutations created by direct DNA strand breaks or indirectly by reactive oxygen species produced by interactions with radiation. The biological complexity is heightened in treatments like stereotactic radiosurgery, in which high doses produce not only cell death among tumor cells but also initiate vascular damage and immune responses that influence cancer development and suppression (Chung, 2025). In addition, ultraviolet radiation, which is beneficial for vitamin D synthesis, is carcinogenic due to its DNA-damaging effect, primarily in skin cells, emphasizing the two-fold character of the biological action of radiation (Terenetskaya, 2018). Explanation of the particular physical interactions and subsequent biological effects is necessary to make radiation therapy more effective while minimizing carcinogenic hazard, similar to the fine boundary in radiation physics and medicine (Figure 2.16).

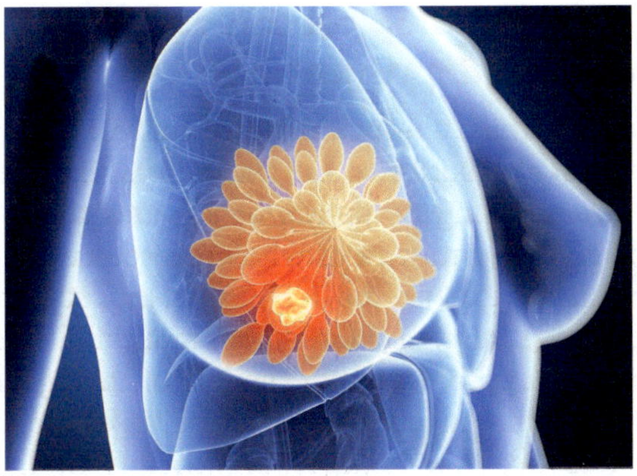

Figure 2.16. Radiation-induced cancer.

Source: https://www.bjmo.be/app/uploads/2022/07/GettyImages-470566383-breast-cancer-1024x768.jpg.

2.3.6. Genetic Effects of Radiation

Radiation's action on living organisms extends beyond immediate cellular damage to involve profound genetic consequences that influence future generations. Ionizing radiation can potentially result in DNA mutations by inducing strand breaks, base changes, and chromosomal aberrations that may lead to inherited genetic alterations. These genetic effects are significant in that they induce increased risks of genetic disorders, cancers, and developmental abnormalities in exposed populations. In addition, awareness of such effects is essential in the assessment of long-term health and ecological impacts, especially with regard to emerging technologies that utilize nanoparticles in medical and environmental applications, where radiation exposure may be coupled with new materials (Shafey, 2020). Moreover, the global scenario of environmental changes, such as those triggered by climate change, underscores the relevance of conducting scientific studies on microbial and genetic radiosensitivity to radiation, given that microorganisms are the major players in biogeochemical cycles and ecosystem stability (Cavicchioli *et. al.*, 2019). The multidisciplinary approach becomes necessary to improve radiation physics better and defend genetic integrity.

2.3.7. Radiation Safety and Protection

The use of safety and protection principles of radiation is necessary in radiation physics practice, particularly in the medical and industrial fields. Medical physicists operate in close collaboration with radiation oncologists and other healthcare workers in a bid to optimize treatment protocols such that there is precise dosimetry with minimal unnecessary exposure of patients as well as medical workers. This responsibility extends beyond clinical duty to include ongoing quality assurance, regulatory compliance, and education, promoting a safety culture in facilities that utilize ionizing radiation (Newhauser *et. al.*, 2022).

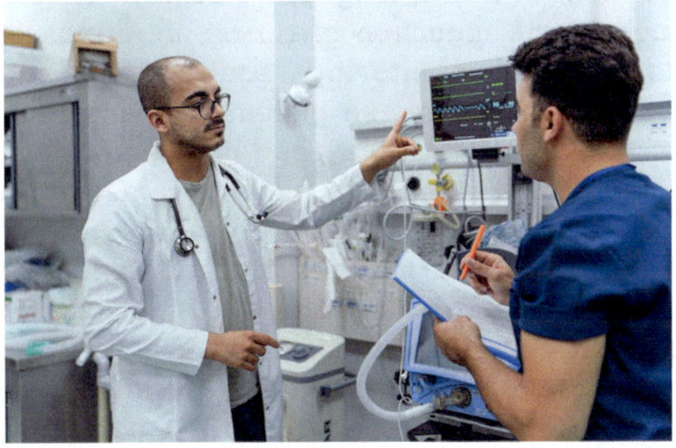

Figure 2.17. Experts in medical physics collaborate closely with radiation oncologists and other healthcare professionals to optimize therapeutic protocols, ensuring accurate dosimetry while minimizing unnecessary exposure to patients and staff.

Source: https://www.edmates.com/wp-content/uploads/2024/12/Medical-Dosimetrist-scaled.jpg.

Similarly, health physicists play a crucial role in protecting workers, the public, and the environment through the assessment of risks and implementation of controls for radiation exposure. Their interdisciplinary knowledge enhances a range of fields, including nuclear energy, healthcare, and emergency preparedness, focusing on prevention as much as response tactics (Michael *et. al.*, 2022). As a group, these professions show the equilibrium between leveraging applications of radiation and mitigating its internal risks in radiation physics (Figure 2.17).

2.3.8. Regulatory Standards for Radiation Exposure

Development of regulatory standards for radiation exposure is important to maximize the medical benefit of interventional and diagnostic procedures relative to any risks associated with them in patients. Guidelines are designed meticulously to avoid tissue reactions as well as long-term stochastic effects, such as the induction of cancer, by imposing dose limits, monitoring requirements, and follow-up measures on patients. For instance, accrediting bodies like The Joint Commission mandate radiation dose index documentation in fluoroscopically guided procedures under which healthcare facilities need to implement policies related to dose notification, patient consent, and post-procedure care to manage high-dose exposures effectively (Fisher *et. al.*, 2022). Similarly, during the COVID-19 pandemic, there was increased use of chest CT scanning. Consequently, advisories were put out regarding proper application in an attempt not to expose patients unnecessarily to radiation, advocating the efficacy of principles of justification and optimization in limiting dose while preserving utility in diagnosis (Garg *et. al.*, 2021). Such stringent regulation assures patient safety by instituting optimum best practices in medical imaging and interventional radiology, scientifically guided and clinically necessitated evolution.

2.3.9. Psychological Effects of Radiation Exposure

Alongside the well-documented physical hazards, radiation exposure also has extreme psychological effects, resulting in mental health and cognitive impairments. Individuals who have been exposed to radiation experience heightened anxiety, post-traumatic stress, and long-term mental illnesses due to the unpredictability and fear of having long-term health consequences. These psychological impacts are particularly significant in high-risk environments such as spaceflight, where radiation exposure is linked with typical stressors affecting astronauts' emotional well-being and performance. Existing research emphasizes the importance of integrating psychosocial factors into radiation risk assessment to facilitate comprehensive protection planning. Furthermore, recent studies give particular emphasis to the role of radiation-induced biological changes, including DNA damage and cellular response pathways, possibly indirectly producing neuropsychological symptoms, revealing the complex interplay between physical and psychological effects (Tan *et. al.*, 2025). Microscopic charge dynamics studies, though more material science-based, give understanding to molecule stability which can similarly inform understanding of radiation's subtle effects on the human body (Andrés *et. al.*, 2024) (Figure 2.18).

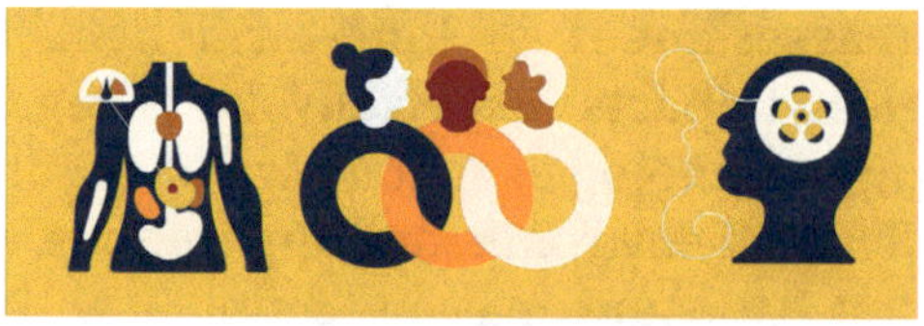

Figure 2.18. Individuals subjected to radiation often experience heightened anxiety, post-traumatic stress, and long-term mental health disorders due to the uncertainty and fear of potential health consequences.

Source: https://cms.wellcome.org/sites/default/files/styles/image_4x3_large/public/2022-03/menta-health-award-funding-call.jpeg?itok=F6IsWG7O.

Test Your Knowledge

1. How does radiation cause damage to living cells?
2. What are the primary biological effects of ionizing radiation?

2.4. Applications of Radiation Physics

Learning Outcome

1. Describe radiation in research and development
2. Discuss environmental monitoring and assessment
3. Discuss nuclear medicine applications
4. Explain radiation therapy for cancer treatment
5. Explain space exploration and radiation
6. Focus on industrial radiography
7. Focus on radiation in food safety
8. Know future trends in radiation applications
9. Understand medical imaging techniques

Advances in radiation physics have impacted the field of practical applications in most fields on the basis of the controlled production and manipulation of particle beams as well as electromagnetic radiation. The advances enable precise investigations of underlying natural processes along with novel technological applications. For example, the creation and control of high-energy beams allow for medical therapeutic development, such as cancer treatment, which selectively target infected tissue with minor damage to surrounding healthy tissue in the affected zone, highlights the essential intersection of physics and medicine (Chattopadhyay *et. al.*, 1994). Laser technology, a subsection of radiation physics, has also revolutionized industry by providing high-accuracy manufacturing tools for part and material production and scientific research. The profound knowledge of laser systems—from optical resonators, excitation, and beam control—has encouraged colossal improvements in quality and efficiency across a broad array of applications (Deneva *et. al.*, 2017). All these applications illustrate how the physics that underlies radiation enables revolutionary techniques with far-reaching social consequences, from medical breakthroughs to state-of-the-art industrial processes.

2.4.1. Medical Imaging Techniques

Medical imaging technology has significantly enhanced diagnostic capabilities with sophisticated radiation physics methods. Among numerous methods, electronic portal imaging devices (EPIDs) are critical for quality assurance and dosimetry, particularly in intensity-modulated radiation therapy (IMRT) and volumetric modulated arc therapy (VMAT). EPIDs make pre-treatment and transit dosimetry possible to a high degree of accuracy, enabling radiation dose verification for individual patients and machine-related faults in the initial stage, hence improving treatment precision and patient safety (Dogan *et. al.*, 2023).

Furthermore, developments in detector materials such as perovskite semiconductors hold potential to further revolutionize radiation detection through the combination of high attenuation coefficients with defect tolerance and high carrier mobility. Such material properties are amenable to enhanced device performance and sensitivity in detecting ionizing radiation, which is pertinent to both medical imaging and therapy applications (Hu *et. al.*, 2022). Combined, these technological developments reflect a widening interface between material science and radiation physics, advancing the frontiers of medical imaging toward enhanced diagnostics and treatments (Figure 2.19).

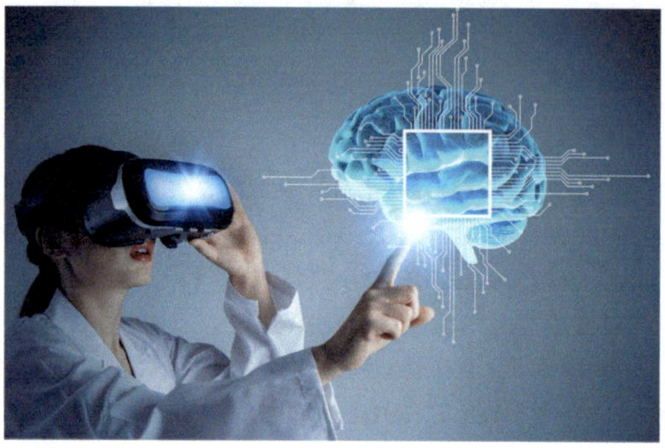

Figure 2.19. Advancements in medical imaging have significantly enhanced diagnostic capabilities through sophisticated radiation physics principles.

Source: https://www.postdicom.com/images/blog-posts/social-media-images/diagnostic-medical-imaging-social.png.

2.4.2. Radiation Therapy for Cancer Treatment

Radiation therapy has undergone significant development in altering cancer treatment through improving precision in dose delivery and minimizing injury to nearby healthy tissues. This advancement is a reflection of the development of traditional external beam radiation to new modalities such as proton therapy. Proton therapy utilizes the physical characteristics of proton beams, particularly the Bragg peak, to provide maximum energy deposition within the tumor with less exposure outside the target. New, up-and-coming treatments, including proton arc therapy and ultrahigh-dose-rate proton FLASH therapy, have been topics of fierce debate regarding their clinical applicability and future importance. Proton arc therapy should provide improved dose conformity with continuous arc delivery, thereby potentially improving the treatment efficacy, while proton FLASH therapy has the potential to transform radiobiological benefits through doses administered at ultrahigh rates that spare normal tissues without sacrificing tumor control. However, both techniques require further evidence for security, effectiveness, and feasibility before they can be practiced on a large scale. Education at the graduate level emphasizes new technologies as core elements of radiation physics education, improving professionals' competency, and making way for further studies to optimize cancer treatment (Burmeister *et. al.*, 2022; Kang *et. al.*, 2023).

2.4.3. Industrial Radiography

The applicability of radiation in industry has greatly enhanced the methods of material integrity evaluation without destroying it. Of all such methods, industrial radiography is a significant non-destructive test that utilizes ionizing radiation to produce clear internal structure images in metals, welds, and composites.

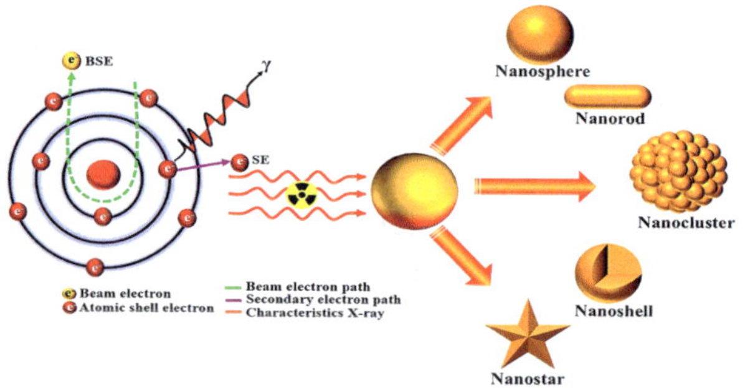

Figure 2.20. The application of radiation in industrial contexts has significantly advanced the methods for evaluating material integrity without causing damage.

Source: https://pub.mdpi-res.com/nanomaterials/nanomaterials-14-02051/article_deploy/html/images/nanomaterials-14-02051-ag.png?1737036757

This is useful to detect hidden flaws such as cracks, voids, or inclusions, which could make the structure unreliable. Rising technology in sensors and analytics has also enhanced the resolution and diagnostic capabilities of radiographic systems, providing more precise assessments required by critical infrastructure and manufacturing sectors (Hassani *et. al.*, 2023). Installation of real-time condition monitoring systems in machinery such as wind turbines is also a way in which radiation-based inspection aids predictive maintenance strategies to ensure operational safety and prolong asset life (Badihi *et. al.*, 2022). Therefore, industrial radiography is a significant tool in radiation physics applications for structural performance maximization and health protection (Figure 2.20).

2.4.4. Nuclear Medicine Applications

Technological innovation in molecular imaging has revolutionized the function of nuclear medicine in the delivery of radiation therapy, namely by leveraging the hybrid mode of positron emission tomography (PET) and CT. The hybrid technique enhances the precision of the radiation treatment planning through appropriate tumor identification and delineation of its borders, reducing exposure of nearby normal tissues, and, in theory, optimizing the efficacy of therapy. By employing numerous radiotracers against specific biochemical targets, PET/CT facilitates better tumor characterization and paves the way for new methods such as biologically-guided and PET-adaptive radiotherapy. However, implementation depends on interdisciplinary collaboration to surmount technical challenges and the biological heterogeneity of underlying imaging information to generate accurate treatment plans. In addition, the use of sophisticated simulation software in medical physics, including the Geant4 Monte Carlo code, serves as a key to validating nuclear medicine applications and optimizing dosimetric calculations for complex clinical cases. Collectively, these developments have led to improved accuracy and performance in cancer treatment within the realm of radiation physics (Arce *et. al.*, 2020; Jacob *et. al.*, 2023).

2.4.5. Radiation in Research and Development

Radiation physics developments have had a profound impact on research and development in other scientific disciplines, making formerly impossible innovations possible. For example, the knowledge of energy exchange processes at the atomic level has been essential in maximizing solid-state laser materials, where the management of atomic interactions with high accuracy has improved the efficiency and spectral parameters of laser emissions. Studies of energy transfer between sensitizer and activator atoms in complex laser materials are a good example of how fundamental radiation interactions lead to technological advancements (Koker *et. al.*, 2025).

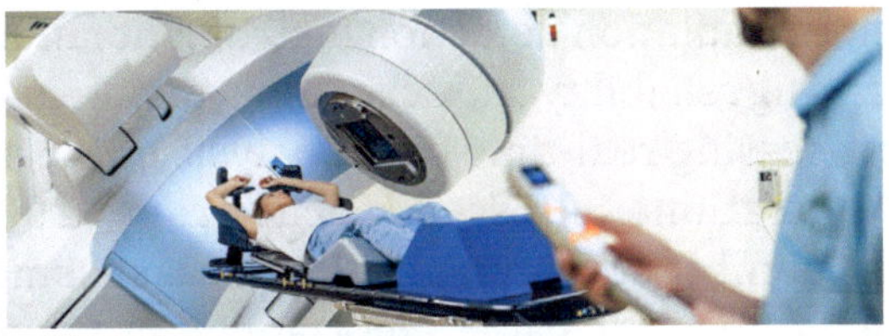

Figure 2.21. Radiation sensing field effect transistors (RADFETs).

Source: https://www.varadis.com/wp-content/uploads/2023/07/medical-radiation.jpg.

Likewise, the design of advanced radiation sensors, like Radiation Sensing Field Effect Transistors (RADFETs), is a good example of where radiation physics meets applied technology. These tools deliver precise, non-destructive dose monitoring in medical radiotherapy, high-energy physics experiments, and space exploration, highlighting their utility and potential in radiation protection and measurement (Jakšić *et. al.*, 2016). In this context, the strategic application of radiation physics principles becomes critical for enhancing experimental accuracy and designing creative solutions in research and development contexts (Figure 2.21).

2.4.6. Environmental Monitoring and Assessment

Successful control of radiation hazards involves precise and continuous monitoring of the environment to assess levels and impacts of ionizing radiation on human health and the environment. Advanced measuring equipment is employed to quantify and analyze radioactive pollutants, enabling early identification of contamination and radiation exposure sources. This cross-disciplinary framework integrates dosimetry application with biological and chemical physics to determine the interaction of radiation with living tissues and environmental matrices (Kaye *et. al.*, 1992). Moreover, the incorporation of prognostic methods into monitoring systems offers the ability to forecast potential radiation detection instrument failures, enhancing reliability and scheduling maintenance by processing real-time data analysis of thermal and operational stresses (Pecht *et. al.*, 2006). Such combined environmental assessment systems are particularly important for regulatory compliance and the effective implementation of radiation protection measures. With the combination of ongoing data collection and sophisticated risk analysis, radiation physics optimizes the capability to shield environmental and public health from radiologic dangers.

2.4.7. Radiation in Food Safety

Progress in radiation physics has facilitated considerable improvement in food safety through the application of ionizing radiation for the elimination of pathogens and shelf life extension. Through careful dosage control of the radiation, undesirable bacteria, molds, and insects can be effectively reduced without compromising nutritional quality or sensory attributes. Such treatments are dependent on the interaction between the radiation and food substance at the molecular level to induce microbial decontamination and spoilage retardation. The principles built in medical physics, such as dosimetry in regard to radiation and safety guidelines, are building blocks that will ensure safe and efficient food irradiation procedures as well as safeguard human health (Newhauser *et. al.*, 2022). The uses of future nano-precursor green synthesis techniques for synthesizing nanoparticles also stand to enhance the targeted delivery and efficacy of radiation-based therapy treatments (Shafey, 2020). Collectively, these interdisciplinary advances demonstrate the central role that radiation physics plays in guaranteeing food security and public health (Figure 2.22).

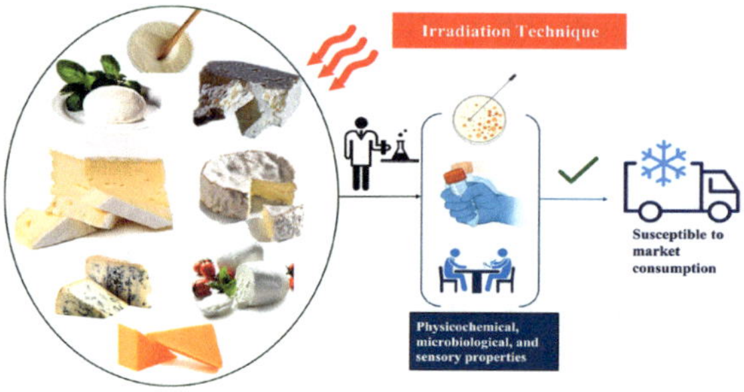

Figure 2.22. Advancements in radiation physics have enabled significant improvements in food safety through the application of ionizing radiation to eliminate pathogens and extend shelf life.

Source: https://media.springernature.com/lw1200/springer-static/image/art%3A10.1007%2Fs13197-024-06190-y/MediaObjects/13197_2024_6190_Fig4_HTML.png.

2.4.8. Space Exploration and Radiation

Traveling outside Earth's shielding atmosphere exposes astronauts to a range of radiation threats that present major challenges to human health and mission success. Space radiation includes primarily galactic cosmic rays and solar particle events, which are significantly different from terrestrial radiation sources because of their high energy and effectiveness in penetrating shields. These ionizing radiations are associated with serious health hazards, such as cancer, cardiovascular disease, and cognitive deficits, that will require stringent mitigation techniques for long-duration missions like those intended for Mars or lunar bases (Zarana *et. al.*, 2020). Devices like the Alpha Magnetic Spectrometer on board the International Space Station are constantly monitoring cosmic ray fluxes, and the information they provide enriches insight into the space radiation environment and supports better protective measures (Aguilar *et. al.*, 2020). These radiation hazards are addressed in a multidisciplinary way through physics, biology, and engineering to protect the health of astronauts and support long-term human exploration of space.

2.4.9. Future Trends in Radiation Applications

Technological advancements in computing and artificial intelligence (AI) will transform radiation applications, especially medical diagnosis and treatment. With the incorporation of AI, precision and personalized treatment plans are being promoted with the overall trend toward personalized medicine. Methods like theranostics, radiomics, and dosiomics are becoming increasingly crucial for enhancing patient outcomes by optimizing the radiation dose and forecasting the response more accurately. Concurrent with these advances, new computational software such as the TRIPOLI-5 Monte Carlo particle transport code is in development to carry out massively parallel calculations, to go beyond reactor physics to shielding and instrumentation of radiation, to be more versatile and efficient in the modeling of radiation. These technological advances are consistent with the direction of increased patient-specific methodology and enhanced simulation capability necessary to optimize safety and effectiveness in the application of radiation. Consequently, future development will most likely focus on precision diagnosis and treatment interventions based on solid computational frameworks (Mancusi *et. al.*, 2024; Sören, 2024) (Figure 2.23).

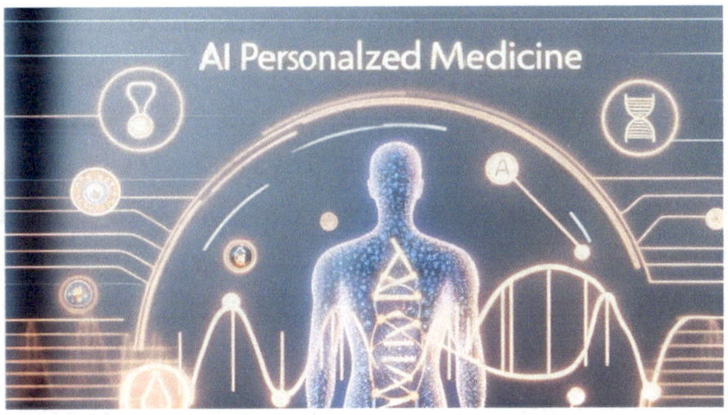

Figure 2.23. The integration of AI facilitates enhanced precision and individualized treatment plans, aligning with the broader shift toward personalized medicine.

Source: https://media.licdn.com/dms/image/v2/D5612AQEdVqqc3dIFKw/article-cover_image-shrink_720_1280/article-cover_image-shrink_720_1280/0/1721190624053?e=2147483647&v=beta&t=e8cPqz2f0IaGvfnhuqAuVJhWc54taZeAayNNb5UtTYg.

Test Your Knowledge

1. What is the role of radiation physics in the sterilization of medical equipment?
2. How is radiation used in industrial radiography for inspecting materials?

SUMMARY

The complex interaction of scientific knowledge and hands-on application in radiation physics underscores the necessity for ongoing interdisciplinary collaboration. Understanding obtained from previous nuclear accidents, such as, the Fukushima Daiichi accident, underscores the necessity for the enhancement of health physics to meet changing societal interests and technological innovations. Addressing these challenges requires a holistic approach that not only prioritizes technical precision but also incorporates regulatory frameworks and safety protocols, particularly in medical contexts like radiotherapy. Developing comprehensive educational models that integrate both scientific principles and legal standards is essential for preparing future professionals capable of managing radiation risks effectively. By fostering collaboration among researchers, educators, and regulatory bodies, the field can ensure the advancement of radiation protection methods grounded in both empirical evidence and sound policy. Ultimately, this integrative effort is fundamental to enhancing public health and safety in the face of ongoing and emerging radiation challenges (Takahara *et. al.*, 2025; Widyaningrum *et. al.*, 2025).

The intricate nature of radiation physics encompasses various fundamental principles governing the behavior and interaction of radiation with matter. Central to this field is understanding how electromagnetic waves and particle emissions propagate and transform energy, which underpins applications ranging from medical imaging to astrophysical observations. The role of topology in wave phenomena, such as those observed in photonic systems, highlights how wave functions are influenced by underlying physical structures, offering insights into stability and invariance under certain conditions (Ozawa *et. al.*, 2019). Additionally, advancements in observational technology, exemplified by projects like the Large Synoptic Survey Telescope, demonstrate how radiation physics facilitates the exploration of cosmic phenomena through precise, high-resolution data collection strategies across broad spectral bands (Željko *et. al.*, 2019). Together, these key points underscore the interdisciplinary nature and technological progression within radiation physics, which continue to expand our understanding of both fundamental physics and practical applications.

KEY TERMS FROM THIS CHAPTER

- Amplitude
- Electromagnetic radiation
- Frequency
- Non-Hermitian systems
- Propagation
- Wavefront
- Conserve energy
- Electromagnetic waves
- Matter
- Polarization
- Radiation channels

CRITICAL THINKING QUESTIONS

1. **Which type of radiation is used in diagnostic radiology?**
   a. Alpha particles
   b. Beta particles
   c. Gamma rays
   d. X-rays
2. **The unit of absorbed radiation dose is:**
   a. Becquerel (Bq)
   b. Sievert (Sv)
   c. Gray (Gy)
   d. Curie (Ci)
3. **What is the primary interaction responsible for image formation in diagnostic X-ray imaging?**
   a. Compton scattering
   b. Photoelectric effect
   c. Pair production
   d. Bremsstrahlung
4. **Ionizing radiation is capable of:**
   a. Heating tissues only
   b. Vibrating atoms in molecules
   c. Removing tightly bound electrons from atoms
   d. Emitting sound waves
5. **Which of the following is not a characteristic of X-rays?**
   a. They are a form of electromagnetic radiation
   b. They have no mass and no charge
   c. They travel slower than visible light
   d. They can ionize atoms

Short Answer Questions

1. What is ionizing radiation, and how does it differ from non-ionizing radiation?
2. Describe the photoelectric effect and its relevance in diagnostic imaging.
3. What are the main types of radiation used in medical imaging?
4. What is the difference between alpha, beta, and gamma radiation in terms of penetration and hazard?
5. Explain the process of X-ray generation in an X-ray tube.
6. How is patient dose minimized in diagnostic radiology?

Answers to Critical Thinking Questions

1.(d); 2.(c); 3.(b); 4.(c); 5.(c)

REFERENCES

1. Abada, A., Abbrescia, M., AbdusSalam, S., Abdyukhanov, I. M., Abelleira Fernandez, J., Abramov, A., Aburaia, M., *et. al.* (2019). FCC-ee: The lepton collider. *The European Physical Journal Special Topics, 228*(261–623). https://doi.org/10.1140/epjst/e2019-900045-4.
2. Penny Jeggo, Martin F Lavin (2009). Cellular radiosensitivity: How much better do we understand it? Int J Radiat Biol. 2009 Dec;85(12):1061-81. doi: 10.3109/09553000903261263.
3. Aguilar, M., Cavasonza, L. A., Ambrosi, G., Arruda, L., Attig, N., Barão, F., Barrin, L., *et. al.* (2020). The Alpha Magnetic Spectrometer (AMS) on the international space station: Part II–Results from the first seven years. *Physics Reports, 894*, 1–116. https://doi.org/10.1016/j.physrep.2020.09.003.
4. Allison, J. E., Amako, K., Apostolakis, J., Arce, P., Asai, M., Aso, T., Bagli, E., *et. al.* (2016). Recent developments in Geant4. *Nuclear Instruments and Methods in Physics Research Section A: Accelerators, Spectrometers, Detectors and Associated Equipment, 835*, 186–225. https://doi.org/10.1016/j.nima.2016.06.125.
5. Almayah, B. A. (2019). Use of gamma radiation techniques in peaceful applications. *IntechOpen eBooks*. https://doi.org/10.5772/intechopen.78481.
6. Antonsen, E. L., Bayuse, T. M., Blue, R. S., *et. al.* (2019). Limitations in predicting radiation-induced pharmaceutical instability during long-duration spaceflight. https://core.ac.uk/download/pdf/288485198.pdf (accessed on 30 May 2025).
7. Arce, P., Bolst, D., Bordage, M. C., Brown, J. M. C., Cirrone, P., Cortés-Giraldo, M. A., Cutajar, D., *et. al.* (2020). Report on G4-Med, a Geant4 benchmarking system for medical physics applications developed by the Geant4 Medical Simulation Benchmarking Group. *Medical Physics, 48*, 19–56. https://doi.org/10.1002/mp.14226.
8. Atakişi, H., Conger, L., Moreau, D., & Thorne, R. (2019). Resolution and dose dependence of radiation damage in biomolecular systems. *IUCrJ, 6*, 1040–1053. https://doi.org/10.1107/s2052252519008777.
9. Atri, D., Griessmeier, J. M., & Hariharan, B. (2013). Galactic cosmic ray induced radiation dose on terrestrial exoplanets. http://arxiv.org/abs/1307.4704 (accessed on 30 May 2025).
10. Auclair, P., Blanco-Pillado, J. J., Figueroa, D. G., Jenkins, A. C., Lewicki, M., Sakellariadou, M., Sanidas, S. A., *et. al.* (2020). Probing the gravitational wave background from cosmic strings with LISA. *Journal of Cosmology and Astro Particle Physics, 2020*(04), 034. https://doi.org/10.1088/1475-7516/2020/04/034.
11. Chancellor, J.C., Blue, R.S., Cengel, K.A. *et. al.* Limitations in predicting the space radiation health risk for exploration astronauts. *npj Microgravity* **4**, 8 (2018). https://doi.org/10.1038/s41526-018-0043-2.
12. Badihi, H., Zhang, Y., Jiang, B., Pillay, P., & Rakheja, S. (2022). A comprehensive review on signal-based and model-based condition monitoring of wind turbines: Fault diagnosis and lifetime prognosis. *Proceedings of the IEEE, 110*, 754–806. https://doi.org/10.1109/jproc.2022.3171691.
13. Başar, E., Di Renzo, M., de Rosny, J., Debbah, M., Alouini, M. S., & Zhang, R. (2019). Wireless communications through reconfigurable intelligent surfaces. *IEEE Access, 7*, 116753–116773. https://doi.org/10.1109/access.2019.2935192.

14. Benkhali, F. A., Hofmann, W., Rieger, F., & Chakraborty, N. (2019). Evaluating quasi-periodic variations in the γ-ray light curves of Fermi-LAT blazars. *Astronomy and Astrophysics, 634*, A120. https://doi.org/10.1051/0004-6361/201935117.

15. Beyea, J. (2024). False and misleading claims of scientific misconduct in early research into radiation dose-response: Part 1. Overlooking key historical text. *Health Physics*. https://www.semanticscholar.org/paper/34ce9c0ad38a3f0a439a65b9053a8d41b043461b (accessed on 30 May 2025).

16. Boschini, M. J., Consolandi, C., Gervasi, M., *et. al.* (2010). Nuclear and non-ionizing energy-loss for Coulomb scattered particles from low energy up to relativistic regime in space radiation environment. http://arxiv.org/abs/1011.4822 (accessed on 30 May 2025).

17. Burgos-Caminal, A., Vale, B. R. C., Fonseca, A. F. V., Collet, E. P. P., Hidalgo, J. F., García, L., Watson, L., *et. al.* (2024). Selective tracking of charge carrier dynamics in CuInS2 quantum dots. https://www.semanticscholar.org/paper/df74b00930b4a476c3feeabd62cfbb54b3fc42be (accessed on 30 May 2025).

18. Burmeister, J., Busse, N. C., Cetnar, A. J., Howell, R. R., Jeraj, R., Jones, A. K., King, S. H., *et. al.* (2022). Academic program recommendations for graduate degrees in medical physics: AAPM Report No. 365 (Revision of Report No. 197). *Journal of Applied Clinical Medical Physics, 23*. https://doi.org/10.1002/acm2.13792.

19. Cavicchioli, R., Ripple, W. J., Timmis, K. N., Azam, F., Bakken, L. R., Baylis, M., Behrenfeld, M. J., *et. al.* (2019). Scientists' warning to humanity: Microorganisms and climate change. *Nature Reviews Microbiology, 17*, 569–586. https://doi.org/10.1038/s41579-019-0222-5.

20. Chattopadhyay, S. (1994). Advances in beam physics and technology: Colliders of the future. https://core.ac.uk/download/484309908.pdf (accessed on 30 May 2025).

21. Choudhuri, A. (2024). The interaction of matter and radiation: The physics of C. V. Raman, S. N. Bose, and M. N. Saha. Part 2: Physics highlights. *Resonance*. https://www.semanticscholar.org/paper/c86d88b70f177e8a84b46881773a0d20b20341f1 (accessed on 30 May 2025).

22. Choudhuri, A. (2024). The interaction of matter and radiation: The physics of C. V. Raman, S. N. Bose, and M. N. Saha. *Resonance*. https://www.semanticscholar.org/paper/080620c88d823b35384265bd835c9577dc2cb087 (accessed on 30 May 2025).

23. Chung, H. T. (2025). Physics and radiobiology of radiosurgery. *Neurofunction*. https://www.semanticscholar.org/paper/f50a6fc6a53602acf11019661a463b962b6cec60 (accessed on 30 May 2025).

24. Cicoli, M., Conlon, J. P., Maharana, A., Parameswaran, S., Quevedo, F., & Zavala, I. (2024). String cosmology: From the early universe to today. *Physics Reports, 1059*, 1–155. https://doi.org/10.1016/j.physrep.2024.01.002.

25. Cohen, A., Schmaltz, M., Katz, E., Rebbi, C., Glashow, S. L., Brower, R. C., & Pi, S. Y. (2016). Topics in theoretical physics. https://doi.org/10.2172/1327249.

26. Das, D. K., Hok, C. I., Lewis, C. E., *et. al.* (1988). Circular 64. https://core.ac.uk/download/162574814.pdf (accessed on 30 May 2025).

27. de Salas, P. F., Gariazzo, S., Mena, O., Ternes, C. A., & Tórtola, M. (2018). Neutrino mass ordering from oscillations and beyond: 2018 status and future prospects. *Frontiers in Astronomy and Space Sciences, 5*. https://doi.org/10.3389/fspas.2018.00036.

28. Deneva, H., Lazov, L. K., Narica, P., *et. al.* (2017). LASER technologies–Master's program between two European universities of applied sciences from Latvia and Germany. https://core.ac.uk/download/386141014.pdf (accessed on 30 May 2025).

29. Di Mitri, S. (2011). Machine design and electron beam control of a single-pass linac for free electron laser: The FERMI@Elettra case study. https://core.ac.uk/download/pdf/12956174.pdf (accessed on 30 May 2025).

30. Di Renzo, M., Zappone, A., Debbah, M., Alouini, M. S., Yuen, C., de Rosny, J., & Tretyakov, S. (2020). Smart radio environments empowered by reconfigurable intelligent surfaces: How it works, state of research, and the road ahead. *IEEE Journal on Selected Areas in Communications, 38*, 2450–2525. https://doi.org/10.1109/jsac.2020.3007211.

31. Dogan, N., Mijnheer, B. J., Padgett, K. R., Nalichowski, A., Wu, C., Nyflot, M. J., Olch, A. J., *et. al.* (2023). AAPM Task Group Report 307: Use of EPIDs for patient-specific IMRT and VMAT QA. *Medical Physics, 50*. https://doi.org/10.1002/mp.16536.

32. El Shafey, A. M. (2020). Green synthesis of metal and metal oxide nanoparticles from plant leaf extracts and their applications: A review. *Green Processing and Synthesis, 9*, 304–339. https://doi.org/10.1515/gps-2020-0031.

33. Fisher, R., Applegate, K. E., Berkowitz, L. K., Christianson, O., Dave, J. K., DeWeese, L., Harris, N., *et. al.* (2022). AAPM Medical Physics Practice Guideline 12.a: Fluoroscopy dose management. *Journal of Applied Clinical Medical Physics, 23*. https://doi.org/10.1002/acm2.13526.

34. Fletcher, S. M., He, S., & Rimal, A. (2025). Factors affecting consumer negative perceptions about beef irradiation. https://core.ac.uk/download/pdf/6563884.pdf (accessed on 30 May 2025).

35. Garg, M., Prabhakar, N., & Bhalla, A. S. (2021). Cancer risk of CT scan in COVID-19: Resolving the dilemma. *The Indian Journal of Medical Research, 153*, 568. https://doi.org/10.4103/ijmr.ijmr_1476_21.

36. George, T. F., Nánai, L., Robinson, C. T., *et. al.* (2015). Investigation of building materials and the street's surface radioactive emission. https://core.ac.uk/download/236293030.pdf (accessed on 30 May 2025).

37. Gonzalez, A. J. (2002). The debate on the health effects attributable to low radiation exposure. https://core.ac.uk/download/72052597.pdf (accessed on 30 May 2025).

38. Grazioso, F. (2015). Introduction to quantum information theory and outline of two applications to physics: The black hole information paradox and the renormalization group information flow. *ArXiv, abs/1507.00957*. https://www.semanticscholar.org/paper/fd06b03951d0d6398fd73ae5f18a81c31a37caf9 (accessed on 30 May 2025).

39. Hassani, S., & Dackermann, U. (2023). A systematic review of advanced sensor technologies for non-destructive testing and structural health monitoring. *Sensors, 23*, 2204. https://doi.org/10.3390/s23042204.

40. Hernandez Montesinos, D., Baron, S., Biereigel, S., Hazell, P., Kulis, S., Vicente Leitao, P., Moreira, P., *et. al.* (2024). Overview of the production and qualification tests of the lpGBT. *Journal of Instrumentation, 19*. https://www.semanticscholar.org/paper/8b44e025607e9c239ae15f34a94ccc79b1bbf3e5 (accessed on 30 May 2025).

41. Hespeels, B., Heuskin, A. C., Perrot, A., *et. al.* (2023). Adineta vaga under fire: Simulating the

impact of radiation. https://core.ac.uk/download/581157251.pdf (accessed on 30 May 2025).

42. Hinrikus, H., Bachmann, M., & Lass, J. (2018). Understanding physical mechanism of low-level microwave radiation effect. *International Journal of Radiation Biology, 94*, 877–882. https://doi.org/10.1080/09553002.2018.1478158.

43. Hossain, M. K., Raihan, G. A., Akbar, M. A., Rubel, M. H. K., Ahmed, M. H., Khan, M. I., Hossain, S., *et. al.* (2022). Current applications and future potential of rare earth oxides in sustainable nuclear, radiation, and energy devices: A review. *ACS Applied Electronic Materials, 4*, 3327–3353. https://doi.org/10.1021/acsaelm.2c00069.

44. Hu, H., Niu, G., Zheng, Z., Xu, L., Liu, L., & Tang, J. (2022). Perovskite semiconductors for ionizing radiation detection. *EcoMat, 4*. https://doi.org/10.1002/eom2.12258.

45. Incatasciato, A., Khochfar, S., & Oñorbe, J. (2023). Modelling the cosmological Lyman-Werner background radiation field in the early Universe. *Monthly Notices of the Royal Astronomical Society*. https://www.semanticscholar.org/paper/f8b3edfac3d9e39e32440d2a05131105f90755ca (accessed on 30 May 2025).

46. Ivezić, Ž., Kahn, S. M., Tyson, J. A., Abel, B., Acosta, E. E., Allsman, R. A., Alonso, D., *et. al.* (2019). LSST: From science drivers to reference design and anticipated data products. *The Astrophysical Journal, 873*, 111. https://doi.org/10.3847/1538-4357/ab042c.

47. Jakšić, A., Stanković, S., & Vasović, N. (2016). Sensitivity of standard and stacked RADFET dosimeters. https://core.ac.uk/download/603272980.pdf (accessed on 30 May 2025).

48. Kamel, R. J., Karim, S. N., Musa, M. M., *et. al.* (2024). Advancements in medical imaging technologies: Ultrasound, X-ray, and MRI. https://core.ac.uk/download/620857181.pdf (accessed on 30 May 2025).

49. Kang, M., Ding, X., & Rong, Y. (2023). FLASH instead of proton arc therapy is a more promising advancement for the next generation proton radiotherapy. *Journal of Applied Clinical Medical Physics, 24*. https://doi.org/10.1002/acm2.14091.

50. Karlovets, D., Baturin, S., Geloni, G., Sizykh, G., & Serbo, V. (2023). Role of postelection in generating vortex states of particles of arbitrary mass, spin, and energy. *SSRN Electronic Journal*. https://www.semanticscholar.org/paper/3aca435064bf42842d47912991a46ff171ca66d8 (accessed on 30 May 2025).

51. Kathren, R. L. (2002). Historical development of the linear no threshold dose-response model as applied to radiation. https://core.ac.uk/download/72053007.pdf (accessed on 30 May 2025).

52. Kaye, S. V. (1992). Health and safety research division progress report for the period April 1, 1990–September 30, 1991. https://core.ac.uk/download/216778388.pdf (accessed on 30 May 2025).

53. Koker, E. B. (2025). The determination of energy transfer rates in the Ho:Tm:Cr:YAG laser material. https://core.ac.uk/download/pdf/42830176.pdf (accessed on 30 May 2025).

54. Kozhevnikova, M. F., Levenets, V., Lonin, O., Omelnik, O., & Shchur, A. O. (2024). Identification of heavy metals pollution sources in the territory adjacent to NSC "Kharkiv Institute of Physics & Technology" by PMF method. *East European Journal of Physics*. https://www.semanticscholar.org/paper/6c1019a58b4ef22cbe4a08f0bcee2497275c5882 (accessed on 30 May 2025).

55. Lemke, M., Hölter, A., & Weinzierl, S. (2025). Physics-informed identification and interpolation of the directivity of sound sources. *IEEE Transactions on Audio, Speech and Language Processing, 33*, 372–385. https://www.semanticscholar.org/paper/0b9351eae35804e57429547de3cbc3f2a046dcba (accessed on 30 May 2025).

56. MacLachlan, A. J., Robertson, C. W., Konoplev, I. V., Cross, A. W., Phelps, A. D. R., & Ronald, K. (2019). Resonant excitation of volume and surface fields on complex electrodynamic surfaces. *Physical Review Applied, 11*. https://doi.org/10.1103/physrevapplied.11.034034.

57. Maes, S. (2023). Multi-folds in Yang Mills Feynman diagrams. https://doi.org/10.31219/osf.io/y8fpd.

58. Mancusi, D., Brun, E., Dechenaux, B., Fröhlicher, K., Gonçalves, T., Jinaphanh, A., Kowalski, M., *et. al.* (2024). Overview of TRIPOLI-5, a Monte Carlo code for HPC. *EPJ Nuclear Sciences & Technologies*. https://www.semanticscholar.org/paper/dba24c342ee99c15f4d00e9c0ebcda2652e36473 (accessed on 30 May 2025).

59. Matsuya, Y., Kai, T., Sato, T., Ogawa, T., Hirata, Y., Yoshii, Y., Parisi, A., *et. al.* (2021). Track-structure modes in particle and heavy ion transport code system (PHITS): Application to radiobiological research. *International Journal of Radiation Biology, 98*, 148–157. https://doi.org/10.1080/09553002.2022.2013572.

60. Matthews, C., Labouré, V., DeHart, M. D., Hansel, J., Andrš, D., Wang, Y., Ortensi, J., *et. al.* (2021). Coupled Multiphysics simulations of heat pipe microreactors using Dire Wolf. *Nuclear Technology, 207*, 1142–1162. https://doi.org/10.1080/00295450.2021.1906474.

61. Mattsson, S. (2024). Current developments in medical radiation physics and radiation protection. Medical physics–the current status, problems, the way of development. *Innovation Technologies*. https://www.semanticscholar.org/paper/0d3308fbb261f9e15edc18550f5c6f8357404659 (accessed on 30 May 2025).

62. Modarai, B., Haulon, S., Ainsbury, E. A., Böckler, D., Vañó-Carruana, E., Dawson, J., Farber, M. A., *et. al.* (2022). Editor's choice–European Society for Vascular Surgery (ESVS) 2023 clinical practice guidelines on radiation safety. *European Journal of Vascular and Endovascular Surgery, 65*, 171–222. https://doi.org/10.1016/j.ejvs.2022.09.005.

63. Newhauser, W., Gress, D. A., Mills, M., Jordan, D. W., Sutlief, S. G., Martin, M., & Jackson, E. F. (2022). Medical physics workforce in the United States. *Journal of Applied Clinical Medical Physics, 23*. https://doi.org/10.1002/acm2.13762.

64. Noska, M. A., Borrás, C., Holahan, E. V., Dewji, S., Johnson, T. E., Hiatt, J. W., Newhauser, W., *et. al.* (2022). Health physics workforce in the United States. *Journal of Applied Clinical Medical Physics, 23*. https://doi.org/10.1002/acm2.13757.

65. Omer, H. (2021). Radiobiological effects and medical applications of non-ionizing radiation. *Saudi Journal of Biological Sciences, 28*, 5585–5592. https://doi.org/10.1016/j.sjbs.2021.05.071.

66. Ozawa, T., Price, H. M., Amo, A., Goldman, N., Hafezi, M., Lü, L., Rechtsman, M. C., *et. al.* (2019). Topological photonics. *Reviews of Modern Physics, 91*. https://doi.org/10.1103/revmodphys.91.015006.

67. Patel, Z. S., Brunstetter, T., Tarver, W. J., Whitmire, A., Zwart, S. R., Smith, S. M., & Huff, J. L. (2020). Red risks for a journey to the red planet: The highest priority human health risks for a mission to Mars. *npj Microgravity, 6*. https://doi.org/10.1038/s41526-020-00124-6.

68. Pecht, M., & Vchare, N. (2006). Enabling electronic prognostics using thermal data. https://core.ac.uk/download/15488695.pdf (accessed on 30 May 2025).

69. Rasheed, A., San, O., & Kvamsdal, T. (2020). Digital twin: Values, challenges and enablers from a modeling perspective. *IEEE Access, 8*, 21980–22012. https://doi.org/10.1109/access.2020.2970143.

70. Roßbach, J., Schneider, J. R., & Würth, W. (2019). 10 years of pioneering X-ray science at the free-electron laser FLASH at DESY. *Physics Reports, 808*, 1–74. https://doi.org/10.1016/j.physrep.2019.02.002.

71. Samei, E., & Mills, M. (2018). Medical physics 3.0, physics for every patient. *Journal of Applied Clinical Medical Physics, 19*, 4, 5. https://www.semanticscholar.org/paper/824364c29b8eb6556812b6020cfb2048dc26890d (accessed on 30 May 2025).

72. Sato, T., Iwamoto, Y., Hashimoto, S., Ogawa, T., Furuta, T., Abe, S., Kai, T., *et. al.* (2018). Features of Particle and Heavy Ion Transport Code System (PHITS) version 3.02. *Journal of Nuclear Science and Technology, 55*, 684–690. https://doi.org/10.1080/00223131.2017.1419890.

73. Schaye, J., Crain, R. A., Bower, R. G., Furlong, M., Schaller, M., Theuns, T., Dalla Vecchia, C., *et. al.* (2014). The EAGLE project: Simulating the evolution and assembly of galaxies and their environments. *Monthly Notices of the Royal Astronomical Society, 446*, 521–554. https://doi.org/10.1093/mnras/stu2058.

74. Shahid, B. (2023). Solar photovoltaics for design engineers. https://core.ac.uk/download/622362128.pdf (accessed on 30 May 2025).

75. Shultis, J. K., & Faw, R. E. (2016). *Fundamentals of Nuclear Science and Engineering*. CRC Press. https://doi.org/10.1201/9781315183183.

76. Steigman, G. (2012). Neutrinos and Big Bang nucleosynthesis. https://core.ac.uk/download/193432018.pdf (accessed on 30 May 2025).

77. Sukharev, M., & Nitzan, A. (2017). Optics of exciton-plasmon nanomaterials. *Journal of Physics: Condensed Matter, 29*, 443003. https://doi.org/10.1088/1361-648x/aa85ef.

78. Takahara, S., Iimoto, T., Igarashi, T., & Kawabata, M. (2025). Review of articles related to the accident at the Fukushima Daiichi nuclear power station published in the Japanese Journal of Health Physics: Opinion and others (Secondary publication). *Journal of Radiation Protection and Research*. https://www.semanticscholar.org/paper/76564227db79810d3ad89d63c798de23023bcb76 (accessed on 30 May 2025).

79. Tan, J., Zhou, Z., Zheng, H., Li, Y., Wang, H., Yang, Q., Tian, H., *et. al.* (2025). Emerging themes and future directions in space radiation health research: A bibliometric exploration from 2013 to 2022. *Radiation and Environmental Biophysics*. https://www.semanticscholar.org/paper/29e57cd126a63d465b2dc3ec56b8a4605f91112f (accessed on 30 May 2025).

80. Tene, T., Bonilla García, N., Coello-Fiallos, D., Borja, M., & Vacacela Gomez, C. (2024). A systematic review of immersive educational technologies in medical physics and radiation physics. *Frontiers in Medicine, 11*. https://www.semanticscholar.org/paper/0f53f1f6825828bac1a74adcf5f29c1b72d05cf3 (accessed on 30 May 2025).

81. Terenetskaya, I. (2018). How to measure the Vitamin-D-synthetic activity of UV lamps used in phototherapy? *Integrative Molecular Medicine, 5*. https://www.semanticscholar.org/paper/3bd3fd9c4bb48126c7c13e8773728cca955e7b6f (accessed on 30 May 2025).

82. Thubab, A. A. A., Ogdi, K. M., Hezam, S. N., Otaif, A. A., Ogdi, A. M., Al Masoud, S. A., Hamad, M. I., *et. al.* (2024). Challenges and solutions in radiation protection for X-ray procedures. https://core.ac.uk/download/616775622.pdf (accessed on 30 May 2025).

83. Tolasa, D. (2025). The physics of semiconductor devices: Principles, applications, and innovations. *American Journal of Physics and Applications*. https://www.semanticscholar.org/paper/0f4002e8a554dc36a678c62d492ffe791c719866 (accessed on 30 May 2025).

84. Tomalak, O., & Hill, R. J. (2020). Theory of elastic neutrino-electron scattering. *Physical Review D, 101*. https://doi.org/10.1103/physrevd.101.033006.

85. Trotter, J. W., Pantel, A. R., Teo, B. K., Escorcia, F. E., Li, T., Pryma, D. A., & Taunk, N. K. (2023). Positron emission tomography (PET)/computed tomography (CT) imaging in radiation therapy treatment planning: A review of PET imaging tracers and methods to incorporate PET/CT. *Advances in Radiation Oncology, 8*, 101212. https://doi.org/10.1016/j.adro.2023.101212.

86. Wald, P. (2016). Introduction to physical hazards. https://www.semanticscholar.org/paper/2f7c2d88507c89cb6fde9299270491ac6a3f4609 (accessed on 30 May 2025).

87. Widyaningrum, R., Nofik, K., Masruroh, A., & Hernawati, S. (2025). Integration of health law and radiation safety aspects in the medical physics curriculum for radiotherapy treatment. *Schrödinger: Journal of Physics Education*. https://www.semanticscholar.org/paper/b1f1f1d6c729fe397d6cf2d893cc47f9f9f2aafe (accessed on 30 May 2025).

88. Yin, X., & Peng, C. (2020). Manipulating light radiation from a topological perspective. *Photonics Research, 8*, B25–B25. https://doi.org/10.1364/prj.403444.

89. Yokoyama, S., Nabatame, K., Suzuki, A., & Iimoto, T. (2024). Review of articles related to the accident of TEPCO's Fukushima Daiichi nuclear power station published in the Japanese Journal of Health Physics: Overview (Secondary publication). *Journal of Radiation Protection and Research*. https://www.semanticscholar.org/paper/af75947896ff8299f322bd81ad3cbd9959f54828 (accessed on 30 May 2025).

RADIATION PROTECTION AND SAFETY

3

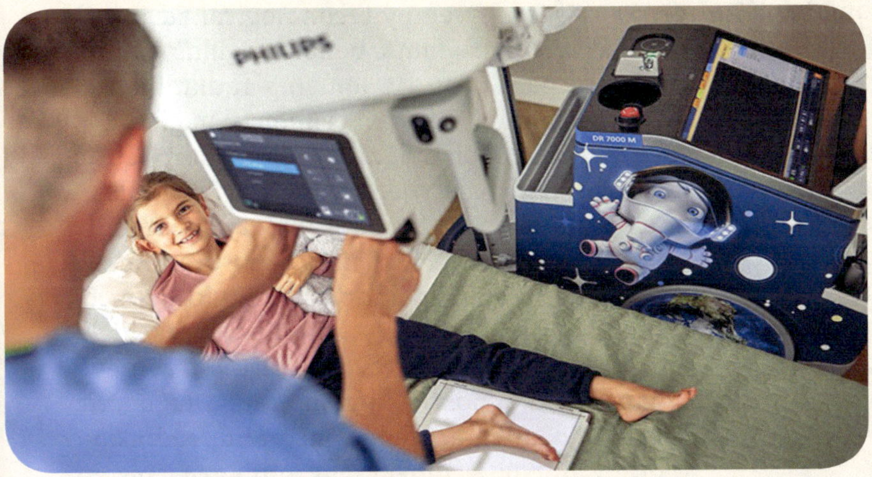

LEARNING OBJECTIVES

After studying this chapter, you will be able to:

1. Explain principles of radiation protection
2. Know safety protocols and guidelines
3. Focus on challenges and innovations in radiation safety

Introduction

The addition of ionizing radiation to medical imaging has transformed medicine to facilitate precise imaging and planning for treatment, thereby enhancing patient outcomes significantly. However, the benefits brought about by these technologies come at the risk intrinsically linked to exposure to radiation, necessitating strict safety protocols. During the last hundred years, diagnostic radiology, nuclear medicine, and radiation therapy have become invaluable modalities in all medical specialties, emphasizing the imperative need to balance diagnostic effectiveness and protection of the patient (Donya et. al., 2014). Radiation protection requires knowing both the physics of ionizing radiation and possible biological consequences of exposure, specifically stochastic and deterministic hazards. Overexposure events, often the byproduct of inadequate training, procedural errors, or faulty apparatus, underscore the necessity of systematic safeguarding by checklists, dose monitoring, and written safety policies to constrain damage and enhance patient safety (Damilakis et.

al., 2017). This introduction is intended to set the stage for a close examination of the strategy for maximum radiation protection and safety in diagnostic practice.

Importance of Radiation Protection

Medical imaging modalities that utilize ionizing radiation are now a crucial tool for accurate diagnosis and therapy planning, but have inherent risks that necessitate rigorous radiation protection systems. Short-term and long-term exposure outcomes can be damaging to both patients and medical workers, meaning full-spectrum protective measures are necessary. Despite advancements in technology, increased usage of diagnostic imaging has created an overall radiation dose that poses human health risks. Proper radiation protection practices, including quality assurance testing and continued medical staff training, are essential in minimizing unwarranted exposure while maintaining diagnostic performance.

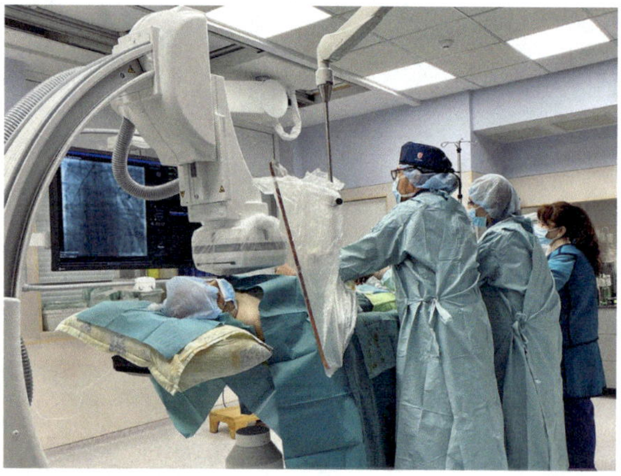

Figure 3.1. Importance of radiation protection in medical imaging.

Source: https://www.iaea.org/sites/default/files/img-3398.jpg.

Secondly, the establishment of regulatory institutions or self-regulatory organizations can significantly assist in maintaining safety standards and checks in healthcare institutions, particularly where there is no official monitoring agency. Ultimately, awareness promotion and emphasis on radiation safety are compatible with good medical practice and public health requirements (Budošová et. al., 2021) (Figure 3.1).

Historical Context of Radiation Use in Medicine

The history of medical treatments has been progressively driven by technological advances that balance therapeutic benefits against injury. Over the past century, ionizing radiation use has been refined from experimental beginnings to a backbone of diagnostic and therapeutic medicine. Early uses were crude and incomplete, and included inadequate safety protocols resulting in unwanted harmful exposures. But as information about radiation's biological effects expanded, the medical community increasingly emphasized reducing the hazard to achieve maximum diagnostic information. Diagnostic radiology, nuclear medicine, and radiation therapy are now universally indispensable in hospitals, underpinned by principle guidelines for radiation protection and safety. These advances illustrate an aware appreciation of the high risk/benefit ratio associated with the application of radiation, highlighting ethical decision-making and rigorous control systems to counteract risk exposures (Donya *et. al.*, 2014). While specifically aimed toward earth medicine, a grasp of radiation impact is translatable to related disciplines as well, such as regulating radiation safety in space flight missions, which necessitates rigorous controls on dosages to protect biological systems.

Relevance to Healthcare Professionals

Medical practitioners play a crucial role in ensuring radiation protection and safety in the course of diagnosis, since they are the initial contact between technology and the treatment of the patient. Their understanding of radiation dangers and ability to relay relevant information to patients concerning radiation risks play a pivotal role in raising awareness among patients and ensuring compliance with safety measures. Despite having information pamphlets, studies indicate that a knowledge gap in understanding radiation exposure among patients, suggesting that health professionals must enhance educational campaigns to meet the gap (Drey *et. al.*, 2020). This emphasizes the need for ongoing education and updated guidelines, particularly for health professionals, to maximize patient interaction and guard against excessive doses of radiation. In addition, adherence to regulations and ethical standards necessitates that healthcare professionals be aware of the current radiation safety best practices to ensure diagnostic dividends are achieved while potential harms are reduced. Even though evidence for these educational interventions is incomplete (Kitsiou *et. al.*, 2013), more emphasis on patient-centered care points to the central role healthcare professionals can assume in instilling a culture of radiation safety (Figure 3.2).

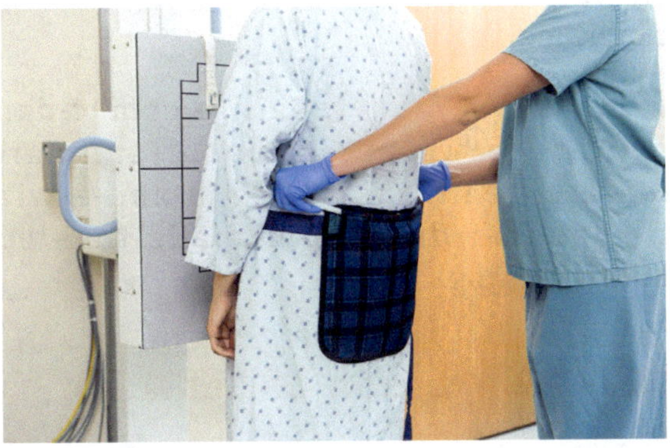

Figure 3.2. Healthcare professionals play a critical role in ensuring radiation protection and safety during diagnostic procedures, as they are the primary interface between technology and patient care.

Source: https://www.statnews.com/wp-content/uploads/2020/05/AdobeStock_58769027.jpeg.

Public Perception of Radiation Safety

Despite enhanced diagnostic imaging technology and stringent safety protocols, public apprehension and confusion over radiation safety persist. Many people oversimplify the risks of diagnostic radiation, fueled by sensationalized reporting by the media or uncertain explanations by healthcare providers. Such apprehension could discourage individuals from receiving the appropriate medical imaging tests, thereby potentially compromising early diagnosis and treatment. Educational initiatives that attempt to demystify radiation exposure and emphasize the strict protective procedures adopted in clinics are required to alleviate such concerns. Further, frank disclosure of scientific findings and safety measures can facilitate patient-clinician trust. Historical documentation of research activities, as reported in NASA technical information systems, emphasizes the evolutionary character of knowledge about radiation safety and the necessity of continuous public engagement and education on the topic. Public opinion is thus an integral part of effective and adequate radiation protection in diagnostics.

3.1. Principles of Radiation Protection

Learning Outcome

1. Discuss the justification of radiation use
2. Explain the optimization of radiation dose
3. Limit exposure to patients and healthcare workers
4. Learn the use of protective equipment
5. Explain the role of shielding in diagnostics
6. Monitor radiation exposure
7. Discuss education and training for staff
8. Know the importance of safety protocols

Effective radiation protection in diagnostic settings depends on the consistent application of fundamental principles to avoid exposure to risk for patients and healthcare workers alike. The principles of time, distance, and shielding have each been established to reduce the amount of ionizing radiation absorbed. Decreasing the time of exposure decreases the radiation dose, decreasing the distance from the source, decreasing intensity, and the use of appropriate shielding materials further decrease unnecessary transmission of radiation. Despite the stringent demands of these practices, compliance and clinician awareness vary widely. For instance, research from dental offices in Khorramabad indicates that specialist dentists possess sufficient knowledge of X-ray protection. In contrast, general dentists demonstrate average knowledge with suboptimal overall compliance with safety precautions (Asgharani *et. al.*, 2025). Similarly, workers dealing with radiation in Mazandaran province display overall satisfactory practices related to radiation protection but indicate areas of inadequacy in ongoing training and practice (Seifi *et. al.*, 2025). These results underline that establishing continuous education and close surveillance is imperative for ensuring radiation safety standards in diagnostic environments.

3.1.1. Justification of Radiation Use

Imaging patient safety involves thorough consideration of the benefits and risks of radiation exposure. Diagnostic imaging departments need to adopt systematic approaches to measuring radiation doses and transparently informing patients about them in order to ensure informed decision-making. Transparent talk about radiation risk, predicated on accurate dose measurement and contextualized by a sense of clinical necessity, is a key component of facilitating any radiographic procedure (Felemban, 2024). Most especially in dental radiography, where exposure is often low but has potential biological effects, justification is crucial to prevent unnecessary radiation, as advocated by the International Commission for Radiological Protection (Thomas, 2023). However, the variable level of knowledge among healthcare providers, such as dental assistants, shows that more education on radiation protection principles is necessary. Coupling extensive training with stringent compliance for justification procedures guarantees that all imaging procedures are medically justified and optimized to minimize exposure and provide maximal diagnostic yield, thereby increasing diagnostic radiology safety protocols (Felemban, 2024; Thomas, 2023) (Figure 3.3).

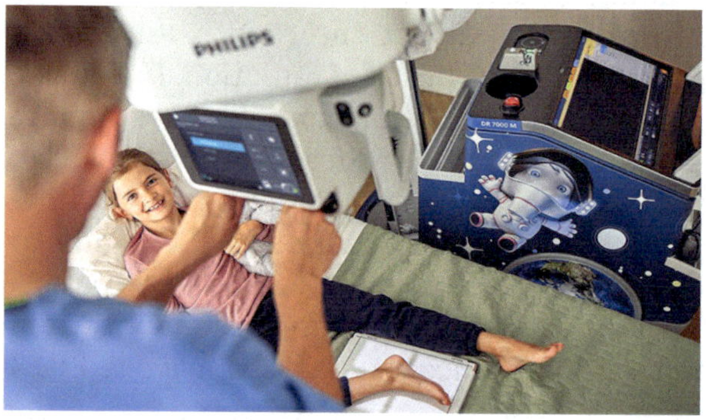

Figure 3.3. Medical imaging facilities must adopt systematic approaches to quantify radiation doses and effectively communicate these to patients, thereby fostering informed decision-making.

Source: https://www.philips.com/c-dam/corporate/newscenter/global/standard/resources/healthcare/2024/q-and-a-with-atul-gupta-md/dr-7000-m-application-tech-pediatric-eth.jpg.

3.1.2. Optimization of Radiation Dose

Patient safety in the process of diagnostic imaging has to balance between obtaining high-quality images and keeping radiation exposure low. Balancing this has been made possible with technological advances, primarily by applying artificial intelligence (AI) in imaging protocols that enable the reduction of radiation doses without compromising the quality of the diagnosis. Artificial intelligence techniques such as deep learning and convolutional neural networks optimize image reconstruction through reduced noise and artifacts, thereby facilitating reduced exposure levels of radiation with maintained image resolution. Optimizing this is crucial because preventable or excessive exposure to ionizing radiation can impose high health risks, especially where effective dose control fails or imaging protocols are unnecessarily repeated. Regulatory frameworks highlight the necessity of selecting the best protection measures appropriate to a particular exposure context, maximizing diagnostic techniques, and minimizing harm as much as possible. Continuing integration of AI into tailored imaging protocols promises to continue improving radiation protection and create safer diagnostic surroundings (Adeleke *et. al.*, 2025; Wróbel *et. al.*, 2017).

3.1.3. Limiting Exposure to Patients

Effective radiation protection in the case of a successful measure calls for the reduction of patient exposure through the application of established safety principles, such as ALARA, ALADA, and ALADAIP, that aim at reducing radiation to diagnostically acceptable and patient-individual values as low as possible. Hand-held X-ray devices present opportunities and challenges in limiting patient exposure. While these devices enhance access across a variety of clinical circumstances, their setup increases the danger of elevated operator and patient doses unless properly regulated. Appropriate practices, including the use of rectangular collimators, backscatter shields, and providing enough distance at the time of exposure, are necessary in keeping unnecessary radiation to a minimum (Martins *et. al.*, 2023). Additionally, rules restricting the use of portable equipment to specific environments emphasize the need to manage exposure without diminishing diagnostic capability. Enforcing the consistent use of such protective measures is needed in order to safeguard patients while maintaining the quality of diagnostic imaging (Figure 3.4).

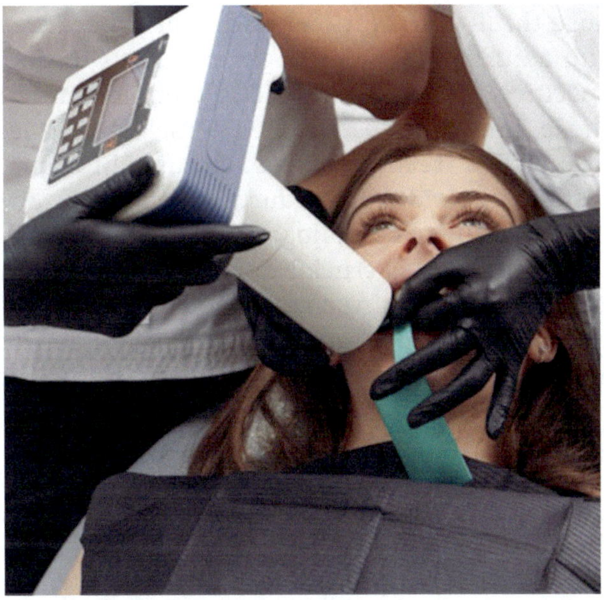

Figure 3.4. The use of portable hand-held X-ray devices presents both opportunities and challenges in limiting patient exposure.

Source: https://img.drbicuspid.com/files/base/smg/all/image/2021/06/drb.2021_06_07_23_43_8829_dental_x-ray_portable_400.png?auto=format%2Ccompress&q=70&w=400.

3.1.4. Limiting Exposure to Healthcare Workers

In contemporary imaging diagnostics, protection of health workers from avoidable exposure to radiation is still an important but frequently neglected issue. Although the unequivocal benefits and extensive use of ionizing radiation in healthcare diagnostics are evident, numerous health professionals receive limited radiation safety training, creating possible cumulative dose risks in the long term. This knowledge deficit reflects the urgent need for improved education and strict adherence to protection rules on radiation to lower job-related risks

(Budošová *et. al.*, 2021). In addition, more advanced technologies, such as AI monitoring systems and new imaging modalities, present potential avenues towards minimizing radiation dose through the rationalization of procedures and adjustment of imaging parameters to case specifics (Adadzi *et. al.*, 2024). Implementing these innovations together with traditional preventive techniques—such as shielding, distancing, and time reduction—is necessary in decreasing the radiological load of healthcare staff. Finally, it is crucial to create a culture of safety that arises from continuous training and technological application for the protection of medical staff without losing diagnostic efficacy.

3.1.5. Use of Protective Equipment

Effective protection against radiation in diagnostic settings is largely contingent upon effective use of protective equipment, which forms an essential barrier against harmful exposure to ionizing radiation. Though there is overall recognition of its importance, usage is not consistent, as indicated by findings with wide disparities in the availability and servicing of equipment. For instance, although lead rubber aprons are consistently in stock and utilized by medical imaging technologists, nearly 59% have never undergone integrity tests, nullifying their protective functions (Maina *et. al.*, 2019). Moreover, essential equipment like radiation-measuring instruments and immobilizing devices is typically scarce or underutilized, also nullifying safety interventions. The value that the healthcare industry places on occupational and environmental hazards accentuates the need for stringent control of radiation protective devices alongside other specialized chemicals and medical imaging-specific procedures (Davies *et. al.*, 2025). Closing administrative loopholes and implementing periodic equipment inspections are key steps towards ensuring the safety culture and minimizing exposure to radiation effectively (Figure 3.5).

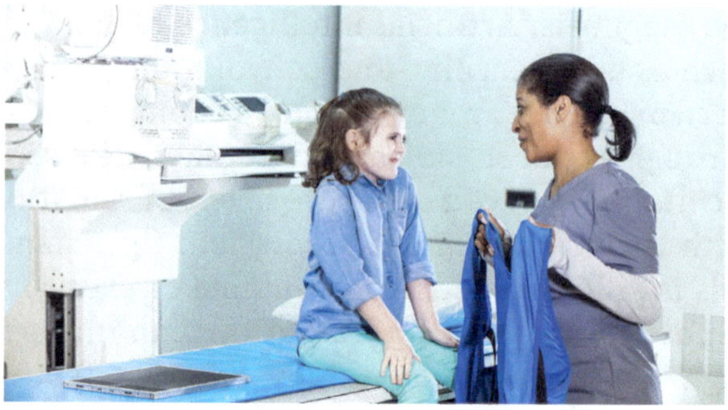

Figure 3.5. Effective radiation protection in diagnostic settings relies heavily on the appropriate use of protective equipment, which serves as a critical barrier against harmful exposure to ionizing radiation.

Source: https://radetco.com/wp-content/uploads/2023/03/BLOG-banner-Protective-Aprons-Shields.png.webp.

3.1.6. Role of Shielding in Diagnostics

Patient protection from unnecessary exposure to radiation is a fundamental principle of diagnostic imaging, with the balance between diagnostic benefit and risk threat still being of concern. Shielding of radiosensitive organs such as the gonads, thyroid, and eyes has been a standard practice with the intent to minimize the dose of radiation. However, recent evidence questions the utility of patient shielding in certain diagnostic applications, suggesting that it may be less effective or even harmful via image quality disruption or by causing repeated imaging. This advancement highlights the need for more balanced and evidence-based radiation protection strategies, favoring optimization instead of routine shielding. In addition, changing guidelines suggest identifying dose or risk thresholds to ascertain when patient shielding is appropriate, thereby preventing an overestimation of radiation risks that can cause unwarranted patient anxiety. In general, the function of shielding in diagnostics is changing as part of an overall radiation protection policy that includes justification, optimization, and technology improvement to guarantee patient safety and diagnostic success (James *et. al.*, 2020; Madan *et. al.*, 2021).

3.1.7. Monitoring Radiation Exposure

Optimal radiation exposure management in diagnostic procedures involves proper monitoring and adherence to guidelines to prevent accompanying risks. Healthcare facilities should have formal policies laid out defining the roles and responsibilities, wherein equipment operation and optimization techniques are well-trained for everyone working within them. Equipment such as checklists, pre-procedure time-outs, and real-time dose alerts is utilized to provide critical protection against overexposure, most particularly in interventional radiology, where tissue reactions to high skin doses can occur (Damilakis *et. al.*, 2017).

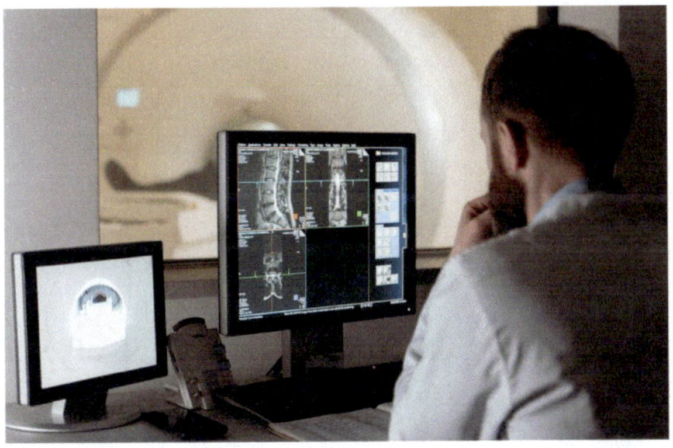

Figure 3.6. Effective management of radiation exposure in diagnostic procedures necessitates meticulous monitoring and adherence to established guidelines to minimize associated risks.

Source: https://raybloc.com/wp-content/uploads/2023/09/healthcare-workers-radiation-protection.jpg.

In addition, generic and individualized dose estimations allow for proper evaluation of organ and effective doses during overexposures, providing informed decision-making. Professional associations like the American Association of Physicists in Medicine emphasize compliance with practice guidelines on safe use of diagnostic radiation and promote the review process and consensus standards as a means to foster greater patient safety and quality of service (Seibert *et. al.*, 2018). Through extensive monitoring systems, risks of stochastic and deterministic effects can be significantly minimized in diagnostic imaging (Figure 3.6.

3.1.8. Education and Training for Staff

Ensuring safety for patients and radiological workers alike involves large-scale education and training in the areas of radiation protection. As diagnostic quality improves with developing technologies, exposure to ionizing radiation grows, and with it comes the problem of cumulative doses and biological effects. The majority of healthcare professionals lack adequate knowledge of radiation safety principles, and this inefficiency takes away from efforts toward protection. This lack highlights the urgent need for systematized training that bridges the theoretical and applied gaps and a culture of safety in healthcare settings. On-the-job training, augmented by specialized courses, akin to those available for other advanced interdisciplinary careers, can make important contributions toward equipping workers with needed competencies (Barletta *et. al.*, 2012). In addition, continuous education for the evolving aspect of radiation use and health effects is essential in order to provide high levels of security and compliance with good medical practice (Budošová *et. al.*, 2021).

3.1.9. Importance of Safety Protocols

It requires strict adherence to guidelines formulated to reduce dangers from exposure to radiation. Not only are safety measures required for avoiding instant danger, but also for prevention from long-term health risks from cumulative doses of radiation, a point emphasized by novel evidence about the lingering impact of contrast media and ionizing radiation (Adadzi *et. al.*, 2024). Their incorporation with advanced imaging technology and AI-driven surveillance programs complements these safety functions by enabling real-time optimization of dose and tailored diagnostic methods, both of which reduce unnecessary radiation without compromise to image quality (Adadzi *et. al.*, 2024). They are further augmented with systematic safety guidelines that guarantee consistent risk management in a broad array of clinical settings, reducing human factors such as human error and equipment abuse that would otherwise enhance radiation hazards. Lastly, strictness in enforcing the safety precautions is most essential in establishing an environment in which diagnostic efficiency and radiation protection harmonize perfectly, safeguarding both the patients and medical professionals (Figure 3.7).

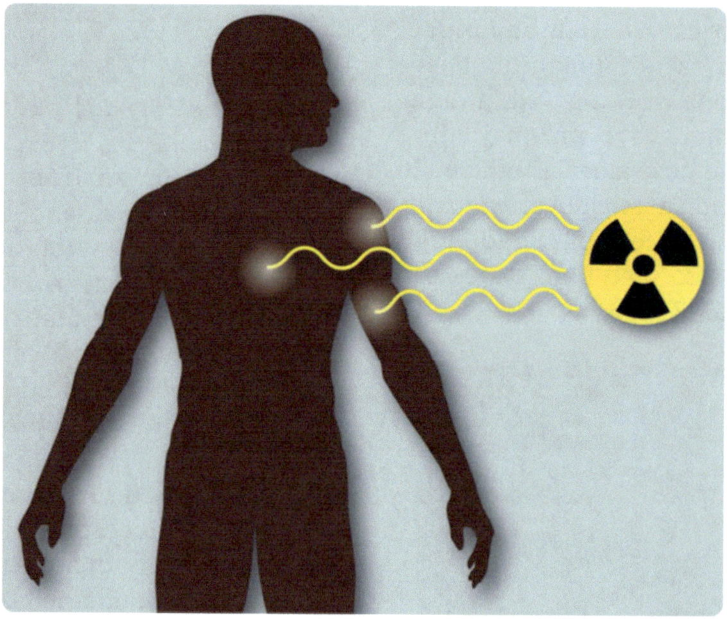

Figure 3.7. Safety protocols are essential not only for reducing immediate harm but also for preventing long-term adverse health effects caused by cumulative radiation doses.

Source: https://www.cdc.gov/radiation-emergencies/media/images/infographics-vector/workplace_radiation_health_effects.png.

Test Your Knowledge

1. How do lead aprons contribute to radiation protection during X-ray and fluoroscopy procedures?
2. What is the significance of using proper shielding in radiology departments?

3.2. Safety Protocols and Guidelines

Learning Outcome

1. Understand national and international guidelines
2. Focus on institutional radiation safety policies
3. Discuss patient consent and information
4. Perform risk assessment procedures
5. Describe emergency procedures for radiation incidents
6. Learn quality assurance in imaging practices
7. Know the role of radiologists in safety
8. Explain collaboration with medical physicists
9. Explain continuous improvement in safety measures

To protect the safety of patients and healthcare providers in diagnostic imaging, strict adherence to established guidelines and procedures is necessary to minimize radiation exposure while maintaining image quality. Optimization of such protocols includes quality assurance, equipment maintenance, and continuous education of the radiology team to prevent excessive doses of radiation, as evidenced by studies indicating high doses of radiation in some diagnostic departments due to the lack of optimization (Abubakar *et. al.*, 2021). Implementation of such a practice reduces the likelihood of re-imaging, which will ultimately enhance the cumulated radiation burden. Advances in technology, primarily the integration of AI, have also enhanced protection with low-dose imaging techniques, maintaining diagnostic quality at much lower exposure to radiation (Adeleke *et. al.*, 2025). Current guidelines emphasize patient-specific imaging protocols tailored to patient needs, real-time evaluation, and dose minimization, reflecting an adaptive strategy to radiation protection that maximizes both clinical efficacy as well as patient safety in the diagnostic setting.

3.2.1. National and International Guidelines

Effective protection and safety of the patient through radiation during diagnostic procedures is basically ensured through adherence to established national and international standards that harmonize diverse regulatory practices to ensure patient and practitioner safety. These rules are guided by evolving trade and health requirements that reflect the dynamics of the international marketplace, particularly in regions such as the European Union and the United States, where standards are regulated by organizations such as the Global Harmonization Task Force and ISO (Maghiar *et. al.*, 2025).

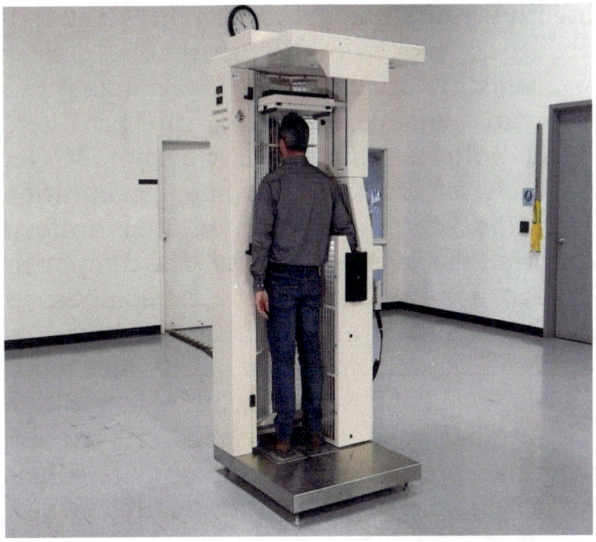

Figure 3.8. Effective radiation protection and safety in diagnostic procedures are fundamentally upheld through adherence to established national and international guidelines.

Source: https://mirion.imgix.net/cms4_ mirion/files/images/learning- center/general-product-videos/Argos-3-5-Whole-Body- Contamination-Monitors_ TN.png?auto= compress%2Cformat&fit= clip&q= 80&w=2084&s=5c6fdec1290375874fc5e6aeda6da8cb.

Also, the incorporation of new diagnostic and treatment technologies, such as theranostics, demands close observation to maintain regional balance in regulation in line with global best practices. This emphasis on compliance and innovation underlines the necessity for extensive guidelines providing a consistent approach to safety, considering the growing use of radioligand therapies, as well as the complexity of their application across different health systems. Thus, these standards are an important resource for limiting the risks of radiation and enhancing diagnostic efficiency internationally (Figure 3.8).

3.2.2. Institutional Radiation Safety Policies

Effective radiation protection in diagnostic settings depends on robust institutional policies governing the use of radiologic technology and protecting patients and health care providers. These policies must have clearly outlined protocols for training, equipment calibration, and exposure tracking to enforce uniform conformity to safety guidelines. One component of such a program is the establishment of multidisciplinary monitoring committees to review risk, allocate resources, and foster interdepartmental communication. In addition, institutional support for specialized training programs enhances proficiency, particularly in new fields such as theranostics, where enhanced knowledge is essential to guarantee safe practice (Al-Ibraheem *et. al.*, 2024; de Reynies *et. al.*, 2009). In coordinating policies with new technological advancements and international standards, institutions promote a culture of safety that minimizes radiation exposure risks and ensures diagnostic quality. This governance model, combining technical infrastructure with continuous education and rigorous quality control, must be used to ensure adequate radiation protection across healthcare facilities.

3.2.3. Patient Consent and Information

Effective patient-provider communication is key in ensuring ethical and safe use of diagnostic radiation. Patients need to be appropriately informed of the risks, benefits, and potential radiation exposure before undergoing any radiologic procedure to enable them to provide informed consent. It not only manifests respect for patient autonomy but also trust and compliance with safety practice. Evidence indicates a wide gap in patient as well as in healthcare staff perception of radiation doses and attendant risks, necessitating widespread education to enable informed decision-making (Alsharif, 2024). Additionally, information tailored to the profile of individual patients as well as to local diagnostic reference levels (DRLs) can assist in localizing the risk with emphasis on protection mechanisms to restrict exposure (Alhujaili *et. al.*, 2024). Accordingly, open communication and comprehensive patient education are essential factors in shielding against radiation, rendering patients partners for their management as well as diagnostic safety in general (Figure 3.9).

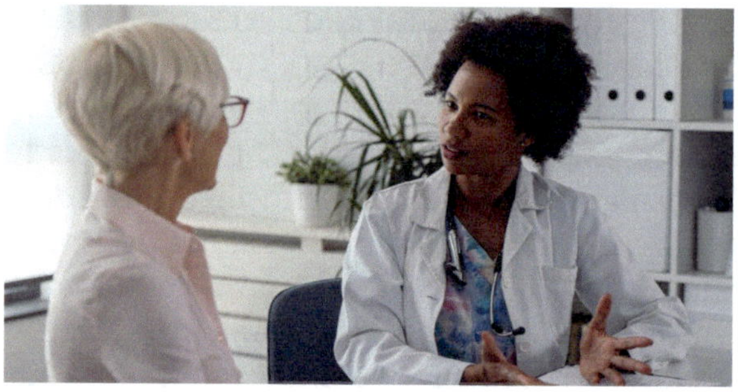

Figure 3.9. Effective communication between healthcare providers and patients is essential in ensuring the ethical and safe use of diagnostic radiation.

Source: https://www.sermo.com/wp-content/uploads/2023/02/effective-communication-img3-min-1050x555.jpg.

3.2.4. Risk Assessment Procedures

Effective radiation exposure control in diagnostic settings relies on adequate risk assessment policies that identify and curb potential hazards to patients as well as health practitioners. Such policies involve ascertaining the overall radiation dose, considering certain patient characteristics, and ensuring adherence to current safety standards. These evaluations are prompted by the widespread use of ionizing radiation in medical diagnosis, which, as useful as it is in enabling superior diagnostic precision, poses in itself intrinsic biological risks that cannot be discounted (Budošová *et. al.*, 2021). Risk assessment also demands continued education of healthcare professionals to supplement knowledge in areas related to the safety of radiation, which can eliminate unnecessary exposure. Moreover, the inclusion of reproducible and accurate measurement techniques, such as those calibrated in different diagnostic environments, enhances risk stratification and accuracy of exposure estimations (Tomei *et. al.*, 2015). In conclusion, proper risk assessment protocols are the bedrock for effective radiation protection measures to provide safe diagnostic procedures and safeguard public health.

3.2.5. Emergency Procedures for Radiation Incidents

Effective management of hazardous incidents in the diagnostic setting involves a holistic strategy that incorporates synergistic technology and well-defined procedures. In radiation accidents, prompt detection and containment can avoid exposure and environmental contamination to a large degree. Recent advancements validate the capability of autonomous robotic systems to carry out high-risk inspection and maintenance tasks, including fire and gas monitoring, on unmanned structures, thereby reducing human exposure and enhancing response efficiency in emergencies (Grytøyr *et. al.*, 2020). In addition, the remoteness control and oversight capability of complex facilities by dispersed teams of experts also enhances decision-making and intervention velocity in radiation emergencies (Czarapata *et. al.*, 2002). Emergency procedures, therefore, must incorporate both technological innovation and coupled communication networks to support the rapid detection, separation, and management of radiation hazards. Such coupling not only improves patient and staff safety but also supports evolving trends in radiation protection and safety within diagnostic processes, with an emphasis on proactive readiness and robust response systems (Figure 3.10).

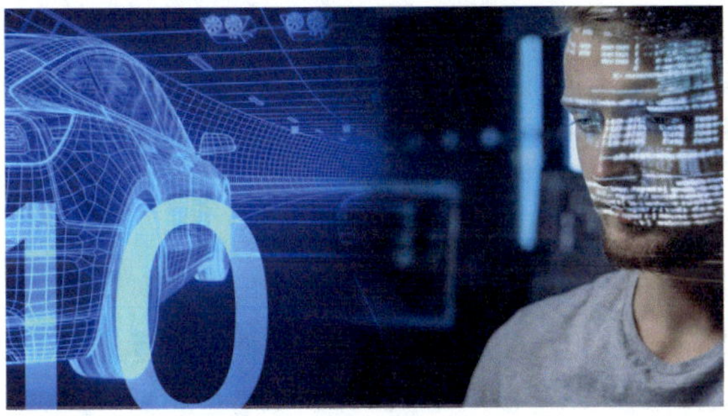

Figure 3.10. Effective management of hazardous scenarios in diagnostic settings necessitates a comprehensive approach that integrates advanced technology and well-defined protocols.

Source: https://media.licdn.com/dms/image/v2/D4D12AQHcx96beHPVbw/article-cover_image-shrink_720_1280/article-cover_image-shrink_720_1280/0/1736061067366?e=2147483647&v=beta&t=CDL0u-WYyYCpqq4qYxtir-ZBHAKcJenroL60f9mbChI.

3.2.6. Quality Assurance in Imaging Practices

Patient safety during imaging diagnosis is ensured through close monitoring of equipment performance and procedure standards. Assurance programs are crucial in maintaining the reliability and accuracy of imaging systems and minimizing radiation exposure. These programs include routine calibration, performance testing, and radiation dose monitoring for identification of drifts likely to degrade the image quality or increase unwarranted patient risk. Regulatory bodies, for instance, conducting periodic inspections and maintaining dose registries, encourage compliance with safety standards and facilitate reporting of incidents to sustain improvement (Venelampi *et. al.*, 2023). The inclusion of advances in radiation physics and biology within the quality assurance procedures allows practitioners to balance the diagnostic benefits against potential biological harm, as discussed in recent studies exploring the optimization of dose reduction without compromising image quality (Thubab *et. al.*, 2024). Thus, systematic quality control underpins both the validity of diagnostic findings and patient safety from unwarranted radiation, outlining its indispensable place in diagnostic safety.

3.2.7. Role of Radiologists in Safety

Patient and healthcare worker protection during diagnostic imaging involves a multidisciplinary approach, where radiologists play an crucial role. Besides their diagnostic skill, radiologists are important professionals applying radiation protection principles, for example, justification and optimization of imaging studies to minimize unnecessary exposure. They operate closely with technologists and medical physicists to implement DRLs and use advanced imaging protocols that provide optimal image quality at the minimum dose. Radiologists also aid in educating referring physicians and patients about the harms and benefits of radiation, supporting well-informed decision-making. They must advocate for adherence to requirements and standards, encourage adoption of emerging technology like AI to support dose optimization, and facilitate accurate diagnosis and treatment planning. With the complexity of cumulative radiation exposure and evolving standards of safety, proactive involvement by radiologists is crucial in maintaining a culture of safety within medical imaging facilities (Madan *et. al.*, 2021; Modarai *et. al.*, 2022) (Figure 3.11).

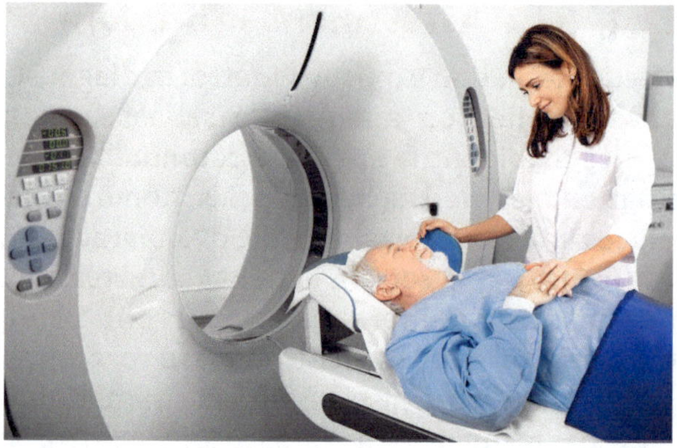

Figure 3.11. Ensuring the safety of patients and healthcare personnel during diagnostic imaging necessitates a multidisciplinary approach, where radiologists play a pivotal role.

Source: https://hdc1984.com/wp-content/uploads/2023/07/AdobeStock_249817238.jpeg.

3.2.8. Collaboration with Medical Physicists

Radiation safety and protection in diagnostic imaging must be ensured through a multidisciplinary approach, with medical physicists playing a key role in the process. They apply their overall knowledge of physics, engineering, and computational science to optimize imaging protocols, minimize patient and staff exposure, and ensure standards of equipment performance. Their input is essential in creating and developing safety controls that are in line with technological advancements, which are advancing rapidly and becoming more complex. However, the medical devices and safety measures can be optimally utilized and their misuse reduced to minimal harm only when there is free communication and coordination among medical physicists and medical professionals for the best use and reduction of risk resulting from misuse. This interaction also creates sustained education and quality assurance essential for the maintenance of high standards in radiation safety (Barletta *et. al.*, 2012; Caruana *et. al.*, 2006). Accordingly, interaction with medical physicists is paramount in improving diagnostic safety and protecting patients from undue radiation risks.

3.2.9. Continuous Improvement in Safety Measures

The evolving nature of diagnostic radiology demands constant vigilance and creativity for enhancing the safety of patients and staff. While technology innovations result in better imaging, safety protocols need to be updated in harmony with that so as to reduce exposure to radiation without compromising the diagnostic value. Enhanced performance involves thorough evaluation and incorporation of new evidence-based clinical procedures, hence putting a spotlight on adaptive learning within clinical environments. For example, novel cancer treatment strategies in oncology emphasize the use of targeted radiation with reduced collateral damage, a process validating the rationale for more stringent safety upgrades within diagnostic settings (Iyengar *et. al.*, 2017). In addition, integrating rigorous risk assessments considering patient-specific factors, such as age and comorbidities, can further enhance the protection measures to a greater extent, as put forth in research on differential demographic vulnerabilities (Alexander *et. al.*, 2022). Lastly, a sustained commitment to education, technological advancement, and process refinement forms a safety culture that is the cornerstone of all activities in diagnostic medicine and radiation protection (Figure 3.12).

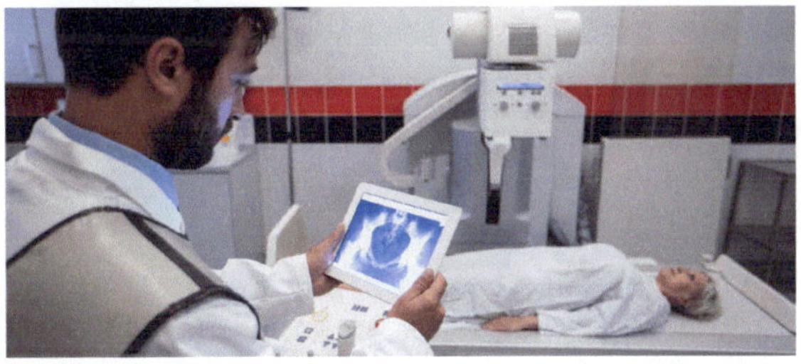

Figure 3.12. Continuous improvement involves systematic evaluation and incorporation of new evidence-based practices, highlighting the importance of adaptive learning within clinical environments.

Source: https://www.mavenimaging.com/hubfs/which-x-ray-system-is-right-for-me-min.png.

Test Your Knowledge

1. What are the guidelines for performing a safe radiological exam on pregnant women?
2. Which regulatory bodies set the safety standards for radiation protection in the workplace?

3.3. Challenges and Innovations in Radiation Safety

Learning Outcome

1. Balance diagnostic benefits and risks
2. Understand the public health implications of radiation exposure
3. Explain technological innovations in radiation safety
4. Address misconceptions about radiation
5. Research on alternative imaging methods
6. Explain global disparities in radiation safety practices
7. Know the impact of regulatory changes
8. Learn case studies of radiation incidents
9. Describe future challenges in radiation safety

Medical diagnostic and imaging technology innovations have enormously enhanced healthcare, but simultaneously pose advanced challenges to radiation safety that need innovative solutions. Radiation protection needs to be improved continuously to mitigate risks of occupational exposure, patient protection, and environmental radiation. Of special interest is the fact that new technologies demand new paradigms that balance safety standards and diagnostic effectiveness, both locally and globally, in radiological protection terms. Technologies such as lower dose technologies, DRLs, and system-based safety cultures are central to optimizing the application of radiation while delivering quality care. Nevertheless, the profession faces the need for long-term investment in research, improved leadership, and broader stakeholder involvement, including active patient participation in safety practices. These multi-purpose activities are included in a holistic approach that unifies benefits and risks, with a view to achieving sustainable development in radiation protection consistent with broader public health and environmental goals (Dauer, 2015; Garnier-Laplace *et. al.*, 2025).

3.3.1. Balancing Diagnostic Benefits and Risks

Medical imaging has transformed diagnostic capabilities, allowing for earlier disease detection and more accurate treatment planning. The advantages of these are accompanied by risks inherent in exposure to radiation. Radiation protection in diagnostics at its best requires a delicate balance between optimizing clinical benefits while limiting potential harm to the patient. The challenge is to render each radiological intervention justifiable by making its diagnostic yield of more value than the possible ill effects, i.e., the cumulative dose of radiation inducing a higher risk of cancer. Optimization of dose, use of alternative modalities with no ionizing radiation, and adherence to safety guidelines are important.

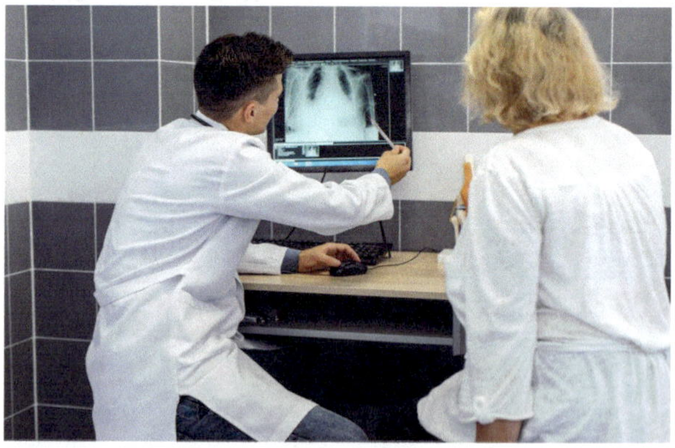

Figure 3.13. Optimal radiation protection in diagnostics necessitates a careful balance between maximizing clinical benefits and minimizing potential harm to patients.

Source: https://orthomiami.com/wp-content/uploads/2023/07/young-doctor-showing-radiography-min-1024x683.jpg.

Also, patient-related factors like age, sex, and underlying disease must inform personalized risk stratification to avoid inappropriate exposures (Alexander *et. al.*, 2022). In the case of an emerging infectious disease outbreak, such as COVID-19, where imaging is a key component of diagnosis, the urgent need for effective diagnosis must be weighed against avoiding excess radiation exposure in vulnerable populations (Pascarella *et. al.*, 2020). Balancing these components is critical to the progression of safe and effective diagnostic procedures (Figure 3.13).

3.3.2. Public Health Implications of Radiation Exposure

Progress in diagnostic imaging has measurably enhanced clinical results, yet, in turn, instigated concern over patient exposure to radiation and its public health implications. With increasing recurrence rates of imaging, cumulative effective doses to patients approach levels linked with elevated stochastic risks such as cancer induction, instigating special concern over radiation protection programs (Madan *et. al.*, 2021). The challenge is to weigh diagnostic benefit against potential long-term risks, calling for measured planning and combining clinical history and dose measurement to ensure maximum safety to the patient.

Moreover, vulnerable groups, such as immunocompromised individuals, may also be at a higher risk, demanding the application of tailored techniques and effective follow-up protocols (Keohane *et. al.*, 2020). The public health significance extends beyond patients, with a plea for joint efforts by healthcare providers, regulating bodies, and manufacturers to engineer safer imaging equipment, enhance justification practices, and implement stringent education and surveillance programs. Navigating these complexities is necessary in minimizing radiation-related health effects while sustaining diagnostic imaging's life-preserving merits.

3.3.3. Technological Innovations in Radiation Safety

New imaging diagnostic techniques have significantly enhanced radiation safety by integrating sophisticated technologies. Technologies such as photon-counting CT scanners reduce doses of radiation with improved image quality, thereby subjecting patients to minimal doses of radiation without compromising diagnostic quality. AI further contributes by personalizing imaging protocols to individual patients and facilitating real-time monitoring to optimize the radiation use, customized to the patient's precise needs. These advances are supplemented by professional guidelines that emphasize the value of specialized education and adherence to prescribed safety procedures for generating effective radiation protection (Seibert *et. al.*, 2018).

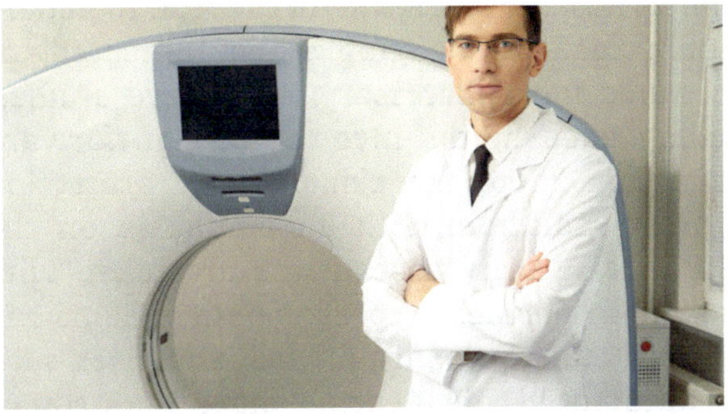

Figure 3.14. Innovations such as photon-counting computed tomography scanners reduce radiation doses while improving image resolution, thereby minimizing patient exposure without compromising diagnostic quality.

Source: https://irp.cdn-website.com/c47c802a/dms3rep/multi/5.png.

Furthermore, non-ionizing imaging techniques, including elastography and photoacoustic imaging, present promising alternatives to ionizing radiation, limiting additional potential health consequences. In addition to clinical benefits, the application of energy-efficient imaging technologies and biodegradable contrast media addresses environmental concerns associated with imaging procedures (Adadzi *et. al.*, 2024). Both of these technological developments mark a multifaceted response to radiational safety improvement, making diagnostic conditions safer for patients and medical professionals alike (Figure 3.14).

3.3.4. Addressing Misconceptions About Radiation

Despite the improvements in medical technology, myths about radiation often cloud effective communication about its risks and benefits when employed for diagnosis. The vast majority of the population mistakenly equates all exposure to radiation with adverse effects and dismisses the fact that diagnostic radiation doses are tightly controlled and optimized to generate the lowest amount of risk with the greatest clinical advantage. This myth can lead to patient fear, refusal of imaging when indicated, or demands for unnecessary alternative studies. Curing such myths involves straightforward education about the principles of protection against radiation, with an emphasis on the fact that security precautions are taken with maximum alertness to protect both patients and medical staff. Secondly, just as industries such as automotive engineering place importance on rigorous testing and security to prevent system breakdown (Prathap *et. al.*, 2013), diagnostic radiology is continuously evolving safety measures based on scientific evidence. Building patient trust and education about radiation can increase adherence to suggested imaging and eventually result in better health outcomes (Chukwueke *et. al.*, 2019).

3.3.5. Research on Alternative Imaging Methods

Advances in diagnostic imaging are being driven ever more by the need to minimize exposure of patients and operators to ionizing radiation. New research has focused on substitute technologies for imaging that are as effective diagnostically but enhance safety procedures. Ultrasound and magnetic resonance imaging (MRI) modalities provide non-ionizing options that reduce cumulative doses of radiation, useful particularly in at-risk groups. For instance, echocardiography has been demonstrated to be very useful with adaptations for higher infection control measures in the time of the COVID-19 pandemic, in line with its broader importance in imaging within safe practice (James *et. al.*, 2020). Moreover, technology like cone beam computed tomography (CBCT) enables specialized imaging with decreased radiation exposure in comparison to traditional computed tomography, with improved procedural guidance in vascular intervention (Modarai *et. al.*, 2022). These advances confirm the supreme balance of diagnostic performance and radiation protection, demanding ongoing research in refining existing technologies and developing new methodologies that further prioritize staff and patient safety in clinical diagnosis (Figure 3.15).

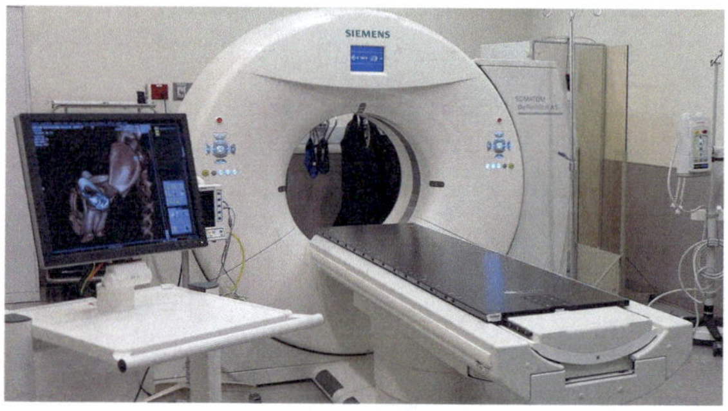

Figure 3.15. Advancements in diagnostic imaging are increasingly driven by the need to minimize patient and operator exposure to ionizing radiation.

Source: https://www.iaea.org/sites/default/files/ctscanner_3.jpg.

3.3.6. Global Disparities in Radiation Safety Practices

Despite advancements in diagnostic imaging technologies and artificial intelligence-led developments with reduced exposure to radiation, broad worldwide inequalities remain in radiation safety guidelines. These inequalities are typically founded on differences in healthcare facilities, availability of resources, and regulations between high-income and low- to middle-income countries. While some regions utilize state-of-the-art technology like photon-counting CT scanners and artificial intelligence-enabled low-dose imaging protocols that provide maximal patient protection and diagnostic accuracy, others continue to employ antiquated equipment with poorer safety characteristics and hence a higher risk of harmful effects of radiation exposure. Environmental and economic factors also contribute to inconsistency in the utilization of radiation protection factors in a broad array of environments (Adadzi *et. al.*, 2024). While AI presents promising solutions in the reduction of exposure by enhancing the quality of images, barriers such as limited technological access, professional skill, and ethical morality hinder its universal application (Adeleke *et. al.*, 2025). Balancing these disparities requires concerted global initiatives toward harmonization of radiation safety methods and concordance of innovative technologies among all healthcare systems.

3.3.7. Impact of Regulatory Changes

Technological advancements in protection against radiation have increasingly been led by shifting regulatory requirements that focus on quality assurance and patient safety. The regulations have ensured rigorous training procedures, dose monitoring, and the utilization of instrumentation to limit harmful exposure during diagnostic examinations. Particularly, professional guidelines by authoritative bodies emphasize the necessity of clearly defined roles and standardized methods to ensure compliant performance by medical institutions. For example, adherence to practice guidelines in medical physics, which have been strenuously put through consensus and public review processes, shows an interest in preserving standards based on expert agreement and scientific evidence (Seibert *et. al.*, 2018). In addition, regulatory changes have promoted the adoption of procedural safeguards such as dose alerts and checklists, which are central to preventing inadvertent overexposure and procedural errors in interventional radiology (Damilakis *et. al.*, 2017). Collectively, these legislative advances reduce the risks associated with radiation, enhance the reliability of diagnoses, and establish a culture for sustained safety enhancement in radiological facilities (Figure 3.16).

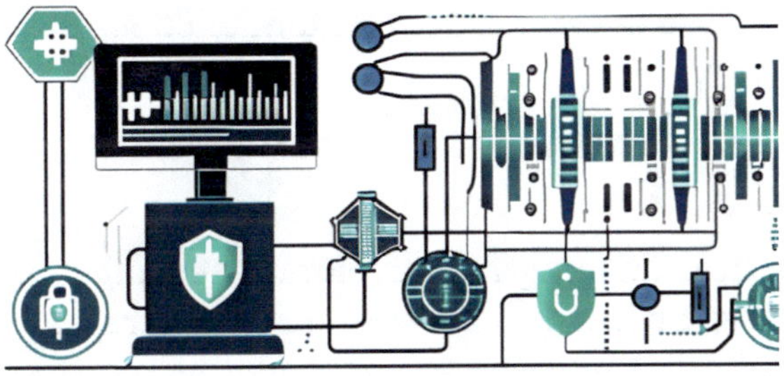

Figure 3.16. Advancements in radiation protection have increasingly been shaped by evolving regulatory frameworks that emphasize patient safety and quality assurance.

Source: https://bluegoatcyber.com/wp-content/smush-webp/2024/02/img_65c58cf5092fa.png.webp.

3.3.8. Case Studies of Radiation Incidents

A historical overview of medical diagnostic radiation accidents emphasizes gross deficits in protection protocols that have resulted in serious patient and operator harm. For example, long fluoroscopy times for complex endovascular procedures have resulted in deterministic injuries such as skin radiation injuries, underscoring the importance of dose monitoring and procedure optimization. These case studies suggest the way in which the absence of operator awareness and inadequate adherence to safety principles—justification, optimization, and dose limitation—may enhance risks both to patients and to health workers, who may suffer cumulative occupational exposure over the long term (Modarai *et. al.*, 2022). In addition, accidents arising from the aging of equipment or non-use of dose-reduction technologies reveal system vulnerabilities that underscore the value of continuous education, strict quality assurance, and adherence to regulatory standards. Recent case studies demonstrate that, despite advances in imaging technology, there remains a risk of stochastic effects, such as malignancies, reinforcing further that radiation protection should continue to be a live issue in diagnostics (Alexander *et. al.*, 2022).

3.3.9. Future Challenges in Radiation Safety

Medical imaging has revolutionized diagnosis, but it brings in complex issues of radiation safety that must be solved urgently. Increasing episodes of repeated imaging have led to elevated cumulative doses of radiation in patients, raising issues of long-term risk and adequacy of present protection measures. Including patient-centered solutions that account for cumulative exposure history, along with clinical need, is a necessity to balance diagnostic benefit against potential radiation damage. In addition, advancements in technology must find ways of inventing imaging modalities that are of diagnostic quality but minimize dose, supported by improved dose monitoring systems to facilitate clinical decision-making more optimally (Madan *et. al.*, 2021). Professional ethical standards of healthcare providers mandate adherence to evolving guidelines and regulatory specifications that guarantee patient safety without compromising the quality of care (François *et. al.*, 2019). Future strategies will have to resolve uncertainties in dose-risk relationships simultaneously, encourage interdisciplinarity, and reinforce teaching in radiation protection in an effort to counter the potential risks of diagnostic radiology.

Test Your Knowledge

1. How does the use of protective lead shields reduce radiation exposure?
2. How do radiology technologists protect themselves while operating radiologic equipment?

SUMMARY

Patient safety and radiation exposure reduction remain of utmost concern in diagnostic imaging, especially with continuous technological advancements. Evidence underscores the need for dose optimization, as evidenced in varying radiation strengths in various diagnostic centers, which are likely to exceed recommended international norms (Abubakar *et. al.*, 2021). Technologies such as photon-counting CT and AI-based imaging protocols have high potential for reducing unnecessary radiation while increasing diagnostic performance, eventually leading to better patient outcomes and workflow optimization (Adadzi *et. al.*, 2024). Furthermore, long-term activities towards professional education, quality assurance, and preventive maintenance will have to be undertaken to provide safety standards and prevent dose buildup due to equipment malfunction or incorrect usage (Abubakar *et. al.*, 2021). The combination of new technology and the tried and tested safety principles can adequately address the trade-off between diagnostic benefit and radiation damage. Ultimately, a multidisciplinary method of combining technology innovation, continuing education, and rigorous quality control is needed to enhance radiation protection and safety in diagnosis.

Effective radiation protection and safety in diagnostic procedures rely on an integrated system that adheres to stringent environmental and patient-based regulations. Understanding the mechanisms of action through which radionuclides affect the environment as well as human health is essential, as seen through the studies of radionuclide transport via food production and soil contamination surrounding research facilities (Barkauskas *et. al.*, 2021). Additionally, theranostic advances point to the mounting need for harmonized safety requirements as they integrate diagnostics with targeted radioligand therapy, requiring specialized infrastructure and rigorous regulatory adherence. These advances reinforce the importance of forging robust guidelines and best practices that can adapt to local variability while maintaining global safety levels. Last, but not least, the safety of both healthcare providers and patients demands continuous education, thorough planning, and collective regulatory action to minimize radiation exposure and optimize the diagnostic utility of imaging technologies.

KEY TERMS FROM THIS CHAPTER

- Computed tomography scanners
- Infectious diseases
- Occupational exposure
- Photon
- Real-time monitoring
- Stakeholder
- Continuous improvement
- Leadership
- Patient safety
- Public health
- Risk assessments

CRITICAL THINKING QUESTIONS

1. Which of the following is the primary principle of radiation protection?

a. Maximizing radiation exposure for diagnostic purposes

b. Minimizing radiation exposure to the patient and staff

c. Using the highest possible dose to ensure accurate results

d. Ensuring that radiation is only used in critical cases

2. What is the ALARA principle in radiation protection?

a. Always limit the amount of radiation exposure to the minimum level necessary

b. Avoid using radiation in medical procedures altogether

c. Apply the same radiation dose to all patients

d. Increase radiation dose to enhance image quality

3. Which of the following is most commonly used as shielding material in radiology departments?

a. Lead

b. Concrete

c. Glass

d. Wood

4. The unit of measurement for radiation dose equivalent is:

a. Gray (Gy)

b. Sievert (Sv)

c. Becquerel (Bq)

d. Curie (Ci)

5. Which of the following radiation protection measures is used to reduce exposure during fluoroscopic procedures?

a. Increase the fluoroscopy time

b. Use the highest possible radiation dose

c. Employ lead aprons for the patient and staff

d. Decrease the image quality

Short Answer Questions

1. What is the primary goal of radiation protection in medical imaging?
2. Explain the ALARA principle and its importance in radiation safety.
3. What is the difference between radiation protection for patients and healthcare workers?
4. Why is radiation safety crucial during fluoroscopic procedures?
5. What is the role of a radiation safety officer in a healthcare setting?
6. Why is it important to reduce the exposure time during diagnostic radiology procedures?

Answers to Critical Thinking Questions

1.(b); 2.(a); 3.(a); 4.(b); 5.(c)

REFERENCES

1. Abubakar, T. S., Anzaku, E. P., Bichi, T. S., Durumin, I. Y., *et. al.* (2021). Evaluation of computed tomography doses in three medical diagnostic centers in Kano. https://core.ac.uk/download/490646822.pdf (accessed on 30 May 2025).

2. Kerna, N. A., Ngwu, D. C., Kadivi, K., Carsrud, N. V., Pruitt, K. D., Flores, J. V., Holets, H. M., Jomsky, B. M., Chawla, S., Azi, C. I., McKee, D., Nwokorie, U., Anderson II, J., Dugeri, J. L., Hammam, H. S. H., Chiedozie, O. B., Nnake, I., David, C. O., & Adadzi, J. (2024). Transformative Advancements in Diagnostic Imaging: Reducing Risks, Enhancing Accuracy, and Promoting Sustainability. *European Journal of Medical and Health Research*, *2*(5), 153-172. https://doi.org/10.59324/ejmhr.2024.2(5).16

3. Adeleke, S., Adeleke, S., Akpan, A. O., Akpan, *et. al.* (2025). AI-driven advances in low-dose imaging and enhancement—A review. https://core.ac.uk/download/647986101.pdf (accessed on 30 May 2025).

4. Alhujaili, S., Alshabibi, A. S., Alafer, F., Alrowaili, Z., Salah, H., Sulieman, A., Subahi, M., *et. al.* (2024). Establishment of local diagnostic reference levels for head CT imaging in the Madina Region, Saudi Arabia. *Diagnostics, 14*. https://www.semanticscholar.org/paper/7cd54639f13de0d90dd4ddf96776ea75d01f8bc8 (accessed on 30 May 2025).

5. Al-Ibraheem, A., Baum, R. P., Ben-Haim, S., Blay, *et. al.* (2024). Guiding principles on the education and practice of theragnostic. https://core.ac.uk/download/611825231.pdf (accessed on 30 May 2025).

6. Alsharif, A. (2024). Assessment of radiation exposure and safety practice in CT unit in a general hospital. *Journal of King Abdulaziz University: Engineering Sciences*. https://www.semanticscholar.org/paper/d7c83cf51a59c5b2da94410a0ef936801265feb2 (accessed on 30 May 2025).

7. Aroesty, J., Logan, J., & Zimmerman, R. (2025). Human support issues and systems for the space exploration initiative: Results from Project Outreach. https://core.ac.uk/download/pdf/42812273.pdf (accessed on 30 May 2025).

8. Asadi Asgharani, F., Alizad, M., Mahdavi, M., & Rashidi, R. (2025). Assessment of dentists' knowledge and performance regarding radiation protection principles in dental offices in Khorram-Abad, Iran 2023. *Jundishapur Journal of Health Sciences*. https://www.semanticscholar.org/paper/78f2ddc08761c77ad6964c9762a91322525eeadb (accessed on 30 May 2025).

9. Baatout, S., Baselet, B., Belmans, N., *et. al.* (2021). Radiobiological risks following dentomaxillofacial imaging: Should we be concerned? https://core.ac.uk/download/543617172.pdf (accessed on 30 May 2025).

10. Barkauskas, V., Bernhardsson, C., Eriksson Stenström, K., *et. al.* (2021). Evaluation of the region-specific risks of accidental radioactive releases from the European Spallation Source. https://core.ac.uk/download/483934860.pdf (accessed on 30 May 2025).

11. Barletta, W. A., Chattopadhyay, S., & Seryi, A. (2012). Educating and training accelerator scientists and technologists for tomorrow. *arXiv*. http://arxiv.org/abs/1207.3065 (accessed on 30 May 2025).

12. Budošová, D., Bárdyová, Z., Horváthová, M., *et. al.* (2021). The importance of public health in radiology and radiation protection. https://core.ac.uk/download/388907612.pdf (accessed on 30 May 2025).

13. Caruana, C. J. (2006). The role of biomedical physics-engineering in the development of medical device education for the healthcare professions. https://core.ac.uk/download/200846833.pdf (accessed on 30 May 2025).
14. Chukwueke, U. N., Hervey-Jumper, S. L., Lee, E. Q., *et. al.* (2019). Barriers to accrual and enrollment in brain tumor trials. https://www.zora.uzh.ch/id/eprint/176128/1/Lee_SNO_RANO_trials_FINAL_VERSION_to_Neuro-Oncology_05-07-2019.pdf (accessed on 30 May 2025).
15. Czarapata, P., Hartill, D., Myers, S., *et. al.* (2002). Status report of the inter-laboratory task force on remote operation. https://core.ac.uk/download/25330848.pdf (accessed on 30 May 2025).
16. Martin CJ, Vassileva J, Vano E, Mahesh M, Ebdon-Jackson S, Ng KH, Frush DP, Loose R, Damilakis J. Unintended and accidental medical radiation exposures in radiology: guidelines on investigation and prevention. J Radiol Prot. 2017 Jan;37(4):883-906. doi: 10.1088/1361-6498/aa881e. PMID: 28836506.
17. Dauer, L. (2015). Radiological safety and quality: Paradigms in leadership and innovation. *Health Physics*. https://www.semanticscholar.org/paper/a9cda1fa0ab02ccb9cd2bca87fa4f0c38e8c88ea (accessed on 30 May 2025).
18. Davies, J. C., & Lowe, A. (2025). Environmental implications of the health care service sector. https://core.ac.uk/download/pdf/9307987.pdf (accessed on 30 May 2025).
19. De Paoli P. Institutional shared resources and translational cancer research. J Transl Med. 2009 Jun 29;7:54. doi: 10.1186/1479-5876-7-54. PMID: 19563639; PMCID: PMC2711056.
20. Donya, M., ElGuindy, A., Firmin, D., Radford, *et. al.* (2014). Radiation in medicine: Origins, risks and aspirations. https://core.ac.uk/download/77008838.pdf (accessed on 30 May 2025).
21. Drey, N., Husson, O., May, K. A., *et. al.* (2020). Radiation exposure awareness from patients undergoing nuclear medicine diagnostic 99mTc-MDP bone scans and 2-deoxy-2-(18F) fluor-D-glucose PET/computed tomography scans. https://core.ac.uk/download/305120002.pdf (accessed on 30 May 2025).
22. Economou, G., Kandarakis, I., Panagiotakis, G., Vlachos, I., & Sklavounos, P. (2022). Principles of ultrasound technology in medical imaging of non-ionization images. *Periapex Indian Journal of Research*. https://www.semanticscholar.org/paper/13e0445705a91ec536033500f6fccabc4a176b0a (accessed on 30 May 2025).
23. Felemban, D. (2024). Radiological safety perspectives among undergraduate dental students, interns, and dental assistant certificate students at Taibah University Dental College and Hospital, Saudi Arabia. *Saudi Journal for Health Sciences*. https://www.semanticscholar.org/paper/030c96045fefaf05c158a45b78dff928d7144fe2 (accessed on 30 May 2025).
24. Garnier-Laplace, J., Gariel, J., Vanhavere, F., Rauser, F., Wojcik, A., Ainsbury, E. A., Bouffler, S., *et. al.* (2025). The vital role of radiation protection research in Europe's future: A PIANOFORTE white paper. *Journal of Radiological Protection: Official Journal of the Society for Radiological Protection*. https://www.semanticscholar.org/paper/daad7b3bc9a15530d5b1beee396604b8a2ba18ed (accessed on 30 May 2025).
25. Giammarile, F., Knoll, P., Kunikowska, J., Paez, D., Estrada Lobato, E., Mikhail-Lette, M., Wahl, R. L., *et. al.* (2024). Guardians of precision: Advancing radiation protection, safety, and quality systems in nuclear medicine. *European Journal of Nuclear Medicine and Molecular Imaging, 51*, 1498–1505. https://www.semanticscholar.org/paper/ba4d477a381f2da0df6fce2b8d911cea6808681d (accessed on 30 May 2025).

26. Grytøyr, C. (2020). Design implications for robotized testing and inspection of fire and gas detectors. https://core.ac.uk/download/646178405.pdf (accessed on 30 May 2025).

27. Hwang, H. (2017). Knowledge, attitude and perception on radiation imaging among children's caregivers in the pediatric dental clinic. https://open.bu.edu/bitstream/2144/23797/5/Hwang_bu_0017N_12842.pdf (accessed on 30 May 2025).

28. Ivanova, E., Petrova, D., Uzunov, A., Valchev, *et. al.* (2017). The effect of X-ray radiation on the human body–pros and cons. Radiation protection in medical imaging and radiotherapy. https://core.ac.uk/download/389005933.pdf (accessed on 30 May 2025).

29. Iyengar, P., Wardak, Z., Gerber, D. E., Tumati, V., Ahn, C., Hughes, R., Dowell, J. E., *et. al.* (2017). Consolidative radiotherapy for limited metastatic non–small-cell lung cancer. *JAMA Oncology, 4*, e173501. https://doi.org/10.1001/jamaoncol.2017.3501.

30. Kant, P., Khan, A. A., & Priya, K. (2024). Protection of radiosensitive organs with diagnosable image maximizing radiation protection for radiosensitive organs during CT. *International Journal of Innovative Science and Research Technology (IJISRT)*. https://www.semanticscholar.org/paper/98c40238ed10936ea9499dd856d8b27fb4598f39 (accessed on 30 May 2025).

31. Keohane, S., Botting, J., Budny, P. G., Dolan, O. M., Fife, K., Harwood, C. A., Mallipeddi, R., *et. al.* (2020). British Association of Dermatologists guidelines for the management of people with cutaneous squamous cell carcinoma 2020*. *British Journal of Dermatology, 184*, 401–414. https://doi.org/10.1111/bjd.19621.

32. Kirkpatrick, J. N., Mitchell, C., Taub, C., Kort, S., Hung, J., & Swaminathan, M. (2020). ASE statement on protection of patients and echocardiography service providers during the 2019 novel coronavirus outbreak: Endorsed by the American College of Cardiology. *Journal of the American Society of Echocardiography, 33*, 648–653. https://doi.org/10.1016/j.echo.2020.04.001.

33. Kitsiou, A., Caforio, A. L. P., Porta-Sanchez, A., Vahanian, A., Iung, B., Carrera, C., Szymanski, C., *et. al.* (2013). *ESC Core Curriculum for The General Cardiologist (2013)*. https://core.ac.uk/download/55756305.pdf (accessed on 30 May 2025).

34. Lyon, A. R., López-Fernández, T., Couch, L. S., Asteggiano, R., Aznar, M. C., Bergler-Klein, J., Boriani, G., *et. al.* (2022). 2022 ESC guidelines on cardio-oncology developed in collaboration with the European Hematology Association (EHA), the European Society for Therapeutic Radiology and Oncology (ESTRO), and the International Cardio-Oncology Society (IC-OS). *European Heart Journal, 43*, 4229–4361. https://doi.org/10.1093/eurheartj/ehac244.

35. Mach, F., Baigent, C., Catapano, A. L., Koskinas, K. C., Casula, M., Badimón, L., Chapman, M. J., *et. al.* (2019). 2019 ESC/EAS guidelines for the management of dyslipidemias: Lipid modification to reduce cardiovascular risk. *European Heart Journal, 41*, 111–188. https://doi.org/10.1093/eurheartj/ehz455.

36. Maghiar, T. T., Straciuc, O., Uivarosan, D., & Unita, L. (2025). The EU import requirements for medical devices by comparison with the USA and the GHTF guidelines. https://core.ac.uk/download/pdf/6304072.pdf (accessed on 30 May 2025).

37. Maina, P. M. (2019). Availability and utilization of radiation protection and safety measures by medical imaging technologists in Rwandan hospitals. https://core.ac.uk/download/323341136.pdf (accessed on 30 May 2025).

38. Martins, G. C., Rocha, T. G., Azeredo, T. L., Domingos, A. C., Visconti, M., & Villoria, E. (2023). Hand-held dental X-ray device: Attention to correct use. *Imaging Science in Dentistry, 53*, 265–266. https://www.semanticscholar.org/paper/56b773eb197956179a26064d7f77ee983c6566af (accessed on 30 May 2025).

39. Modarai, B., Haulon, S., Ainsbury, E. A., Böckler, D., Vañó-Carruana, E., Dawson, J., Farber, M. A., *et. al.* (2022). Editor's choice – European Society for Vascular Surgery (ESVS) 2023 clinical practice guidelines on radiation safety. *European Journal of Vascular and Endovascular Surgery, 65*, 171–222. https://doi.org/10.1016/j.ejvs.2022.09.005.

40. Newhauser, W., Gress, D. A., Mills, M., Jordan, D. W., Sutlief, S. G., Martin, M., & Jackson, E. F. (2022). Medical physics workforce in the United States. *Journal of Applied Clinical Medical Physics, 23*. https://doi.org/10.1002/acm2.13762.

41. Oliveira, A., Lacerda, I., & Germano, M. V. (2025). Radiation protection and quality control in radiography services: A comparative study between national and international standards. *Brazilian Journal of Radiation Sciences*. https://www.semanticscholar.org/paper/d8dfa2d0abd9bcc526bdb546fe8eeee133e7103c (accessed on 30 May 2025).

42. Pascarella, G., Strumia, A., Piliego, C., Bruno, F., Del Buono, R., Costa, F., Scarlata, S., *et. al.* (2020). COVID-19 diagnosis and management: A comprehensive review. *Journal of Internal Medicine, 288*, 192–206. https://doi.org/10.1111/joim.13091.

43. Prathap, V., & Rachumallu, A. (2013). Penetration testing of vehicle ECUs. https://core.ac.uk/download/622410642.pdf (accessed on 30 May 2025).

44. Rehani, M. M., & Brady, Z. (2021). Contemporary issues in radiation protection in medical imaging: Introductory editorial. *British Journal of Radiology, 94*. https://doi.org/10.1259/bjr.20219004.

45. Clements JB, Baird CT, de Boer SF, Fairobent LA, Fisher T, Goodwin JH, Gress DA, Johnson JL, Kolsky KL, Mageras GS, Marsh RM, Martin MC, Parker B, Pavord DC, Schell MC, Anthony Seibert J, Stevens DM, Tarver RB, Waite-Jones CG, Wingreen N. AAPM medical physics practice guideline 10.a.: Scope of practice for clinical medical physics. J Appl Clin Med Phys. 2018 Nov;19(6):11-25. doi: 10.1002/acm2.12469. Epub 2018 Oct 19. PMID: 30338913; PMCID: PMC6236822.

46. Seifi, D., & Khorrami, A. (2025). Assessment of staff's knowledge, attitude, and practice on radiation protection measures in Mazandaran Province, Iran. *Frontiers in Biomedical Technologies*. https://www.semanticscholar.org/paper/5d4a2cb139c2eaea6d07d5dd3bfd3b35124b0f62 (accessed on 30 May 2025).

47. Sevalnev, A. I., Kutsak, A. V., Sharavara, L. P., & Volkova, Y. V. (2021). A look at the problem of exposure of the population caused by X-ray diagnostics: Approaches to analysis and forecasting. https://core.ac.uk/download/493174937.pdf (accessed on 30 May 2025).

48. Thomas, P. (2023). Quantifying and communicating radiation dose and risk from imaging procedures. *Journal of Medical Radiation Sciences, 70*, 11–12. https://www.semanticscholar.org/paper/73a09d349b34e3bd75d5b100653a0823624452a5 (accessed on 30 May 2025).

49. Thubab, A. A. A., Ogdi, K. M., Hezam, S. N., Otaif, A. A., Ogdi, A. M., Al Masoud, S. A., Hamad, M. I., *et. al.* (2024). Challenges and solutions in radiation protection for X-ray procedures. https://core.ac.uk/download/616775622.pdf (accessed on 30 May 2025).

50. Tomei, E., Zaccagna, F., Rodacki, K., Marinelli, E., Martino, M., Semelka, R. C., *et. al.* (2015). Accuracy of MRI skeletal age estimation for subjects 12–19: Potential use for subjects of unknown age. https://core.ac.uk/download/54248856.pdf (accessed on 30 May 2025).

51. Venelampi, E. (2023). Radiation practices: Annual report 2022. https://core.ac.uk/download/590276802.pdf (accessed on 30 May 2025).

52. Vlachos, I. (2022). Principles of magnetic resonance technology in medical imaging of non-ionization images. *Periapex Indian Journal of Research*. https://www.semanticscholar.org/paper/14ef09988b793617134fa9d43c5a1d5921840d99 (accessed on 30 May 2025).

53. Wittenburg, K. (2013). Specific instrumentation and diagnostics for high-intensity hadron beams. http://arxiv.org/abs/1303.6767 (accessed on 30 May 2025).

54. Wróbel, G. P. (2017). Selected aspects of patient health in nuclear medicine. https://core.ac.uk/download/587242016.pdf (accessed on 30 May 2025).

55. Zainuddin, Z. I. (2018). Towards holistic radiation protection: Lessons from the literatures. https://core.ac.uk/download/300470758.pdf (accessed on 30 May 2025).

56. Zeppenfeld, K., Tfelt-Hansen, J., Riva, M., Winkel, B. G., Behr, E. R., Blom, N. A., Charron, P., *et. al.* (2022). 2022 ESC guidelines for the management of patients with ventricular arrhythmias and the prevention of sudden cardiac death. *European Heart Journal, 43*, 3997–4126. https://doi.org/10.1093/eurheartj/ehac262.

57. Zhang, S., Zhu, Z., Yu, Z., Sun, H., Sun, Y., Huang, H., Xu, L., *et. al.* (2025). Effectiveness of AI for enhancing computed tomography image quality and radiation protection in radiology: Systematic review and meta-analysis. *Journal of Medical Internet Research, 27*. https://www.semanticscholar.org/paper/b13c560bae13ace7a0854079a0e42c590852644f (accessed on 30 May 2025).

RADIOBIOLOGY

4

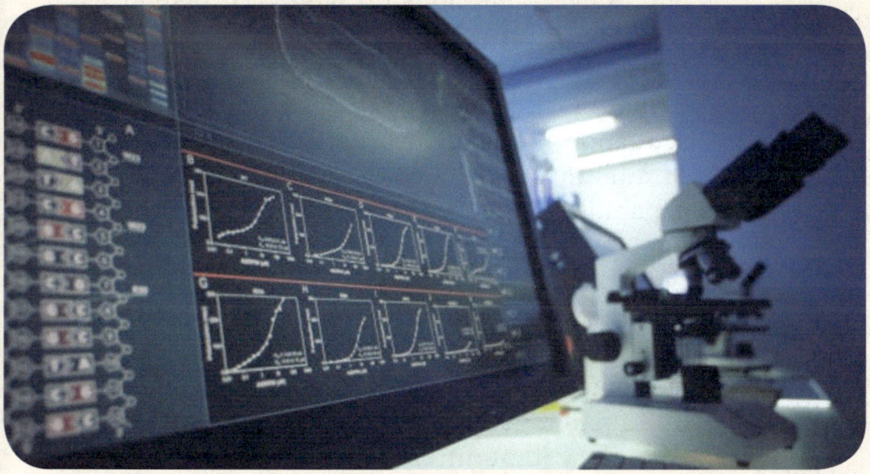

Introduction

Understanding the interaction between ionizing radiation and biological tissue lies at the heart of developing cancer therapy and radiation protection. Radiobiology, as a science of understanding such interactions, provides useful information regarding the mechanism of radiation interaction with cell structures, DNA, and biosystems. Radiobiology bridges the gap between scientific principles and their application, enabling the development of radiation therapy techniques and the maximization of patient outcomes. The complexity of radiation effects also requires not only a rigorous knowledge of physical principles but also an intimate knowledge of biological responses to varying doses of radiation. For instance, expertise in significant concepts such as beam divergence and inverse-square law is cardinal to provide secure and efficient clinical use in radiation therapy, emphasizing pedagogical challenges among students and experts in the field (Engel-Hills *et. al.*, 2018). Also, spontaneous cancers in pet animals, like dogs, provide valuable comparative models that facilitate translational research for the

LEARNING OBJECTIVES

After studying this chapter, you will be able to:

1. Understand mechanisms of radiation interaction with biological systems
3. Explain radiobiological effects on human health
4. Know applications of radiobiology

benefit of both veterinary and human oncology (Boss *et. al.*, 2019).

Definition of Radiobiology

The study of ionizing radiation interactions with living organisms provides a fundamental background for understanding radiation biological effects and risks perception. Radiobiology unites the study of the damage caused by radiation at the molecular, cellular, tissue, and organ levels, and repair processes and resulting health consequences. This science not only addresses the fundamental mechanisms through which radiation acts upon the biology of living organisms but also provides insights into applied applications, such as radiation protection and medicine. In space exploration, radiobiology takes on a special importance for the assessment of risks to astronauts exposed to the unique and multidimensional radiation environment beyond Earth's atmosphere. Efforts by organizations such as NASA focus on developing a broad scientific foundation for radiation protection, with an emphasis on cancer risk estimation and the molecular interactions of radiation with biological systems. Such efforts underscore understanding radiation effects so that mitigation of the effects can be planned for future interplanetary missions (Auñón-Chancellor *et. al.*, 2018) (Figure 4.1).

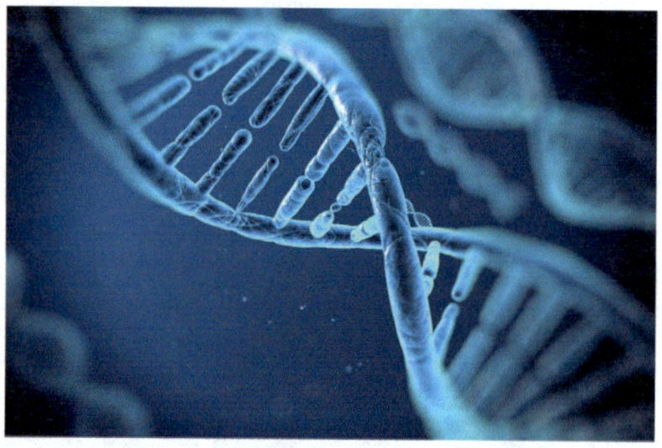

Figure 4.1. Radiobiology.

Source: https://www.sckcen.be/sites/default/files/styles/half_lg/public/files/2020-01/iStock-450853983.jpg?itok=WoALTdqQ.

Historical Background of Radiobiology

Radiobiology's history has been impacted by key advances that revealed the complex interrelations between ionizing radiation and tissues of living organisms. Initial investigations initially focused on the deleterious effects of radiation on cells, which were the basis for its clinical uses. Over the years, the field expanded to explore the influence of dose modification and delivery methods on biological responses. Recent findings with ultrahigh-dose rate therapies, such as FLASH radiotherapy, reflect a landmark development, through extreme reduction in normal tissue damage at the cost of tumor control, transforming therapeutic capabilities (Charles *et. al.*, 2023). Beyond that, ongoing work on dose rate effects highlights the delicate character of the interface between radiation variables and biological outcomes, necessitating multidisciplinary studies spanning from molecular to clinical levels (Lowe *et. al.*, 2022). All together, they form a broad historical trajectory that intertwines experiment with discovery and clinical advances and further refines our understanding and use of radiation in medicine.

Importance of Studying Radiobiology

Advances in technology for human space exploration have put a greater emphasis on the need for unraveling the complex interplay between space radiation and living organisms, especially highlighting the significance of radiobiology. This study is important because it highlights the biological consequences of space radiation, which pose significant health risks like tissue damage and cancer to deep-space explorers. Through the demystification of the fundamental processes of radiation interaction at the cellular and molecular levels, radiobiology opens the way for the establishment of effective protective schemes and radiation shielding methods. Already, agencies such as NASA have recognized this importance, having funded large programs of investigation to establish a firm scientific foundation for radiation risk assessment and planetary exploration protection. Secondly, the overall research of radiobiology provides us with more information regarding broader biomedical applications, informing medical treatment and safety measures in the environment exposed to ionizing radiation (Rowe *et. al.*, 2025). Hence, radiobiology is not only required for space travel development but also to safeguard human health in radiation-risky environments (Figure 4.2).

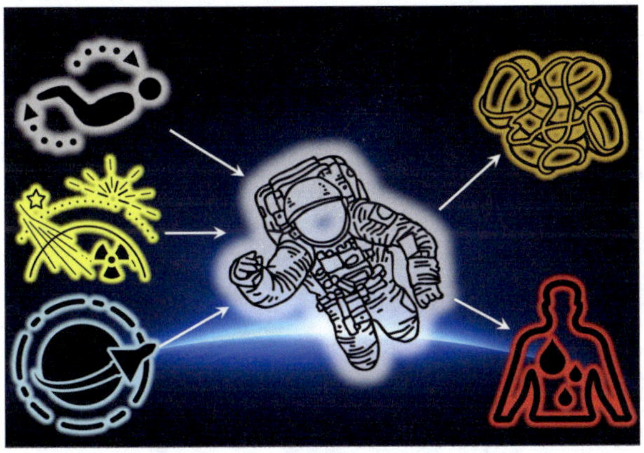

Figure 4.2. Advancements in human space exploration have heightened the need to understand the complex interactions between radiation and living organisms, emphasizing the critical role of radiobiology.

Source: https://www.ahajournals.org/cms/10.1161/ATVBAHA.123.318783/asset/40be2365-7361-46e3-9ee9-034be5b19592/assets/graphic/atvbaha.123.318783.fig02.jpg.

Applications of Radiobiology in Medicine

Advancements in radiobiology have largely contributed to medical interventions, particularly cancer diagnosis and treatment. The development of sophisticated models of *in vitro* systems, such as scaffold-free and organ-on-a-chip systems, has enabled researchers to appreciate better the influence of ionizing radiation on cancer cells at the molecular level, thereby enhancing therapeutic strategies to maximize the killing of tumor cells while minimizing damage to normal tissues (Akolawala *et. al.*, 2025). In addition, improvements in positron emission tomography (PET) and nuclear medicine have expanded the clinical applications of radiobiology to provide more precise imaging and therapeutic radiation pharmaceutical targeting. These developments not only enhance the sensitivity for diagnostic purposes but also facilitate personalized treatment planning, enabling optimal dose delivery based on the patient's nature (Teresińska *et. al.*, 2024). Together, they emphasize the critical significance of radiobiology in the advancement of progressive medical technologies and methods, driving the advancement toward more effective, personalized, and safer therapies in oncology and other areas.

Key Concepts in Radiobiology

Understanding the fundamental laws governing the interaction between ionizing radiation and biological tissues is required for the formulation of theoretical knowledge and practical applications in radiobiology. These include radiation dose-response relationship features and the statistical nature of cell damage. Cell survival curves illustrate how randomness in biology and chance events influence the degree of radiation damage, with specific parameters such as the mean inactivation dose and variance providing information about this complex interaction (Kellerer *et. al.*, 1989). Moreover, knowledge of threshold concepts like the inverse-square law and beam divergence is critical for safe handling of radiation in clinical settings, as these concepts define the way intensity of the radiation decreases with distance and spreads out in tissue (Engel-Hills *et. al.*, 2018). These ideas collectively constitute a scientific paradigm that not only raises our knowledge of radiation effects at the cellular level but also raises the precision and safety in cancer therapy in oncology.

Research Methodologies in Radiobiology

Radiobiology research growth has been strongly impacted by integrative and multidisciplinary approaches combining experimental, computational, and clinical methods. Past observation quantitatively of tumor responses to radiation has controlled treatment policies, but contemporary research increasingly relies on sophisticated mathematical models and computer-based biologically informed simulations to optimize therapy. These models, through partnerships between radiobiologists, clinicians, physicists, and data scientists, are designed to forecast individual patient responses and allow for adaptive radiotherapy protocols, making it possible for personalized treatment planning. An example is the use of spontaneously occurring pet dog cancers, which are very valuable translational models due to similarities in their physiology with humans and the same environment, yielding insights that connect preclinical and clinical studies (Boss *et. al.*, 2019). Further, activities like ESTRO DREAM workshop have laid out methodologies for rigorous model validation and interdisciplinarity research on collaboration that emphasize the point that integrated methodologies play a pivotal role in propelling radiobiology towards adaptive and biologically targeted radiotherapy (Alber *et. al.*, 2024) (Figure 4.3).

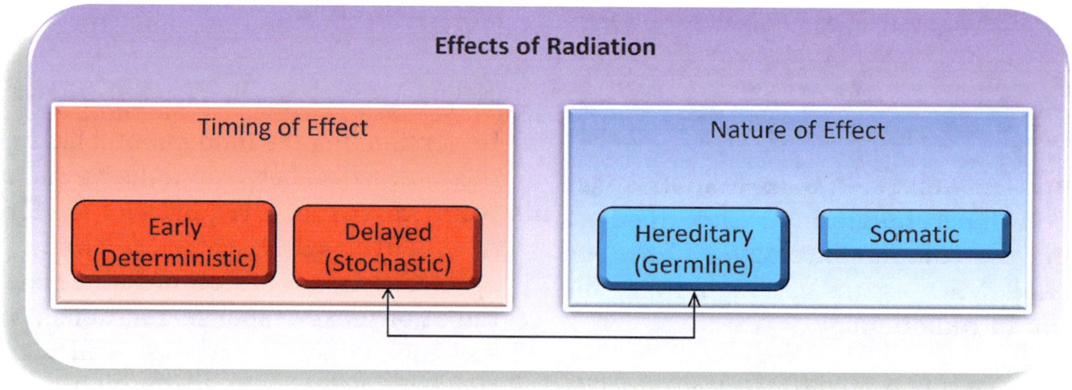

Figure 4.3. Advancements in radiobiology research have been profoundly shaped by integrative and multidisciplinary methodologies that combine experimental, computational, and clinical approaches.

Source: https://pub.mdpi-res.com/biology/biology-13-00098/article_deploy/html/images/biology-13-00098-g001.png?1707029496

Future Directions in Radiobiology

The evolving radiobiology paradigm needs novel approaches to enhance both the knowledge and application of radiation effects in medicine and biology. Emerging research trends point to the integration of contemporary computational methods, such as the use of machine learning (ML) for anomaly detection, in tackling high-level biological data with increased accuracy and efficiency (Haland *et. al.*, 2025). This convergence could contribute to making the detection of weak radiation-induced cellular changes more accurate and enhancing therapy regimens. Furthermore, technical advances in rectification of analytical biases, exemplified by better range restriction correction methods, offer better radiobiological data analysis, namely in clinical and experimental evaluations (Le *et. al.*, 2025). Future advances include individualized radiotherapy on the basis of genetic and molecular identification, enabling therapy tailored to the patient's radiosensitivity. Collectively, these interdisciplinarian approaches aim to propel radiobiology toward more predictive, effective, and patient-specific outcomes, ultimately making radiation-based diagnostics and therapies more targeted and safer.

4.1. Mechanisms of Radiation Interaction with Biological Systems

Learning Outcome

1. Explain the direct and indirect effects of radiation
2. Focus on DNA damage and repair mechanisms
3. Know cellular response to radiation
3. Describe radiation-induced mutations
4. Focus on apoptosis and cell cycle effects
5. Understand the radiation sensitivity of different cell types
6. Discuss the role of free radicals in radiation damage
7. Identify mechanisms of radiation protection

Its comprehension of how radiation acts on biological systems is the cornerstone of radiobiology, as it forms the basis for understanding the effects of exposure on cellular and molecular organization. When ionizing radiation traverses the tissues of organisms, it causes ionization and molecule excitation, mainly water, which results in the production of reactive oxygen species (ROS) that cause damage to DNA, proteins, and lipids. This indirect action is accountable for most biological damage, with direct interactions causing breaks in the genomic integrity of DNA strands. The complexity of these interactions dictates cellular response, including repair mechanisms, apoptosis, or carcinogenesis. The processes underlying these pathways have been a research target, particularly in environments where exposure to radiation poses serious health risks to astronauts. The Space Radiation Health Program recognizes the need to learn about these processes in order to assess cancer risks and to effect protective measures for space missions, using advanced instrumentation and multi-institutional coordination of research efforts. Detailed analyses, such as those reported in the USSR Space Life Sciences Digest, enable these endeavors by categorically placing radiation-biology interactions (Hooke & Teeter, 2025).

4.1.1. Direct Effects of Radiation

Comprehending the biological impact of radiation requires meticulous attention to the initial interactions that occur at the cellular stage. The direct effects of radiation are primarily ionizing particles depositing energy directly into the DNA and essential cellular machinery, causing direct molecular injury. This energy deposition can result in strand breaks or chemical alterations that threaten the reproductive potential of the cell, often resulting in cell death or dysfunction. Such direct damage caused by ionization is contrasted with indirect action through ROS, underlining the significance of microdosimetry to measure energy distribution at microscopic scales of measurement for precise prediction of biological response (Knopf *et. al.*, 2024). The cell capacity for repair after direct DNA damage is also in tandem with tyrosine kinase-mediated signaling pathways, the inhibition of which impacts radiation therapy response (Sokol, 2021). Effective cancer treatments thus depend on the understanding and exploitation of these direct effects to obtain optimal killing of tumor cells while sparing normal tissue (Figure 4.4).

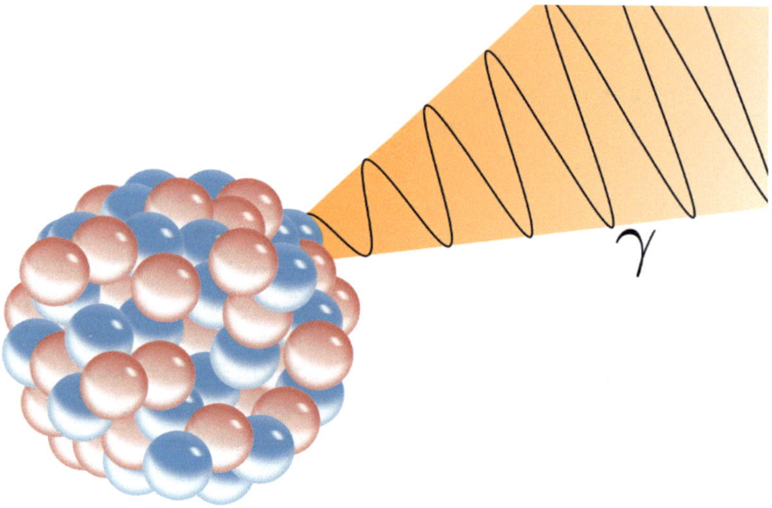

Figure 4.4. Understanding the biological consequences of radiation requires a thorough examination of the initial interactions occurring at the cellular level.

Source: https://upload.wikimedia.org/wikipedia/commons/thumb/c/c2/Gamma_Decay.svg/1200px-Gamma_Decay.svg.png.

4.1.2. Indirect Effects of Radiation

Radiation exposure initiates a multi-dimensional cascade of biological responses, including direct damage to DNA, as well as indirect effects that have significant roles in cellular consequences. The indirect effects are primarily through water radiolysis, which produces ROS that later induce oxidative damage on nearby macromolecules, including nucleic acids, proteins, and lipids. This process complicates the dose-effect relationship traditionally defined in terms of cell survival curves, as stochastic deposition of energy and biological heterogeneity alter the quantity and quality of damage. Cell repair mechanisms then encounter changing burdens of lesions, which could induce repair overload or misrepair and also impact the overall biological effect of radiation exposure (Kellerer *et. al.*, 1989). It is particularly challenging to comprehend these indirect effects in space radiation due to the multi-dimensional nature of the radiation environment and poor analog models, highlighting the imperative for advanced predictive means to assess risks for long-term human missions (Auñón-Chancellor *et. al.*, 2018). This highlights the significant importance of indirect radiation effects in radiobiology and the difficulty in countering their influence.

4.1.3. DNA Damage and Repair Mechanisms

Cellular ionizing radiation response is typified by complex interactions between the induction of DNA damage and repair, which play a critical role in determining survival cell outcomes. Ionizing radiation leads to a spectrum of lesions that include single- and double-strand breaks, whose repair efficiency determines cell fate. Traditional models that attempt to describe the survival of cells after exposure to radiation have faced the uncertainties of biological heterogeneity and microdosimetric heterogeneity, which affect the shape and slope of the survival curve.

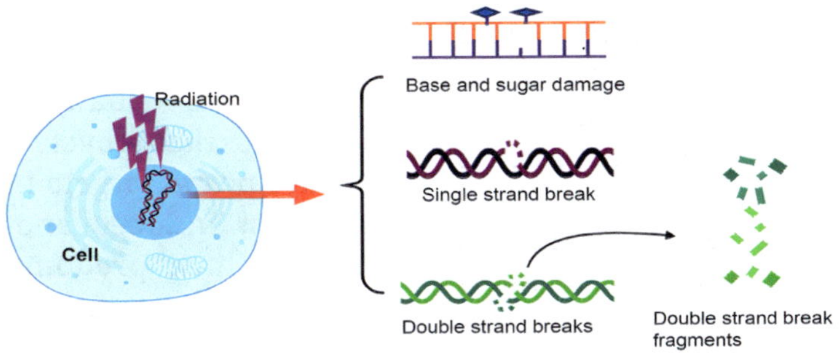

Figure 4.5. The cellular response to ionizing radiation involves complex interactions between DNA damage induction and subsequent repair processes, which are critical in determining cell survival outcomes.

Source: https://media.springernature.com/full/springer-static/image/art%3A10.1038%2Fs41392-020-0150-x/MediaObjects/41392_2020_150_Fig1_HTML.png.

These stochastic factors verify the insufficiency of traditional parameters and show the necessity of including stochastic processes in models describing the repair of DNA damage (Kellerer *et. al.*, 1989). Current theoretical advancement, such as the target cumulating model, achieves greater predictability by incorporating molecular-level interaction and sensitivity parameters, thereby accounting for phenomena like dose rate effects and low-dose hypersensitivity, which earlier models failed to adequately explain (Shixiu *et. al.*, 2009). Such findings also highlight further the pivotal role played by DNA repair mechanisms in radiobiology and their implication for radiation therapy success (Figure 4.5).

4.1.4. Cellular Response to Radiation

Understanding the intricate radiation effects on biological cells involves the examination of both direct and indirect forms of injury. Historically, ionizing radiation was believed to directly impact DNA in the cellular nucleus, leading to cell damage and death, but current studies recognize that radiation produces advanced biological changes beyond direct DNA damage. Interestingly, non-irradiated cells could also exhibit deep impacts through bystander signaling and genomic instability that imply the involvement of extracellular mediators and intercellular communication in radiation response (Alatas *et. al.*, 2015). Computational modeling has also demonstrated how varying doses of radiation impact the cellular kinetics in varying manners, with low doses producing cell killing similar to any radiation, and high doses have dose- and linear energy transfer (LET)-dependent effects (Tavares *et. al.*, 2012). The observations support reformulating traditional radiobiological models to encompass both targeted and non-targeted effects in order to enhance therapeutic strategies and risk estimations involving ionizing radiation.

4.1.5. Radiation-induced Mutations

Radiation impact on the genetic material is important since ionizing and ultraviolet radiation have the capacity to induce different types of mutations that alter cellular function and are amenable to disease processes. These kinds of mutations induced by radiation include single-nucleotide substitutions, tandem mutations, and DNA fragment deletions that together compromise the genomic integrity. Experiments involving whole-genome sequencing have identified that ultraviolet light causes non-random patterns of mutations based on surrounding nucleotide sequences, which determine frequency and type of mutation, such as adenine-cytosine transitions and transversions (Huang *et. al.*, 2024).

In radiotherapy, epigenetic alterations such as differential patterns of DNA methylation have been linked to patient-specific responses and side effects, a reflection of the complexities of genomic alterations induced by radiation and their biological consequences (Lopez-Pleguezuelos *et. al.*, 2025). In general, the evidence points to the complicated mechanisms of radiation-induced mutagenic damage with the inference that personalized measures in radiobiology are crucial in a bid to mitigate hazards and optimize therapeutic gain (Figure 4.6).

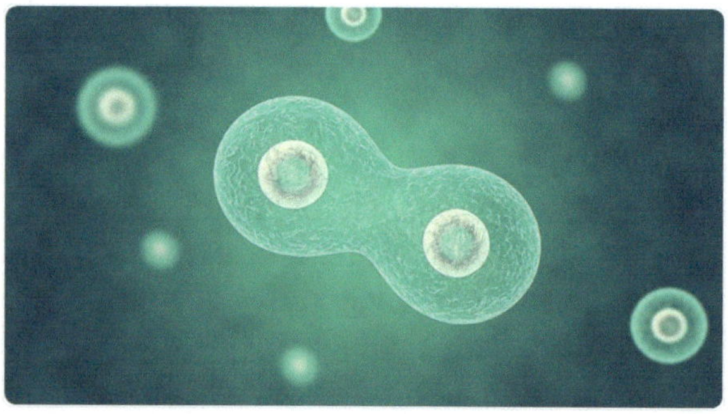

Figure 4.6. The impact of radiation on genetic material is profound, as ionizing and ultraviolet radiation can induce a variety of mutations that alter cellular function and contribute to disease processes.

Source: https://d2jx2rerrg6sh3.cloudfront.net/image-handler/picture/2018/4/shutterstock___By_janez_volmajer.jpg.

4.1.6. Apoptosis and Cell Cycle Effects

Tumor cells usually manifest dysregulated pathways that govern survival and growth, and are prime targets in radiobiology. Ionizing radiation induces apoptosis and cell cycle arrest, which predominantly involves G2-M phase arrest, to disrupt the growth potential of cancer cells to proliferate and grow. However, the response to radiation of cancer stem cells is very different from that of bulk tumor cells, wherein these stem-like cells have a lesser production of ROS and an attenuated apoptotic response after exposure, resulting in radio resistance. Particularly, breast cancer stem cells (CD44+CD24+ phenotype) express lower levels of ROS and exhibit lower apoptotic rates following irradiation, as expected from a failure of typical G2-M arrest observed in non-stem cancer cells. These findings underscore the complexity of targeting radiotherapy against tumor heterogeneity and the importance of modulating cell cycle checkpoints and apoptotic pathways to overcome resistance. Moreover, epigenetic modifiers such as HDAC6 affect apoptosis and cell cycle proteins and, therefore, alter tumor growth and response to treatment, suggesting the potential for combinatory therapies employing HDAC inhibitors and immune checkpoint blockade (Banik *et. al.*, 2017; Yan *et. al.*, 2014).

4.1.7. Radiation Sensitivity of Different Cell Types

Recognition of variable cell responses to ionizing radiation is a principal feature of radiobiology, having implications for both radiation therapy and radioprotection. Certain cells are rendered more sensitive due to their proliferative status, DNA repair potential, and cell cycle position. For example, actively dividing cells, such as those of bone marrow or gastrointestinal epithelium, are much more sensitive than more differentiated, resting cells. This differential sensitivity is the basis of tissue-specific radiation effects as well as the therapeutic window employed in cancer treatment. Inherent radiosensitivity is not only tissue-specific but also cell population-specific within a shared tissue environment, complicating predictions of damage and recovery. Research documented in comprehensive reports of space life sciences extends this information by exploring wide-ranging biological effects under varying exposures of radiation, like microgravity, and thus emphasizing the need for an integrative approach in evaluating cellular radiosensitivity (Rowe *et. al.*, 2025) (Figure 4.7).

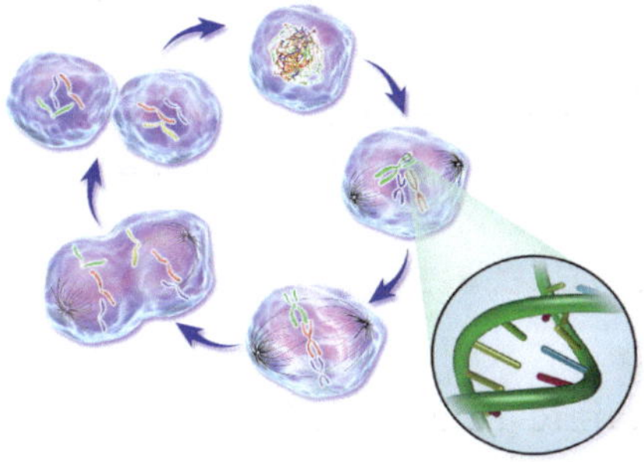

Figure 4.7. Certain cell types exhibit heightened sensitivity due to their proliferative activity, DNA repair capacity, and stage within the cell cycle.

Source: https://upload.wikimedia.org/wikipedia/commons/a/a4/Normal_Cell_Life_Cycle.png.

4.1.8. Role of Free Radicals in Radiation Damage

The biological effect of ionizing radiation is generally mediated through the formation of free radicals, which are the cause of radiation-induced tissue damage. Radiation, in its interaction with cells, yields highly reactive species, predominantly through the ionization of water molecules, giving rise to hydroxyl radicals, which cause extensive damage to DNA as well as other biopolymers. This indirect form of damage is accountable for the induction of single- and double-strand breaks in DNA, double-strand breaks are particularly cell-lethal, and potentially trigger apoptosis, mutagenesis, or carcinogenesis. Moreover, free radicals disrupt cellular redox homeostasis to trigger oxidative stress and associated metabolic alterations that result in acute cytotoxicity and chronic tissue injury, such as fibrosis and inflammation. Understanding how such radicals affect cell death and genomic instability is at the heart of radiobiology, as it determines ways to minimize normal tissue damage in the interest of optimizing tumor control (David *et. al.*, 2015; Pathak *et. al.*, 2015).

4.1.9. Mechanisms of Radiation Protection

Radiobiological advances have increasingly revealed the complex mechanisms of protection at cellular and tissue levels against radiation. One shining future direction is the phenomenon known as the FLASH effect, whereby ultra-high dose rate irradiation preferentially spares normal tissues without losing tumoricidal effectiveness. This effect, observed at doses up to 109 Gy/s, is suggested to be mediated through reduced ROS production and enhanced DNA repair mechanisms, promising an avenue toward preventing radiation-induced damage during therapy (Metzkes-Ng *et. al.*, 2023). Augmenting these findings, the long-debated linear no-threshold model continues to be the norm for describing our understanding of radiation risk, with recent radiobiological evidence continuing to support its applicability at low doses. Notwithstanding the complications brought by non-mutational biological reactions to risk assessment, linearity at doses as low as 10 mGy justifies the use of the model in radiation protection policy to obtain conservative but effective management of risks (Laurier *et. al.*, 2023). Together, all these results refine mechanisms to shield normal tissues, resulting in better therapeutic success and radiological safety.

Test Your Knowledge

1. Define direct and indirect action of radiation on biological molecules.
2. What types of DNA damage can ionizing radiation induce?

4.2. Radiobiological Effects on Human Health

Learning Outcome

1. Understand acute radiation syndrome
2. Explain the long-term health effects of radiation exposure
3. Identify cancer risk associated with radiation
4. Focus on radiation therapy and its effects
5. Discuss occupational exposure to radiation
6. Describe environmental radiation exposure
7. Understand risk assessment in radiobiology
8. Explain epidemiological studies in radiobiology
9. Identify public health policies regarding radiation

An insight into human health consequences of ionizing radiation includes a comprehensive study of its cellular and systemic consequences. Radiation induces damage to DNA, and this may lead to mutations, carcinogenesis, or cell death, depending on the dose and duration of exposure. High-dose acute exposure typically produces immediate tissue damage, while chronic exposure to low doses may induce long-term effects such as cancer and genetic disorders. Also, the sensitivity of different tissues differs, and unique vulnerabilities necessitate special research.

Advances in radiobiology have given improved models of prognosis for such effects, reconciling data from dissimilar biological systems to maximize protection strategies. In spite of claims by some authors of enormous research into these phenomena, technical difficulties remain in accessing all the required data (Chmelevsky *et. al.*, 1986; Hooke & Teeter, 2025). Therefore, there is a need for constant interdisciplinary research to prevent radiation hazards, inform medical treatments, and apply safety standards that protect against harmful radiobiological impacts on human health.

4.2.1. Acute Radiation Syndrome (ARS)

The dynamic relationship between radiation dose and biological effect is the foundation of the clinical syndrome of acute radiation syndrome (ARS), an illness produced by high doses of ionizing radiation accumulated over a short time period. ARS predominantly affects tissue with a high rate of cell division, the hematopoietic system, gastrointestinal tract, and central nervous system, leading to symptoms ranging from nausea and vomiting to severe immunosuppression and multiorgan failure. Current radiobiological research emphasizes the challenge of accurately modeling and predicting human ARS outcomes due to these problems, required by the impossibility of extrapolating animal model data to humans and replicating space radiation environments on the ground (Auñón-Chancellor *et. al.*, 2018).

Besides, new approaches such as protective wounding show efficient mitigation through enhanced hematopoietic recovery by cytokine modulation, promising medical countermeasures that can increase survival even when used after exposure (Dynlacht *et. al.*, 2017). This underlines the dynamic nature of radiobiological science in dealing with ARS and supports ongoing efforts in developing beneficial interventions (Figure 4.8).

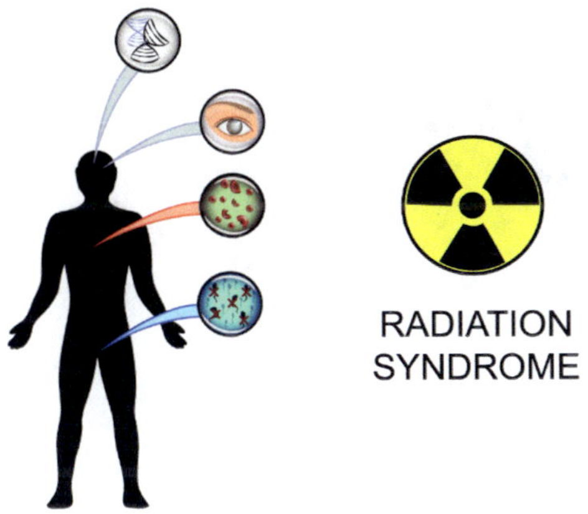

Figure 4.8. Acute radiation syndrome.

Source: https://www.bioworld.com/ext/resources/BWS/BWS-library/Radiation-exposure-syndrome.png?1677685994

4.2.2. Long-term Health Effects of Radiation Exposure

Advancements in radiobiology have progressively highlighted the intricacy of the long-term health effects resulting from radiation exposure, particularly in circumstances that mimic real-world environmental and occupational exposures. Sickness due to acute radiation is well characterized, but long-term effects such as carcinogenesis, cardiovascular disease, and neurologic impairment pose a significant challenge for scientists and clinicians alike.

New technology, including accelerator-based particle microbeam systems, has improved the sensitivity of radiobiological studies to enable more refined understanding of phenomena like the radiation-induced bystander effect and cellular radiosensitivity (Xu *et. al.*, 2016). Furthermore, the space radiation environment offers an unmatched risk environment for long-duration space travelers, where current models on Earth cannot precisely model the multidimensional exposure patterns encountered outside Earth's atmosphere. The difference between clinical outcomes and experimental findings accentuates the imperative of enhanced methodologies to foresee and reverse such long-term health impacts (Auñón-Chancellor *et. al.*, 2018). Finally, complete understanding and innovative solutions remain paramount in managing radiation's enduring impact on human health.

4.2.3. Cancer Risk Associated with Radiation

Understanding the long-term biological effects of ionizing radiation is critical in making risk judgments about radiation exposure. Low-dose rates of chronic exposure have been linked with systemic immune alterations, including dysfunction of neutrophilic granulocytes, which are vital for anti-tumor immunity. This dysregulation of immunity may result in increased rates of malignancies as well as cardiovascular disease (CVD), as observed in subjects exposed to environmental radiation over extended periods (Kodintseva *et. al.*, 2024).

Further, while radiotherapy is an established cornerstone of cancer treatment, bystander damage to normal tissues is complicated by radiation-induced toxicity. Experimental therapies like BNCT try to minimize these risks by hitting cancer cells specifically and minimizing exposure to normal tissue. More investigations on the cellular and molecular response to the therapy are necessary to optimize the effectiveness and reduce adverse effects, a reflection of the complex relationship between radiation, DNA damage, and the onset of cancer (Leah *et. al.*, 2024) (Figure 4.9).

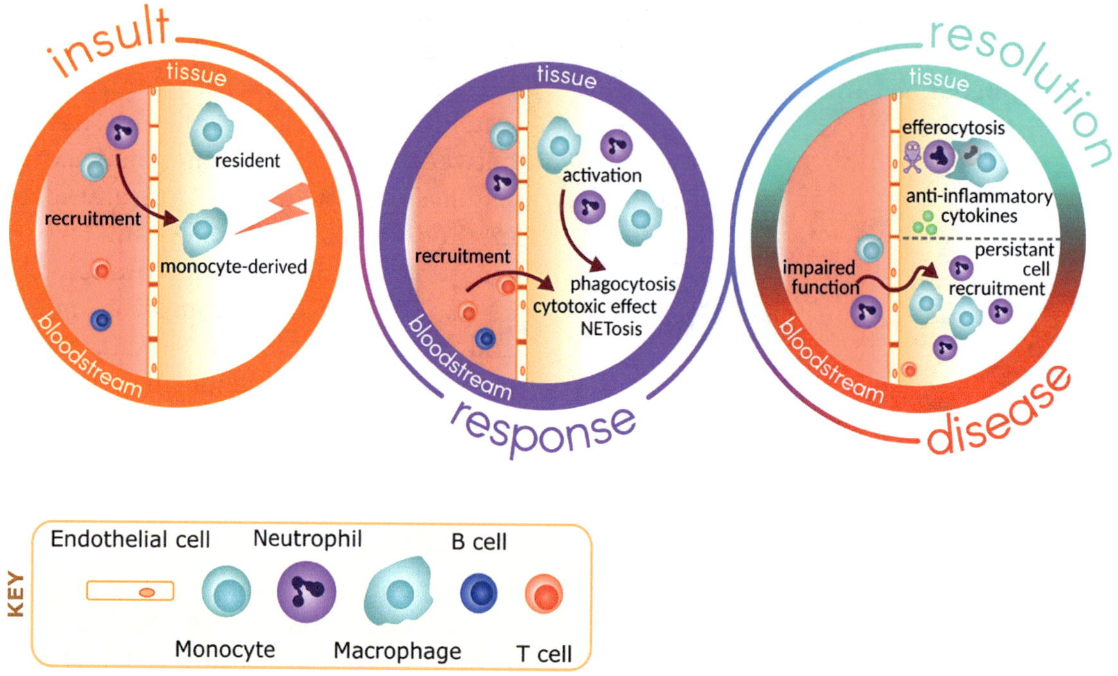

Figure 4.9. Chronic exposure, even at low dose rates, has been linked to systemic immune alterations, including impaired function of neutrophilic granulocytes, which are crucial for anti-tumor immunity.

Source: https://www.frontiersin.org/files/Articles/704173/fimmu-12-704173-HTML/image_m/fimmu-12-704173-g001.jpg.

4.2.4. Radiation Therapy and its Effects

Advances in treating cancer have led to a growing concern with the precision and biological impact of radiation therapy employing ionizing radiation to kill cancer cells while causing negligible damage to nearby healthy tissues. Radiation's therapeutic efficacy is not only dependent on the total dose but also on the exact fractionation influenced by the four R's of radiobiology: Repair, Reoxygenation, Reassortment, and Repopulation. These principles underlie a model to account for cellular radiation response and treatment schedule optimization, particularly in prostate cancer, where multiple treatments with androgen deprivation can double treatment toxicities affecting patients' quality of life. Physical and psychological consequences must be addressed by clinicians, ensuring there is complete patient care through frequent monitoring and personalized self-management plans (Paterson *et. al.*, 2020). Apart from that, emerging technologies such as proton and heavy ion therapy are more spatially selective, depositing a higher dose in tumors and a lower dose in normal tissue, thus enhancing cure rates with fewer side effects compared to conventional electron and photon radiation therapies (Bolton *et. al.*, 2014).

4.2.5. Occupational Exposure to Radiation

In environments where ionizing radiation is prevalent, such as nuclear reactors, medical imaging facilities, and space environments, understanding the impact of occupational exposure is critical to maintaining health and safety. Workers in these sectors are exposed to low-dose chronic radiation with potential cumulative biological effects, necessitating vigilant monitoring and protective measures. The complexities of the space radiation exposures, in particular, introduce the challenge of assessing risk considering the variable and unique forms of radiation available beyond Earth's atmosphere (Auñón-Chancellor *et. al.*, 2018). Occupational radiobiological studies must therefore account for different radiation qualities, durations of exposure, and individual-specific sensitivity to adequately predict potential health outcomes. Recent developments in research have emphasized increasing dosimetry and radioprotection techniques to minimize long-term effects such as carcinogenesis and tissue injury (Rowe *et. al.*, 2025). Thus, occupational radiation exposure is a critical subsection in radiobiology with the need for research expansion to enhance safety protocols both on Earth and off-Earth workplaces (Figure 4.10).

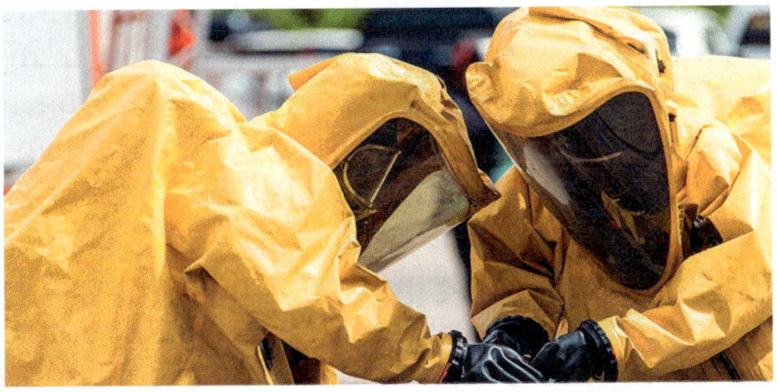

Figure 4.10. Occupational exposure to radiation.

Source: https://nucleus.iaea.org/sites/orpnet/training/orphighexposure/SiteAssets/SitePages/Home/oef_-_emergency_workers.jpg.

4.2.6. Environmental Radiation Exposure

Understanding of the biological consequences of exposure to low-dose and low-dose-rate radiation continues to be a radiobiological priority, especially in the context of relevance to public health and environmental protection. Chronic environmental radiation exposure, expressed in the form of elevated frequencies among populations residing near contaminated sites, has been linked to increased risks for malignancies and CVD, in part through chronic effects on immune function. Most notably, chronic radiation exposure disrupts the function of neutrophilic granulocytes, which are key cells in tumor immunity and inflammation, and may induce carcinogenesis along with cardiovascular disease as a consequence of impaired phagocytic activity. To address these shortcomings, initiatives like the Canadian Organization on Health Effects from Radiation Exposure aim at the intersection of molecular and epidemiological research to bring together pertinent areas of knowledge gaps for occupational and public settings. Through focusing on early molecular events and enhancing risk assessments, such cooperative efforts contribute to the enhancement of radiation protection frameworks and augmenting risk communication to at-risk communities (Kodintseva *et. al.*, 2024; Randhawa *et. al.*, 2024).

4.2.7. Risk Assessment in Radiobiology

Excellent risk estimation in radiobiology involves an intensive assessment mechanism that considers the multi-aspect nature of radiation exposure and its biological consequences. It involves evaluating the probability and magnitude of potential harmful health consequences, including DNA damage, carcinogenesis, and ARS. Traditional models of risk rely to a significant extent on historical data and empirical information, but technological and methodological progress are enabling more advanced assessments that include mechanistic insights and probabilistic estimations. The nature of radiobiological systems requires objective multi-parameter weighting to rank risk factors adequately, a method akin to multi-criteria decision-making approaches used in environmental hazard assessment (Mahmoodi *et. al.*, 2023). Moreover, engineering risk assessment courses emphasize the necessity of creating strong standards and evidence-based practice in order to forecast unwarranted exposures or failures within radiological uses, such as with the changing needs in autonomous machinery safety testing (Shutske *et. al.*, 2023). The extensive risk assessment process is indispensable for the development of efficient protective measures and regulation policies within radiobiology (Figure 4.11).

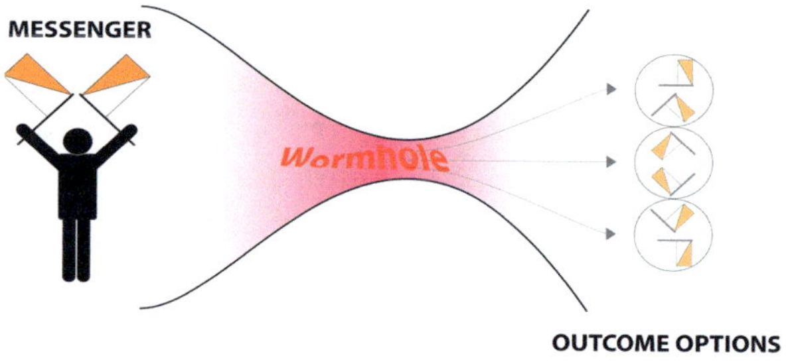

Figure 4.11. Effective risk assessment in radiobiology necessitates a comprehensive evaluation framework that accounts for the multifaceted nature of radiation exposure and its biological consequences.

Source: https://pub.mdpi-res.com/ijms/ijms-23-11118/article_deploy/html/images/ijms-23-11118-ag.png?1664868433

4.2.8. Epidemiological Studies in Radiobiology

Recognition of the risks of ionizing radiation exposure has been a long-standing part of radiobiology, and epidemiological studies have played a central role in cancer risk assessment. These studies trace cohorts receiving varying doses of radiation, offering empirical data that informs safety regulations and guidelines. It is, however, complicated by the low-dose exposures ubiquitous in environmental and occupational exposures, where evidence is not definitive. The U.S. National Research Council supports the linear no-threshold model of risk estimation, stating that all doses of radiation entail some risk, but other scientific associations question this model, indicating inconsistencies between epidemiologic evidence and the found biological mechanisms (Ulsh *et. al.*, 2012). Space radiation studies are an example, wherein efforts are being made to delineate danger from new cosmic radiation types while traveling in space, such that protection of astronauts' health demands integrative approaches that harmonize epidemiology and mechanism-based investigations. Hence, epidemiological studies are still necessary but must be highly cautious, combined with biological data to refine radiobiological models to assess risk.

4.2.9. Public Health Policies Regarding Radiation

Effective management of radiation exposure entails the implementation of overarching public health policy in balancing technological advancement with human security. Over time, regulation has evolved to address the many sources of ionizing radiation by attempting to contain risk through dose limitation, monitoring, and emergency preparedness. These policies are founded on radiobiological research that recognizes the origin of radiation damage and tolerances for acceptable exposure. Interdisciplinary action, as explained by the TEMPUS project, is education and training from an environmental, food quality, and societal perspective, highlighting the complex nature of radiation safety in contaminated environments. Public health systems also consist of surveillance systems and risk communication arrangements designed to protect vulnerable groups and consider the complex interrelationship between radiation and health effects. Hence, public policy in the area of radiation combines scientific information with proactive community action to lower risks and improve longer-term resilience (Figure 4.12).

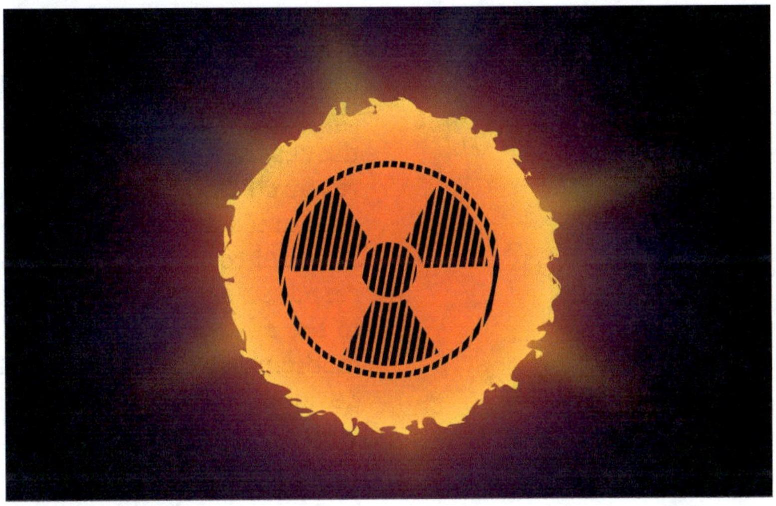

Figure 4.12. Effective management of radiation exposure necessitates the implementation of comprehensive public health policies that balance technological advances with human safety.

Source: https://www.toptenz.net/wp-content/uploads/2020/03/nuclear2.jpg.

Test Your Knowledge

1. What are the major factors influencing the severity of radiation effects on human health?
2. How does high-dose radiation affect rapidly dividing tissues such as bone marrow and gastrointestinal lining?
3. How does long-term radiation exposure increase the risk of cancer?

4.3. Applications of Radiobiology

Learning Outcome

1. Explain radiotherapy in cancer treatment
2. Focus on diagnostic imaging techniques
3. Learn radiation safety and protection
4. Know the use of radiobiology in space exploration
5. Explain radiobiology in nuclear medicine
6. Describe research in radiation biology
7. Discuss the development of radioprotective agents
8. Understand the role of radiobiology in bioterrorism preparedness
9. Know future technologies in radiobiology

Advances in radiation technology have significantly expanded the beneficial uses of radiobiology, particularly in medicine and space research. Radiotherapy cancer therapies, such as proton and heavy ion therapy, exploit the selective deposition of doses of radiation in tumors, sparing adjacent normal tissues and enhancing treatment efficacy. This technique, evolved over decades, has good potential benefits over traditional electron and photon radiation therapy due to its improved spatial resolution and deposition of dose (Bolton *et. al.*, 2014). Radiobiology also helps establish the impact of cosmic radiation on human physiology, a critical parameter for long-duration spaceflight. Research collected under space life sciences presents the effects of radiation on biology beyond Earth's environment and guides protection against radiation for astronauts (Hooke & Teeter, 2025). Combined applications of these research studies present how basic radiobiological principles drive innovation in clinical oncology as well as aerospace medicine, discovering an essential interaction between radiation science and applied health problems.

4.3.1. Radiotherapy in Cancer Treatment

Cancer treatment has, over time, focused more on the use of accurate and efficient therapeutic methods. Radiotherapy, specifically, has been at the forefront of oncological therapy because it can destroy malignant cells while leaving normal tissues intact. One of the most thrilling fields of research in radiotherapy studies is the use of spontaneously occurring tumours in pet dogs as a model to enhance our knowledge of tumour response and to maximize treatment protocols to the advantage of both veterinary and human medicine (Boss *et. al.*, 2019). Another is the development of novel modalities such as proton and heavy ion therapy that offer enhanced spatial selectivity and tissue-sparing relative to standard photon and electron treatments. The use of these particle treatments, driven in part by improvements in laser technology, will transform radiotherapeutic modalities by delivering more dose to the tumor site with less collateral injury (Bolton *et. al.*, 2014). These radiotherapy advances underscore the essential interface between radiobiologic insight and clinical application to maximize cancer outcome (Figure 4.13).

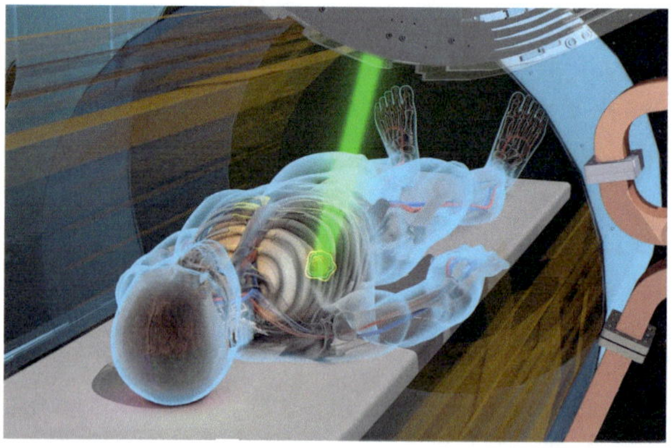

Figure 4.13. Radiotherapy in cancer treatment.

Source: https://media.assettype.com/thenewsminute%2F2024-03%2F0f59a916-bea8-4fe3-99b5-008e7e28de56%2Fradiationtherapy.jpg.

4.3.2. Diagnostic Imaging Techniques

Technological advancements in medicine have revolutionized the methods used in visualizing internal structures and significantly enhanced diagnostic capability in radiobiology. Among them, imaging techniques such as magnetic resonance imaging (MRI) provide accurate anatomical and functional details that are invaluable in outlining the impact of radiation on tissues. The emergence of new computational models, including Vision Transformers with Shifted Patching Techniques supplementation, has improved insight from brain MRI scans by outlining complex spatial and contextual relationships difficult to envision using conventional analysis (Habib *et. al.*, 2025). Not only does this imaging analysis advancement assist in precise disease detection, but it also assists with the creation of targeted treatment strategies by implementing radiation-induced alterations on the cellular level. In addition, the application of ML to longitudinal health records supports imaging through allowing for the prediction and intervention of disease at an earlier time, ultimately enhancing clinical outcomes in radiation therapy settings (Swinckels *et. al.*, 2023). Collectively, these developments underscore the significance of diagnostic imaging techniques as they propel radiobiological inquiry and patient management.

4.3.3. Radiation Safety and Protection

Effective management of occupational ionizing radiation exposure demands systemic knowledge and conformity to safety standards. Despite the extensive use of radiation in diagnosis and therapy in medicine, knowledge deficits among health care workers, particularly nurses, can overcome preventive measures. Findings indicate that, prior to focused training initiatives, nurses are not well aware of radiation safety, and this awareness significantly improves following structured interventions meant to raise awareness and enhance practices (Wahab *et. al.*, 2025). Similarly, research among health workers in various specialties identifies that while overall knowledge, attitude, and practice (KAP) towards protection from radiation are satisfactory, disparities still exist, especially based on gender and years of working experience, more so than on educational attainment (Seifi *et. al.*, 2025). These findings highlight the need for ongoing, consistent training on varied healthcare roles to promote safer practice, prevent exposure to the risks of radiation, and thereby safeguard both patients and practitioners in the clinical setting (Figure 4.14).

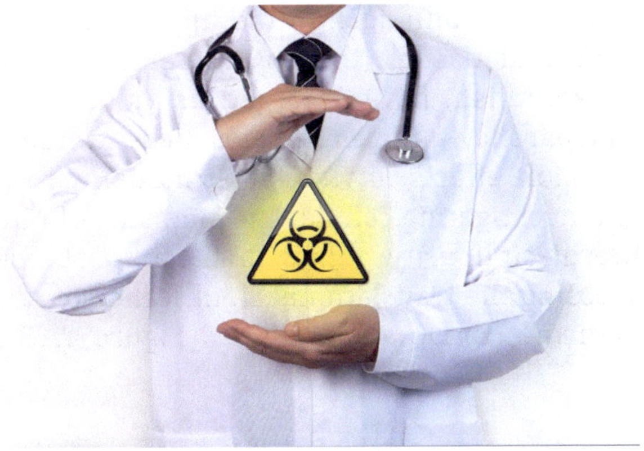

Figure 4.14. Effective management of occupational exposure to ionizing radiation demands comprehensive understanding and adherence to safety protocols.

Source: https://www.safetystratus.com/wp-content/uploads/2022/09/Picture1-1.jpg.

4.3.4. Use of Radiobiology in Space Exploration

Space exploration achievements increasingly have highlighted the crucial role of radiobiology in safeguarding the health of astronauts on long-duration missions. The multifaceted character of space radiation, composed of high-energy particles and involving intricate exposure patterns, poses deep-seated challenges to elucidating biological dangers comprehensively and instituting suitable protective measures. Terrestrial experimentation, although useful, is typically short in replicating the sophisticated space environment and therefore the direct transferability of results from experiment to human spaceflight. In filling these gaps, certain radiobiological studies are directed towards clarifying cellular and molecular responses to cosmic radiation to forecast potential clinical consequences such as carcinogenesis and tissue deterioration. NASA's Space Radiation Health Program is a prime example of this strategy by linking basic radiation biology research with technological breakthroughs to enable precise measurement and mitigation strategies (Auñón-Chancellor *et. al.*, 2018). Not only does this multidisciplinary research enlighten risk reduction, but it also guides the development of countermeasures that are critical for safe future lunar and interplanetary missions.

4.3.5. Radiobiology in Nuclear Medicine

Medical physics advancements have been critical in establishing awareness and application of radiobiology in nuclear medicine, with more precise and effective diagnostic and therapeutic modalities. The combination of radiobiology and nuclear medicine has resulted in the development of targeted radionuclide therapy, which optimizes dose distribution with a minimum of damage to normal tissues, thereby increasing patient benefit. Moreover, novel animal models, such as the zebrafish, have emerged as valuable research tools in radiobiological studies due to their transparency and genetic closeness to human beings, thus allowing sophisticated investigation of radiation effects *in vivo*. Such models are relevant in radiopharmaceutical response assessment and investigating cellular mechanisms of radiation exposure in nuclear medicine applications. Such interdisciplinarity points to the importance of continuous research and technological progress, stressing the translational significance of radiobiology from the basic to the clinical level in nuclear medicine (Bravo *et. al.*, 2011) (Figure 4.15).

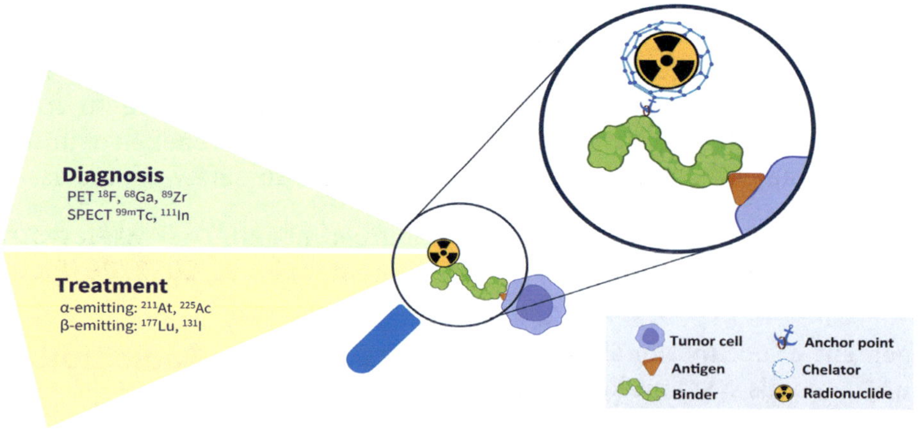

Figure 4.15. The integration of radiobiological principles with nuclear medicine has facilitated the development of targeted radionuclide therapies that optimize dose distribution while minimizing damage to healthy tissues, thereby improving patient outcomes.

Source: https://www.frontiersin.org/files/Articles/911080/fimmu-13-911080-HTML/image_m/fimmu-13-911080-g001.jpg.

4.3.6. Research in Radiation Biology

Advances in understanding the biological effects of radiation have been spurred by coordinated research efforts in many fields, with significant advances resulting from missions into space. The investigation into the basic processes of radiation damage at the cellular and molecular levels has been instrumental in providing explanations for how radiation induces carcinogenesis and tissue damage. These studies have been instrumental in the development of shielding strategies for humans exposed to ionizing radiation, especially within the challenging environment of long-duration space flight. NASA's Life Sciences Division operated at the center by funding studies that explore radiation interactions with living beings, enhancing risk evaluation and mitigation planning. This includes collaborative initiatives involving universities, research institutions, and national laboratories to facilitate measurements and biological understanding. Furthermore, comprehensive overviews of pertinent investigations, including the research documented in overseas scientific digests, have provided informative insights into radiobiology, and this has benefited a global database that sustains ongoing studies and operational safety (Rowe *et. al.*, 2025).

4.3.7. Development of Radioprotective Agents

Since the early days of radiobiology, intense efforts have been directed towards minimizing the damaging effects of ionizing radiation on biological systems. The foundational works revealed that cysteine was the initial chemical radioprotector, setting the stage for subsequent studies towards free radical scavengers, oxygen modulators, antioxidants, and immune response regulators. Despite extensive research, most radioprotective drugs have exhibited poor clinical effectiveness, highlighting the nature of radiation-induced cell damage and the complexity of multiple mechanisms of protection. More recent studies have investigated the ability of drugs like 6-propyl-2-thiouracil (PTU) to elevate intracellular cAMP concentrations and improve cell survival after irradiation in thyroid and cancer cells. This means that modulation of signal cascades is likely to provide a promising avenue for advancing radioprotection. Research today increasingly determines structure-activity relationships and maximizes combinatorial therapy in an attempt to develop more efficient agents with lower toxicity and higher applicability across cell types (Casal *et. al.*, 2010; Dwarakanath *et. al.*, 2005) (Figure 4.16).

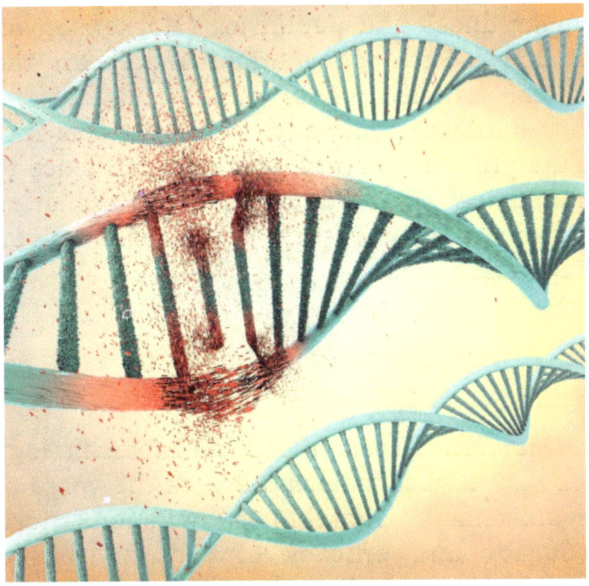

Figure 4.16. Throughout the history of radiobiology, significant efforts have been dedicated to mitigating the damaging effects of ionizing radiation on biological systems.

Source: https://letstalkscience.ca/sites/default/files/2019-10/Damage_to_DNA.jpg.

4.3.8. Role of Radiobiology in Bioterrorism Preparedness

Successful preparedness for bioterrorism is a multidisciplinary endeavor with specialized knowledge and expertise from various areas, including radiobiology. An understanding of the mechanisms of interaction of radiation with biological processes allows one to develop specific countermeasures against damage in case of exposure to radiological agents. Radiobiology provides essential information on dose estimation, symptomatology, and treatment, which is important for emergency planning and medical management. Besides, the creation of evidence-based guidelines ensures that vulnerable populations, such as children, are given adequate care tailored to their unique physiological responses in radiological emergencies, as has been noted by recent attempts at consensus among experts in disaster preparedness and pediatrics (Markenson *et. al.*, 2004). Such contributions underscore the central contribution of radiobiology to the illumination of policy and clinical protocol and, in the process, to optimizing total resilience to radiological hazard in bioterrorism scenarios and optimizing results by science-driven preparation steps.

4.3.9. Future Technologies in Radiobiology

Technological developments in nanotechnology and biointerface materials are on the verge of revolutionizing radiobiology with enhanced accuracy and efficacy of radiation-based treatments and diagnostics. For instance, surface-enhanced Raman spectroscopy (SERS) developments have significantly improved molecular detection sensitivity, enabling real-time single-molecule-level monitoring of cellular radiation responses. These developments allow for whole-body metabolic phenotyping and liquid biopsy, with potential for personalized radiotherapy and toxicity monitoring at an early stage (Lin *et. al.*, 2025). In addition, hydrogel-based use in human–machine interfaces holds promise for developing wearable biosensors that can monitor continuously radiation-induced physiological changes, enabling timely intervention and improved patient outcomes. The designing of hydrogel properties through innovative manufacturing techniques also further increases their applicability for *in vivo* applications and clinical translation (Ullah *et. al.*, 2025). Collectively, these emerging technologies underscore the potential for an era in which radiobiology takes advantage of sophisticated sensing and interface materials to advance our knowledge of radiation effects and optimize therapeutic modalities (Figure 4.17).

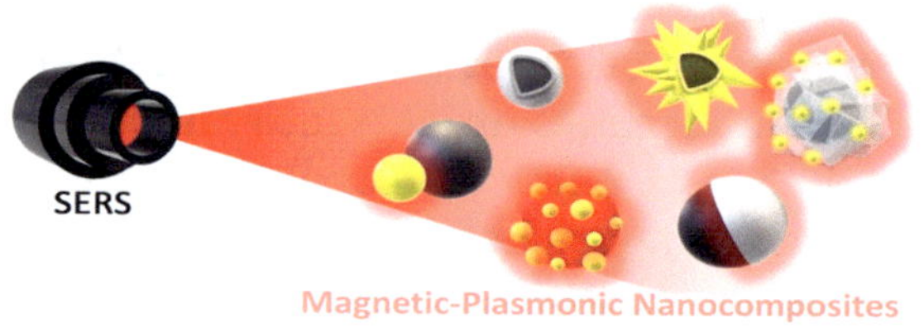

Figure 4.17. Advancements in surface-enhanced Raman spectroscopy (SERS).

Source: https://chemistry-europe.onlinelibrary.wiley.com/cms/asset/efc371d4-a9c2-458e-8565-f8f60dc66f05/chem202303987-toc-0001-m.jpg.

Test Your Knowledge

1. How do radiobiological principles guide the use of radiosensitizers in oncology?
2. How does radiobiology help in assessing the risks from low-dose radiation exposure?

SUMMARY

Advances in radiobiology have immensely advanced our understanding of the interaction between radiation and biological systems, making way for improved therapeutic management and estimation of risks. Synthesis of genetic and molecular data has highlighted the intricacies of DNA damage and repair processes, cellular responses, and the impact of individual genetic variation on radiosensitivity. These advances emphasize the importance of individualized therapy regimens to achieve maximum efficacy with minimal side effects. Additionally, the identification of putative biomarkers and pathogenic variants through genomic profiling underscores the role of multidisciplinary coordination that harmonizes radiobiology with genomics and clinical practice to enhance patient outcomes. Exploration of novel agents and natural products, including recent studies on antifungal leaf extracts combating infection caused by radiation, further indicates radiobiology's expanding therapeutic potential (In *et. al.*, 2025). Furthermore, detection of potential pathogenic germline variants in cancer patients underscores the imperative necessity of integrating genetic counseling with traditional oncologic practice, further consolidating the practice's transition towards precision medicine (Franco *et. al.*, 2024).

A realization of the difference between high and low-LET radiations is critical to an understanding of the actions of radiation on the biological system since they influence the nature of the severity and the ability to repair biochemical lesions. High-LET radiation induces more complex and difficult-to-repair lesions at the molecular and cellular levels with more marked biological implications. This heterogeneity of damage is quantified in biochemical relative biological effectiveness (RBE) values, which depend on radiation quality and energy (Wiley *et. al.*, 1972). In addition, the dose-effect relationships, studied with consideration, are highlighted in cell survival curves and stress the cooperation between the stochastic variables of biological variation and microdosimetric fluctuations in energy deposition. They show characteristic sigmoid dose responses and point to the limitations of simplistic mechanistic models of repair or misrepair. Global indicators like the coefficient of variance and mean inactivation dose provide a better description of radiation effects than do conventional measures (Kellerer *et. al.*, 1989).

KEY TERMS FROM THIS CHAPTER

- Astronauts
- Clinicians
- Environments
- Microdosimetric heterogeneity
- Physicists
- Radiobiologists
- Biomedical
- Data scientists
- Ionizing radiation
- Microdosimetry
- Positron emission tomography
- Reactive oxygen species

CRITICAL THINKING QUESTIONS

1. **What is the primary effect of ionizing radiation on living cells?**
   a. Heat generation
   b. Ionization of atoms and molecules
   c. Change in color of tissues
   d. Increase in cellular growth
2. **Which of the following is the most radiosensitive part of a cell?**
   a. Nucleus
   b. Cytoplasm
   c. Plasma membrane
   d. Mitochondria
3. **The term "radiation dose" refers to:**
   a. The energy deposited in a biological system
   b. The amount of ionizing radiation produced in a machine
   c. The total energy absorbed by all tissues
   d. The frequency of X-ray emissions
4. **The primary target for radiation-induced damage in a cell is:**
   a. Water molecules
   b. DNA
   c. Proteins
   d. Lipids
5. **Which of the following effects is typically observed at high radiation doses?**
   a. Stochastic effects
   b. Deterministic effects
   c. Chromosomal mutations
   d. Reduced tissue healing

Short Answer Questions

1. Define radiobiology, and why is it important in understanding radiation safety?
2. What is the main factor that determines the extent of biological damage caused by radiation?
3. What is the most common type of damage caused by ionizing radiation to DNA?
4. What is the primary biological response of cells exposed to low doses of radiation?
5. Describe the process of radiation-induced cell death.

Answers to Critical Thinking Questions

1. (b); 2. (a); 3. (a); 4. (b); 5.(b)

REFERENCES

1. Akolawala, Q., & Accardo, A. (2025). Engineered cell microenvironments: A benchmark tool for radiobiology. *ACS Applied Materials & Interfaces, 17*, 5563–5577. https://www.semanticscholar.org/paper/2eaa77be60cc534bcfcf002bfcc7d481066be6e4 (accessed on 30 May 2025).
2. Alatas, Z. (2015). A paradigm shift in low dose radiation biology. https://media.neliti.com/media/publications/57035-EN-a-paradigm-shift-in-low-dose-radiation-b.pdf (accessed on 30 May 2025).
3. Alber, M., Bahn, E., Brualla, L., Böhlen, *et. al.* (2024). A joint physics and radiobiology DREAM team vision–Towards better response prediction models to advance radiotherapy. https://core.ac.uk/download/611825281.pdf (accessed on 30 May 2025).
4. Chancellor, J.C., Blue, R.S., Cengel, K.A. *et. al.* Limitations in predicting the space radiation health risk for exploration astronauts. *npj Microgravity* **4**, 8 (2018). https://doi.org/10.1038/s41526-018-0043-2
5. Banik, D., Hadley, M., Kim, J., Knox, T., Nair, J., Kozikowski, A., Shen, S., *et. al.* (2017). Abstract 4854: Evaluating HDAC6 as a causal factor in metastatic breast cancer to develop immunotherapy. *Cancer Research, 77*, 4854–4854. https://www.semanticscholar.org/paper/7300876c611459c769bde1bdffac2bdc18d8c6f2 (accessed on 30 May 2025).
6. Bolton, P. R., Ledingham, K. W. D., Ma, C. M., *et. al.* (2014). Towards laser driven hadron cancer radiotherapy: A review of progress. https://core.ac.uk/download/211698981.pdf (accessed on 30 May 2025).
7. Nolan MW, Kent MS, Boss MK. Emerging Translational Opportunities in Comparative Oncology With Companion Canine Cancers: Radiation Oncology. Front Oncol. 2019 Nov 22;9:1291. doi: 10.3389/fonc.2019.01291. PMID: 31824863; PMCID: PMC6883487.
8. Lemos, Joana, *et. al.* (2011). Zebrafish and nuclear medicine methods and techniques: An each-day improving partnership. http://hdl.handle.net/10400.22/6445
9. Casal, M., Dagrosa, M. A., Juvenal, G. J., *et. al.* (2010). Study of 6-propyl-2-thiouracil as a radioprotector for the thyroid gland. https://core.ac.uk/download/558794019.pdf (accessed on 30 May 2025).
10. Chmelevsky, D., Gössner, W., Kellerer, A. M., *et. al.* (1986). Bone sarcoma cumulative tumor rates in patients injected with 224Ra. https://core.ac.uk/download/12169633.pdf (accessed on 30 May 2025).
11. Dwarakanath, B. S., Mathew, T. L., Ravindranath, T., *et. al.* (2005). Chemical radioprotectors. https://core.ac.uk/download/333720365.pdf (accessed on 30 May 2025).
12. Dynlacht, J. R., Garrett, J., Joel, R., *et. al.* (2017). Further characterization of the mitigation of radiation lethality by protective wounding. https://core.ac.uk/download/187423791.pdf (accessed on 30 May 2025).
13. Engel-Hills, P., Hudson, L., & Winberg, C. (2018). Threshold concepts in radiation physics underpinning professional practice in radiation therapy. https://core.ac.uk/download/229874374.pdf (accessed on 30 May 2025).
14. Franco, P. I., Que, F. V., Andal, J., & Ang, D. (2024). Abstract 6461: Prevalence and implications of potentially pathogenic germline variants among adult patients in the Philippines with solid malignancies who underwent tumor genomic profiling: A multi-institutional, cross-sectional

study. *Cancer Research*. https://www.semanticscholar.org/paper/713984809ba14fe3399603873d2618b996cc29bf (accessed on 30 May 2025).

15. Habib, G., Malik, I. A., Qureshi, S., Ra, I. H., Singh, S., & Sharma, S. (2025). Harnessing the power of attention for patch-based biomedical image classification. *IEEE Access, 13*, 36760–36774. https://www.semanticscholar.org/paper/cc91020efb35f685fbc6eca998f128022a169b90 (accessed on 30 May 2025).

16. Haland, C., & Granmo, A. (2025). Machine learning for anomaly detection: Insights into data-driven applications. *International Journal of Data Science and Machine Learning*. https://www.semanticscholar.org/paper/adad31a3e5ed9c1805987fcba3e4e7f89d0856f5 (accessed on 30 May 2025).

17. Hooke, L. R., & Teeter, R. (2025). USSR Space Life Sciences Digest: Index to issues 1–4. https://core.ac.uk/download/pdf/42841024.pdf (accessed on 30 May 2025).

18. Horowitz, D. H., Gross, C., Frank, R., Hsu, A. R., Diaz, A., & Gitelis, S. (2015). External beam radiation therapy for orthopaedic pathology. *The Journal of the American Academy of Orthopedic Surgeons, 23*(8), e9, e10. https://www.semanticscholar.org/paper/0b8101f12d44a2d5d1792e91ae9b5fd3911929c7 (accessed on 30 May 2025).

19. Huang, Q., Han, X., Tong, Z., Deng, Y., Xie, L., Liu, S., Xie, B., *et. al.* (2024). A comprehensive assessment of ultraviolet-radiation-induced mutations in *Flammulina filiformis* using whole-genome resequencing. *Journal of Fungi, 10*. https://www.semanticscholar.org/paper/17c8b218c3ff79f5046ffaafc0b04a0d98c057a5 (accessed on 30 May 2025).

20. Kellerer, A. M., Kellerer, A. M., Kellerer, A. M., Kellerer, A. M., Kellerer, A. M., Kellerer, A. M., Kellerer, A. M., *et. al.* (1989). Studies of the dose-effect relation. https://core.ac.uk/download/12166962.pdf (accessed on 30 May 2025).

21. Knopf, M., Barna, S., Radmanovac, D., Bergauer, T., Hirtl, A., & Magrin, G. (2024). Exploring offline pileup correction to improve the accuracy of microdosimetric characterization in clinical ion beams. https://www.semanticscholar.org/paper/30a7ea9879c9e548c041a846bdd85230e01a4568 (accessed on 30 May 2025).

22. Kodintseva, E., & Akleyev, A. (2024). Phenotypic heterogeneity of the neutrophilic granulocytes in terms of the pathogenesis of the late effects of the chronic radiation exposure. *Radiation and Risk: Bulletin of the National Radiation and Epidemiological Registry*. https://www.semanticscholar.org/paper/f004fa5a4d963b9f1fd4216a0a6810b51334e717 (accessed on 30 May 2025).

23. Laurier, D., Billarand, Y., Klokov, D., & Leuraud, K. (2023). The scientific basis for the use of the linear no-threshold (LNT) model at low doses and dose rates in radiological protection. *Journal of Radiological Protection, 43*. https://www.semanticscholar.org/paper/8173f4635614bdba84cfd66b8401e909ff632fce (accessed on 30 May 2025).

24. Le, H., Oh, I. S., Roth, P. L., & Schmidt, F. L. (2025). Range restriction corrections in personnel selection: A mixed range restriction correction approach to overcome a key limitation in applying Case V. *The Journal of Applied Psychology*. https://www.semanticscholar.org/paper/88554825b62cfbfa0c3b3d5b07e49b418cc0950d (accessed on 30 May 2025).

25. Limoli, C. L., & Vozenin, M. C. (2023). Reinventing radiobiology in the light of FLASH radiotherapy. *Annual Review of Cancer Biology, 7*, 1–21. https://doi.org/10.1146/annurev-cancerbio-061421-022217.

26. Lin, L. L., Alvarez-Puebla, R. A., Liz-Marzán, L. M., Trau, M., Wang, J., Fabris, L., Wang, X., *et. al.* (2025). Surface-enhanced Raman spectroscopy for biomedical applications: Recent advances and future challenges. *ACS Applied Materials & Interfaces.* https://www.semanticscholar.org/paper/0f8233469b92498835d714d00ad1c414fe134826f (accessed on 30 May 2025).

27. Lopez-Pleguezuelos, C., Aguado-Barrera, M. E., Carballo-Castro, A. M., Peleteiro, P., Calvo-Crespo, P., Taboada-Valladares, B., Lobato-Busto, R., *et. al.* (2025). Epigenome-wide analysis reveals potential biomarkers for radiation-induced toxicity risk in prostate cancer. *Clinical Epigenetics, 17.* https://www.semanticscholar.org/paper/e3b06a873b9df6c168a493b4fd42f483ee38b444 (accessed on 30 May 2025).

28. Lowe, D., Roy, L., Tabocchini, M. A., Rühm, W., Wakeford, R., Woloschak, G. E., & Laurier, D. (2022). Radiation dose rate effects: What is new and what is needed? *Radiation and Environmental Biophysics, 61*, 507–543. https://doi.org/10.1007/s00411-022-00996-0.

29. Mahmoodi, E., Azari, M., & Dastorani, M. (2023). Comparison of different objective weighting methods in a multi-criteria model for watershed prioritization for flood risk assessment using morphometric analysis. *Journal of Flood Risk Management, 16.* https://www.semanticscholar.org/paper/5cc3aea252815e8cb2a5546edf8f71eec3261f7b (accessed on 30 May 2025).

30. Markenson, D., & Redlener, I. E. (2004). Pediatric terrorism preparedness national guidelines and recommendations: Findings of an evidence-based consensus process. https://core.ac.uk/download/161444205.pdf (accessed on 30 May 2025).

31. Metzkes-Ng, J., Brack, F., Kroll, F., Bernert, C., Bock, S., Bodenstein, E., Brand, M., *et. al.* (2023). The Dresden platform is a research hub for ultra-high dose rate radiobiology. *Scientific Reports, 13.* https://www.semanticscholar.org/paper/85757358be98f410bb90cff5bcdf618065a9a57f (accessed on 30 May 2025).

32. Pande Putu, K. C., Made Jawi, G. A., *et. al.* (2025). Synergistic antifungal effects of *Gardenia augusta* and *Averrhoa bilimbi* leaf extracts against *Candida albicans*: Implications for the treatment of oral candidiasis *in vitro* study. *Open Access Indonesian Journal of Medical Reviews.* https://www.semanticscholar.org/paper/7fe09293f115ca321f40c13b22c140409e69cba4 (accessed on 30 May 2025).

33. Paterson, C., & Roberts, C. (2020). An exploration of the Rs of radiobiology in prostate cancer. https://core.ac.uk/download/328731150.pdf (accessed on 30 May 2025).

34. Pathak, R., Cheema, A., Boca, S., Krager, K., Hauer-Jensen, M., & Aykin-Burns, N. (2015). Modulation of radiation response by the tetrahydrobiopterin pathway. *Antioxidants, 4*, 68–81. https://www.semanticscholar.org/paper/6ae4dbd81e98ed48be3d1b234a2464400b8084fb (accessed on 30 May 2025).

35. Punshon, L. D., Fabbrizi, M., Phoenix, B., Green, S., & Parsons, J. L. (2024). Current insights into the radiobiology of boron neutron capture therapy and the potential for further improving biological effectiveness. *Cells, 13.* https://www.semanticscholar.org/paper/47e3ea3fa88b7935b7d2f2f12d8e20867e42bf16 (accessed on 30 May 2025).

36. Randhawa, K., Wilkins, R., Burtt, J., Lane, R. S. D., Ivanova, A., Leblanc, J., Sadi, B., *et. al.* (2024). Canadian Organization on Health Effects from Radiation Exposure (COHERE): Strengthening co-operation within the Canadian Government on radiation research. *Annals of the ICRP.* https://www.semanticscholar.org/paper/c82027ca34697112349e0e6a4c618b41aa62e215 (accessed on 30 May 2025).

37. Rowe, J., Stone, L. R., & Teeter, R. (2025). Digest of Russian Space Life Sciences, issue 33. https://core.ac.uk/download/pdf/42807398.pdf (accessed on 30 May 2025).

38. Seifi, D., & Khorrami, A. (2025). Assessment of staff's knowledge, attitude, and practice on radiation protection measures in Mazandaran Province, Iran. *Frontiers in Biomedical Technologies*. https://www.semanticscholar.org/paper/5d4a2cb139c2eaea6d07d5dd3bfd3b35124b0f62 (accessed on 30 May 2025).

39. Shutske, J., Sandner, K. J., & Jamieson, Z. (2023). Risk assessment methods for autonomous agricultural machines: A review of current practices and future needs. *Applied Engineering in Agriculture*. https://www.semanticscholar.org/paper/d9bf6648ed8e0d7a1c94a5653d79cac6ae7a4696 (accessed on 30 May 2025).

40. Sokol, G. (2021). Radiation/drug interactions and the combinational effects of tyrosine kinase inhibitors and radiation therapy in the treatment of cancer. *Advances in Clinical Toxicology*. https://www.semanticscholar.org/paper/06ffb60a093de65258c84b98730d459a4012585e (accessed on 30 May 2025).

41. Swinckels, L., Bennis, F., Ziesemer, K. A., Scheerman, J., Bijwaard, H., de Keijzer, A., & Bruers, J. (2023). The use of deep learning and machine learning on longitudinal electronic health records for the early detection and prevention of diseases: Scoping review. *Journal of Medical Internet Research, 26*. https://www.semanticscholar.org/paper/bbb3bd1ff203e5707eb29234cb5666cb68c0a264 (accessed on 30 May 2025).

42. Tavares, A. A. S., & Tavares, J. M. R. S. (2012). Computational modeling of cellular effects post-irradiation with low- and high-LET particles and different absorbed doses. https://core.ac.uk/download/32435331.pdf (accessed on 30 May 2025).

43. Teresińska, A., Mikołajczak, R., Jarząb, B., Królicki, L., Płachcińska, A., Braziewicz, J., Kostkiewicz, M., *et. al.* (2024). Current state and prospects for the development of nuclear medicine in Poland. *Nuclear Medicine Review. Central & Eastern Europe, 27*(0), 42–52. https://www.semanticscholar.org/paper/bb7e465bfd57932c260c637ae701843fc82791d1 (accessed on 30 May 2025).

44. Ullah, A., Kim, D. Y., Lim, S. I., & Lim, H. R. (2025). Hydrogel-based bio interfaces: Recent advances, challenges, and future directions in human–machine integration. *Gels, 11*. https://www.semanticscholar.org/paper/e13f6aa43866f58a534a2f45d8dbea024b565217 (accessed on 30 May 2025).

45. Ulsh, B. A. (2012). The new radiobiology: Returning to our roots. https://core.ac.uk/download/32435527.pdf (accessed on 30 May 2025).

46. Wahab, M. A., & Younis, N. M. (2025). Efficacy of an educational program-based intervention in improving nurses' knowledge toward radiation protection measures: A randomized controlled trial. *Salud, Ciencia y Technology–Serie de Conferenciers*. https://www.semanticscholar.org/paper/c99031010a509b2a7d12325d3e179422b163e3de (accessed on 30 May 2025).

47. Wiley, A., Jr. (1972). A review: Some biological effects of high LET radiations. https://core.ac.uk/download/pdf/10297185.pdf (accessed on 30 May 2025).

48. Wu, S., Xie, C., Zhang, L., & Zhao, L. (2009). A new mathematical model for radiation cell killing mechanism: Target cumulating model. https://core.ac.uk/download/pdf/288301.pdf (accessed on 30 May 2025).

RADIOLOGICAL ANATOMY

5

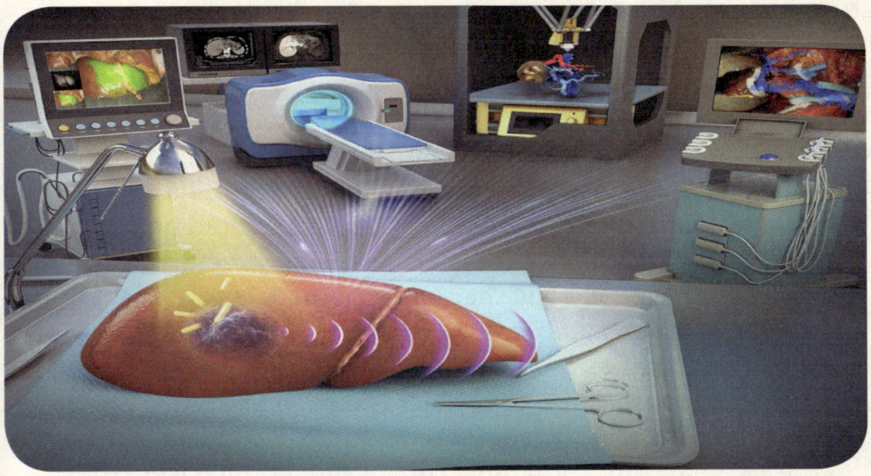

LEARNING OBJECTIVES

After studying this chapter, you will be able to:

1. Understand anatomical structures in radiology
2. Explain applications of radiological anatomy
3. Focus on challenges and limitations

Introduction

The intricate interplay between anatomical structures and how they are visualized has been a cornerstone of both medical education and practice for many years. Advances in radiological imaging, such as computed tomography (CT) and magnetic resonance imaging (MRI), have rendered in vivo observation of human anatomy a revolutionary field of research with previously unattainable levels of detail. Such imaging modalities need a stringent understanding of spatial arrangements in the body, which is crucial for effective diagnosis and treatment planning. To enhance this understanding, sophisticated training systems have been designed to simulate actual cases, offering a structured and interactive learning experience based on well-delineated image description paradigms (Azevedo *et. al.*, 2000). Moreover, the integration of formal anatomical ontologies, such as the Foundational Model of Anatomy, enhances these systems by providing semantic context and spatial reasoning capability, and allowing for automatic annotation and interpretation of complex radiological data (Folz *et. al.*, 2009). This synthesis of technology and anatomical data serves to underscore the significant role that radiological anatomy plays in modern medicine.

Definition of Radiological Anatomy

An understanding of the inner arrangements of the human body that are not visible to the naked eye requires specialized imaging techniques offering anatomical details in situ. Radiological anatomy is a field of anatomy concerned with the examination of body part organization and interrelationships using imaging modalities, such as X-rays, CT, and MRI. This region combines classical anatomy with modern technology in a way that allows clinicians to visualize bones, soft tissue, and organs without penetrating them, thereby enhancing diagnostic rates and planning for treatment.

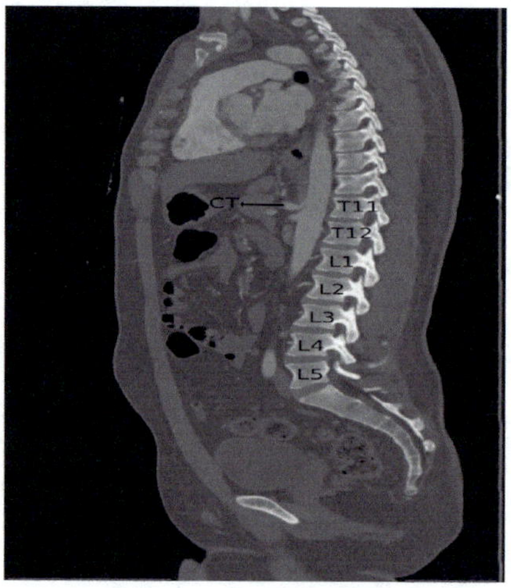

Figure 5.1. Radiological anatomy is the branch of anatomy that focuses on studying the organization and relationships of body parts through imaging modalities.

Source: https://www.mdpi.com/applsci/applsci-14-12033/article_deploy/html/images/applsci-14-12033-g004.png.

For instance, the evaluation of complex spinal disorders in conditions like Mucopolysaccharidosis IVA relies heavily on radiological anatomy to detect abnormalities and guide surgery (Goel *et. al.*, 2013). Visual data, including radiographic high-resolution images and digital files, improve our knowledge of anatomical variation and pathological changes. Radiological anatomy thus complements traditional anatomical information by including image data, which is essential for contemporary medical practice (Figure 5.1).

Importance in Medical Imaging

Technological advancements in imaging have revolutionized medical diagnostics with significantly improved accuracy of anatomical representation. Radiological anatomy, founded on several imaging modalities, plays a significant role in the diagnosis of pathological changes and treatment guidance. Sophisticated imaging ability allows clinicians to assess structures non-invasively, and thus enhances patient care by way of early and accurate diagnosis. Pediatric imaging signifies the need for personalized radiological approaches, especially where finances are tight and costly equipment and specialized skills are unavailable. This issue emphasizes the requirement for a global initiative to provide efficient imaging technology and professional advice, specifically targeting vulnerable groups afflicted with infectious diseases and trauma (Brandt *et. al.*, 2011). Also, integration of high-tech imaging systems has enhanced the quality and availability of radiological services, promoted better anatomical understanding, and fostered advances in medical education and patient care.

Role in Diagnosis and Treatment

The incorporation of radiological anatomy into clinical care has significantly improved the precision of diagnosis and the effectiveness of treatment planning. Radiological imaging is a critical device for the visualization of anatomical structures in vivo, enabling clinicians to identify pathological changes that might not be apparent through physical examination alone.

For instance, in pediatric patients, execution of specialized radiological protocols intended to restrict ionizing radiation utilization is crucial, especially in resource-limited nations with a great deal of infectious diseases and trauma (Brandt *et. al.*, 2011). In addition, evidence-based recommendations in imaging, such as those for the diagnosis of rhinosinusitis, emphasize the importance of careful use of radiological resources to balance diagnostic benefit against cost, as well as radiation risks (Borg-Xuereb *et. al.*, 2013). Radiological anatomy, as a whole, not only facilitates precise anatomical location and assessment but also supports clinical decision-making by providing critical pathologic information into disease processes, thereby maximizing patient outcomes through targeted treatment approaches (Figure 5.2).

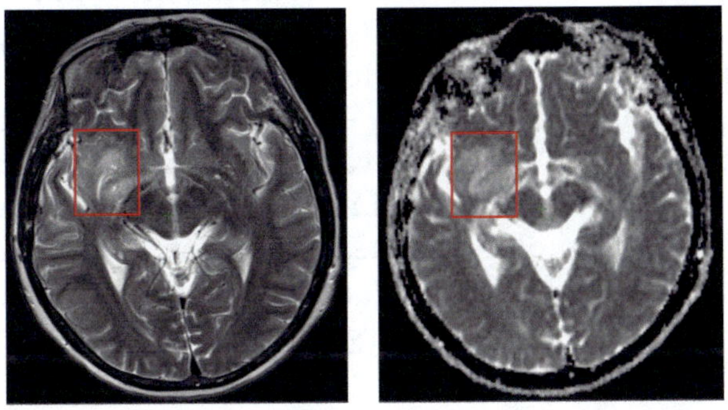

Figure 5.2. Radiological imaging serves as a vital tool for visualizing anatomical structures *in vivo*, allowing clinicians to detect pathological changes that may not be evident through physical examination alone.

Source: https://www.frontiersin.org/files/Articles/764665/fonc-11-764665-HTML/image_m/fonc-11-764665-g001.jpg.

Interdisciplinary Nature of Radiological Anatomy

Radiological anatomy necessitates a cooperative interaction of multiple fields, bridging the appreciation of traditional anatomy with contemporary technology and physics. Sophisticated imaging modalities such as MRI, CT, and ultrasound, firmly rooted in medical physics principles, are widely relied upon by radiologists to effectively visualize internal structures. Medical physicists play a key role in maximizing imaging techniques, protecting patients, and adjusting equipment to yield precise diagnostic results, besides their involvement in radiation treatment planning and follow-up (Newhauser *et. al.*, 2022). Besides, emerging technologies like artificial intelligence (AI) are revolutionizing image analysis by enhancing diagnostic quality and workflow productivity, highlighting the necessity to integrate computer science expertise in radiology (Najjar, 2023). This blending of anatomy, physics, engineering, and computer science thus reinforces the interdisciplinary nature of radiological anatomy, furthering its evolution from a descriptive science into a technologically driven, dynamic specialty positioned at the heart of today's healthcare diagnostics and treatment planning.

Scope of Radiological Anatomy

Advances in imaging technologies have tremendously expanded the arena of applications for radiological anatomy so that more precise morphological entities and functional activities of the human body can now be visualized with higher accuracy. New techniques, such as molecular fluorescence imaging and three-dimensional (3D) visualization, offer detailed anatomical knowledge that guides surgical interventions, particularly in complex operations, such as liver tumor hepatectomy. This integration not only assists in preoperative planning but also intraoperative decision-making by delineating tumor margins and detecting residual disease at a molecular level, as with the use of indocyanine green (ICG) imaging technology (Digital *et. al.*, 2019). Secondarily, the use of AI in radiologic interpretation is an exemplar for the union of computational imaging and anatomical imaging that facilitates improved diagnostic power and modeling for prediction in pathological inspection (Mulliqi *et.*

al., 2025). Cumulatively, these innovations mark the widening scope of radiological anatomy past fundamental imaging to its central role in precision medicine and customized patient care (Figure 5.3).

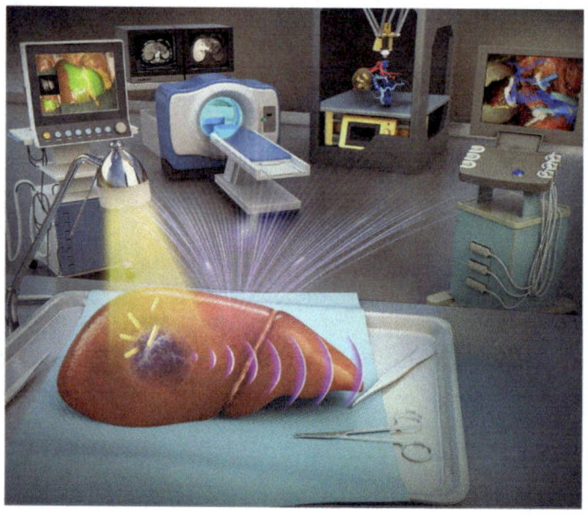

Figure 5.3. Modern techniques such as molecular fluorescence imaging and three-dimensional (3D) visualization offer detailed anatomical insights that guide surgical interventions, particularly in complex procedures like liver tumor hepatectomy.

Source: https://www.thelancet.com/cms/10.1016/j.ebiom.2019.02.017/asset/45ed26fc-d48e-4b05-9457-7fda695c7752/main.assets/gr1_lrg.jpg.

5.1. Anatomical Structures in Radiology

Learning Outcome

1. Understand the skeletal system
2. Explain the muscular system
3. Discuss the cardiovascular system
4. Focus on the respiratory system
5. Learn the digestive system
6. Describe the nervous system
7. Explain the endocrine system
8. Discuss the urinary system
9. Describe the reproductive system

Technological advances in imaging have significantly enhanced anatomical structure visualization and understanding, generating more insight critical for medical education and clinical practice. The integration of CT and MRI is applied to obtain precise three-dimensional reconstructions of difficult-to-delineate anatomical regions, such as the human brain, with ease, facilitating the easy delineation of neuroanatomical and vascular structures. These computer models, generated by high-level software packages like 3D Slicer, are far superior to traditional pedagogical tools in that they consist of dynamic, interactive representations that facilitate a deeper spatial understanding. Moreover, subjecting students to manual segmentation of these radiological images has been shown to significantly improve visuospatial skills, with a correlation to better performance in anatomy exams and validating the promise of active learning methodologies in radiological anatomy education (Karstens *et. al.*, 2024). These innovations underscore the utility of multimodal imaging and interactive digital technologies in learning anatomy, which is important for the accurate radiological interpretation and surgical planning (Ou *et. al.*, 2023).

5.1.1. Skeletal System

Improvements in radiological anatomy have significantly improved the visualization and management of complex skeletal injuries, particularly fractures of load-bearing vital structures. Thorough imaging techniques give good visualization of fracture morphology and differences in anatomy, which are essential for optimal fixation methods. Distal femur fractures, for instance, present significant challenges due to their proximity to the knee joint and susceptibility to comminuted bone along with soft tissue damage, complicating surgery. Utilization of locking compression plates with less invasive stabilizing devices has been shown to show positive outcomes in restoring function and alignment, as revealed by improved healing times and minimal malalignment in recent clinical studies (Nizar *et. al.*, 2024). Additionally, pelvic morphology differences directly affect the success of percutaneous fixation procedures, where a newly developed anatomy-based sacroiliac joint classification system assists surgeons in preoperative planning to decrease the risk of malposition and improve outcomes (Lee *et. al.*, 2023). These technology-driven approaches emphasize the intersection of anatomical intricacy and technology in the evolution of skeletal system management (Figure 5.4).

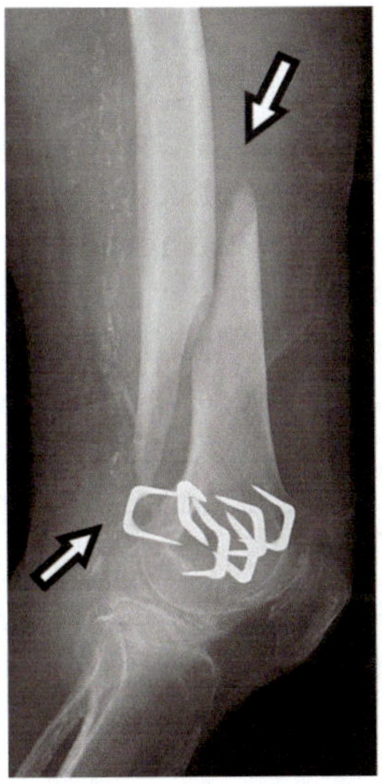

Figure 5.4. Precise imaging techniques enable detailed visualization of fracture patterns and anatomical variations, which are crucial for optimal fixation strategies.

Source: https://www.mdpi.com/anatomia/anatomia-02-00026/article_deploy/html/images/anatomia-02-00026-g001.png.

5.1.2. Muscular System

Understanding complex variations in the anatomy of muscles is crucial for accurate radiological interpretation, particularly in the clinical setting where accurate diagnosis determines effective therapy. Anomalies of muscles, such as accessory or supernumerary bellies, are difficult to diagnose unless they are known. For instance, the adductor brevis muscle occasionally develops additional bellies, a variation that is optimally identified by advanced imaging technologies, like CT and MRI. Such a realization allows radiologists to differentiate between anatomical variation and pathological mass, and hence avoid misdiagnosis. Moreover, detection of these variations in muscles facilitates easier surgical planning and reconstruction, emphasizing the importance of close anatomical familiarity in radiology practice (Vandana *et. al.*, 2011). While disorders of the orbital muscles also need diligent imaging evaluation, the wide range of potential pathologies necessitates integration of clinical information to effectively shortlist differential diagnoses (Brennan *et. al.*, 2014). Thus, understanding the fine muscular anatomy through radiological anatomy enhances diagnostic efficiency and patient management.

5.1.3. Cardiovascular System

Imaging technological innovations have revolutionized the exploration of complex anatomical structures with unprecedented three-dimensional presentations. The cardiovascular system, with its sensitive network of chambers, vessels, and valves, is particularly well-served by such innovation. Traditional two-dimensional representations seldom capture the spatial relationship critical to accurate diagnosis and treatment. Procedures of radiological anatomy in the recent past have utilizedCT, MRI, and ultrasound to build high-definition three-dimensional reconstructions that model the in vivo heart anatomy with precision. Interactive digital models allow researchers and clinicians to visualize internal structures from several perspectives, offering improved understanding of both normal and disease states. Furthermore, this technology enhances preoperative planning and intraoperative navigation for surgical and endovascular therapies, ultimately leading to better patient outcomes and education. These digital images also allow for integration into extended reality platforms, which enhances immersive learning and precise procedural guidance, emphasizing the evolving impact of radiological anatomy in cardiovascular medicine (Hunt *et. al.*, 2024; Petrov *et. al.*, 2024).

5.1.4. Respiratory System

The complexity of the respiratory system is underscored by its multi-dimensional interplay with the rest of the organs and pathologies, for which radiological anatomy gives meaning. An example is the identification of rare congenital malformations such as communicating bronchopulmonary foregut malformations, providing critical information on impaired communication between the respiratory and gastrointestinal systems, which indicates the importance of precise radiological description in planning clinical treatment (Shama *et. al.*, 2021).

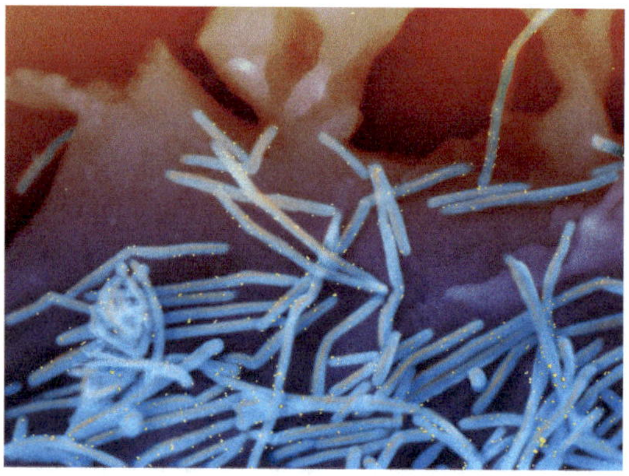

Figure 5.5. Respiratory syncytial virus (RSV) infections.

Source: https://upload.wikimedia.org/wikipedia/commons/d/d6/Human_Respiratory_Syncytial_Virus_%28RSV%29_%2833114415716%29.jpg.

Moreover, radiologic imaging is paramount for the diagnosis and identification of disease processes impacting the adult respiratory airway. Studies of the respiratory syncytial virus (RSV) infections demonstrate how radiologic findings correspond with clinical severity and distinguish them from other respiratory infections like influenza, particularly among elderly patients whose symptoms are confounded by comorbidities (Symes *et. al.*, 2025). Hence, application of radiological anatomy is of utmost importance not only for the diagnosis of structural abnormalities but also for the assessment of functional impairment and planning of treatment in the respiratory system (Figure 5.5).

5.1.5. Digestive System

The complexity of the gastrointestinal tract becomes particularly evident when viewed from the radiological anatomy's point of view, especially in the context of postoperative complications and oncologic treatments. Radiologic imaging is pivotal in the identification of complications such as hemorrhage following biliary surgery, where deformed anatomical structures may preclude traditional endoscopic interventions. For instance, CT angiography has proven to be invaluable in the identification of active sites of bleeding in biliary-digestive anastomoses, guiding interventional radiology in the provision of customized embolization therapy that improves the patient's outcome despite risk factors like cirrhosis and antiplatelet therapy (Vincenzi *et. al.*, 2024). Further, the digestive system's proximity to pelvic organs indirectly renders it part of radiation therapy complications, which typically include neighboring urinary structures but can spread to the integrity of the digestive tract. These are complexities that call for thorough anatomical understanding in order to adequately treat and counteract untoward effects and avoid life-threatening outcomes, highlighting the responsibility of radiological anatomy in diagnosis and treatment in the intricate anatomy of the digestive tract (Chorbi *et. al.*, 2021).

5.1.6. Nervous System

Advances in radiological imaging have revolutionized the examination of complex anatomical structures, enabling detailed visualization of areas previously accessible only by invasive means. The central nervous system, in particular, presents particular challenges due to the complicated orientation of nerve fibers. In the past, direct dissection was needed to see these tracts of nerves; however, MRI technology today can allow for three-dimensional tractography non-invasively, offering high resolution on structures such as the corticospinal tract. While this modality can revolutionize, it faces issues of image distortion and interpretive limitations that impair its utility and accuracy in use, especially in neurosurgical planning (Mujika *et. al.*, 2018). Further, nervous system pathology cannot be conceptualized using imaging alone; newer paradigms accentuate the biopsychosocial model, recognizing that psychosocial factors and nervous system sensitization play a big role in symptom presentation and response to treatment, emphasizing the value of integrative clinical assessment coupled with radiological anatomy (Sharma *et. al.*, 2022) (Figure 5.6).

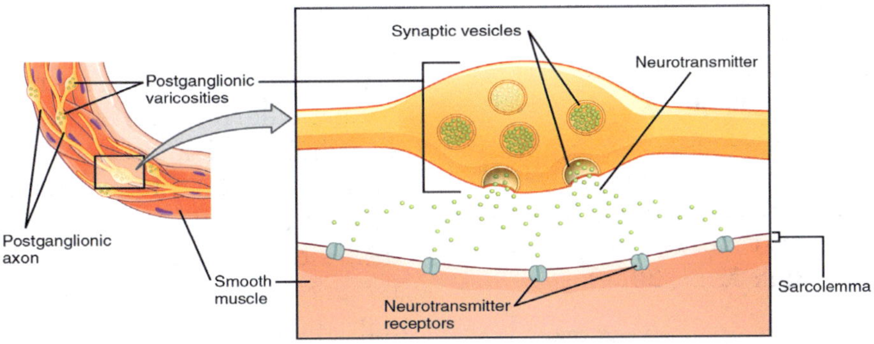

Figure 5.6. The nervous system, particularly the central nervous system, presents unique challenges due to the intricate arrangement of nerve fibers.

Source: https://open.oregonstate.education/app/uploads/sites/157/2021/02/1504_Autonomic_Varicosities.jpg.

5.1.7. Endocrine System

Understanding the fine anatomy of the human body mandates precise imaging modalities that provide both anatomical and functional data. The endocrine system, composed of glands that secrete hormones, presents peculiar challenges in radiological anatomy due to its diffuse and variable nature on radiography. More advanced imaging techniques, like ultrasound, MRI, and CT scans, have enhanced the visibility of endocrine organs, like the thyroid gland, adrenal glands, and pancreas. Besides, radiological assessment also allows for the diagnosis of pathological changes that may have an effect on hormonal balance, i.e., tumors or hyperplasia, and thus clinical treatment. Recent developments in automatic image analysis, more so in pediatric skeletal assessment, indicate that deep learning can be applied in solving endocrine-related diagnostic challenges, i.e., growth aberrations due to hormonal disorders (Rakhlin *et. al.*, 2018). While such software has, for the most part, been focused on skeletal development, expanding its role to encompass endocrine gland evaluation can revolutionize diagnostic precision. Despite these advancements, complete clinical correlation is always required for proper interpretation and effective treatment planning (Brennan *et. al.*, 2014).

5.1.8. Urinary System

Radiological imaging is especially useful in the appreciation of the complex anatomy and pathology of the urinary tract, particularly when assessing conditions that require precise intervention. The prostatic artery, one of the important vessels for male urinary anatomy, has been found to show considerable anatomical variability, which has been detailed with advanced imaging techniques such as 3D rendering dual-energy CT. Studies have indicated that the majority of prostatic arteries originate from a common source in the internal pudendal artery, with prevailing tortuosity and atherosclerotic changes impairing vascular accessibility during procedures like prostatic artery embolization (Binh *et. al.*, 2024).

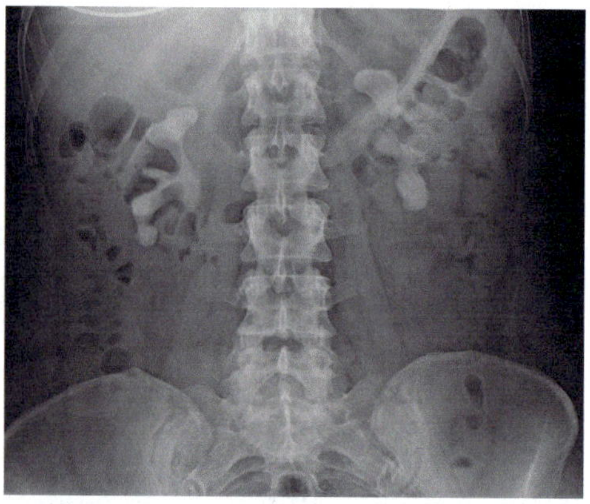

Figure 5.7. Radiological imaging plays a crucial role in understanding the complex anatomy and pathology of the urinary system, particularly when assessing conditions that require precise intervention.

Source: https://www.ajkd.org/cms/10.1053/j.ajkd.2023.03.017/asset/e3f02e39-93da-466d-893c-1e152d384300/main.assets/gr4_lrg.jpg.

Moreover, radiotherapy for pelvic malignancies has a tendency to inadvertently affect the urinary tract due to anatomical proximity, causing severe late complications such as hemorrhagic cystitis and bladder necrosis. These complications are very challenging for diagnosis and treatment, emphasizing the usefulness of careful radiological anatomy in devising treatment and managing post-radiation damage to the urinary tract (Omkaram *et. al.*, 2021) (Figure 5.7).

5.1.9. Reproductive System

The radiological visualization of the intricate anatomy of the human body requires advanced imaging modalities that reveal the fine details of anatomy crucial in diagnosis and therapy. Among all the systems, however, the reproductive system is particularly challenging and challenging to radiological anatomy due to its dynamic nature and distinctive tissue composition. Existing radiologic imaging modalities such as MRI, ultrasonography, and CT scanning allow doctors to visualize reproductive organs with high fidelity, making it possible to identify abnormalities and intercede therapeutically.

Merging imaging data with tissue-specific radiological characteristics enhances accuracy for identifying pathologies of male and female reproductive systems. Also, modifying radiological protection standards guarantees diagnostic imaging minimizes exposure risks while maintaining image quality, consistent with ongoing developments discussed at recent expert gatherings (Laurier *et. al.*, 2024). Such innovations underscore the central role of radiological anatomy in optimizing reproductive health results through precise visualization and intelligent use of imaging modalities (Hunt *et. al.*, 2024).

Test Your Knowledge

1. What is the importance of identifying anatomical structures accurately in radiological images?
2. What are the major anatomical landmarks seen in a standard PA chest X-ray?

5.2. Applications of Radiological Anatomy

Learning Outcome

1. Understand applications of radiological anatomy in diagnostic imaging
2. Explain applications of radiological anatomy in interventional radiology
3. Know applications of radiological anatomy in surgical planning
4. Learn applications of radiological anatomy in oncology
5. Perform trauma assessment
6. Discuss applications of radiological anatomy in pediatric radiology
7. Focus on applications of radiological anatomy in geriatric considerations
8. Describe applications of radiological anatomy in research and development
9. Know applications of radiological anatomy in education and training

Radiological anatomy integration into clinical practice has revolutionized diagnostic precision and intervention treatments. By providing detailed imagery of inner structures, radiological anatomy allows clinicians to assess pathological conditions non-invasively and accurately, leading to better patient outcomes. For instance, the ability to differentiate between tissue types and visualize organ relationship aids in planning surgical intervention and guiding minimally invasive procedures to reduce operative risks. Besides, technological progress in imaging modalities has allowed for extension of applications to dynamic studies, e.g., functional assessment and real-time monitoring of therapies. The heuristic potential of radiological anatomy extends beyond diagnostic use into educational arenas, where it forms a central element for the education of health professionals in anatomy and pathology.

5.2.1. Diagnostic Imaging

In order to understand the intricate internal anatomy of the human body, it is necessary to turn to advanced techniques beyond the traditional training in anatomy. Diagnostic imaging serves as the answer to visualizing in vivo these structures so that clinicians may accurately detect and inspect pathological changes. The X-ray, CT, and MRI modalities provide differing perspectives and levels of resolution and therefore permit detailed anatomical assessment.

The combination of radiological anatomy and diagnostic imaging improves the interpretive value of clinical observations to allow better disease description and treatment. For instance, highly detailed images taken using high-technology X-ray equipment reveal minute anatomical variations that are critical for diagnosis and therapy planning. Moreover, advances in imaging hardware enhance the quality of anatomical visualization and specificity, enhancing the precious synergy between diagnostic imaging and radiological anatomy in modern medicine. This collaboration improves patient outcomes through early and accurate diagnosis (Figure 5.8).

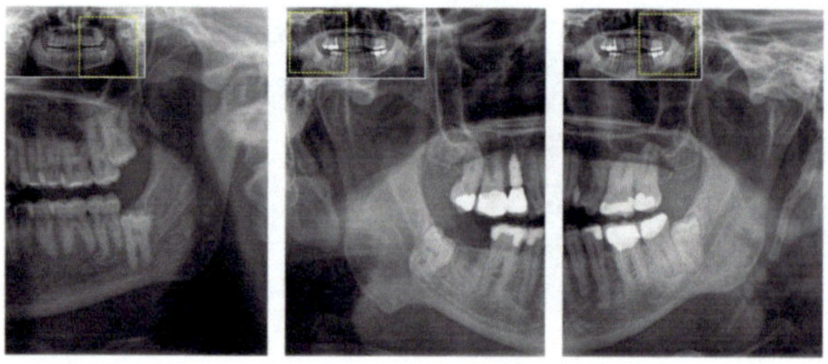

Figure 5.8. Diagnostic imaging plays a pivotal role in visualizing structures *in vivo*, enabling clinicians to identify and analyze pathological changes with precision.

Source: https://www.mdpi.com/jcm/jcm-12-07688/article_deploy/html/images/jcm-12-07688-g001.png.

5.2.2. Interventional Radiology

Technological advancements in medical fields have revolutionized the way vascular disease is diagnosed and treated with an emphasis on minimal invasion. Intervisional radiology exploits meticulous understanding of radiological anatomy to navigate complex vascular systems with image guidance, thus enabling precise therapeutic intervention. This specialty is endovascular in nature, which accesses target areas through blood vessels, reducing patient trauma and recovery periods with localized therapy such as targeted chemotherapy or embolization. Challenges still exist due to the intricate and personalized nature of vascular anatomy, issues related to the accessibility of small vessels, and procedural risks exacerbated by weak or disease-prone vessels. With evolving innovations, like the advancement of miniaturized robotic devices, there is potential for overcoming such limitations with greater accuracy and self-navigating abilities within the vascular system. However, technical and clinical issues remain prior to their applicability on a larger scale, highlighting the importance of continuous research to further develop these instruments in the radiologic anatomical realm (Alshammary & Alwahdani, 2024). Besides, the incorporation of AI in imaging analysis has the potential to optimize intervention performance and planning, particularly in children, where anatomical variability hinders the application of universal protocols, thus optimizing interventional radiology practice with increased diagnostic accuracy and personalized treatment (Kelly *et. al.*, 2024).

5.2.3. Surgical Planning

Radiologic anatomy advancements have significantly enhanced the safety and accuracy of complex surgery through precise preoperative planning. Sophisticated surgery planning integrates high-resolution imaging information in the generation of personalized three-dimensional models, allowing surgeons to precisely mimic osteotomies and screw placement.

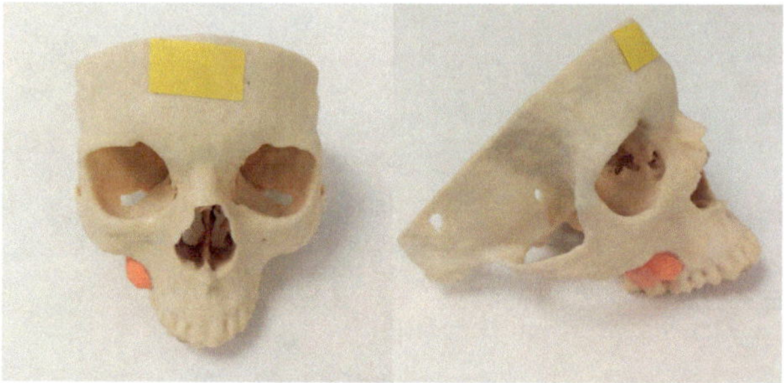

Figure 5.9. Modern surgical planning integrates high-resolution imaging data to create personalized three-dimensional models, allowing surgeons to simulate osteotomies and screw placement with remarkable accuracy.

Source: https://www.mdpi.com/jcm/jcm-11-02385/article_deploy/html/images/jcm-11-02385-g001.png.

This approach is especially effective in the correction of severe spinal deformities, where using 3D-printed guidance templates, created from individualized digital simulations, has indicated a correction rate over 90% and has greatly reduced the surgical risks associated with screw misplacement and osteotomy errors (Ding *et. al.*, 2023). Similarly, highly complex surgical sites such as the skull base benefit from precise radiological examination of anatomical variation, confirming significant neurovascular structures and maintaining them in the course of endoscopic surgery. CT provides key measurements that guide the safest surgical corridors based on precise anatomical landmarks, reducing intraoperative complications and improving patient outcomes (Edouard *et. al.*, 2022). Thus, planning of surgery from radiological anatomy is a paradigm towards personalized, safer, and more effective operations (Figure 5.9).

5.2.4. Oncology

Advances in radiologic anatomy have significantly enhanced the diagnosis and treatment of oncologic disease, providing precious information regarding tumor form and body spatial anatomy. Reliable imaging technologies allow clinicians to visualize the dimensions of cancerous tumors, making precise staging and affecting curative therapy. For instance, high-resolution radiographic techniques reflect acceptable anatomical variations that might signify initial neoplastic change, thereby adding diagnostic sensitivity. In addition, radiological anatomy of different tissues is a must in outlining the margins of the tumor, an aspect of utmost significance in surgery and radiation treatment planning. The combination of high-resolution anatomy imaging with oncologic assessment contributes to individualized treatment regimens, achieving maximum outcome with minimal damage to normal tissues. As well, progressive improvements in imaging modalities continue to provide improvements in distinguishing between benign and malignant lesions, thus reinforcing the role of radiological anatomy in enhancing oncologic care.

5.2.5. Trauma Assessment

Adequate evaluation of trauma is crucial in the diagnosis and treatment of injuries; accordingly, it is particularly important where radiological anatomy is of core importance. Preliminary imaging techniques such as X-rays and CT scans are important to identify fractures and internal injuries that are not externally visible by physical examination alone. For instance, clavicle fractures that affect 5% to 10% of all fractures require careful radiographic evaluation to guide the treatment, especially in the event of surgical intervention such as open reduction and internal fixation (ORIF) to provide optimal healing and restitution of function (Ramalingam *et. al.*, 2023). Moreover, trauma assessment must also be wary of strange presentations that can disguise themselves as other processes; a typical case was an obtunded massive hemothorax that was initially imaged but later identified as large empyema after insertion of the chest drain, which emphasizes the importance of correlating clinical and radiological characteristics in trauma patients (Ghaffar *et. al.*, 2023). Such integration aids enhanced diagnostic precision and directs early and prudent interventions (Figure 5.10).

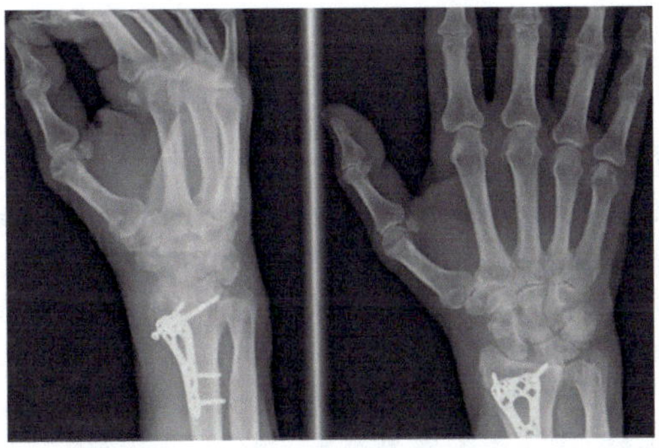

Figure 5.10. Initial imaging techniques such as X-rays and CT scans are indispensable for identifying fractures and internal injuries that might not be immediately evident through physical examination alone.

Source: https://www.central-health.com/wp-content/uploads/Common-Hand-Wrist-blog-1-1024x683.jpg.webp.

5.2.6. Pediatric Radiology

Advances in technology have added significantly to diagnostic capability in pediatric medicine, particularly in the field of abdominal pathology. Emerging ultrasound techniques like contrast-enhanced ultrasound, microvascular ultrasound, elastography, and fat quantification have demonstrated bright promise not just to complement conventional practices but also to reduce reliance on more invasive or radiation-dependent modalities like CT and MRI in children. These new technologies offer dynamic, real-time assessment with improved tissue characterization in the context of pediatric patients, whose smaller anatomy presents unique imaging challenges. Furthermore, when complicated procedures like pediatric liver transplantation are in question, ultrasound continues to be the cornerstone of preoperative evaluation of anatomical structures, with CT and MRI playing adjunctive roles based on specific clinical questions. Yet, imaging protocol diversity across centers highlights the imperative for standard protocols to improve surgical planning and patient outcomes in pediatric radiology (Davis *et. al.*, 2024; Herrmann *et. al.*, 2023).

5.2.7. Geriatric Considerations

Advances in radiological anatomy have significantly altered the treatment of fractures and tumors in aging patients, with a need for an individualized approach responsive to geriatric physiology and comorbidities. In orthopedic surgery, such as the fixation of intertrochanteric fractures, proximal femoral nail anti-rotation (PFNA) implants have been advantageous through shorter operating times and less blood loss with no compromise on postoperative functional outcomes, which is important given the limited physiological reserves found in older patients (Bhardwaj *et. al.*, 2024). Moreover, risk stratification of neurosurgical interventions for intracranial meningiomas is supplemented with grading systems like SKALE, CRGS, and GSS, which incorporate radiological parameters alongside clinical variables to effectively predict postoperative complications. They allow the clinician to better predict risks in patients > 75 years, thus optimizing surgical selection and maximizing patient outcomes (Lee *et. al.*, 2022). Therefore, incorporating certain radiological evaluations with clinical considerations of age is essential when treating older patients, providing interventions that are both effective and minimize morbidity in this compromised group (Figure 5.11).

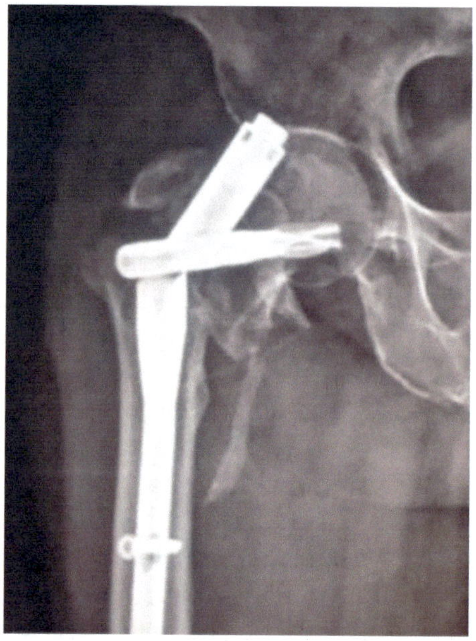

Figure 5.11. Proximal femoral nail anti-rotation (PFNA) implants.

Source: https://www.tandfonline.com/cms/asset/1dfd4a8f-27c8-47ea-8d60-ad31f6233fd7/gcmb_a_1964488_f0001_c.jpg.

5.2.8. Research and Development

Medical imaging advancements have widely transformed the study of human anatomy by enabling visualization of interior structures in depth without resorting to invasive methods. This is largely driven by continued research and development in radiological anatomy, where new imaging technologies such as CT and MRI have been fine-tuned to improve resolution and yield diagnostic information. The technologies support precise mapping of anatomical structures, facilitating enhanced clinical decision-making and educational methodology. Further R&D effort is also focused on enhancing image contrast and reducing exposure to radiation, improving safety while enhancing the likelihood of earlier disease detection. The R&D process has also been towards integrating digital image processing and AI to automate anatomy recognition and analysis, further streamlining clinical workflows. These developments illustrate the central role of research and development in the advancement of radiological anatomy, ultimately bringing together classical anatomical knowledge with modern diagnostic capabilities.

5.2.9. Education and Training

Advances in technology have overhauled the medical education field, particularly radiological anatomy, which cannot be practiced using old methods. The integration of three-dimensional imaging modalities like CT and MRI with anatomy teaching gives a clearer vision into complex spatial relationships that are essential for accurate diagnosis and treatment planning. Combining radiological images with anatomy classes enhances students' application of theoretical concepts to clinical scenarios, facilitating enhanced spatial visualization and appreciation of dynamic anatomy. Moreover, new learning tools such as 3D-printed models based on radiological imaging facilitate a haptic and visual learning experience, bridging the gap between virtual and physical anatomy. These models, rendered accessible for learning and research purposes, maximize active learning and cross-disciplinary teamwork. These changes highlight the importance of initial and ongoing exposure to radiological anatomy during education and training to equip future clinicians with the skills to meet contemporary clinical demands (Todor *et. al.*, 2025) (Figure 5.12).

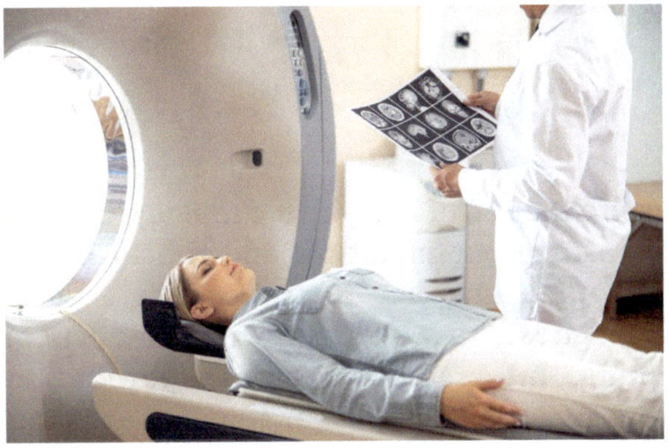

Figure 5.12. The integration of three-dimensional imaging techniques like CT and MRI with anatomical education allows for a deeper understanding of complex spatial relationships that are essential for accurate diagnosis and treatment planning.

Source: https://jayxray.com/wp-content/uploads/2024/04/AdobeStock_283195217.jpeg.

Test Your Knowledge

1. Why is it essential for radiologists to recognize normal anatomical variants?
2. How is radiological anatomy incorporated into anatomy curricula for healthcare professionals?

5.3. Challenges and Limitations

Learning Outcome

1. Understand radiation exposure
2. Explain image interpretation errors
3. Focus on the cost of imaging technologies
4. Discuss the accessibility of imaging services
5. Focus on ethical considerations
6. Consider technological limitations
7. Describe patient safety concerns
8. Know variability in anatomical presentation
9. Describe future directions in radiological anatomy

Despite the use of imaging technology, there are several inherent limitations and difficulties with radiological anatomy that affect the accuracy of diagnosis as well as clinical decision-making. Intersecting anatomy, pathological alterations, and complex anatomical variations render clear vision impossible and impede the interpretation process. For instance, in ankylosing spondylitis, osteoporosis, and altered bony anatomy interfere with precise surgical planning and instrumentation of the cervical spine, demonstrating the difficulty of correlating the radiological images with the clinical situation (Alaosta, 2025). In addition, standard imaging biomarkers, like RECIST 1.1 measurements, fail to capture the intricate facet of tumor burden and morphology, thus their failure to be utilized effectively in oncological evaluation. The base on simplified measurement and supervised artificial intelligence models also limits a certain level of versatility towards varied presentations, a reason more sophisticated tools that combine radiologist expertise with enhanced computational algorithms are a requirement (Léo *et. al.*, 2024). These challenges underscore the ongoing necessity to develop imaging techniques, design interactive AI-based models, and enhance interpretive frameworks to overcome the limitations of radiological anatomy.

5.3.1. Radiation Exposure

Knowledge of radiation exposure risk is of utmost relevance in radiological anatomy, as it directly affects patient safety and diagnostic success. Radiological procedures, while being highly beneficial in imaging internal anatomy, involve varying levels of ionizing radiation, potentially causing cellular damage and increasing malignancy risk unless best controlled. Diagnostic benefit-to-harm ratio demands adherence to guidelines and protocols that minimize exposure without affecting the image quality. Enhanced imaging technology and protection practice have notably reduced avoidable radiation, resulting in safer clinical practice. .

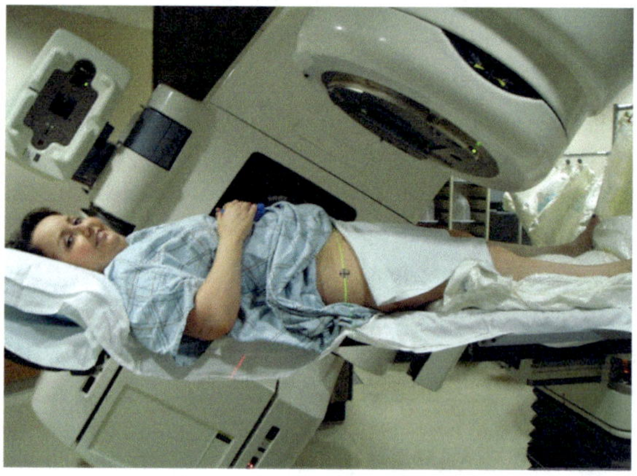

Figure 5.13. Radiological procedures, while invaluable for visualizing internal structures, involve varying degrees of ionizing radiation, which can cause cellular damage and increase the risk of malignancies if not properly managed.

Source: https://upload.wikimedia.org/wikipedia/commons/d/d5/Radiation_therapy.jpg.

Patient-specific factors such as age, comorbidities, and total radiation history must also be considered when planning for diagnostic imaging. With these considerations being included, clinicians are able to optimize diagnostic efficacy while reducing patient safety concerns, as proposed in broader clinical recommendations that may be relevant to anatomical imaging and disease diagnosis (Eric *et. al.*, 2022; Meryl *et. al.*, 2022) (Figure 5.13)

5.3.2. Image Interpretation Errors

Radiological image interpretation error remain a leading issue in diagnostic medicine, typically due to non-uniform image quality, anatomical structure complexity, and observer experience. The nuanced nature of chest CT scans, for instance, demands precise detection of subtle pathological changes; however, recent evidence indicates even advanced AI models such as ChatGPT-4V are of differing diagnostic accuracy, particularly in discriminating between conditions like COVID-19 and non-small cell lung cancer, with constant errors due to limitations in spatial and pathological context comprehension (Dehdab *et. al.*, 2024). Moreover, imaging modalities such as ultrasound introduce additional challenges, with suboptimal contrast and in-built artifacts compromising tissue discrimination, increasing the likelihood of segmentation failure at interpretation. Improved unsupervised deep learning techniques have promise by enhancing semantic segmentation without requiring large quantities of labeled data, potentially reducing human error through more accurately defining tissue boundaries (Tmenova *et. al.*, 2024). These complicated obstacles in radiological anatomy must be overcome to improve diagnostic uniformity and patient care.

5.3.3. Cost of Imaging Technologies

Availability of advanced imaging technology is often limited by considerable economic barriers, particularly in low-resource settings with limited healthcare budgets. Capital investments needed to purchase and install radiologic devices, for example, CT scanners and MRI scanners, are compounded by ongoing costs of maintenance, specialized personnel, and infrastructure accommodations. These economic barriers are especially apparent in developing countries, where pediatric imaging is under-resourced, with high demand due to prevalent illnesses and poor health status (Brandt *et. al.*, 2011). Moreover, the lack of affordable digital solutions impacts the scalability of imaging programs that are required for adequate radiological anatomy assessment. Efforts to produce low-cost, durable technology and international alliances for teleradiology reporting are essential building blocks to bridge the gap and improve diagnostic capability worldwide (Brandt *et. al.*, 2011). The financial challenge is still a primary driver of affordability and quality of radiological anatomical imaging on a global scale (Figure 5.14).

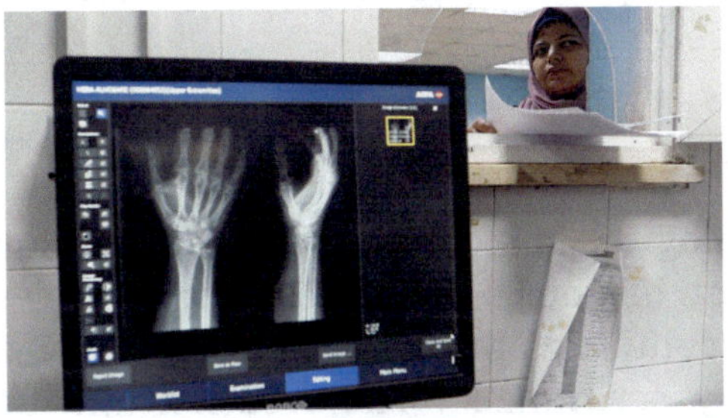

Figure 5.14. The high initial costs of purchasing and installing radiological equipment, such as CT scanners and MRI machines, are compounded by ongoing expenses for maintenance, specialized personnel, and infrastructure adaptations.

Source: https://static.toiimg.com/thumb/msid-112883662,width-1280,height-720,resizemode-4/112883662.jpg.

5.3.4. Accessibility of Imaging Services

Technological developments have considerably enhanced diagnostic abilities in radiological anatomy, yet disparity in access remains an urgent concern. High-resolution modalities such as non-EPI diffusion-weighted MRI have increased sensitivity to offer accurate anatomical evaluation as seen in cholesteatoma assessment, but are still at the mercy of cost and infrastructure constraints for accessibility (Covelli *et. al.*, 2025). Alternatively, CT scans, although more available, overestimate lesion volumes, highlighting the use of complementary applications and better access to sophisticated imaging devices. Educational strategies like interactive three-dimensional programs have exhibited promise in filling gaps in anatomical knowledge through highly accessible and affordable platforms that incorporate radiologic correlates to assist learners in gaining mastery over complicated structures (Saraswathula *et. al.*, 2024). Correction of inequality in the availability of imaging services not only improves diagnosis but also supports huge training in radiological anatomy, which eventually results in better patient outcomes in different health care settings.

5.3.5. Ethical Considerations

Radiological anatomy has indeed transformed medical diagnosis, but with such advances come very complex ethical issues that need to be closely scrutinized. The creation and use of anatomy illustrations, for example, bring massive copyright violations and plagiarism problems, particularly when there are prior images being employed as blueprints for new work without clear guidelines on originality and intellectual property rights (Cornwall *et. al.*, 2025). These moral challenges extend to the incorporation of AI in radiology, where benefits to improved diagnostic potential must be balanced against patient safety, confidentiality, and the reliability of AI-based devices (Adrian *et. al.*, 2024). This intersection of technology and ethics demands tight control and transparent practice, so the benefits of radiological anatomy developments don't reduce legal or ethical standards. Finally, it is important to address these ethical concerns in order to promote responsible innovation, respecting both human rights and scientific integrity (Figure 5.15).

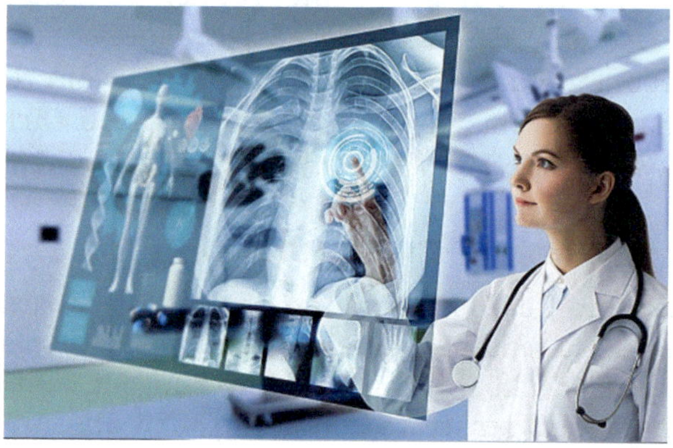

Figure 5.15. Advancements in radiological anatomy have undoubtedly transformed medical diagnostics, yet these innovations bring complex ethical challenges that demand careful scrutiny.

Source: https://www.healthcareradius.in/cloud/2024/11/22/Radiology-images.jpg.

5.3.6. Technological Limitations

Technological advances have significantly enhanced our radiological anatomy knowledge, but technological limitations continue to limit diagnostic and operative precision. A case in point is the utilization of high-resolution CT scanning, often utilized for anatomical size measurement, such as cholesteatoma volume measurement, which is prone to overestimation of size compared to non-echo planar imaging diffusion-weighted MRI, which is still the reigning gold standard. This disparity necessitates compensatory techniques like fusion techniques to increase diagnostic precision (Covelli *et. al.*, 2025). Similarly, minimally invasive surgical procedures rely on fluoroscopic imaging to reach hard-to-reach anatomy regions, yet the lack of direct visualization of neurovascular structures is dangerous for iatrogenic injury. Technological developments such as fluoroscopic heatmaps superimposing significant anatomical routes have the potential for positive direction, yet remain dependent on imaging data quality and interpretation (Karaismailoğlu *et. al.*, 2024). All these drawbacks emphasize the ongoing necessity for the improvement of technology refinements in order to maximize radiological anatomy application in diagnosis and intervention.

5.3.7. Patient Safety Concerns

Patient safety is of paramount concern in radiological anatomy, with the inherent use of ionizing radiation, whose possible health effects are to be contained with suitable control. Accurate anatomical information prevents avoidable exposure by optimizing the imaging angle and technique, thus sparing radiosensitive organs.

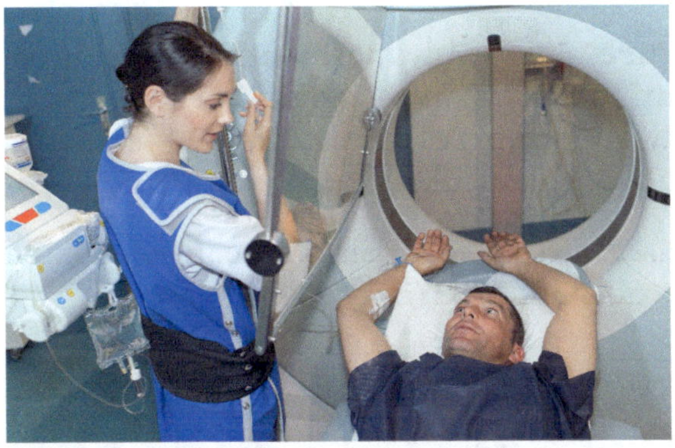

Figure 5.16. Ensuring patient safety within radiological anatomy is paramount, as the inherent use of ionizing radiation poses potential health risks if not carefully managed.

Source: https://www.versantphysics.com/wp-content/uploads/2022/04/AdobeStock_262422665.jpeg.

Moreover, faulty positioning or misinterpretation can lead to repeated scanning, which increases the cumulative dose of radiation and the associated risk of tissue damage or increased risk of cancer. Modern imaging protocols today concentrate on dose reduction strategies, preserving diagnostic quality, emphasizing the greatest possible need to preserve a delicate balance between extensive anatomical representation and patient safety. Continuous education of radiologists in anatomical variation and radiological safety protocols enhances awareness of patient-related factors potentially leading to increased risk. This is further validated by studies showing that adherence to standardized protocols significantly reduces radiation errors and enhances patient outcomes. Besides, the inclusion of technological innovations such as automated monitoring of dose enhances responsibility and vigilance in radiology work (Figure 5.16).

5.3.8. Variability in Anatomical Presentation

Technical developments in imaging have significantly enhanced the capability to diagnose and interpret anatomical variation, underpinning the requirement to recognize variability in anatomical presentation in radiological anatomy. Anatomical structures often deviate from standard descriptions due to genetic, developmental, or disease-related factors, thus complicating diagnosis and planning treatment. Aorta diseases, for instance, occur clinically in a broad variety of phenotypes that need personalized imaging approaches and careful surveillance to successfully treat the range of symptomatic and asymptomatic states (Eric *et. al.*, 2022).

Moreover, the use of AI in medical imaging has revolutionized the identification and interpretation of such diversity, which also overcomes some limitations, like sparse labeling and interpretability by sophisticated deep neural networks (Zhou *et. al.*, 2021). These technologies not only improve diagnostic accuracy but also make personalized medicine by accommodating individual anatomical differences. It is thus important that radiologists are aware of and take into account anatomical variability to optimize diagnostic performance and treatment efficacy in clinical settings.

5.3.9. Future Directions in Radiological Anatomy

Technological advancements continue to reshape medical specialties, creating new opportunities for radiological anatomy to evolve in revolutionary ways. One such promising future direction involves enhancing spatial understanding through integrating formal ontologies, such as the Foundational Model of Anatomy (FMA), with a comprehensive schema for describing the spatio-structural relationships that exist in human anatomy. Research is geared to take advantage of these ontologies to improve computer-assisted parsing of complex 3D imaging information from MRI and CT scans, enabling precise and quicker interpretation of radiologic images. Another role is the development of semantic annotation using ontology concepts that facilitate enhanced search capability within extensive collections of medical images, with the potential to revolutionize diagnostic work flows and education (Folz *et. al.*, 2009). Moreover, as technology in imaging develops, further improvement in the precision and detail of radiological data is critical, with the assistance of innovation in imaging hardware and computer software programs that generate improved images with reduced exposure risks. Together, they portend an age where radiological anatomy is inextricably bound up with computational facilities to improve both clinical and educational outcomes (Figure 5.17).

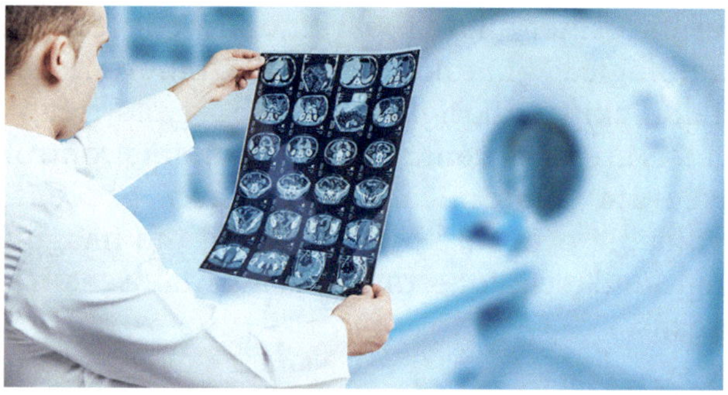

Figure 5.17. Advancements in technology continue to reshape medical fields, creating new opportunities for radiological anatomy to evolve dramatically.

Source: https://medicalbuyer.co.in/wp-content/uploads/2023/02/Xray.jpg.

Test Your Knowledge

1. What are the common challenges in accurately interpreting radiological images?
2. What are the resolution limitations of different imaging modalities?

SUMMARY

The incorporation of radiological anatomy in practice is essential in diagnostic correctness and effective treatment planning. The development of technology in imaging has rendered more diagnostic information of fine anatomical detail visible, which has improved diagnostic accuracy. However, the variability in radiological interpretation indicates the presence of expertise and continuous training in the discipline. Studies of radiologic proficiency point out that experience has a vital impact on diagnostic competence, and thus training programs need to emphasize the cultivation of perceptual ability as well as in-depth anatomical knowledge in order to minimize error rates and enhance outcomes (Taylor *et. al.*, 2007). In addition, the use of CBL platforms may aid the development of expert-level proficiency by exposing participants to varied cases and solidifying pattern recognition. Lastly, a deeper understanding of radiological anatomy and sophisticated training aids will enhance radiologic performance and quality of patient care. This development not only enhances medical imaging but also enhances confidence in clinical decision-makingbased on solid anatomical knowledge.

It is vital to have an understanding of the basic aspects of radiological anatomy in providing precise diagnosis and effective clinical treatment. Advanced imaging techniques such as cone-beam computed tomography (CBCT) provide high-resolution data with respect to anatomical features such as the maxillary sinus, enabling effective assessment of variation in morphology with age and gender, which can be utilized for surgical planning and the avoidance of complications in implant dentistry (Gargi *et. al.*, 2025). In addition, the integration of ML models with radiological and laboratory data has been promising in predicting patient outcomes in complex diseases like poor-grade aneurysmal subarachnoid hemorrhage. The prediction methods apply traditionally acquired radiological metrics to enhance prognostication, thus allowing for personalized treatment protocols (Bangash *et. al.*, 2025). Comprehensively, these findings underscore the importance of correlating radiological findings with clinical parameters to enhance both anatomical insight and patient care outcomes. Lastly, embracing radiological anatomy technological innovations promotes precision medicine and optimizes therapy decision-making.

KEY TERMS FROM THIS CHAPTER

- Artificial intelligence
- Diagnostic accuracy
- Molecular fluorescence imaging
- Predictive modeling
- Spondylitis
- Visualization
- Clinical decision-making
- Indocyanine green (ICG) imaging technology
- Monitoring
- Radiation therapy
- Trauma

CRITICAL THINKING QUESTIONS

1. **Which imaging modality provides the best soft tissue contrast?**
   a. X-ray
   b. Ultrasound
   c. CT scan
   d. MRI
2. **On a chest X-ray, which structure is typically seen as the most radiopaque?**
   a. Lungs
   b. Heart
   c. Ribs
   d. Diaphragm
3. **In a normal axial CT scan of the brain, the ventricles are located:**
   a. In the anterior portion
   b. Within the gray matter
   c. Centrally, surrounded by white matter
   d. Posterior to the cerebellum
4. **What structure appears darkest (most radiolucent) on a standard X-ray?**
   a. Bone
   b. Air in the lungs
   c. Blood
   d. Muscle
5. **In abdominal CT imaging, the liver is usually located:**
   a. In the left upper quadrant
   b. In the right lower quadrant
   c. In the right upper quadrant
   d. Midline below the diaphragm

Short Answer Questions

1. What is radiological anatomy, and how does it differ from gross anatomy?
2. How are anatomical structures typically visualized on an X-ray?
3. Which imaging modality is most useful for viewing soft tissues like the brain or liver?
4. How does the appearance of air, bone, and soft tissue differ on a CT scan?
5. What is the significance of knowing anatomical planes (axial, coronal, sagittal) in radiological imaging?

Answers to Critical Thinking Questions

1.(d); 2.(c); 3.(c); 4.(b); 5.(c)

REFERENCES

1. Alaosta, A. M. S. (2025). Assessment of cervical spine surgery in ankylosing spondylitis. *South Eastern European Journal of Public Health*. https://www.semanticscholar.org/paper/eed46e8548358acf7f09cfb1bfda98de0aa08913 (accessed on 30 May 2025).
2. Alshammary, N. S., & Alwahdani, M. N. (2024). The effectiveness of interventional radiology procedures in minimally invasive treatments: (Critical review). *The Medical Journal of Cairo University*. https://www.semanticscholar.org/paper/52ab4ba46159f2bb6ffbac2e68b73e57342dedad (accessed on 30 May 2025).
3. Audenaert, E., Mahieu, P., Pattyn, C., Van Hoof, *et. al.* (2010). Soft tissue structure modelling for use in orthopedic applications and musculoskeletal biomechanics. https://core.ac.uk/download/55761253.pdf (accessed on 30 May 2025).
4. Bangash, A. H., Toledo, J., Essibayi, M. A., Haranhalli, N., De la Garza Ramos, R., Altschul, D. J., Tjoumakaris, S., *et. al.* (2025). State-of-the-art for automated machine learning predicts outcomes in poor-grade aneurysmal subarachnoid hemorrhage using routinely measured laboratory & radiological parameters: Coagulation parameters and liver function as key prognosticators. *Neurosurgical Review, 48*. https://www.semanticscholar.org/paper/e979c1d1b0a89cc33946921b1aa427878a9f86a2 (accessed on 30 May 2025).
5. Bhardwaj, S., Sakale, H., Agrawal, A. C., Kar, B., Dash, R. N., Rai, A., & Garg, A. (2024). A comparison of the clinic radiological outcomes of intertrochanteric fractures treated using proximal femoral nail and proximal femoral nail anti-rotation. *Cureus, 16*. https://www.semanticscholar.org/paper/de2da8530e7d5d7defd8f730cfc3d62d2300267d (accessed on 30 May 2025).
6. Bogdanov, T. G., Hikov, T., Sabit, Z. A., Tafradzhiyska-Hadzhiolova, R., & Pencheva, D. (2025). Development of a 3D-printed Wistar rat model from digital imaging and communications in medicine (DICOM) data for medical education and research applications. *Cureus, 17*. https://www.semanticscholar.org/paper/af9d2ae1d0d362c5c1eb32029fd1dc8f66dc8848 (accessed on 30 May 2025).
7. Borg-Xuereb, H. K., Grech, S., & McKearney, R. M. (2013). Audit on the use of radiological investigations in the management of rhinosinusitis. https://core.ac.uk/download/46602404.pdf (accessed on 30 May 2025).
8. Brady, A. P., Allen, B., Chong, J. J. R., Kotter, E., Kottler, N., Mongan, J., Oakden-Rayner, L., *et. al.* (2024). Developing, purchasing, implementing and monitoring AI tools in radiology: Practical considerations. A multi-society statement from the ACR, CAR, ESR, RANZCR & RSNA. *Insights into Imaging, 15*. https://www.semanticscholar.org/paper/0eb0e917f7698dd90c6dbf7d03f844a8a8250022 (accessed on 30 May 2025).
9. Brandt, A., Malkin, A. A., Zanoni, B., Khoury, B., Stuckler, D., Krupinski, E. A., Patton, G. C., *et. al.* (2011). Pediatric radiology seen from Africa. Part I: Providing diagnostic imaging to a young population. https://core.ac.uk/download/pdf/10674304.pdf (accessed on 30 May 2025).
10. Brennan, P., Galvin, P. L., Grech, R., *et. al.* (2014). Imaging of adult ocular and orbital pathology–a pictorial review. https://core.ac.uk/download/323186424.pdf (accessed on 30 May 2025).

11. Chorbińska, J., Krajewski, W., & Zdrojowy, R. (2021). Urological complications after radiation therapy—Nothing ventured, nothing gained: A narrative review. *Translational Cancer Research, 10*, 1096–1118. https://www.semanticscholar.org/paper/7251f2903c91024c4a3b8b88e057fd85f7e5ec18 (accessed on 30 May 2025).

12. Cornwall, J., White, R., Pennefather, P., Hildebrandt, S., Gregory, J., Smith, H. F., Organ, J. M., *et. al.* (2025). Legal and ethical considerations around the use of existing illustrations to generate new illustrations in the anatomical sciences. *Anatomical Sciences Education, 18*, 289–300. https://www.semanticscholar.org/paper/7fefccc7ada091b5eff6c07c3e61323a4210f411 (accessed on 30 May 2025).

13. Covelli, E., Bozzao, A., Meliante, P., Filippi, C., Pizzolante, S., Elfarargy, H. H., Romano, A., *et. al.* (2025). Decoding cholesteatoma radiological dimensions: Unveiling the discrepancy between CT and MRI imaging and development of a predictive model based on CT and MRI volume comparison. *Acta Oto-Laryngological.* https://www.semanticscholar.org/paper/7ca3e6943007e7ba3ee75b16dc9475e679a5c0fe (accessed on 30 May 2025).

14. Davis, L. M., Martinez-Correa, S., Freeman, C., Adams, C., Sultan, L. R., Le, D. Q., Lemessa, N. F., *et. al.* (2024). Ultrasound innovations in abdominal radiology: Techniques and clinical applications in pediatric imaging. *Abdominal Radiology (New York), 50*, 1744–1762. https://www.semanticscholar.org/paper/384926c5227775a5ff44582cb2924f7566a01039 (accessed on 30 May 2025).

15. Dehdab, R., Brendlin, A. S., Werner, S., Almansour, H., Gassenmaier, S., Brendel, J. M., Nikolaou, K., *et. al.* (2024). Evaluating ChatGPT-4V in chest CT diagnostics: A critical image interpretation assessment. *Japanese Journal of Radiology, 42*, 1168–1177. https://www.semanticscholar.org/paper/f866397509357b3da9cff9afded4e80ec2a988f2 (accessed on 30 May 2025).

16. Ding, H., Hai, Y., Zhou, L., Liu, Y., Zhang, Y., Han, C., & Zhang, Y. (2023). Clinical application of personalized digital surgical planning and precise execution for severe and complex adult spinal deformity correction utilizing 3D printing techniques. *Journal of Personalized Medicine, 13*. https://www.semanticscholar.org/paper/9a02d999afe744ec4770f8e5cd1855ea2a61bb64 (accessed on 30 May 2025).

17. Edouard, A., Ibrahim, A. A., Shama, S., Abdelnabi, M. M., Birindwa, P. B., & Elwany, S. (2022). Radiological anatomy of foramen rotundum and its surgical implications. *The Egyptian Journal of Otolaryngology, 38*. https://www.semanticscholar.org/paper/7587527f7b7ba48c99647f6dd5ce7ff71bd5e5f3 (accessed on 30 May 2025).

18. Folz, C., Mö, M., Sintek, M., Wennerberg, P., & Seifert, S. (2009). Extending the foundational model of anatomy with automatically acquired spatial relations. https://core.ac.uk/download/pdf/288617.pdf (accessed on 30 May 2025).

19. Gargi, V., Bhadage, C. J., & Bhoosreddy, A. (2025). Radiological analysis of maxillary sinus anatomy in the 1st molar region in different ages and genders—A cone beam CT study. *SRM Journal of Research in Dental Sciences.* https://www.semanticscholar.org/paper/2370da693a8957f5dc3b617d12e61b155865b620 (accessed on 30 May 2025).

20. Ghaffar, A., Gillani, S. A. J., & Imam, S. F. (2023). Unmasking the unforeseen: A case of radiological tension empyema mimicking a traumatic hemothorax. *Cureus, 15*. https://www.semanticscholar.org/paper/4bd74c522f59f5d1bc0ded04be01c0d360d64851 (accessed on 30 May 2025).

21. Goel, A., McDonald, A., Madawi, A. A., Brooks, A. L., McLaughlin, A. M., Montano, A. M., Ransford, A. O., *et. al.* (2013). Spinal involvement in mucopolysaccharidosis IVA (Morquio-Brailsford or Morquio A syndrome): Presentation, diagnosis and management. https://core.ac.uk/download/323073297.pdf (accessed on 30 May 2025).

22. Herrmann, J., Ording-Müller, L., Franchi-Abella, S., Verhagen, M. V., McGuirk, S., Dammann, E., Bokkers, R., *et. al.* (2023). European Society of Pediatric Radiology survey of perioperative imaging in pediatric liver transplantation: (1) pre-transplant evaluation. *Pediatric Radiology, 54*, 260–268. https://www.semanticscholar.org/paper/8e6834b06415de7127e9f1758b40fb0db0cf1be8 (accessed on 30 May 2025).

23. Hunt, L., Annibali, F., Cuillandre, J., Ferguson, A., Jablonka, P., Larsen, S., Marleau, F., *et. al.* (2024). Euclid: Early release observations–Deep anatomy of nearby galaxies. https://www.semanticscholar.org/paper/ef5d9e808cc4b92c645de104c1212c75630c8271 (accessed on 30 May 2025).

24. Isselbacher, E. M., Preventza, O., Black, J. H., Augoustides, J., Beck, A. W., Bolen, M. A., Braverman, A. C., *et. al.* (2022). 2022 ACC/AHA guideline for the diagnosis and management of aortic disease: A report of the American Heart Association/American College of Cardiology Joint Committee on Clinical Practice Guidelines. *Circulation, 146*. https://doi.org/10.1161/cir.0000000000001106.

25. Karaismailoğlu, B., Peiffer, M., Raduan, F., Hollander, J., Knebel, A., Kwon, J. Y., Bejarano-Pineda, L., *et. al.* (2024). Heatmaps on radiological safety in minimally invasive midfoot fusion: A cadaver study. *Foot & Ankle Orthopedics, 9*. https://www.semanticscholar.org/paper/5422a8fba71eb1376d56fcf4c96680f5e0e4d009 (accessed on 30 May 2025).

26. Karstens, J., Boer, L., Maal, T., & Henssen, D. (2024). The possible impact of segmenting radiological images on students' spatial abilities. *Discover Education*. https://www.semanticscholar.org/paper/266a9910647c8e2a53566f43844d0a6c1b94ebd9 (accessed on 30 May 2025).

27. Kelly, B. S., Clifford, S., Judge, C., Bollard, S. M., Healy, G. M., Hughes, H., Colleran, G. C., *et. al.* (2024). A survey of pediatric radiology artificial intelligence. https://www.semanticscholar.org/paper/5ec047b4f22be5d5a9b1ed458234de88da54f84d (accessed on 30 May 2025).

28. Laurier, D., Schneider, T., *et. al.* (2024). Workshop on the future of radiological protection. *Radioprotection*. https://www.semanticscholar.org/paper/2a2cd4c506004989f0233d758289da685f28d55d (accessed on 30 May 2025).

29. LeBoff, M. S., Greenspan, S. L., Insogna, K., Lewiecki, E. M., Saag, K. G., Singer, A., & Siris, E. S. (2022). The clinician's guide to prevention and treatment of osteoporosis. *Osteoporosis International, 33*, 2049–2102. https://doi.org/10.1007/s00198-021-05900-y.

30. Lee, K., Lin, J., Lynch, J., & Smith, P. (2023). Radiological classification of the pelvis: A tool for trauma surgery planning. *Orthopedic Proceedings*. https://www.semanticscholar.org/paper/c262f950a43d24f11677352401e673a9c9bdb3be (accessed on 30 May 2025).

31. Lee, Y. J., Hong, J. H., Kim, Y. J., Lee, T. K., Jung, T., Kim, I. Y., Jung, S., *et. al.* (2022). Comparison of scoring systems for the prediction of complication rates in intracranial meningioma resection of the elderly. *Journal of Korean Skull Base Society*. https://www.semanticscholar.org/paper/fae1700a01e5ed7fa93f9a289bde1ba421bca8e6 (accessed on 30 May 2025).

32. Machado, L., Philippe, H., Ferreres, É., Khlaut, J., Dupuis, J., Le Floch, K., Gatenyo, D. H., *et. al.* (2024). ONCOPILOT: A promotable CT foundation model for solid tumor evaluation. *ArXiv*. https://www.semanticscholar.org/paper/1c95fcdb19c2402b5d3e49b67750178c5477d9f0 (accessed on 30 May 2025).

33. Medical Association of Chinese Medical Association Digital, Intelligent Surgery Committee of Chinese Research Hospital Ass Digital, C. C. O. C. M. D. A. Liver, Precise Medicine Professional Committee Clinical, Imaging and Equipment Professional Committee of China Grap Medical, Imaging Professional Committee of China Biophysical Societ Molecular. (2019). Guidelines for application of computer-assisted indocyanine green molecular fluorescence imaging in diagnosis and surgical navigation of liver tumors (2019). *Nan Fang Yi Ke Da Xue Xue Bao = Journal of Southern Medical University, 39*(10), 1127–1140. https://www.semanticscholar.org/paper/c296821c685874c7952aaa9ea7051f38bb070ac4 (accessed on 30 May 2025).

34. Mujika, K. M., Méndez, J. A. J., & Framiñán, A. (2018). Software applications for the digital management of radiological images in the study of the corticospinal tract. Proceedings of the Sixth International Conference on Technological Ecosystems for Enhancing Multiculturality. https://www.semanticscholar.org/paper/f044fed26b32dacde86dcc0e50bd71629f1b4d47 (accessed on 30 May 2025).

35. Mulliqi, N., Blilie, A., Ji, X., Szolnoky, K., Olsson, H., Boman, S. E., Titus, M., *et. al.* (2025). Foundation models–A panacea for artificial intelligence in pathology? https://www.semanticscholar.org/paper/516d76eb4547667ff9191853afc407fedb0564e4 (accessed on 30 May 2025).

36. Najjar, R. (2023). Redefining radiology: A review of artificial intelligence integration in medical imaging. *Diagnostics, 13*, 2760. https://doi.org/10.3390/diagnostics13172760.

37. Newhauser, W., Gress, D. A., Mills, M., Jordan, D. W., Sutlief, S. G., Martin, M., & Jackson, E. F. (2022). Medical physics workforce in the United States. *Journal of Applied Clinical Medical Physics, 23*. https://doi.org/10.1002/acm2.13762.

38. Nguyen, B., Thien, L., Huyen, D., Ngo, Q. D., Nguyen, T. H. A., Dung, L., & NguyenCuong, H. (2024). Assessment of radiological anatomy of prostatic artery on 3D DECT in symptomatic benign prostatic hypertrophy. *Acta Informatica Medica, 32*, 107–111. https://www.semanticscholar.org/paper/0ac4d38ba9f6aa6f49aaccc0f33968fd1edc50dd (accessed on 30 May 2025).

39. Nizar, A. M., & Subash, Y. (2024). A short-term study of 18 cases of distal femur fractures managed by locking compression plate (LCP) using a less invasive skeletal stabilization system (LISS). *South Eastern European Journal of Public Health*. https://www.semanticscholar.org/paper/33bc647fcb52df7196936ac6793c7af7b88c42c5 (accessed on 30 May 2025).

40. Omkaram, K., Nalabolu, M. R., Galeti, E., Reddy, V., Reddy, B., & Galeti, A. (2021). A rare case of post radiation urinary bladder necrosis in a patient with carcinoma cervix. *Annals of Urologic Oncology*. https://www.semanticscholar.org/paper/9f728945cd5015c2f862ab04be43ca3e97519e9e (accessed on 30 May 2025).

41. Ou, Y., Chen, Q., Xu, D., Gong, J., Li, M., Tang, M., Wu, D., *et. al.* (2023). Anatomical digital twins for medical education: A stepwise guide to create perpetual multimodal three-dimensional reconstruction of digital brain specimens. *Quantitative Imaging in Medicine and Surgery*. https://www.semanticscholar.org/paper/b054bf50a6a5750256f5f00a340084eef5e00fbe (accessed on 30 May 2025).

42. Petrov, V., & Pankiv, M. (2024). Application of three-dimensional digital technologies to display the structure of the heart. *Eastern Ukrainian Medical Journal*. https://www.semanticscholar.org/paper/6d0c075c554063c01c23a4c0ef8e0a3ec193b4ff (accessed on 30 May 2025).

43. Vandana, M., Suri, R., Ravi, S., Vandana, D., & Gayatri, R. (2011). Clinical submission of supernumerary head of adductor brevis muscle. https://core.ac.uk/download/11490057.pdf (accessed on 30 May 2025).

44. Rakhlin, A., Kalinin, A. A., Spampinato, C., Thodberg, H. H., Tanner, J., Ronneberger, O., Gilsanz, V., *et. al.* (2018). Pediatric bone age assessment using deep convolutional neural networks. http://arxiv.org/abs/1712.05053 (accessed on 30 May 2025).

45. Ramalingam, S., Kumar, K., Dhivaakar, V., & Santhosh, M. S. (2023). Functional outcome of surgical management of mid-diaphyseal clavicle fractures treated by plate osteosynthesis. *Journal of Orthopedics, Traumatology and Rehabilitation*. https://www.semanticscholar.org/paper/8ee71b9f97d859ceafe315b3e705b4fdd3d0e325 (accessed on 30 May 2025).

46. Saraswathula, A., Huang, E. Y., Li, S., Garcia, J. R., & Rowan, N. (2024). Improving the educational accessibility of sinonasal and skull base anatomy: A novel virtual tool for otolaryngology trainees. *Eye & ENT Research*. https://www.semanticscholar.org/paper/9bdde35f042dc5bae9afd577e0f2b400f82c5cba (accessed on 30 May 2025).

47. Shama, N., Mathai, J., Rai, E., & Kodiatte, T. (2021). Elucidating the anatomy of a rare communicating bronchopulmonary foregut malformation (CBPFM) in a preschool child. *BMJ Case Reports, 14*. https://www.semanticscholar.org/paper/0d52222df48317cc8ed1ab6cbefb4c9810c83548 (accessed on 30 May 2025).

48. Sharma, N., Chitapure, T., & Bhalerao, A. (2022). A narrative review of anatomy and clinical biopsychosocial assessment of sacroiliac joint pain. *Journal of Clinical and Diagnostic Research*. https://www.semanticscholar.org/paper/a7a011a6b20d4e4c5b758dc10ec966d3e9d5e41a (accessed on 30 May 2025).

49. Sharples, M., Jeffery, N. P., du Boulay, B., Teather, B. A., Teather, D., & du Boulay, G. H. (2000). Structured computer-based training in the interpretation of neuroradiological images. *International Journal of Medical Informatics, 60*(3), 263–280. https://doi.org/10.1016/s1386-5056(00)00101-5.

50. Symes, R., Keddie, S. H., Walker, J., McKeever, T., Ahmad, S., Arnold, D., Evans, C. M., *et. al.* (2025). Estimating the disease burden of respiratory syncytial virus (RSV) in older adults in England during the 2023/24 season: A new national hospital-based surveillance system. https://www.semanticscholar.org/paper/46cc949c37444336e0b7469239dc7b20ec447f14 (accessed on 30 May 2025).

51. Taylor, P. M. (2007). A review of research into the development of radiologic expertise: Implications for computer-based training. https://core.ac.uk/download/1673134.pdf (accessed on 30 May 2025).

52. Tmenova, O., Velikova, Y., Saleh, M., & Navab, N. (2024). Deep spectral methods for unsupervised ultrasound image interpretation. *arXiv preprint* abs/2408.02043. https://www.semanticscholar.org/paper/2a3fd79fcaee04a5521f83c206c665c58bb22fe5 (accessed on 30 May 2025).

53. Tobias, J. (2015). Pediatric airway anatomy may not be what we thought: Implications for clinical practice and the use of cuffed endotracheal tubes. *Pediatric Anesthesia, 25*. https://

www.semanticscholar.org/paper/12d3dc641a46e7f1dc07775ddefd31b47dd8a3fc (accessed on 30 May 2025).

54. Vincenzi, M., Rigoni, B., Manuppelli, C., Mazzoli, M., & Balestriero, G. (2024). Endovascular embolization of a biliary-digestive loop bleeding. *Journal of Medical Imaging and Interventional Radiology*. https://www.semanticscholar.org/paper/c56501b730dd7f535c2bb430ec61fcde503a32f4 (accessed on 30 May 2025).

55. Wojciechowski, T. (2023). Radiologic anatomy of the middle ear and inner ear in computed tomography images. *Polski Przegląd Otorynolaryngologiczny*. https://www.semanticscholar.org/paper/d83eec875bfa28dc0cee235c90c7d760c6bf80a3 (accessed on 30 May 2025).

56. Zhou, S. K., Greenspan, H., Davatzikos, C., Duncan, J. S., van Ginneken, B., Madabhushi, A., Prince, J. L., *et. al.* (2021). A review of deep learning in medical imaging: Imaging traits, technology trends, case studies with progress highlights, and future promises. *Proceedings of the IEEE, 109*, 820–838. https://doi.org/10.1109/jproc.2021.3054390.

CHEST RADIOLOGY

6

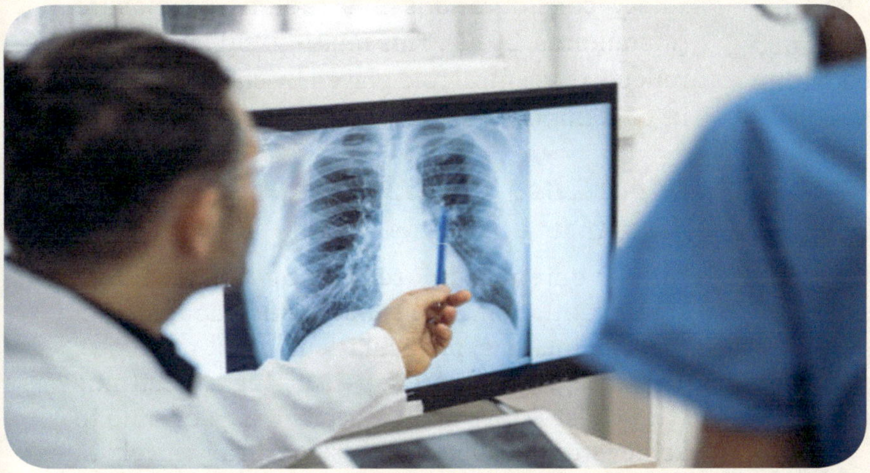

LEARNING OBJECTIVES

After studying this chapter, you will be able to:

1. Identify imaging techniques in chest radiology
2. Explain common chest conditions diagnosed
3. Discuss the interpretation of chest radiographs
4. Focus on clinical applications and guidelines

Introduction

Advancements in medical imaging technologies have significantly impacted thoracic disease diagnosis and treatment, and offered clinicians useful tools for the investigation of lung pathology with accuracy. Among these technologies, chest radiology remains a cornerstone for investigating pulmonary disease due to its ease, speed, and cost-effectiveness. Imaging modalities such as chest X-ray, computed tomography (CT), and ultrasonography (EUS) provide critical information about a broad spectrum of chest pathology, from infectious diseases such as pneumonia to congenital abnormalities in the pediatric population. The diagnostic value of these techniques is brought to light in emergent circumstances such as the COVID-19 pandemic, where common radiological features such as ground glass opacities and consolidations contribute to early diagnosis and quantification of disease severity (Rahman *et. al.*, 2025). Along with this, new imaging protocols for children help in achieving a balance between diagnostic quality and minimizing exposure to radiation, addressing the specific challenges in neonatal and pediatric chest pathology (Lovrenski *et. al.*, 2025). This background sets the context for a detailed review of the role of chest radiology in clinical practice.

Definition of Chest Radiology

Progress in medical imaging has revolutionized the diagnosis and management of thoracic disease to supply never-before-seen information on pulmonary and cardiovascular disease. Chest radiology is one of the medical imaging techniques and is a group of methods intended to radiograph the body structures housed within the thoracic cage, such as the lungs, heart, and related tissues. Its principal function is to detect, characterize, and follow up illnesses such as infection, tumor, and vascular malformations.

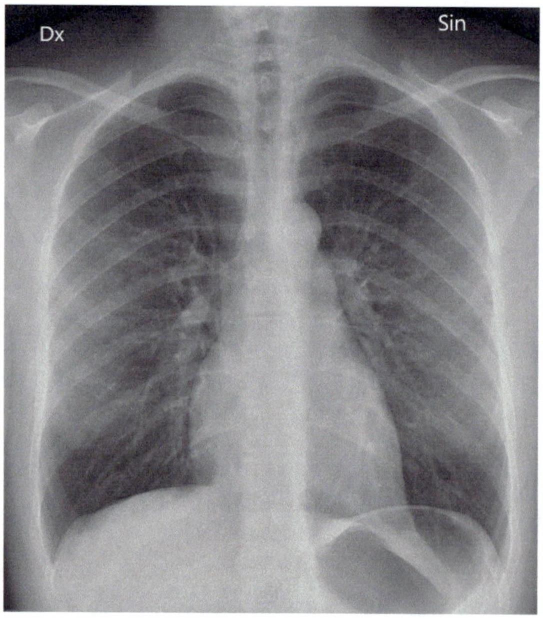

Figure 6.1. Chest radiology, a specialized branch within medical imaging, encompasses various techniques aimed at visualizing the structures within the thoracic cavity, including the lungs, heart, and surrounding tissues.

Source: https://upload.wikimedia.org/wikipedia/commons/a/a1/Normal_posteroanterior_%28PA%29_chest_radiograph_%28X-ray%29.jpg.

For example, CT scans allow for the precise assessment of lung nodules that may be indicative of underlying pathologies like neuroendocrine tumors or ectopic hormone-secreting lesions, as seen in advanced diagnostic challenges of Cushing syndrome (Han *et. al.*, 2016). Whole chest radiology integrates clinical evaluation with evidence-based imaging techniques for maximizing patient outcomes and resource utilization, while ensuring accuracy against safety considerations like radiation exposure (Matamoros, 2012). This multi-disciplinary focus reflects the central role played by chest radiology in contemporary medicine (Figure 6.1).

Importance of Chest Radiology in Medicine

Improvements in technology have also significantly enhanced diagnostic capability in medical imaging, particularly in chest radiology. The integration of deep learning algorithms with chest X-rays and CT scans has been able to achieve up to 90% and 98% accuracy levels in detecting potentially life-threatening conditions such as pneumonia and COVID-19, respectively. Explainable Artificial Intelligence (XAI) systems are increasingly being deployed to explain these decisions, encouraging greater clinical trust and transparency. While practitioner sentiment towards such systems has proven positive in their opinion, technical challenges and limited general understanding still limit their effective use in healthcare settings. In addition, chest radiology remains an integral component of neonatology, including chest radiographs and lung ultrasonographies, to largely contribute to early and accurate diagnoses of conditions like Transient Tachypnoea of the Newborn, facilitating timely interventions. These are some of the areas that attest to the pivotal role chest radiology plays in diverse clinical practices, enhancing patient outcomes and more informed clinical decision-making (Izegbua *et. al.*, 2024; Kumar *et. al.*, 2024).

Historical Background of Chest Radiology

The evolution of chest radiology is closely tied to the grand development of medical imaging technologies and diagnostic strategies. Early progress centered around the use of X-rays, discovered by Wilhelm Conrad Roentgen in 1895, that quickly transformed clinical practice by enabling non-surgical imaging of the chest cavity. As radiographic technology advanced, clinicians were able to obtain valuable data on pulmonary structure and disease, greatly enhancing infection diagnosis, such as tuberculosis (TB) and pneumonia. Subsequent advances in resolution and contrast resolution expanded diagnostic capability. More recently, the intersection of computational methods, notably deep learning and convolutional neural networks, revolutionized chest radiology by enabling computerized image analysis and improved diagnostic performance. These biologically derived neural network architecture-based machine learning (ML) algorithms learn adaptively from large data sets to identify subtle patterns that may be elusive to human detection, representing a revolutionary path that bridges traditional radiologic methods with state-of-the-art data-driven diagnostics (Chartrand *et. al.*, 2017; Raghu *et. al.*, 2020).

Role of Radiologists in Diagnosis

The successful detection of chest diseases greatly relies on the expertise of radiologists interpreting sophisticated imaging tests, such as chest X-rays and high-resolution computed tomography (HRCT) scans. Their role is more than simply ,identifying abnormalities; radiologists integrate clinical and imaging information to optimize diagnostic accuracy. For instance, in idiopathic pulmonary fibrosis, interpretation of HRCT requires careful communication between pulmonologists and radiologists to put radiologic findings into the context of the clinical history of the patients so that a more accurate diagnosis can be made and further multidisciplinary discussion if necessary (Chung *et. al.*, 2018). Additionally, radiologists are important in resource-constrained settings where TB and pneumonia are prevalent diseases via the provision of specialized pediatric imaging expertise responding to certain challenges of radiation protection and the need for individualized diagnostic processes (Brandt *et. al.*, 2011). This interdisciplinary and cooperative approach emphasizes the unique role of radiologists in chest radiology's diagnostic pathway (Figure 6.2).

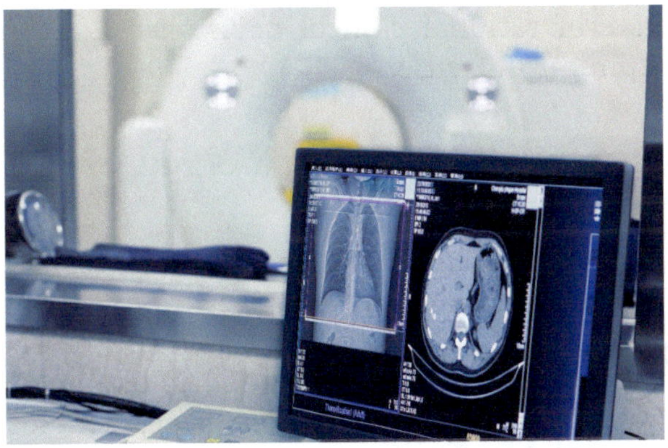

Figure 6.2. The accurate diagnosis of chest diseases relies heavily on the expertise of radiologists who interpret complex imaging studies, such as chest X-rays and high-resolution computed tomography (HRCT) scans.

Source: https://www.touchstoneimaging.com/wp-content/uploads/2023/01/iStock-520128028-scaled.jpg.

Common Conditions Diagnosed with Chest Radiology

The function of chest radiology is a critical one in the detection of a variety of thoracic pathologies, often first because of its presence and speed. Pneumothorax, pneumonia, lung mass, and mediastinal disease are some of the abnormalities that may otherwise be undetected until more severe symptoms arise. For instance, secondary pneumothorax, a common clinical emergency, can be readily diagnosed alongside pneumomediastinum complications using chest X-rays, enabling immediate and potentially life-saving interventions (Bhatia *et. al.*, 2012). Additionally, subtle findings such as early infiltrates or small-sized pleural effusions are frequently recognized during routine examinations, guiding the choice of additional testing or therapeutic interventions. The importance of chest radiology is highlighted in cases where clinical assessment by itself is not satisfactory and radiological findings become an essential requirement for optimal diagnosis and management. Imaging thus becomes the pillar of rational clinical decision-making in respiratory disease.

Advances in Chest Radiology Technology

The evolution of imaging technologies has increased diagnostic accuracy and patient care in chest radiology to a significant extent. Improved digital radiography and CT equipment now capture higher resolution images with less radiation dose, allowing doctors to detect subtle pulmonary and mediastinal diseases earlier than before. Some newer technologies include enhancements in detector sensitivity and sophisticated image post-processing algorithms to allow better visualization of delicate anatomical structures. In addition, integration with AI algorithms facilitates automation of high-priority case prioritization and anomaly detection, thereby enhancing workflow and reducing diagnostic errors. These developments herald a move away from traditional film-based imaging towards newer, more dynamic and adaptive digital modalities that provide for rapid image capture and real-time analysis. Visual demonstration of such current imaging facilities puts on display the tremendous progress that has been made in this field, as can be contrasted with research of old and new modalities. Such advancements illustrate the pivotal role that technology assumes in enhancing the practice of chest radiology (Figure 6.3).

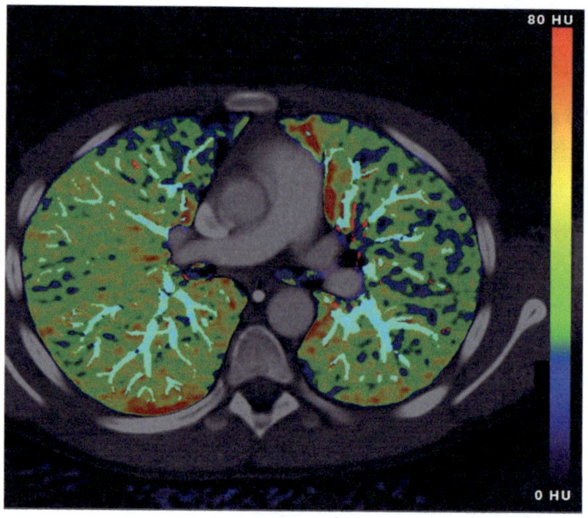

Figure 6.3. Enhanced digital radiography and computed tomography systems now offer higher resolution images with reduced radiation exposure, allowing clinicians to detect subtle pulmonary and mediastinal abnormalities earlier than before.

Source: https://ajronline.org/cms/10.2214/AJR.23.29244/asset/images/large/23_29244_02d_cmyk.jpeg.

Challenges in Chest Radiology

Technology has progressed remarkably in medical imaging, but chest radiology faces certain challenges that make accurate diagnosis and interpretation challenging. The most prominent among them is the complex thoracic anatomy, where interposed structures create subtle signs of pathology, which are difficult to identify. Also, variable use of imaging techniques and patient positioning influence image quality and uniformity. AI application in chest radiology has potential solutions, but current AI models require large, task-specific annotated data, which is scarce and costly to obtain. Emerging paradigms like generalist medical AI are attempting to solve these problems through self-supervised learning across multiple datasets, thus enhancing flexibility and diagnostic performance (Moor *et. al.*, 2023). Despite these advances, deep learning approaches also have to counteract issues such as noisy labels, interpretability, and uncertainty quantification in order to ensure clinical reliability in chest imaging tasks (Zhou *et. al.*, 2021). These issues underscore the need for continued innovation to improve diagnostic accuracy in chest radiology.

6.1. Imaging Techniques in Chest Radiology

Learning Outcome

1. Explain X-ray imaging
2. Discuss computed tomography (CT) scans
3. Focus on magnetic resonance imaging (MRI)
4. Describe ultrasound in chest imaging
5. Understand positron emission tomography (PET)
6. Learn fluoroscopy in chest radiology
7. Know contrast agents in imaging
8. Identify 3D imaging techniques
9 Know future trends in imaging technologies

Advances in imaging technology have significantly enhanced diagnostic capabilities in chest radiology, particularly with development in CT. Iterative reconstruction (IR) algorithms are now an invaluable tool with better picture quality through reduction of noise and artifacts, thus facilitating easier visualization of thoracic anatomy. IR algorithms involve cyclic image processing, which goes beyond using filtered back projection methods, allowing reduced doses of radiation without diminishing diagnosis. The efficiency of IR techniques varies according to the specific algorithm applied, but in all cases, results in improved chest imaging outcomes. Furthermore, routine chest radiography remains fundamental, supplemented by developments in digital processing and detector technology that enhance image resolution and contrast (Bastarika *et. al.*, 2015). Alongside these advances, high-resolution imaging and advanced software visualization enhance more precise assessment of pulmonary pathologies, mediastinal disease, and vascular illness, thereby increasing the clinical responsibility of chest radiology.

6.1.1. X-Ray Imaging

Machine learning (ML) advancements have significantly improved the effectiveness of X-ray imaging in chest radiology, addressing age-old challenges such as the requirement for large annotated datasets and model interpretability in diagnostic models. Recent studies have introduced new solutions, including Ensemble-CAM, an ensemble framework based on class activation mapping using weakly supervised learning to conduct effective thoracic disease detection with reduced reliance on strongly annotated data.

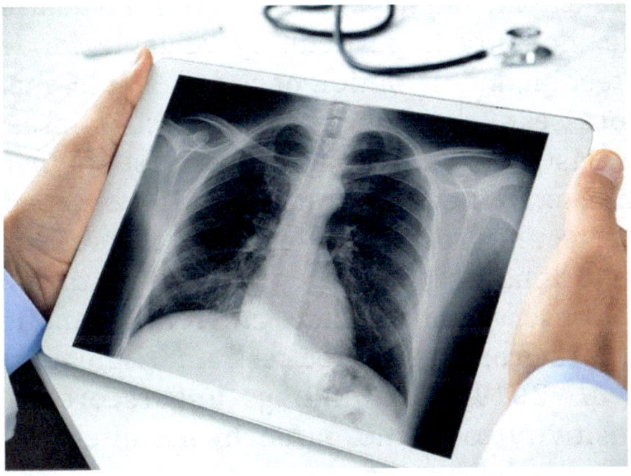

Figure 6.4. X-ray imaging in chest radiology.

Source: https://media.post.rvohealth.io/wp-content/uploads/2020/08/chest-x-ray_thumb-1-732x549.jpg.

This approach not only improves diagnostic accuracy but also provides a graphical depiction of the disease localization, which increases the confidence level of doctors regarding the results (Aasem *et. al.*, 2024). Furthermore, deep learning architectures such as ResNet-50 have been successfully used to accurately demarcate cardiac regions on chest X-rays by employing complex preprocessing and augmentation techniques to make the model insensitive enough to perform across different clinical conditions (Rathod *et. al.*, 2024). Together, they point to the growing potential of AI-assisted X-ray imaging for improving the speed of diagnosis, especially in environments where professional examination may not be immediately available (Figure 6.4).

6.1.2. Computed Tomography (CT) Scans

Advances in imaging technology have significantly enhanced the diagnostic capabilities in chest radiology, most significantly by way of CT scans. Compared to routine radiographs, CT provides high-resolution cross-sectional imaging that allows for detailed visualization of lung parenchyma, airways, and adjacent structures. The modality is particularly valuable for the detection and definition of complex pulmonary processes such as idiopathic pulmonary fibrosis. For instance, a study of awake West Highland white terriers demonstrated that CT was capable of detecting ground glass opacities and reticular alterations of pulmonary fibrosis with high interobserver concordance and reduced motion artifacts from specialized restraint (Holopainen *et. al.*, 2019). The findings underscore CT's sensitivity to subtle parenchymal alterations that can be missed on planar images. Also, advances in dual-slice and helical scanning techniques have improved the speed and quality of chest CTs, achieving maximum patient comfort and diagnostic capability. Therefore, CT is a diagnostic mainstay in modern-day chest radiology.

6.1.3. Magnetic Resonance Imaging (MRI)

Technical advances in imaging have had a significant effect on diagnostic precision and patient care, especially in chest radiology. MRI provides superior soft tissue contrast without the use of ionizing radiation, making it extremely useful for the characterization of complex thoracic masses and distinguishing benign from malignant disease. Advances in speed and resolution in MRI have augmented its clinical role in the assessment of mediastinal masses, chest wall disease, and cardiovascular disease. Furthermore, the intersection of XAI and deep learning in MRI processing promises to enhance the delicacy of image interpretation so that more accurate and precise diagnoses are possible in chest pathology (Bas et al., 2022). Safety considerations, nevertheless, regarding gadolinium-based contrast media remain in the spotlight, and the work goes on with a view to limiting risks associated with tissue retention of gadolinium (Val *et. al.*, 2021). Thus, MRI continues to evolve as a needed tool in chest radiology, balancing the fine line of technological advancement and patient safety to optimize diagnostic returns.

6.1.4. Ultrasound in Chest Imaging

Technological advances in imaging technology have drastically changed diagnostic avenues available for thoracic pathology, and ultrasound has emerged as a valuable tool to complement routine chest X-ray. Unlike X-rays or CT scans, ultrasound allows dynamic imaging without ionizing radiation, and thus is a superior choice in some clinical scenarios, especially for bedside evaluation of pleural effusions, pneumothorax, and chest wall masses. Its mobility and dynamic imaging capability allow for rapid assessment and immediate interventional procedures, such as thoracentesis.

However, the efficiency of ultrasound is limited by air interference and inability to penetrate bone, which restricts its application in pleural and superficial lung diseases but not deep pulmonary diseases. New developments in high-frequency probes and better image algorithms have increased resolution and diagnostic sensitivity, and resulted in a more advanced characterization of chest diseases.

Such developments highlight the growing relevance of ultrasound in chest radiology as a verification of its status as a valuable commodity alongside more established modalities (Figure 6.5).

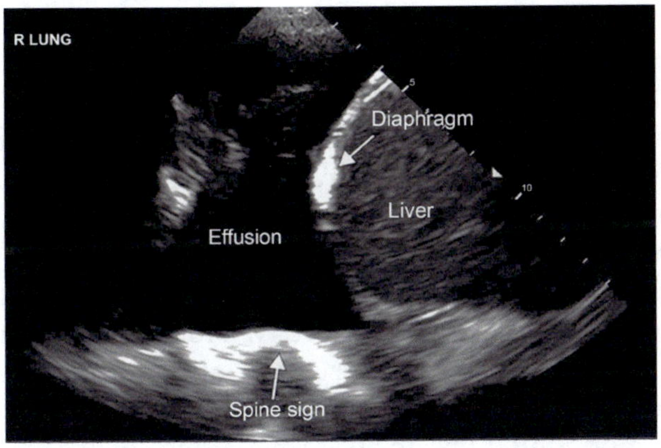

Figure 6.5. Unlike X-rays or CT scans, ultrasound offers real-time visualization without exposure to ionizing radiation, making it preferable in certain clinical scenarios, especially for bedside assessment of pleural effusions, pneumothorax, and chest wall abnormalities.

Source: https://pubs.rsna.org/cms/10.1148/ryct.2021200564/asset/images/medium/ryct.2021200564.fig8.gif.

6.1.5. Positron Emission Tomography (PET)

Medical imaging technologies have played critical roles in diagnostic technology for chest radiology, particularly through the integration of functional imaging modalities. Of these, Positron Emission Tomography (PET) has unparalleled information by imaging metabolism rather than anatomy in isolation, providing critical information in the evaluation of thoracic cancers and inflammatory diseases. The use of radiotracers, such as fluorodeoxyglucose (FDG), enables PET to identify hypermetabolic lesions more specifically, distinguishing malignant tumors from benign lesions. This functional imaging complements conventional radiographic and CT imaging and enables more accurate staging and treatment planning. In addition, PET has also been shown to be useful in assessing response to therapy and detecting recurrence and has emerged as an essential tool in patient management. While valuable, the limitations of relatively low spatial resolution compared to CT and radiation exposure necessitate its use as a part of a multimodal imaging protocol, rather than as an individual isolated examination.

6.1.6. Fluoroscopy in Chest Radiology

Advances in imaging technology have significantly expanded the scope of diagnostic tools available to chest radiology, with fluoroscopy playing a vital role in dynamic thoracic structure evaluation. Compared to static X-ray, fluoroscopy provides real-time imaging, enabling physicians to observe respiratory mechanics, swallowing dynamics, and circulation within the chest. However, this real-time imaging technique has the underlying aspect of extended exposure to radiation, necessitating cautious precautions to avoid harm.

Use of dose alerts and procedural checklists is now a necessity in minimizing patient radiation burden and preventing tissue reactions related to cumulative doses, as described in contemporary guidelines for radiological safety (Damilakis *et. al.*, 2017). Fluoroscopy's utility is not confined to guidance of interventional procedures in which precision is critical. Its utility must be pursued while keeping in mind equipment controls and the requirement for optimizing technique to avoid unnecessary overexposures. Proper use of fluoroscopy thus balances diagnostic advantages against prudent control of the radiation, underlined by ongoing education and adherence to best practice (Damilakis *et. al.*, 2017) (Figure 6.6).

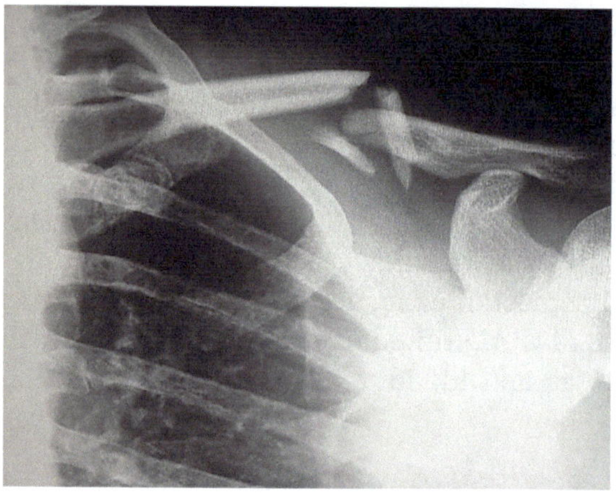

Figure 6.6. Technological advancements in imaging have significantly enhanced the diagnostic capabilities available to chest radiology, with fluoroscopy playing a pivotal role in dynamic assessment of thoracic structures.

Source: https://www.glmi.com/static/sitefiles/blog/glmixrays_thumb1_thumb.png.

6.1.7. Contrast Agents in Imaging

Technological advances in chest radiology have significantly enhanced diagnostic validity, partly due to the development and use of contrast agents to visualize. Contrast agents increase the clarity between anatomical and pathological processes by altering the attenuation or signal characteristics within the chest cavity. Iodinated contrast agents, for example, are used regularly in CT to enhance vascular and soft tissue definition, providing critical information on such conditions as pulmonary embolism or neoplastic disease. The same applies to gadolinium agents in magnetic resonance imaging (MRI), which maximize the visualization of mediastinal masses and chest wall extension. Their selection and administration must be properly determined based on the provision of patient safety, renal function, and potential allergic sensitivity. Besides, there are new contrast media emerging continuously with greater specificity and fewer toxicities, all of which contribute to elevating the levels of chest imaging analysis. All these advances highlight the pivotal role of contrast media in contemporary chest radiology.

6.1.8. 3D Imaging Techniques

Technical advances in medical imaging have also significantly enhanced the scope of diagnostic capability in chest radiology, particularly through the development of three-dimensional (3D) imaging modalities. Compared to conventional two-dimensional radiographs, 3D imaging offers volumetric information that affords higher resolution visualization of thoracic anatomy for better evaluation of complex anatomical relationships and pathology. Modalities such as CT and 3D reconstruction allow clinicians to identify lesions, vascular disease, and airway remodeling more accurately, making earlier and more accurate diagnoses possible.

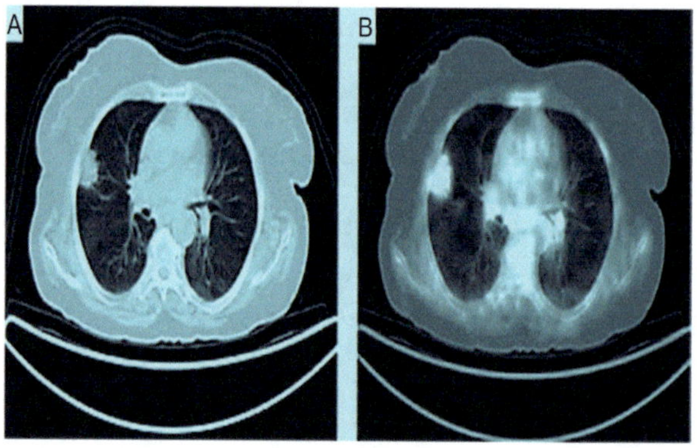

Figure 6.7. Modalities such as computed tomography (CT) and 3D reconstruction allow clinicians to identify lesions, vascular abnormalities, and airway changes with greater precision, aiding in earlier and more accurate diagnoses.

Source: https://media.springernature.com/lw1200/springer-static/image/art%3A10.1186%2Fs12880-024-01192-w/MediaObjects/12880_2024_1192_Fig7_HTML.png.

Use of foundation models trained on large datasets has further enhanced these approaches since AI algorithms can now assist with the interpretation of intricate image patterns, improve the quality of images, and provide contextual reasoning without involving substantial retraining (Azad *et. al.*, 2023). This union of advanced imaging and ML improves diagnostic confidence and the ability to reduce invasive testing. Therefore, ongoing refinement of 3D chest imaging is a significant step forward for patient care (Figure 6.6).

6.1.9. Future Trends in Imaging Technologies

Advances in imaging technologies will, in the years to come, significantly transform the practice of chest radiology, promoting diagnostic capability and patient outcomes. The integration of AI in modalities such as CT and MRI is particularly auspicious, enabling enhanced image assessment and generation as well as maximized image quality with the aid of sophisticated ML algorithms. These technological advancements have also witnessed the lowering of acquisition dose and time, especially for CT scans, which addresses some of the conventional issues concerning safety. Moreover, the transition from old film-based radiographs to digital image systems necessitates the updating of training and interpretation standards, such as with initiatives like the AIR Pneumo program for long-term proficiency in diagnosing pneumoconiosis in Asia. These developments emphasize the paramount importance of technology not only in image acquisition but also in harmonizing diagnostic criteria throughout the world so that radiologists can optimally utilize sophisticated instruments for the evaluation of thoracic diseases (Kantarcı *et. al.*, 2025; Tungsagunwattana *et. al.*, 2025).

Test Your Knowledge

1. What are the limitations of chest X-rays compared to CT scans?
2. How does contrast-enhanced CT help in evaluating vascular structures in the chest?

6.2. Common Chest Conditions Diagnosed

Learning Outcome

1. Understand pneumonia, tuberculosis, and lung cancer
2. Explain chronic obstructive pulmonary disease (COPD)
3. Focus on pulmonary embolism
4. Describe interstitial lung disease
5. Know pleural effusion
6. Define mediastinal masses
7. Discuss congenital anomalies of the chest

Radiologic evaluation lies at the heart of the diagnosis of many different diseases in the chest, and provides valuable information that guides clinical management. It is one of the most frequent conditions diagnosed, including pulmonary nodules, inflammatory conditions such as pneumonia, and heart disease. High-density lesions on lung imaging typically represent a diagnostic challenge and necessitate differential diagnoses between benign and malignant conditions, inflammatory and deposition diseases (Jaramillo *et. al.*, 2024). The overlapping clinical features of inflammatory conditions of the heart, like myocarditis, pericarditis, and endocarditis, are resolved using specialized imaging techniques like cardiac magnetic resonance. This modality offers improved tissue characterization and the ability to pick up mild myocardial inflammation, the effect of which plays a key role in guiding patient management decisions (Dominici *et. al.*, 2024). Therefore, correlating the clinical presentation with radiologic findings is important in order to accurately diagnose ordinary chest diseases and attain the best therapeutic outcomes.

6.2.1. Pneumonia

Technical innovations in imaging have significantly enhanced the diagnosis and treatment of pulmonary disease, the most important being pneumonia due to its life-threatening nature. Early detection of pneumonia is crucial since timely intervention can transform patient outcomes dramatically. Chest radiology, particularly digital chest X-rays, remains a primary diagnostic tool, but the addition of new approaches such as deep learning algorithms has increased classification accuracy between bacterial and viral pneumonias to 98% or more for differentiating normal from pneumonia cases (Chowdhury *et. al.*, 2020).

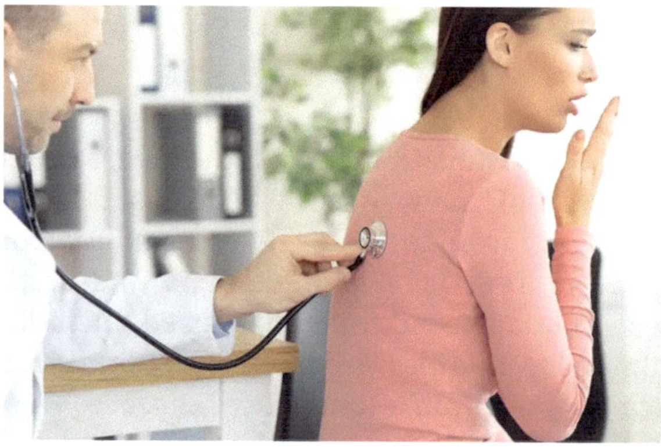

Figure 6.8. Early and accurate identification of pneumonia is essential, as timely intervention can drastically improve patient outcomes.

Source: https://thumbnails.icloudhospital.com/tr:w-1536,f-webp,q-75/1-e6b2eac9-f6b5-4076-a0cb-ace2b8376600.webp.

Additionally, MRI is acting as a true alternative or adjunct, especially in children, yielding complete morphological and functional lung information without irradiation (Hebestreit *et. al.*, 2011). While MRI is now more of an ancillary tool in the diagnosis of pneumonia, its potential to provide better diagnostic information can alter future clinical practice and allow for more individualized and effective treatment in chest radiology (Figure 6.8).

6.2.2. Tuberculosis (TB)

Advances in chest radiology have significantly enhanced the detection and treatment of pulmonary diseases, and TB is a significant area of interest due to its widespread prevalence across the globe and its varied radiographic appearance. Chest X-rays are a dominant screening agent for TB, but may be hard to interpret due to overlapping imaging features from other diseases of the lung. Recent integration of artificial intelligence, such as deep learning algorithms like convolutional neural networks, has shown promising potential to improve diagnostic accuracy and consistency by reading chest radiographs and computed tomographic scans more accurately than traditional methods. AI algorithms can rapidly identify faint radiographic signs of TB, allowing earlier interventions and better patient outcomes, especially in low-resource environments where specialist radiologists can be scarce. However, clinical uptake of success relies on surmounting the obstacle of data variability, model interpretability, and workflow embedding to attain dependability as well as bolster clinician trust in AI-based diagnosis (Ahmad *et. al.*, 2024; Bartoszek *et. al.*, 2025).

6.2.3. Lung Cancer

Advances in chest radiology have made a significant contribution to early diagnosis and delineation of lung cancer, a leading cause of cancer mortality worldwide. Imaging by radiography, particularly HRCT, is the cornerstone of the detection of pulmonary nodules and differentiation between malignant and benign lesions. The subtle patterns revealed by imaging tests give precise staging, which is most important for prognostic establishment and therapeutic decisions. Furthermore, the integration of radiologic findings with clinical information enables intensive assessment of tumor aggressiveness and dissemination, enabling specifically targeted interventions. New imaging technologies continue to bring enhanced visualization of minute abnormalities, enhancing diagnostic performance and enabling earlier intervention. These advances continue to highlight the importance of chest radiology in multidisciplinary lung cancer treatment, evidenced by recent advances published in the field. This evolving setting carries the potential for improved patient outcomes from early and accurate diagnosis (Figure 6.9).

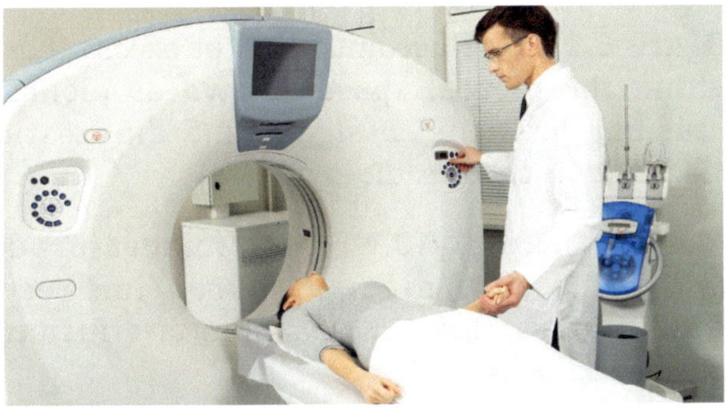

Figure 6.9. Radiographic imaging, particularly high-resolution computed tomography (CT), plays a pivotal role in identifying pulmonary nodules and distinguishing malignant from benign lesions.

Source: https://irp.cdn-website.com/c47c802a/dms3rep/multi/1-6d21bd49.png.

6.2.4. Chronic Obstructive Pulmonary Disease (COPD)

Technological advancements in imaging modalities have significantly enhanced diagnostic sensitivity and understanding of pulmonary diseases. In the case of COPD, chest radiology comes to the forefront in measuring disease severity and progression. Routine X-ray imaging, while available to the majority, is usually insensitive to the detection of mild emphysematous alterations. However, the introduction of new techniques, such as grating-based X-ray dark-field imaging, has also been found to improve projection sensitivity through combining transmission and dark-field signals. The technique is capable of providing high-resolution parametric mapping of emphysema distribution with high correlation with histopathological results, in addition to providing a better evaluation than regular X-rays alone (Achterhold *et. al.*, 2013). Furthermore, MDCT and new MRI techniques enable morphological and functional evaluation of the lung. These methods help in phenotypic characterization and enhance understanding of COPD pathogenesis and hence facilitate insights into individualized therapeutic strategies (Bonomo *et. al.*, 2007).

6.2.5. Pulmonary Embolism

Technical advancements within chest radiology have significantly contributed to the diagnosis and management of most thoracic illnesses, particularly pulmonary embolism (PE). Even though computed tomography pulmonary angiography (CTPA) remains the gold standard for embolus detection in the lungs' circulation, MRI has emerged as a valuable adjunct, especially in patients where minimal radiation exposure is preferred, e.g., pregnant women and adolescents. MRI yields morphologic and functional information through the quantification of regional lung perfusion and respiratory mechanics and is therefore the preferred choice in some clinical contexts. Although there are some limitations regarding availability and expertise, MRI is equally diagnostic compared to conventional modalities with no ionizing radiation exposure and therefore enhances patient safety without diminishing diagnostic yield. This emerging use of MRI in the diagnosis of PE is a testament to its value as an adjunct modality to chest imaging, enabling early and precise intervention in acute presentations and facilitating thorough pulmonary evaluation (Hebestreit *et. al.*, 2011) (Figure 6.10).

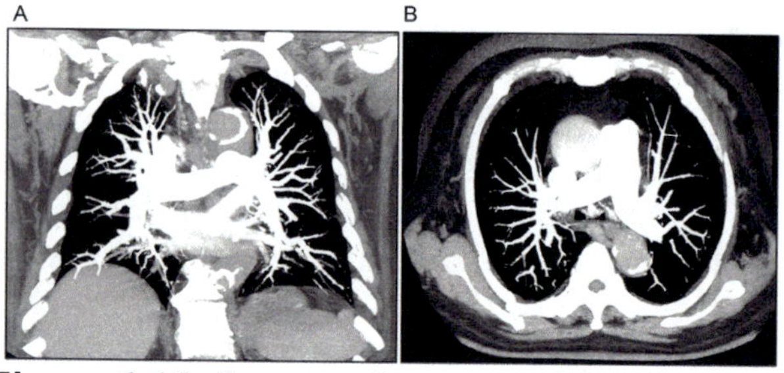

Figure 6.10. Computed tomography pulmonary angiography (CTPA).

Source: https://www.researchgate.net/publication/342383454/figure/fig3/AS:906020771610637@1593023593910/Computed-tomography-pulmonary-angiography-CTPA-A-coronal-B-axial-of-a-77-year-old.ppm.

6.2.6. Interstitial Lung Disease (ILD)

Advances in imaging technologies have significantly enhanced diagnostic possibilities for complex pulmonary conditions, yielding copious information on lung pathology beyond plain radiology. Interstitial Lung Disease (ILD), due to its variable presentation and superimposable imaging characteristics, is difficult to diagnose. Even though HRCT is the gold standard, interest in MRI as an adjunct is rising. MRI is an advantage to provide both morphological and functional information without using ionizing radiation, particularly valuable in young patients and those requiring repeat imaging. Nevertheless, although MRI can be helpful, its clinical application in ILD has not been definitively proven and is reserved for research contexts, rather than standard practice (Hebestreit *et. al.*, 2011). In addition, ultrasound techniques, employed more often in intensive care units, hold promise for assessing lung involvement and disease progression when combined with other imaging methods (Chong *et. al.*, 2020).

6.2.7. Pleural Effusion

Deposition of excess fluid into the pleural space, as described by pleural effusion, is among the significant diagnostic challenges in chest radiology. It has a frequent occurrence across various clinical contexts, including infections like TB and viral pneumonias like COVID-19, whose imaging features might overlap with other pulmonary pathologies.

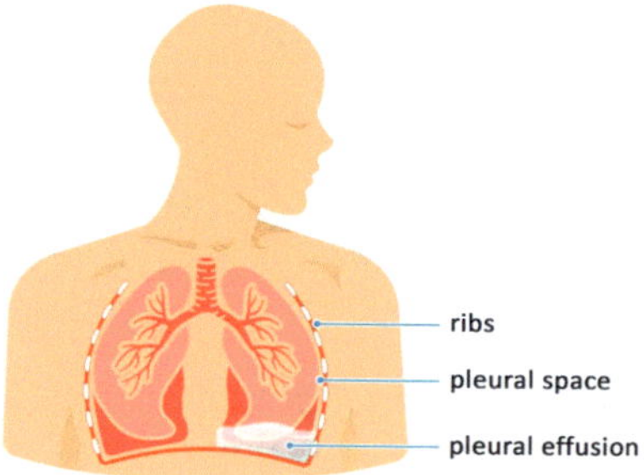

Figure 6.11. The accumulation of excess fluid within the pleural space, known as pleural effusion, presents a significant diagnostic challenge in chest radiology.

Source: https://i0.wp.com/images-prod.healthline.com/hlcmsre*source*/images/topic_centers/fluidinChest_pleural-effusion.jpg?w=1155&h=1497

Radiologic imaging, particularly chest X-ray and CT scan, is central in the detection of pleural effusion, which has characteristic findings such as blunting of costophrenic angles or layering of fluid. Higher imaging and deep learning image analysis have optimized effusion detection, with the ability to distinguish from other pathological processes such as consolidation or ground-glass opacities seen in infectious diseases (Rahman *et. al.*, 2025; Salkade *et. al.*, 2025). Accurate diagnosis of pleural effusion is imperative in guiding appropriate therapeutic maneuvers and maximizing patient outcomes, emphasizing the importance of integrating traditional radiological assessment with new computational technology in modern chest radiology practice (Figure 6.11).

6.2.8. Mediastinal Masses

Diagnosis and characterization of mediastinal masses are highly reliant on advanced imaging modalities in chest radiology since most lesions are clinically nonspecific. CT remains the gold standard to establish the anatomical location, size, and internal composition of mediastinal masses and to differentiate between cystic, solid, and vascular lesions. MRI further enhances the characterization of soft tissue in more complex cases. Although ultrasound has a limited but significant complementary function, especially in guiding percutaneous biopsies, it is an important modality in evaluating chest wall extension and enabling safe tissue sampling to obtain histopathological evidence (Zadeh *et. al.*, 2023). Among mediastinal masses, e.g., lymphangiomas, though rare in adults, need to be considered due to their symptomatology potential and differential diagnostic challenge; curative surgical excision is the rule and emphasizes the importance of proper imaging and clinical correlation (Fatema *et. al.*, 2024). Consistent with this, multimodal imaging integration optimizes diagnostic accuracy and therapeutic decision-making in chest radiology.

6.2.9. Congenital Anomalies of the Chest

Evaluation of congenital anomalies of the chest requires precise imaging methods that can provide detailed anatomical and functional information. Advances in chest radiology, particularly with the use of CTA and MRI, have significantly enhanced the detection and characterization of such anomalies. CTA, using standardized systems like CAD-RADS, improves coronary artery anomaly evaluation accuracy through reproducible stenosis and findings classification, of critical value in the careful treatment of congenital defects of cardiac structures (Razek *et. al.*, 2018). Conversely, fetal MRI is a superior adjunctive tool to ultrasound in prenatal diagnosis, overcoming problems introduced by fetal movement and providing better visualization of thoracic malformations antenatally (Stafrace *et. al.*, 2008). These imaging advances not only make precise diagnosis possible but also facilitate enhanced clinical decision-making, with increased focus on integrating various radiologic approaches in the comprehensive assessment of congenital chest defects (Figure 6.12).

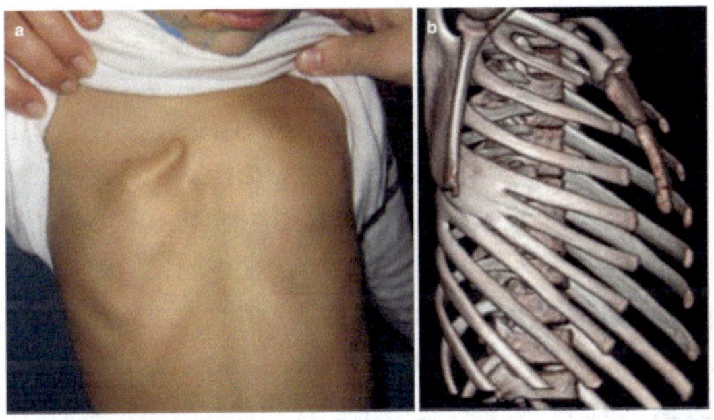

Figure 6.12. Congenital anomalies of the chest.

Source: https://media.springernature.com/lw685/springer-static/image/chp%3A10.1007%2F978-3-319-93534-8_9/MediaObjects/333563_1_En_9_Fig5_HTML.png.

Test Your Knowledge

1. What are the most common chest conditions diagnosed using imaging techniques?
2. How does radiology help differentiate between cardiac and pulmonary causes of chest pain?

6.3. Interpretation of Chest Radiographs

Learning Outcome

1. Understand the anatomy of the chest on radiographs
2. Explain the systematic approach to reading chest x-rays
3. Identify common radiographic signs
4. Focus on differentiating pathologies
5. Know the role of clinical history in interpretation
6. Discuss limitations of chest radiographs
7. Describe the importance of follow-up imaging
8. Learn the use of artificial intelligence in interpretation
9. Discuss case studies in radiographic interpretation

Advances in artificial intelligence, or AI, have begun to transform the reading of chest radiographs with promising potential for improving the accuracy and efficiency of diagnosis. Traditional radiographic review is highly reliant on the experience and individual judgment of radiologists, with the potential to lead to inconsistency and some diagnostic errors. New development in deep learning techniques specifically tailored for chest X-rays has demonstrated excellent potential in identifying complex cardiac defects, such as atrial septal defect and ventricular septal defect, more accurately than some experienced practitioners (Jia *et. al.*, 2024). Besides, automated reporting of complex radiology from chest X-ray images is also gaining popularity, leveraging robust neural network architectures employing attention and transformer models to produce clinically informative stories, potentially reducing workload and accelerating patient management (Dhamanskar *et. al.*, 2024). These developments underscore the evolving role of computer-assisted technology in chest radiology, as a response to the need for continued research solving problems of data quality and interpretive complexity, finally directed toward improving diagnostic accuracy and healthcare delivery.

6.3.1. Anatomy of the Chest on Radiographs

It is important to understand the radiologically visible anatomical landmarks on chest films in order to provide accurate diagnosis and treatment of thoracic disease. The chest X-ray provides a two-dimensional image of complex anatomy, including lungs, heart, mediastinum, and bony chest. Knowledge of normal anatomy, for instance, pulmonary vasculature, diaphragmatic contours, and rib cage alignment, allows clinicians to identify pathological changes more accurately.

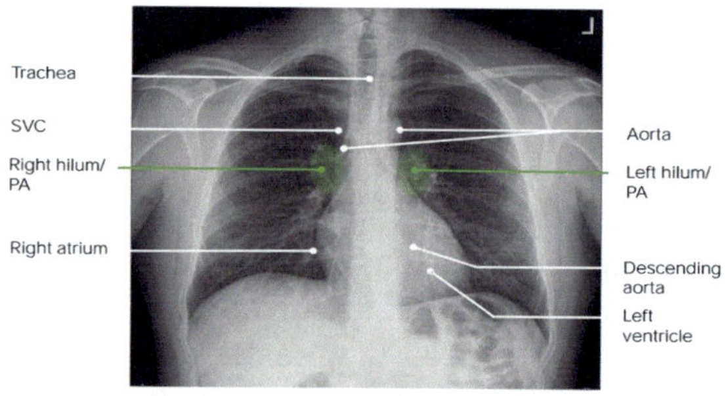

Figure 6.13. The chest X-ray provides a two-dimensional representation of complex structures, including the lungs, heart, mediastinum, and bony thorax.

Source: https://cdn.lecturio.com/assets/Normal-PA-view-chest-X-ray-with-labels-1.jpg.

For instance, air loss situations such as pneumothorax or pneumomediastinum, traditionally diagnosed by disruptions in such anatomical barriers, have been highly prevalent among subjects undergoing invasive ventilation for acute respiratory disease (Goossen *et. al.*, 2023). Moreover, quantifiable radiological involvement, as indicated by chest X-ray scores, can guide clinical decision-making via structural abnormalities' concordance with the severity of the disease and the prognosis, particularly in conditions like COVID-19 (Eroglu *et. al.*, 2021). Therefore, familiarity with chest anatomy on X-rays is the foundation of appropriate radiologic assessment and subsequent patient management in chest radiology (Figure 6.13).

6.3.2. Systematic Approach to Reading Chest X-Rays

A comprehensive evaluation of chest X-rays requires a systematic, disciplined process that minimizes the likelihood of overlooking subtle but clinically significant findings. To begin with, patient information and image check-off are the foundation for accurate interpretation. Then, a systematic examination proceeds from the bony contours and soft tissues through to the lungs, heart, mediastinum, and diaphragm in such a manner that all anatomical structures are examined in an orderly step-by-step fashion. This methodical method helps to detect abnormalities such as infiltrates, masses, or effusions, and also facilitates the detection of abnormalities in normal anatomical relationships. Application of such a method is crucial to offer diagnostic precision as well as reproducibility, especially when slim radiographic findings may be correlated with intricate clinical presentations, such as in situations of immune reconstitution or emerging pulmonary pathology (Bader *et. al.*, 2014; Elze *et. al.*, 2011). Lastly, systematic examination of chest radiographs remains a cornerstone technique in chest radiology which can enable effective clinical decision-making based on thorough and consistent image analysis.

6.3.3. Common Radiographic Signs

Radiographic imaging remains the foundation of the diagnosis of widespread thoracic pathology, with specific findings representing vital signs of underlying disease. Methodical analysis of chest radiographs, for instance, in pediatric chest radiology, enables the differentiation of neonatal lung disease, with specific findings such as diffuse ground-glass opacities or air bronchograms pointing towards respiratory distress syndrome or bronchopulmonary dysplasia (Lovrenski *et. al.*, 2025). In adults, characteristic but subtle chest X-ray patterns reveal congenital heart disease; dilated cardiac silhouettes, increased vascular pulmonary markings, and abnormal contouring lead to diagnosis and management of these challenging conditions (William *et. al.*, 2024). The detection of such common radiographic findings enhances the diagnostic process by correlating imaging observations with clinical presentation Additionally, the integration of patient history information, such as gestational age or prior interventions, further supports interpretation, enabling timely and appropriate treatment planning. Last but not least, proficiency in these radiographic signs is the foundation of successful chest radiology practice for all age groups (Figure 6.14).

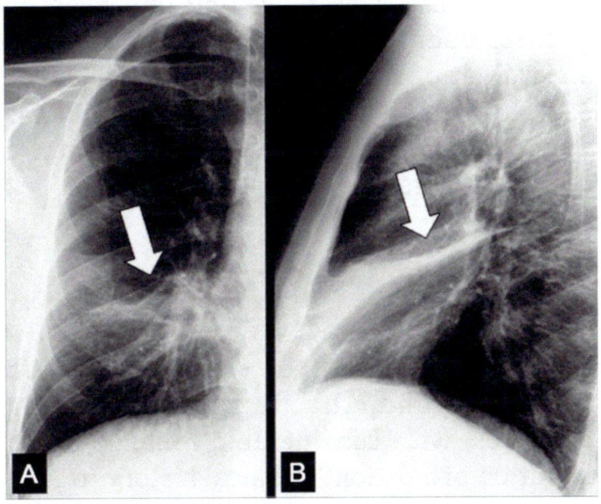

Figure 6.14. Radiographic imaging remains a cornerstone in diagnosing a wide array of thoracic conditions, with specific signs serving as critical indicators of underlying pathology.

Source: https://pubs.rsna.org/cms/10.1148/radiol.232558/asset/images/medium/radiol.232558.fig34.gif.

6.3.4. Differentiating Pathologies

Accurate reading of chest X-rays is critical in the clinical setting since subtle radiologic variation tends to separate severe pathologies such as pneumonia, TB, cardiomegaly, and COVID-19. The marriage of advanced computing systems, especially deep learning algorithms like convolutional neural networks, has enhanced the ability to detect ,subtle patterns in X-rays with accuracy beyond traditional human interpretation. These models leverage massive datasets to teach algorithms that are capable of differentiating between overlapping radiographic features, reducing diagnostic faults, and accelerating timely treatment (Goswami *et. al.*, 2024). Furthermore, the advent of vision-language models has introduced sophisticated multimodal analysis with a fusion of image comprehension and contextual clinical data to create more complete and uncertainty-laden radiology reports. This technique not only improves diagnostic accuracy but also surmounts false confidence and interpretative vagueness traditionally encountered in abnormal scan evaluations (Sharma, 2024). Collectively, these advances focus on a shift toward more uniform and interpretable differentiation of chest pathologies.

6.3.5. Role of Clinical History in Interpretation

Proper interpretation of chest radiographs extends beyond the radiologic findings themselves, with considerable reliance on the integration of a patient's clinical history to assist in diagnostic precision. Clinical information that incorporates symptoms, exposure history, and relevant laboratory values provides context that may differentiate among radiologic patterns that appear to be similar, particularly in complex disorders like ILD. For instance, in idiopathic pulmonary fibrosis, patterns of HRCT must be interpreted within the framework of clinical data to avoid misdiagnosis and to create the necessity further multidisciplinary deliberation by pulmonologists, radiologists, and other experts (Chung *et. al.*, 2018). Secondly, the application of large annotated datasets with clinical complications can increase the ability of ML algorithms to identify subtle radiographic findings, recognizing the relationship between imaging interpretations and patient history (Ball *et. al.*, 2019). Last but not least, clinical history incorporation in radiological results encourages a more precise, accurate, and patient-specific diagnosis of chest radiology (Figure 6.15).

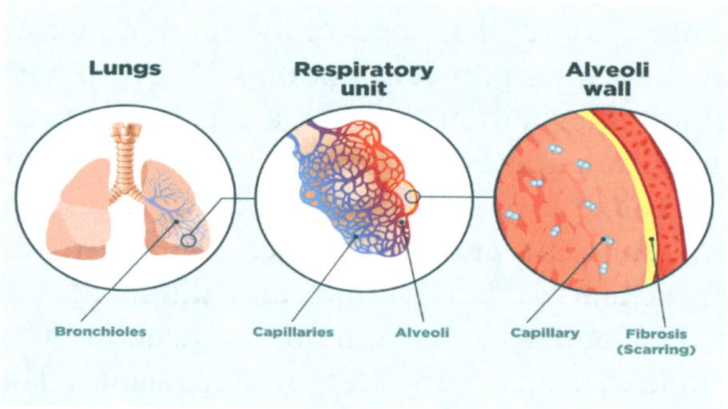

Figure 6.15. Clinical information such as symptoms, exposure history, and relevant laboratory results provides essential context that can differentiate between similar radiologic patterns, particularly in complex diseases like interstitial lung disease.

Source: https://med.stanford.edu/ild/patient-resources/understanding-ild/_jcr_content/main/panel_builder/panel_0/panel_builder/panel_1/image.img.620.high.jpg/ILD-Understanding-fibrosis-stages.jpg.

6.3.6. Limitations of Chest Radiographs

Even if a fundamental diagnostic tool, chest radiographs have a number of inherent limitations that affect precision and clinical utility, one such limitation is the need for large amounts of high-quality data to train advanced ML models that are capable of interpreting such images accurately. Restricted access to datasets available, particularly for rare conditions or poly-ethnic populations, restricts the development of universally relevant algorithms, hence limiting diagnostic precision (Sellergren *et. al.*, 2022). This issue is even exacerbated in pediatric imaging, as the absence of large-scale, publicly available datasets hampers AI advancement and limits automated interpretation to a limited subset of diseases, primarily pneumonia (Padash *et. al.*, 2022). Furthermore, chest radiographs inherently offer two-dimensional representations of three-dimensional anatomy, which can obscure subtle pathologies and overlapping between normal tissues, and hence introduce potential misinterpretations. These hence require appropriate complementary imaging modalities and judicious clinical correlation in order to enhance diagnostic confidence in chest radiology.

6.3.7. Importance of Follow-Up Imaging

In the clinical setting, the initial imaging is often only a snapshot of a patient's state, and follow-up evaluation is necessary to monitor disease progression or response to treatment accurately. Follow-up imaging in chest radiology is necessary to delineate changes over time, distinguish between benign and malignant lesions, and identify potential complications following intervention. It is most important, however, in percutaneous lung biopsy situations, where baseline imaging guides the procedure but sequential scans are essential to recognize complications such as pneumothorax or pulmonary hemorrhage and to evaluate therapeutic outcomes (Andrani *et. al.*, 2017). Early imaging follow-up ensures early detection of recurrence or progression, which significantly influences patient therapy and prognosis. Besides, improvements in imaging technology enable high-resolution visualization, enhancing the accuracy of follow-up diagnostics. Thus, implementation of systematic follow-up imaging protocols in chest radiology plays a pivotal role in optimal patient management (Figure 6.16).

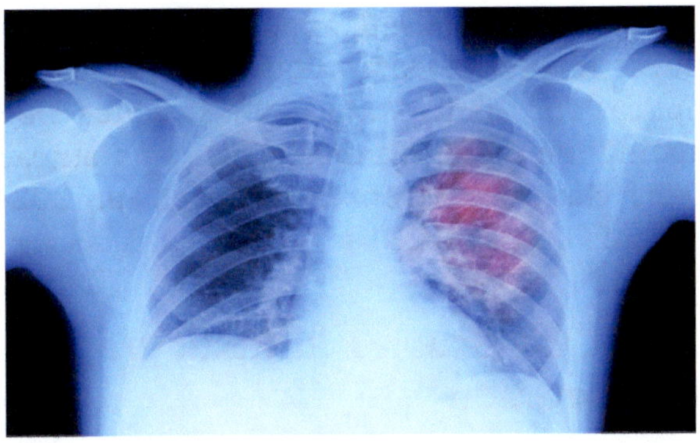

Figure 6.16. Follow-up imaging in chest radiology plays a crucial role in delineating changes over time, distinguishing benign from malignant lesions, and identifying potential complications post-intervention.

Source: https://www.verywellhealth.com/thmb/GSrw3MG3Lkne6xP0YkWpHGTgdd8=/1500x0/filters:no_upscale():max_bytes(150000):strip_icc()/x-ray-of-lung-showing-chest-cancer-103046683-594a631f3df78c537b68ea18.jpg.

6.3.8. Use of Artificial Intelligence in Interpretation

New AI innovations have had a considerable influence on the practice of chest radiology by expanding image interpretation and diagnostic quality. AI-based machine vision algorithms enable automatic chest radiograph and CT scan analysis that is often at least as good as, and sometimes superior to, that of highly skilled radiologists. These technologies are based on highly advanced algorithms, such as convolutional neural networks, to identify anatomical structures and pathological abnormalities with high speed and accuracy. In thoracic imaging, not only is AI able to speed detection of abnormalities, but it also makes the workflow smoother by reducing human error and assisting with challenging decision-making tasks. Furthermore, the use of AI in modalities like ultrasound-guided interventions and airway evaluation demonstrates its growing clinical use beyond static image interpretation.

Despite such promising applications, there are issues, including data requirements, ethical implications, and AI model bias, which need ongoing tuning for maximal safety and efficacy in the clinical environment (Jin *et. al.*, 2024; Lonsdale *et. al.*, 2023).

6.3.9. Case Studies in Radiographic Interpretation

Incorporation of CBL into radiographic reporting has been a major benefit to enhancing diagnostic competency, particularly in chest radiology. Research indicates that students who are exposed to case-based courses in radiology exhibit improved long-term ability to interpret difficult radiographs and produce sound reports, focusing on active learning over traditional lectures (Devine *et. al.*, 2025). This educational method not only builds confidence but also equips students better for clinical problems by mimicking conditions in real life. Furthermore, with developments in AI comes complementary assistance with interpreting chest radiographs by achieving or exceeding the precision of typical radiologists, particularly in low-ambiguity conditions, with high expertise in recognizing normal findings (Ndiaye *et. al.*, 2025). Nevertheless, the limited sensitivity of AI in the detection of abnormalities confirms the necessity of human expertise. Therefore, case studies are still quite crucial in learning interpretive skills, and when combined with AI tools, they can potentially improve diagnostic quality and pedagogic outcomes in chest radiology.

Test Your Knowledge

1. What are the key steps in a systematic approach to interpreting a chest radiograph?
2. What landmarks should be used to assess for patient rotation?

6.4. Clinical Applications and Guidelines

Learning Outcome

1. Learn guidelines for chest imaging in acute care
2. Know screening recommendations for lung cancer
3. Explain the role of chest radiology in preoperative assessment
4. Discuss imaging protocols for specific conditions
5. Focus on patient safety and radiation exposure
6. Describe ethical considerations in chest imaging
7. Understand a multidisciplinary approach in patient management
8. Explain tele-radiology and remote consultations
9. Discuss future directions in clinical applications

Technological advancements in chest radiology have contributed significantly to clinical decision-making by evidence-based standards that maximize patient care. Multidisciplinary professional panels have established more stringent guidelines for ILD diagnosis, including idiopathic pulmonary fibrosis, so that less intrusive transbronchial lung cryobiopsy is recommended in specialist centers without exposing the researchers to unnecessary anti-reflux therapy, thus achieving the dual purpose of diagnostic efficacy and patient safety (Raghu *et. al.*, 2022). The COVID-19 pandemic brought into focus the critical role played by chest CT imaging, especially in establishing severity, guiding management, and predicting long-term complications. According to expert opinion, routine CT usage is not advised due to specificity concerns and resource availability, and it is suggested to be employed primarily in patients with declining respiratory status or uncertain molecular tests (Machnicki *et. al.*, 2021). Standardized reporting systems, including the RSNA classification and CO-RADS scoring, have universalized and predictive chest imaging interpretations, facilitating triage and prognosis. The guidelines collectively represent the progressive alignment of chest radiology with clinical pathways through promotion of evidence-based, adapted interventions (Figure 6.17).

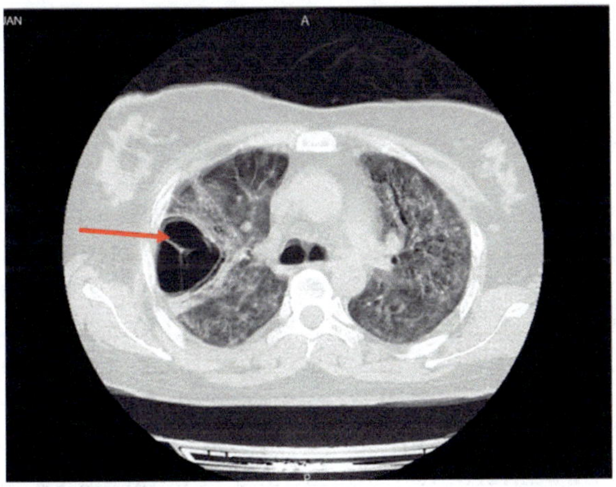

Figure 6.17. The emergence of COVID-19 underscored the critical role of chest CT imaging, especially in assessing disease severity, guiding management, and predicting long-term complications.

Source: https://pub.mdpi-res.com/amh/amh-69-00008/article_deploy/html/images/amh-69-00008-g001.png?1715151046.

6.4.1. Guidelines for Chest Imaging in Acute Care

Prompt and correct diagnosis in an acute setting relies on the best use of chest imaging, where clinical decision-making must balance the urgency of the patient's condition with the appropriateness of imaging modalities. Guidelines for chest imaging in the acute setting address the need for prioritizing imaging modalities that yield rapid, accurate information with minimal redundant exposure and consumption of resources. Chest X-ray remains the initial imaging modality due to its availability, speed, and immediate recognition of significant conditions such as pneumothorax, pulmonary edema, or pneumonia. CT is used as an adjunct modality in cases where chest radiographs are nondiagnostic or when more advanced evaluation of complex pathologies is required. The application of standardized ordering and interpretation guidelines for these imaging tests works to optimize diagnostic yield and improve patient outcomes. Additionally, emergency department imaging order requests and interpretation analysis point to the necessity of complying with guidelines in order to optimize the high value of chest imaging in the acute setting.

6.4.2. Screening Recommendations for Lung Cancer

Prompt diagnosis of lung cancer significantly improves the patient's outcome, justifying the need for appropriate screening in chest radiology. Existing guidelines have attributed much emphasis to the management of solid pulmonary nodules based on specific morphological characteristics identified with low-dose CT. For instance, noncalcified solid nodules with adherent mediastinal or diaphragmatic pleura and smooth edges and sharp triangular or lentiform morphology have essentially zero opportunity for malignancy and merit annual follow-up rather than emergency invasive assessment (Zhu *et. al.*, 2024). This personalization reduces unnecessary procedures while remaining vigilant for malignancy. In addition, AI technology seeks to maximize screening performance by enabling rapid sorting of abnormal chest X-rays for prioritization. Software like qXR applies ML to detect cases with malignancy-defining features, speeding assessment by radiologists and enabling prompt follow-up CT scans (Sean *et. al.*, 2024). These approaches individually exhibit a complex, technology-enabled paradigm for optimizing lung cancer screening referrals in chest radiology (Figure 6.18).

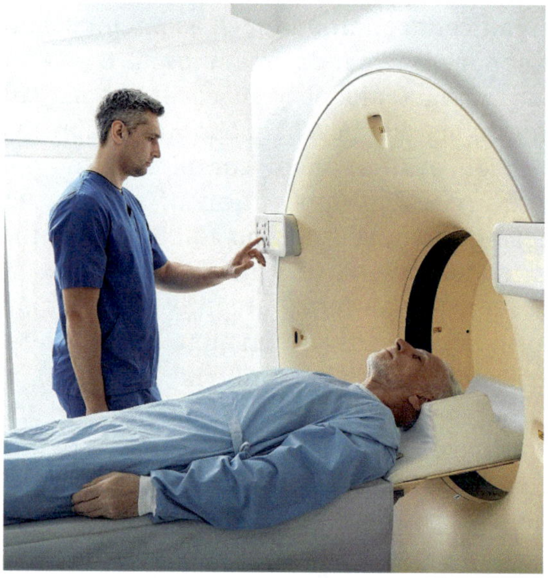

Figure 6.18. Screening recommendations for lung cancer.

Source: https://ctvstexas.com/wp-content/uploads/2024/01/lung-cancer.png.

6.4.3. Role of Chest Radiology in Preoperative Assessment

Appropriate preoperative assessment is vital in minimizing the risks of surgery and optimizing patient outcomes, particularly in thoracic procedures. Correct imaging is a fundamental element in the process of providing valuable anatomical and pathological information, which is essential in directing clinical decision-making. Chest radiology, such as chest X-rays and CT scans, yields invaluable information regarding lung parenchyma, vascular anatomy, and airway anatomy. This imaging is useful for detecting potential complications, such as airway compression or vascular malformations, which may alter surgical planning. For instance, the use of CT and bronchoscopy to diagnose left mainstem bronchus compression has played a pivotal role in planning surgical intervention, e.g., aortopexy (Arcieri *et. al.*, 2016). Chest radiology also aids in cardiopulmonary status assessment and for occult masses or infections, thereby decreasing operative risk. The addition of chest radiology to preoperative evaluation regimens enhances safety and surgical success, solidifying its important position in thoracic patient care.

6.4.4. Imaging Protocols for Specific Conditions

Technical advances in imaging have significantly facilitated protocols for individual chest conditions, optimizing diagnostic performance while minimizing risk to the patient. CT protocols, for instance, have been optimized with IR algorithms that reduce image noise and improve quality so that dose reduction can be achieved without loss of diagnosis—a key consideration in repeat imaging scenarios or in vulnerable populations (Bastarika *et. al.*, 2015). In parallel, MRI is an effective substitute in situations where ionizing radiation is not indicated, such as in pediatric patients, pregnant patients, and patients with cystic fibrosis or PE (Hebestreit *et. al.*, 2011).

Customized MRI protocols employing fast breath-hold techniques and functional imaging sequences provide additional morphological and physiological data that enhance decision-making. Even if MRI is still in its investigative role in ILD, its use as a third imaging modality of the lungs is indicative of the direction toward customized imaging protocols that harmonize efficacy, safety, and patient-specific considerations (Hebestreit *et. al.*, 2011). Condition-specific protocols illustrate the changing scenario of chest radiology (Figure 6.19).

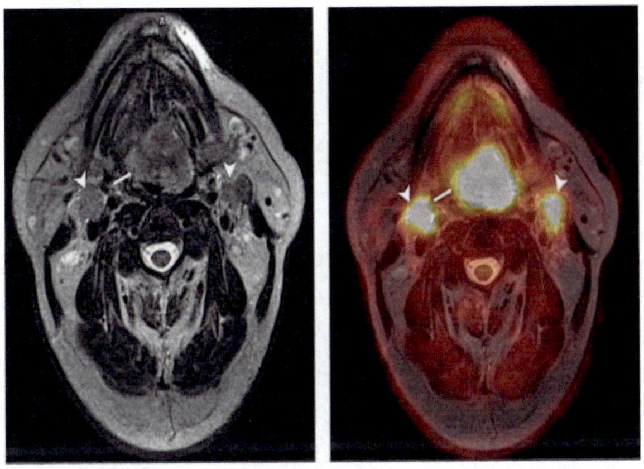

Figure 6.19. Customized MRI protocols, incorporating fast breath-hold techniques and functional imaging sequences, provide complementary morphological and physiological data that enhance clinical decision-making.

Source: https://pub.mdpi-res.com/diagnostics/diagnostics-05-00333/article_deploy/html/images/diagnostics-05-00333-ag-550.jpg?1581018763.

6.4.5. Patient Safety and Radiation Exposure

Protection of patients in chest radiology demands strict regulations to restrict exposure to radiation while maintaining diagnostic efficacy. Overexposure incidents, although rare, can lead to tissue reactions in terms of skin injury, primarily in the event of interventional procedures and CT scans. The majority of these adverse effects are due to a lack of adequate training for staff and improper use of equipment, which further necessitates efficient education and accurate operational procedures. Integration of safety measures like pre-procedure checklists, time-outs, and real-time alerts for doses can significantly minimize radiation dose-related risks. In addition to this, optimization of imaging practices—like modulating protocols of iodinated contrast media and use of newer technology in the form of low tube voltage with IR—can further reduce radiation without compromising image quality. This is particularly important in first-pass studies where individualized contrast injection contributes to safety and tolerability. Systematic reporting of any exposure accidents and official policies is significant in the context of discussing root causes and improving overall radiological practice to better shield patients in chest radiology (Albrecht *et. al.*, 2017; Damilakis *et. al.*, 2017).

6.4.6. Ethical Considerations in Chest Imaging

Technical innovations in imaging have revolutionized chest radiology diagnostic performance, but pose difficult ethical concerns that must be carefully addressed. The application of AI, in the form of convolutional neural networks, enhances sensitivity and specificity but raises interpretability and transparency issues in clinical decision-making.

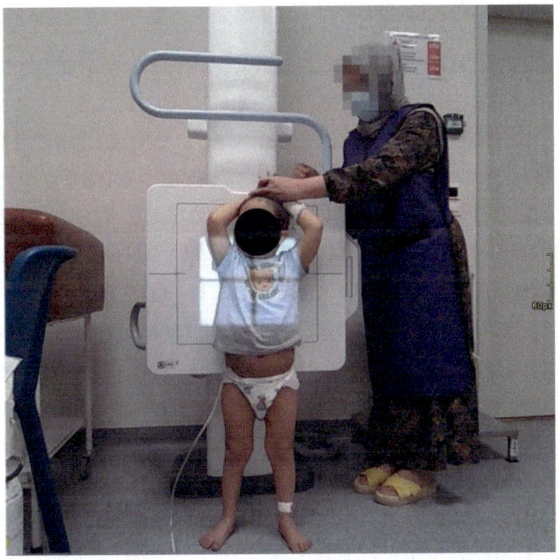

Figure 6.20. Advancements in imaging technology have revolutionized diagnostic accuracy in chest radiology, yet they bring forth complex ethical challenges that must be carefully navigated.

Source: https://media.springernature.com/lw685/springer-static/image/art%3A10.1007%2Fs00247-023-05671-0/MediaObjects/247_2023_5671_Fig1_HTML.png.

Without transparent comprehension, such systems can compromise patient trust and even lead to diagnostic errors if clinicians over-rely on algorithmic results without critical evaluation Keshav Kumar, K., & Narasimham, N. V. S. L. (2023). Ensuring uniform access to sophisticated imaging modalities also remains an urgent matter, as unequal distribution of healthcare resources can prejudicially impact at-risk populations. Patient confidentiality is another significant consideration, especially in the context of increased digitization and sharing of imaging data that necessitates strong safeguards. Therefore, ethical debates must persist on not just technical proficiency but also on justice, responsibility, and informed consent as the foundation for ethical practice of chest imaging technology (Figure 6.20).

6.4.7. Multidisciplinary Approach in Patient Management

Effective patient care in chest radiology now greatly relies on the multi-disciplinary model comprising a convergence of expertise from radiologists, pulmonologists, oncologists, among other specialists, to provide appropriate diagnosis and customized treatment plans. Multi-disciplinary guidance optimizes the interpretation of intricate imaging findings within the total clinical context, which enhances patient outcomes. For instance, multidisciplinary conferences and teleconferencing platforms have been effective in teaching medical students and clinicians about the interconnected roles of various specialties, thereby bettering an integrated perception of radiological information in clinical decision-making (Patel *et. al.*, 2024). Similarly, care management of complex conditions such as Neurofibromatosis Type 1 emphasizes the central function of unit care teams that coordinate multisystem involvement through coordinated care, promoting quality of life through unit's experience (Lalvani *et. al.*, 2024). Combined approaches promote the new paradigm of chest radiology where multilearning is important for correct diagnosis and effective patient-centered care.

6.4.8. Tele-radiology and Remote Consultations

The technological advances in digital technology have significantly influenced the practice of radiology, making diagnostic services more convenient and accessible. Among these technological advances, tele-radiology and remote consultation are now indispensable factors, particularly in chest radiology. Through the application of cloud computing and web-based systems, radiologists can now read imaging studies anywhere in the world, providing timely diagnosis and consultations without geographical limitations.

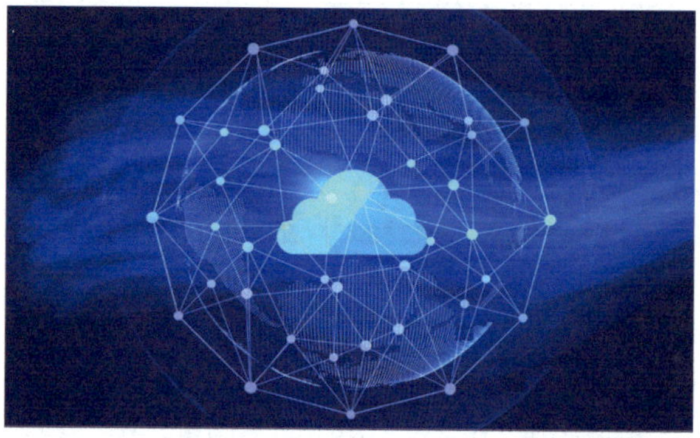

Figure 6.21. By leveraging cloud computing and internet-based platforms, radiologists can now interpret imaging studies from virtually any location, facilitating timely diagnosis and consultation without geographic limitations.

Source: https://dcmsys.com/wp-content/uploads/2020/01/How-Cloud-Computing-is-Transforming-the-Healthcare-Industry-980x610A.png.

This capability not only improves outcomes for patients by accelerating clinical decision-making but also maximizes the utilization of resources, especially in underserved populations where specialists may be less accessible. Additionally, integration with electronic medical records and mature imaging repositories provides a continuous clinical workflow, facilitating continuity of care. Despite these advantages, issues such as data security, image quality, and regulatory compliance are still pertinent. However, ongoing progress in medical imaging informatics highlights the core role of tele-radiology in modern chest radiology practice (Archer *et. al.*, 2014). Furthermore, the ubiquitous use of portable ultrasound devices and remote access also reflects the change in paradigm to decentralized real-time imaging diagnosis (Chai *et. al.*, 2021) (Figure 6.21).

6.4.9. Future Directions in Clinical Applications

The evolution in imaging technology continues to revitalize the field of chest radiology, with the potential for revolutionary improvements in diagnostic accuracy and patient benefit. The newer applications of AI and ML are poised to enhance image interpretation and enable subtle pathologies to be detected at an earlier point in time, which traditional means may not detect. Furthermore, progress in low-dose CT is also expected to reduce radiation dosage while ensuring high-quality images necessary for mass screening and follow-up in vulnerable populations. A combination of functional imaging modalities, i.e., perfusion and ventilation scanning, with routine anatomical assessment, will provide a more precise diagnosis of diseases affecting the lungs. This also helps in personalized medicine by allowing the tailoring of treatment protocols based on proper characterization of the disease. With advancing multi-modality imaging systems, collaboration between clinicians and radiologists will increase. Combined, these advances represent a move toward more effective, accurate, and patient-centered chest radiology with the potential for revolutionary enhancement of clinical applications in the very near future.

Test Your Knowledge

1. How can serial chest X-rays be used to monitor disease progression or treatment response?
2. What are the risks of misinterpreting overexposed or underexposed films?

SUMMARY

Chest radiology interpretation demands a fine skill that involves perceptual skill in addition to a clinical background in a way that decreases diagnostic errors. Radiologic experience is achieved through extensive exposure and intensive inspection of numerous instances, which increases a radiologist's potential to distinguish subtle differences that may indicate pathology (Taylor *et. al.*, 2007). This higher-level expertise is critical in high-stakes cases where timely and accurate diagnosis, such as diagnosing the etiology of chest pain in the context of drug abuse, has a direct correlation with patient outcomes (Bandeeri *et. al.*, 2004). With each step in technology and learning methods, attention to training courses promoting perceptual learning and practice case-based grows more important. Last but not least, the usefulness of chest radiology is in bringing top-shelf interpretive ability together with clinical knowledge to render diagnoses precise and timely, with a significant consequential advantage to patient management and care.

Advancements in chest radiology have significantly enhanced diagnostic precision and clinical decision-making, although complications are linked to resource utilization and require specialized skills. Concurrent application of different imaging methods, such as HRCT and MRI, enhances the potential for diagnosis but demands specialized knowledge shared across clinical groups to be utilized at their optimal levels (Maurer *et. al.*, 2020). On top of that, high reporting standards require organized peer review mechanisms that require substantial human resources, time, and trained staff to check for accuracy and reduce interpretive variance (Desai *et. al.*, 2007). As impossible as a total review of all radiology reports may be, targeted quality assurance efforts are crucial for ongoing improvement. Lastly, shared understanding of clinical indications, imaging modalities, and interpretive nuances forms the basis of effective chest radiology practices, balancing technological advances with pragmatic workflow issues to enhance patient care results (Desai *et. al.*, 2007; Maurer *et. al.*, 2020).

KEY TERMS FROM THIS CHAPTER

- Accessibility
- Cushing syndrome
- Explainable Artificial Intelligence (XAI)
- Infections
- Neonatal
- Precision
- Assessment
- Ectopic hormone-secreting lesions
- Heart
- Lung nodules
- Neuroendocrine tumors
- Vascular abnormalities

CRITICAL THINKING QUESTIONS

1. **In a normal posteroanterior (PA) chest X-ray, which side of the diaphragm is usually higher?**
   a. Left
   b. Right
   c. Both are equal
   d. It varies randomly
2. **Which of the following is a radiographic sign of pneumothorax?**
   a. Blunted costophrenic angle
   b. Air bronchogram
   c. Visible pleural line with absence of lung markings beyond
   d. Homogeneous opacity in the lower lung field
3. **What does the silhouette sign on a chest X-ray indicate?**
   a. Air in the pleural space
   b. Loss of normal border due to adjacent pathology
   c. Presence of lung mass
   d. Cardiac enlargement
4. **Which imaging modality is best for evaluating pulmonary embolism?**
   a. Chest X-ray
   b. High-resolution CT (HRCT)
   c. CT pulmonary angiography (CTPA)
   d. MRI
5. **On chest X-ray, which structure forms the right heart border?**
   a. Aorta
   b. Right atrium
   c. Left ventricle
   d. Pulmonary artery

Short Answer Questions

1. What are the key anatomical landmarks evaluated in a normal chest radiograph?
2. How does a lateral chest X-ray complement a PA view?
3. What are the standard views used in chest CT imaging?
4. What are common indications for ordering a chest X-ray?
5. How can you determine the quality and adequacy of a chest X-ray?
6. What does an enlarged cardiac silhouette indicate on a chest X-ray?
7. How do you identify pleural effusion on a chest X-ray?
8. What is the silhouette sign, and how does it help localize pathology?
9. What features suggest consolidation or pneumonia on imaging?

Answers to Critical Thinking Questions

1.(b); 2.(c); 3.(b); 4.(c); 5.(b)

REFERENCES

1. Aasem, M., & Iqbal, M. J. (2024). Toward explainable AI in radiology: Ensemble-CAM for effective thoracic disease localization in chest X-ray images using weak supervised learning. *Frontiers in Big Data, 7*. https://www.semanticscholar.org/paper/f6a29c925fc48177f1b7e2edd1b39c2bfee3474f (accessed on 30 May 2025).
2. Razek Abdel , A., Abdel Khalek, A., Elrakhawy, M. M., Nageb, H. M., *et. al.* (2018). Inter-observer agreement of the Coronary Artery Disease Reporting and Data System (CAD-RADS™) in patients with stable chest pain. https://core.ac.uk/download/160736729.pdf (accessed on 30 May 2025).
3. Achterhold, K., Auweter, S., Bamberg, F., *et. al.* (2013). Diagnosing and mapping pulmonary emphysema on X-ray projection images. https://core.ac.uk/download/12175665.pdf (accessed on 30 May 2025).
4. Ahmad, H. K., Bottrell, G., Brotchie, P., *et. al.* (2024). Machine learning augmented interpretation of chest X-rays: A systematic review. https://core.ac.uk/download/622650105.pdf (accessed on 30 May 2025).
5. Albrecht, T., Aschoff, A. J., Catalano, C., *et. al.* (2017). Low radiation dose in computed tomography: The role of iodine. https://core.ac.uk/download/98341308.pdf (accessed on 30 May 2025).
6. Andrani, F., Anzidei, M., Bezzi, M., *et. al.* (2017). Imaging-guided chest biopsies: Techniques and clinical results. https://core.ac.uk/download/127588220.pdf (accessed on 30 May 2025).
7. Archer, N. P., McClung, A., McKibbon, A., & McMaster eBusiness Research Centre (MeRC) (2014). Novel eHealth trends in the field of radiology: A scoping review. https://core.ac.uk/download/639169329.pdf (accessed on 30 May 2025).
8. Arcieri, L., Assanta, N., Baggi, R., *et. al.* (2016). The role of posterior aortopexy in the treatment of left mainstem bronchus compression. https://core.ac.uk/download/74319435.pdf (accessed on 30 May 2025).
9. Azad, B., Azad, R., Bozorgpour, A., *et. al.* (2023). Foundational models in medical imaging: A comprehensive survey and future vision. *arXiv*. http://arxiv.org/abs/2310.18689 (accessed on 30 May 2025).
10. Bader, P., Ciocarlie, O., Elze, M. C., *et. al.* (2014). Dendritic cell reconstitution is associated with relapse-free survival and acute GVHD severity in children after allogeneic stem cell transplantation.
11. Ball, R., Chute, C., Ciurea-Ilcus, S., Haghgoo, *et. al.* (2019). CheXpert: A large chest radiograph dataset with uncertainty labels and expert comparison. *arXiv*. http://arxiv.org/abs/1901.07031 (accessed on 30 May 2025).
12. Bandeeri, N., Henry, J. A., Meredith, C., *et. al.* (2004). The prevalence of cocaine-associated chest pain in a London hospital. https://core.ac.uk/download/5230488.pdf (accessed on 30 May 2025).
13. Bartoszek, L., Kapłan, W., Kaus, M., *et. al.* (2025). Application of artificial intelligence in radiological image analysis for pulmonary disease diagnosis: A review of current methods and challenges. https://core.ac.uk/download/636386127.pdf (accessed on 30 May 2025).

14. Bastarrika, G., De Cecco, C. N., Geyer, L. L., *et. al.* (2015). State of the art: Iterative CT reconstruction techniques. https://core.ac.uk/download/54522078.pdf (accessed on 30 May 2025).

15. Bhardwaj, B. K., Pullalathu Abraham, J., Murthy, C., & Aiyappa, A. (2024). Ultrasound imaging in the early detection of transient tachypnoea of the newborn: A cross-sectional study. *International Journal of Anatomy Radiology and Surgery*. https://www.semanticscholar.org/paper/30ae399aba49694e75c6f0bfe1dd1b272cd85152 (accessed on 30 May 2025).

16. Sood RG, Sharma S, Mokta JK, Jhobta A, Bhatia V, Panda P. Pneumothorax and Pneumomediastinum in a Sputum Positive Tuberculosis Patient: The Continous Diaphragm Sign. Online J Health Allied Scs. 2012;11(1):16. URL: http://www.ojhas.org/issue41/2012-1-16.htm

17. Sverzellati N, Molinari F, Pirronti T, Bonomo L, Spagnolo P, Zompatori M. New insights on COPD imaging via CT and MRI. Int J Chron Obstruct Pulmon Dis. 2007;2(3):301-12. PMID: 18229568; PMCID: PMC2695207.

18. Brandt, A., Malkin, A. A., Zanoni, B., Khoury, B., Stuckler, D., Krupinski, E. A., Patton, G. C., *et. al.* (2011). Pediatric radiology seen from Africa. Part I: Providing diagnostic imaging to a young population. https://core.ac.uk/download/pdf/10674304.pdf (accessed on 30 May 2025).

19. Chai, H., Li, J., Lin, C., *et. al.* (2021). Point-of-care ultrasound: New concepts and future trends. https://core.ac.uk/download/516418270.pdf (accessed on 30 May 2025).

20. Chang, J. Y., & Makary, M. (2024). Evolving and novel applications of artificial intelligence in thoracic imaging. *Diagnostics, 14*. https://www.semanticscholar.org/paper/119fbb440fc412ee487b609948eb565ec7d1e7cb (accessed on 30 May 2025).

21. Chartrand, G., Cheng, P. M., Vorontsov, E., Drozdzal, M., Turcotte, S., Pal, C., Kadoury, S., *et. al.* (2017). Deep learning: A primer for radiologists. *Radiographic, 37*, 2113–2131. https://doi.org/10.1148/rg.2017170077.

22. Chong, M. D., Weelic, H., Yang, L., *et. al.* (2020). Critical care ultrasonography and its application for COVID-19. https://core.ac.uk/download/322850187.pdf (accessed on 30 May 2025).

23. Rahman, T.; Chowdhury, M.E.H.; Khandakar, A.; Islam, K.R.; Islam, K.F.; Mahbub, Z.B.; Kadir, M.A.; Kashem, S. Transfer Learning with Deep Convolutional Neural Network (CNN) for Pneumonia Detection Using Chest X-ray. *Appl. Sci.* 2020, *10*, 3233. https://doi.org/10.3390/app10093233

24. Chung JH, Goldin JG. Interpretation of HRCT Scans in the Diagnosis of IPF: Improving Communication Between Pulmonologists and Radiologists. Lung. 2018 Oct;196(5):561-567. doi: 10.1007/s00408-018-0143-5. Epub 2018 Aug 10. PMID: 30097721; PMCID: PMC6153593.

25. Martin CJ, Vassileva J, Vano E, Mahesh M, Ebdon-Jackson S, Ng KH, Frush DP, Loose R, Damilakis J. Unintended and accidental medical radiation exposures in radiology: guidelines on investigation and prevention. J Radiol Prot. 2017 Jan;37(4):883-906. doi: 10.1088/1361-6498/aa881e. PMID: 28836506.

26. Desai, S., Franquet, T., Hartman, T., & Wells, A. (2007). Pulmonary imaging: Contributions to key clinical questions. https://www.semanticscholar.org/paper/2c1e35e2aeb1d681309202063c877003bf3307f3 (accessed on 30 May 2025).

27. Devine, E., Hunt, J. A., Mavromatis, M. V., & Anderson, S. L. (2025). An online case-based radiology course improves veterinary students' day one competency in small animal

radiographic interpretation. *The Veterinary Record*. https://www.semanticscholar.org/paper/4cd2204c6a7225ad148ce9faacd3ef546b18ba41 (accessed on 30 May 2025).

28. Dhamanskar, P., & Thacker, C. (2024). A detailed analysis of deep learning-based techniques for automated radiology report generation. *International Journal of Electrical and Computer Engineering (IJECE)*. https://www.semanticscholar.org/paper/9b86d0a9d322ca98ce6c073ee9544bf13bb1d29e (accessed on 30 May 2025).

29. Dominici, L., Marchitelli, L., Ruoli, L., Conia, L., Cundari, G., Pambianchi, G., Catalano, C., *et. al.* (2024). Cardiac magnetic resonance in inflammatory heart disease: A single tool for multiple clinical scenarios. *Journal of Medical Imaging and Interventional Radiology*. https://www.semanticscholar.org/paper/ce30516577db7c1f3ea0aa4a87a6831be0eaa844 (accessed on 30 May 2025).

30. Duncan, S. F., McConnachie, A., Blackwood, J., Stobo, D. B., Maclay, J. D., Wu, O., Germeni, E., *et. al.* (2024). Radiograph accelerated detection and identification of cancer in the lung (RADICAL): A mixed methods study to assess the clinical effectiveness and acceptability of Qure.ai artificial intelligence software to priorities chest X-ray (CXR) interpretation. *BMJ Open, 14*. https://www.semanticscholar.org/paper/0f4e89819fa006b8f6ab35c9e33180132531b315 (accessed on 30 May 2025).

31. Elze, M. C., Gagneur, J., & Tresch, A. (2011). Selective phenotyping, entropy reduction, and the mastermind game. https://core.ac.uk/download/29151719.pdf (accessed on 30 May 2025).

32. Eroglu, S. A., Çağavi, Z., Yıldız, T., & Karakurt, Z. (2021). Can the usage of the chest X-ray scoring during hospitalization in patients with COVID-19 predict the severity of the disease? *Turkish Thoracic Journal, 22*(3), 190–198. https://www.semanticscholar.org/paper/e19a9dc766c1308ed5d416c26a61620018628442 (accessed on 30 May 2025).

33. Goossen, R. L., Verboom, M., Blacha, M. M. J., Smesseim, I., Beenen, L., Meenen, D. V., Paulus, F., *et. al.* (2023). Incidence of air leaks in critically ill patients with acute hypoxemic respiratory failure due to COVID-19. *Diagnostics, 13*. https://www.semanticscholar.org/paper/e9b7172ae28768570ee8ba774fafc09d88ae6fae (accessed on 30 May 2025).

34. Goswami, K. K., Tak, N., Wadhawan, A., Landau, A. B., Bajaj, J., Sahni, J., Iqbal, Z., *et. al.* (2024). Enhancing clinical diagnosis with convolutional neural networks: Developing high-accuracy deep learning models for differentiating thoracic pathologies. *Cureus, 16*. https://www.semanticscholar.org/paper/be1274cd7e27d7ea07824eede86c758a63922830 (accessed on 30 May 2025).

35. Han, S., Kim, B., Jang, H. R., Kim, W. J., Jeon, Y., Kim, S. S., & Kim, I. (2016). Ectopic ACTH syndrome caused by pulmonary carcinoid tumor mimicking long-standing sclerosing hemangioma. *The Korean Journal of Internal Medicine, 31*, 794–797. https://www.semanticscholar.org/paper/c55fcce1db14482bce31a7ce7770bfb60c91158e (accessed on 30 May 2025).

36. Hebestreit, A., Kluge, A., Kluge, A., Kluge, A., Bankier, A. A., Henderson, A. C., Brody, A. S., *et. al.* (2011). MRI of the lung (3/3)–Current applications and future perspectives. https://core.ac.uk/download/28969132.pdf (accessed on 30 May 2025).

37. Holopainen, S., Lappalainen, A. K., Lilja-Maula, L., Lohi, *et. al.* (2019). Thoracic high-resolution CT using the modified VetMousetrap™ device is a feasible method for diagnosing canine idiopathic pulmonary fibrosis in awake West Highland White Terriers. https://core.ac.uk/download/401691652.pdf (accessed on 30 May 2025).

38. Ihongbe, I. E., Fouad, S., Mahmoud, T. F., Rajasekaran, A., & Bhatia, B. (2024). Evaluating explainable artificial intelligence (XAI) techniques in chest radiology imaging through a human-centered lens. *PLOS ONE, 19*. https://www.semanticscholar.org/paper/dda4db58b2c6ee228c461b505e1786b07ace231b (accessed on 30 May 2025).

39. Jaramillo, C., Ferguson, E., Odisio, E., & Ocazionez, D. (2024). High-density pulmonary lesions: Review in chest imaging. *Current Problems in Diagnostic Radiology*. https://www.semanticscholar.org/paper/3b0d074152a62a7edf1c2e3d66ef0ef88b19d12a (accessed on 30 May 2025).

40. Jia, H., Tang, S., Guo, W., Pan, P., Qian, Y., Hu, D., Dai, Y., *et. al.* (2024). Differential diagnosis of congenital ventricular septal defect and atrial septal defect in children using deep learning–based analysis of chest radiographs. *BMC Pediatrics, 24*. https://www.semanticscholar.org/paper/1fdb2059b04a2b735370a069d5eb51a19e7bdfca (accessed on 30 May 2025).

41. Kantarcı, M., Aydın, S., Oğul, H., & Kızılgöz, V. (2025). New imaging techniques and trends in radiology. *Diagnostic and Interventional Radiology*. https://www.semanticscholar.org/paper/227b86e1f579d86cef6ee3988ffa183bf2741b9d (accessed on 30 May 2025).

42. Keshav Kumar, K., & Narasimham, N. V. S. L. (2023). Enhancing radiology diagnosis through convolutional neural networks for computer vision in healthcare. *arXiv*. http://arxiv.org/abs/2311.11234 (accessed on 30 May 2025).

43. Lalvani, S., & Brown, R. (2024). Neurofibromatosis type 1: Optimizing management with a multidisciplinary approach. *Journal of Multidisciplinary Healthcare, 17*, 1803–1817. https://www.semanticscholar.org/paper/14cf93fe44ec819e90934aa0929d0cd2033ac33a (accessed on 30 May 2025).

44. Lonsdale, H., Gray, G. M., Ahumada, L. M., & Matava, C. (2023). Machine vision and image analysis in anesthesia: Narrative review and future prospects. *Anesthesia and Analgesia, 137*(4), 830–840. https://www.semanticscholar.org/paper/6a7facd2180e952fa59e9048f490c8a25371c25f (accessed on 30 May 2025).

45. Lovrenski, J., Raissaki, M., Plut, D., Alexopoulou, E., Görkem, S., Özcan, H. N., Geiger, J., *et. al.* (2025). ESR essentials: Imaging of common pediatric pulmonary diseases—Practice recommendations by the European Society of Pediatric Radiology. *European Radiology*. https://www.semanticscholar.org/paper/ecf92e55cb582e17f59411c4492d47c8c58099c9 (accessed on 30 May 2025).

46. Machnicki, S., Patel, D., Singh, A., Talwar, A., Mina, B., Oks, M., Makkar, P., *et. al.* (2021). The usefulness of chest CT imaging in patients with suspected or diagnosed COVID-19. *CHEST Journal, 160*, 652–670. https://doi.org/10.1016/j.chest.2021.04.004.

47. Matamoros, A. (2012). Evidence-based imaging: Improving the quality of imaging in patient care. *The Journal of Nuclear Medicine, 53*, 660. https://www.semanticscholar.org/paper/a810eaa45e02a14d535581ae7292c27a588f534a (accessed on 30 May 2025).

48. Maurer, M., Brönnimann, M., Schroeder, C., Ghadamgahi, E., Streitparth, F., Heverhagen, J., Leichtle, A., *et. al.* (2020). Time requirement and feasibility of a systematic quality peer review of reporting in radiology. *RöFo–Fortschritte auf dem Gebiet der Röntgenstrahlen und der bildgebenden Verfahren, 193*, 160–167. https://www.semanticscholar.org/paper/e3eb3dcb0dd98eaf49533f566396319dd4d67f10 (accessed on 30 May 2025).

49. Moor, M., Banerjee, O., Hossein Abad, Z. S., Krumholz, H. M., Leskovec, J., Topol, E. J., &

Rajpurkar, P. (2023). Foundation models for generalist medical artificial intelligence. *Nature, 616*(259–265). https://doi.org/10.1038/s41586-023-05881-4.

50. Ndiaye, Y. S., Cramton, P., Chernev, C., Ockenfels, A., & Schwarz, T. (2025). Comparison of radiological interpretation made by veterinary radiologists and state-of-the-art commercial AI software for canine and feline radiographic studies. *Frontiers in Veterinary Science, 12.* https://www.semanticscholar.org/paper/eada01b6c3ace42fdf583c883fc1668d27b1f442 (accessed on 30 May 2025).

51. Padash, S., Mohebbian, M., Adams, S., Henderson, R. D. E., & Babyn, P. (2022). Pediatric chest radiograph interpretation: How far has artificial intelligence come? A systematic literature review. *Pediatric Radiology, 52,* 1568–1580. https://www.semanticscholar.org/paper/3b12d1b25e161a199874933aaf336a2e60294fb4 (accessed on 30 May 2025).

52. Patel, P., Altinmakas, E., Ayas, G., Stanietzky, R., Stewart, M. L., Elshikh, A., Ram, D., *et. al.* (2024). Multidisciplinary approach to diagnostic radiology education: A novel educational intervention for Turkish medical students. *Diagnostic and Interventional Radiology.* https://www.semanticscholar.org/paper/8aa96259242520382c93d0cc051a2aeafcc120a5 (accessed on 30 May 2025).

53. Qaher, F. M., Husain, M. A., Almansoor, M. F., Abdulameer, F. H., & Al-Ammar, A. A. (2024). Adult mediastinal lymphangioma presenting as persistent chest pain: A case report. *Cureus, 16.* https://www.semanticscholar.org/paper/6d857825a643278bef073c0725bbc7ab27ebeae2 (accessed on 30 May 2025).

54. Raghu, G., Rémy-Jardin, M., Richeldi, L., Thomson, C. C., Inoue, Y., Johkoh, T., Kreuter, M., *et. al.* (2022). Idiopathic pulmonary fibrosis (an update) and progressive pulmonary fibrosis in adults: An official ATS/ERS/JRS/ALAT clinical practice guideline. *American Journal of Respiratory and Critical Care Medicine, 205,* e18–e47. https://doi.org/10.1164/rccm.202202-0399st.

55. Raghu, G., Rémy-Jardin, M., Ryerson, C. J., Myers, J. L., Kreuter, M., Vašáková, M., Bargagli, E., *et. al.* (2020). Diagnosis of hypersensitivity pneumonitis in adults: An official ATS/JRS/ALAT clinical practice guideline. *American Journal of Respiratory and Critical Care Medicine, 202,* e36–e69. https://doi.org/10.1164/rccm.202005-2032st.

56. Rahman, N. A., Amin, M., & Rosyid, A. (2025). Imaging techniques in COVID-19 diagnosis: Evaluating the role of chest X-ray, chest CT scan, and lung ultrasound in identifying key radiological features. *Coronaviruses.* https://www.semanticscholar.org/paper/d690b65da459a52d523ef2964b621795f283b4eb (accessed on 30 May 2025).

57. Rathod, N., Awasthi, K., Kostkiewicz, M., Klimeczek, P., & Stępień, E. (2024). Advancing cardiac detection in chest X-ray images using machine learning: A practical application of AI in medical imaging. *Bio-Algorithms and Med-Systems.* https://www.semanticscholar.org/paper/84de0099e5bb61afce367b9fca24518dc561331e (accessed on 30 May 2025).

58. Runge, V. M., & Heverhagen, J. T. (2021). Scientific advances, Investigative Radiology 2020 (and beyond). *Investigative Radiology, 56,* 271–273. https://doi.org/10.1097/rli.0000000000000783.

59. Safai Zadeh, E., Görg, C., Prosch, H., Horn, R., Jenssen, C., & Dietrich, C. (2023). The role of thoracic ultrasound for diagnosis of diseases of the chest wall, the mediastinum, and the diaphragm—Narrative review and pictorial essay. *Diagnostics, 13.* https://www.semanticscholar.org/paper/7502b4e57c3b5acc99a12b105a05de3edb73dd47 (accessed on 30 May 2025).

60. Salkade, S. A., & Rathi, S. (2025). An adaptive convolution neural network model for tuberculosis detection and diagnosis using semantic segmentation. *Polish Journal of Radiology*. https://www.semanticscholar.org/paper/f6f9f884d39560d24d7c5dcc68f42fa0954954e3 (accessed on 30 May 2025).

61. Schiavone, W. A., & Majdalany, D. S. (2024). Chest radiography pearls in select adult congenital heart disease. *Journal of Personalized Medicine, 14*. https://www.semanticscholar.org/paper/f7f2102998adc0e05e9d34bc5122e6043018db5c (accessed on 30 May 2025).

62. Sellergren, A., Chen, C., Nabulsi, Z., Li, Y., Maschinot, A., Sarna, A., Huang, J., *et. al.* (2022). Simplified transfer learning for chest radiography models using less data. *Radiology*. https://www.semanticscholar.org/paper/00a4214c54afd9426997bb91027098b82ce9e1dc (accessed on 30 May 2025).

63. Sharma, N. (2024). CXR-Agent: Vision-language models for chest X-ray interpretation with uncertainty aware radiology reporting. *arXiv* (abs/2407.08811). https://www.semanticscholar.org/paper/371549980121e83042afccdecb575724be2d4827 (accessed on 30 May 2025).

64. Stafrace, S. (2008). Foetal MRI: Advances in the evaluation of the developing fetus. https://core.ac.uk/download/46602180.pdf (accessed on 30 May 2025).

65. Taylor, P. M. (2007). A review of research into the development of radiologic expertise: Implications for computer-based training. https://core.ac.uk/download/1673134.pdf (accessed on 30 May 2025).

66. Tungsagunwattana, S., & Lertrojanapunya, S. (2025). AIR Pneumonia, a project to standardize chest radiograph interpretation of occupational lung diseases in Thailand and ASEAN countries: Challenges and future trends. *The ASEAN Journal of Radiology*. https://www.semanticscholar.org/paper/9415cc1287f3a8d34fc4257a6602a6cb18e96cdb (accessed on 30 May 2025).

67. Van der Velden, B. H. M., Kuijf, H. J., Gilhuijs, K. G. A., & Viergever, M. A. (2022). Explainable artificial intelligence (XAI) in deep learning-based medical image analysis. *Medical Image Analysis, 79*, 102470. https://doi.org/10.1016/j.media.2022.102470.

68. Zhou, S. K., Greenspan, H., Davatzikos, C., Duncan, J. S., van Ginneken, B., Madabhushi, A., Prince, J. L., *et. al.* (2021). A review of deep learning in medical imaging: Imaging traits, technology trends, case studies with progress highlights, and future promises. *Proceedings of the IEEE, 109*, 820–838. https://doi.org/10.1109/jproc.2021.3054390.

69. Zhu, Y., Yip, R., Zhang, J., Cai, Q., Sun, Q., Li, P., Paksashvili, N., *et. al.* (2024). Radiologic features of nodules attached to the mediastinal or diaphragmatic pleura at low-dose CT for lung cancer screening. *Radiology, 310*(1), e231219. https://www.semanticscholar.org/paper/5e35986d4aa80eabcf971eec077ae4937a4ce6ef (accessed on 30 May 2025).

CARDIOVASCULAR IMAGING

7

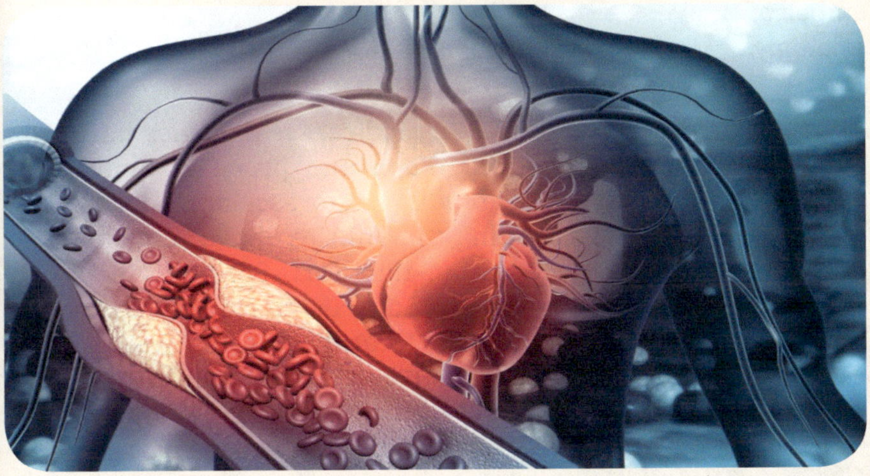

LEARNING OBJECTIVES

After studying this chapter, you will be able to:

1. Understand types of cardiovascular imaging modalities
2. Discuss applications of cardiovascular imaging
3. Know advances in cardiovascular imaging technology
4. Identify challenges and limitations of cardiovascular imaging

Introduction

Innovations in medical technology have dramatically changed the process of diagnosis in cardiology, allowing clinicians to gain accurate information about the structure and function of the heart without undergoing invasive techniques. Among these technological advancements, cardiovascular imaging has proven to be a must-have tool for cardiac pathology evaluation, therapeutic decision-making, and treatment monitoring. Techniques such as cardiovascular magnetic resonance (CMR) possess individual strengths, such as the excellent resolution of images, the ability to see cardiac tissue in additional planes, and a lack of ionizing radiation, thus maintaining patient safety and diagnostic accuracy. The advancement in magnetic field strength and operator skill has made CMR feasible, and through this, its value in the clinic has grown, allowing accurate measurement of structural heart disease. In addition, integrating imaging findings with current guidelines ensures that clinicians make patient-centered decisions following care standards that are continuously evolving (François *et. al.*, 2019;

Situ *et. al.*, 2020). This chapter explores the pivotal role of cardiovascular imaging in modern medicine, tracing its technological origins and clinical importance.

Definition of Cardiovascular Imaging

Advances in medical technology have revolutionized the ability to visualize the vascular anatomy and the heart and acquire crucial information on cardiovascular health. Cardiovascular imaging comprises a number of methodologies to assess cardiovascular anatomy, function, and disease noninvasively.

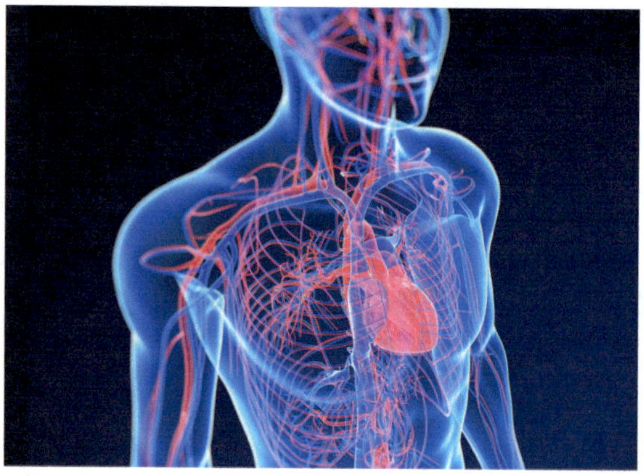

Figure 7.1. Cardiovascular imaging encompasses a range of techniques designed to noninvasively assess the anatomy, function, and pathology of the cardiovascular system.

Source: https://bcen.org/wp-content/uploads/2023/07/Cardiovascular-Heart-Emergency-Medical-Training-Online-Courses-for-Nurses-1.png.

These imaging modalities are echocardiography, magnetic resonance imaging (MRI), computed tomography (CT), and nuclear imaging, all with different advantages for the diagnosis of conditions such as coronary artery disease, heart failure, and congenital heart malformations. Recent progress, such as the use of nuclear magnetic resonance spectroscopy and positron emission tomography-CT, has enhanced the understanding of systemic inflammation and cardiovascular risk, particularly in complex inflammatory disorders (Carrillo, 2024). Besides, the intricate intracellular calcium modulation that is vital in cardiovascular function is now interrogated using improved imaging techniques that capture real-time cellular activity in the cardiovascular system (Moccia *et. al.*, 2023). All these point to the central role of cardiovascular imaging in both research and clinical settings (Figure 7.1).

Importance of Cardiovascular Imaging in Medicine

Recent advances in medical technologies have vastly improved diagnostic precision, most notably in the arena of cardiovascular medicine. Precise imaging modalities have become unavoidable within this area. Cardiovascular imaging must play a crucial role in early diagnosis and risk stratification, as well as treatment of heart ailments, allowing for patient-specific therapeutic interventions. By providing unambiguous imaging of the cardiac structure and vascular disease, imaging technologies allow clinicians to make informed decisions, improving the efficacy of therapy and patient outcomes.

In addition, the integration of emerging fields such as nanomedicine holds promising potential to improve cardiovascular imaging through target delivery of diagnostic and therapeutic agents at the site of interest, increasing accuracy and reducing intervention risk (Patra *et. al.*, 2018). Prevention medicine guidelines and clinical judgment, suggested by institutional organizations, emphasize the significance of cardiovascular imaging, citing its relevance in applying scientific evidence to patient-specific care (François *et. al.*, 2019). Therefore, cardiovascular imaging is also vital not only for diagnostic precision but for enhancing personalized medicine, an indispensable place established in modern medical practice.

Historical Development of Cardiovascular Imaging Techniques

Over the past decades, cardiovascular imaging modalities have developed immensely, driven by the demand for increasingly accurate and non-invasive diagnostic equipment. In the initial years, cardiac structure and function evaluation was largely influenced by invasive catheter-based methods, informative though they were, with procedure risks and therefore limited applicability. The introduction of echocardiography and cardiovascular magnetic resonance towards the end of the 20th century was a revolutionary step, allowing clinicians to define cardiac anatomy and function without resorting to invasive therapeutic procedures. These technologies, albeit mainly provided morphological and functional data, with active disease processes being less available. The introduction of molecular nuclear imaging techniques, such as PET and single-photon emission CT, bridged the gap by enabling visualization at the cellular and molecular level, enhancing disease characterization (Joshi *et. al.*, 2024). Concurrently, the concept of ventricular-arterial coupling in the 1980s and subsequent extension through non-invasive imaging and computational modeling is an exemplary convergence of physiological understanding with imaging technology (Toktarbay *et. al.*, 2024). These developments all point the way to precision medicine via the integration of structural, functional, and molecular information in cardiovascular medicine.

Current Trends in Cardiovascular Imaging

The use of advanced technologies has profoundly influenced cardiovascular imaging, enhancing diagnostic precision and facilitating more effective therapy planning. Deep learning- and ML-based algorithms have been revolutionary in their application, enabling comprehensive analysis of complex imaging data from CT scans and MRI scans to identify blockages, plaques, and abnormal cardiac rhythms with unprecedented accuracy (Reshma *et. al.*, 2024).

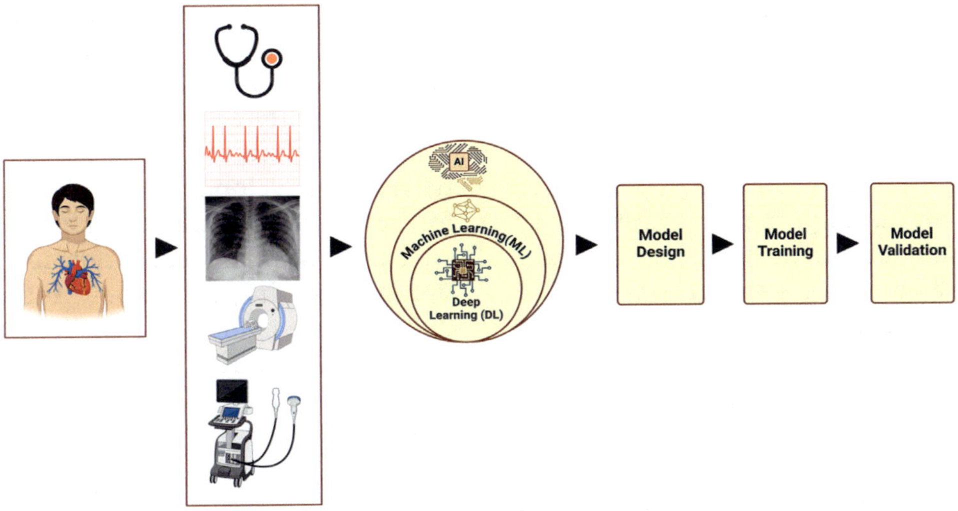

Figure 7.2. Machine learning and deep learning algorithms have emerged as transformative tools, enabling detailed analysis of complex imaging data from CT and MRI scans to identify blockages, plaques, and irregular cardiac patterns with unprecedented accuracy.

Source: https://www.mdpi.com/medicina/medicina-61-00085/article_deploy/html/images/medicina-61-00085-g001.png.

These newer computational algorithms not only allow for more pre-emptive finger-pointing but also aid in predictive modeling of cardiovascular disease progression. Concurrently, intravascular imaging technology such as intravessel ultrasound and optical coherence tomography (OCT) is now essential to fine-tune stent positioning in percutaneous coronary interventions (PCI), reflecting current clinical guideline recommendations (Abubakar *et. al.*, 2023). Promising as these technologies are, they require continued rigorous validation to demonstrate both safety and efficacy across large numbers of patient populations. The overlap of these advances highlights a fundamental shift in cardiovascular imaging toward more patient-specific, data-driven medicine, with the possibility of improved patient outcomes and more individualized therapeutic interventions (Figure 7.2).

Target Audience for Cardiovascular Imaging

Technological advancement in cardiovascular imaging has become increasingly targeted at particular patient populations, reflective of a changing adeptness in diagnosis and treatment. Patients with multi-vessel coronary artery disease, particularly those who have been considered to have high bleeding risk (HBR), are a significant target group for intravascular imaging techniques, as these techniques are better than traditional angiography-guided therapy in clinical outcomes. This subgroup, even if more susceptible to bad cardiovascular events, stands to gain much from the accuracy that cardiovascular imaging brings to the management of percutaneous coronary interventions, lowering the complications of cardiac death and myocardial infarction (Jo *et. al.*, 2025). Further, elderly individuals with no apparent cardiovascular disease but with intrinsic risk factors, such as dyslipidemia and vascular changes with age, can also benefit from cardiovascular imaging modalities like cine cardiovascular MRI, which quantifies pulmonary artery strain and correlates it with metabolic and structural changes (Zhang *et. al.*, 2024). Thus, cardiovascular imaging is used across a broad spectrum, from high-risk patients requiring focused interventional guidance to asymptomatic patients where early detection determines preventive measures.

Challenges in Cardiovascular Imaging

Despite historic advancements in cardiovascular imaging, some limitations hinder its full potential for clinical use. Among the most important challenges is the lack of adequate datasets that are appropriately annotated, limiting the design and evaluation of effective diagnostic algorithms. Standard imaging techniques also lack the ability to image complex cardiac anatomy and dynamic function adequately, with common diagnostic uncertainty. Additionally, the integration of novel technologies like AI in cardiovascular imaging poses questions regarding the reliability of algorithms, cross-platform compatibility, and ease of adoption into practice. While AI-based methods ensure enhanced accuracy and efficiency in diagnosis, their reliability and applicability remain a key concern (Vishwakarma *et. al.*, 2024). In addition, the rapid development of AI technology calls for constant updates to imaging protocols as well as continuing education for clinicians to optimize their utilization (Adertinto *et. al.*, 2024). Overcoming these challenges is essential in advancing cardiovascular imaging towards more personalized and successful treatment of patients.

Future Directions in Cardiovascular Imaging

The continuous evolution of cardiovascular imaging has the potential to transform diagnostic accuracy and therapeutic approaches in cardiology. Advanced mass spectrometry and other new technologies may have the ability to uncover new biomarkers that reflect underlying pathologic mechanisms like plaque morphology, and through such, earlier intervention of coronary artery disease before clinical events occur (Hassan *et. al.*, 2015). Concurrently, the synergy between surgical innovation and minimally invasive imaging modalities allows greater visualization to guide advanced repair techniques, such as those for thoracic and abdominal aortic aneurysms (AAA), to improve patient outcomes with reduced procedural morbidity (Bhogal *et. al.*, 2011). In addition, the future also envisions the incorporation of AI with molecular imaging to provide comprehensive cardiovascular function assessments with structural pathology correlated to biochemical changes. This cross-disciplinary paradigm is predicted to improve individualized treatment regimens, optimize risk stratification, and facilitate the advancement of precision medicine in cardiovascular treatment, in the end improving both prognostic function and therapeutic efficacy (Figure 7.3).

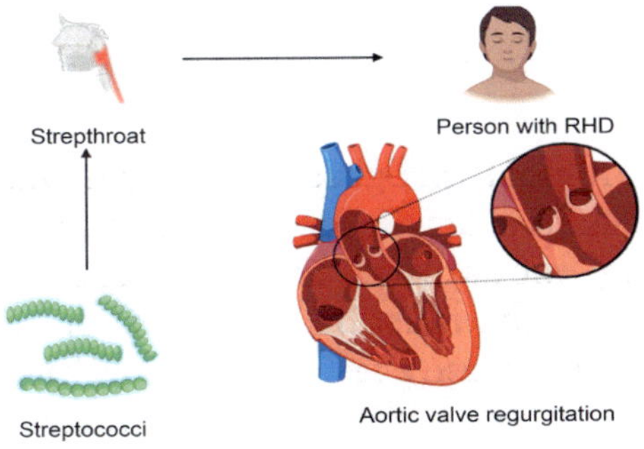

Figure 7.3. Emerging technologies, such as advanced mass spectrometry, hold promise for identifying novel biomarkers that reflect underlying pathological processes like plaque morphology, potentially enabling earlier intervention in coronary artery disease before clinical events occur.

Source: https://www.mdpi.com/cells/cells-13-01471/article_deploy/html/images/cells-13-01471-g006.png.

7.1. Types of Cardiovascular Imaging Modalities

Learning Outcome

1. Understand x-ray imaging
2. Explain computed tomography (CT)
3. Describe magnetic resonance imaging (MRI)
4. Focus on ultrasound imaging
5. Discuss positron emission tomography (PET)
6. Define single photon emission computed tomography (SPECT)
7. Learn angiography
8. Understand echocardiography
9. Describe hybrid imaging techniques

Technological advancement in cardiovascular imaging has significantly broadened diagnostic facilities available to the clinician, facilitating earlier detection and better characterization of cardiac abnormalities. Of greatest prominence among these are transthoracic echocardiography (TTE), cardiac magnetic resonance imaging (CMR), computed tomography (CT), and nuclear imaging techniques, each with its respective advantages and disadvantages. For instance, CMR and TTE are gold standard equipment in cardiac structural and functional abnormality assessment, with the latter being more desirable in providing better tissue characterization with techniques such as T1/T2 mapping and strain measurement, while being crucial in Fabry cardiomyopathy with early sphingolipid deposition before hypertrophy (Roy *et. al.*, 2022). Besides, new approaches integrate sophisticated ML algorithms tailored to specific imaging data to boost predictive accuracy for various cardiovascular diseases (CVD), depending on selecting appropriate models as a function of disease pathology and imaging modality (Toma *et. al.*, 2024). Such multimodal imaging combined with computational analysis, represents a paradigm shift toward more individualized and precise cardiovascular care.

7.1.1. X-Ray Imaging

Technological innovation in cardiovascular imaging has significantly enhanced the diagnosis and therapy of heart disease, yet each modality differs in terms of its strengths and weaknesses. Of all these, X-ray imaging, particularly invasive X-ray angiography, is a standby modality due to the ability to produce high-quality images of coronary arteries and allow interventional therapies. Despite the introduction of non-invasive modalities such as cardiovascular magnetic resonance and CT, X-ray angiography offers an unparalleled real-time imaging necessary for intervention planning and hemodynamic status determination. However, radiation and invasiveness-related issues fuel ongoing interest in new technologies. In the treatment of congenital heart disease, for example, non-invasive modalities are increasingly mainstream, but X-ray remains indispensable for its functional data acquisition during catheter therapies (Muthurangu *et. al.*, 2017). Although new technologies are emerging, the persistent use of X-ray imaging in cardiovascular medicine attests to its role as a crucial tool for gap-filling in alternative modalities and management of complex clinical cases (Kitsiou *et. al.*, 2013) (Figure 7.4).

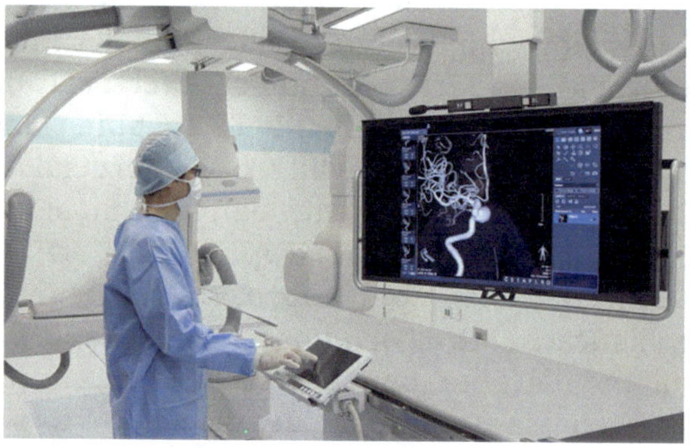

Figure 7.4. X-ray angiography.

Source: https://global.canon/en/technology/img/frontier/sp/head_img33.jpg.

7.1.2. Computed Tomography (CT)

Medical imaging has played a tremendous role in CVD diagnosis and treatment, and CT is a breakthrough technology. CT delivers high-resolution cross-sectional images, enabling precise visualization of blood vessels and the heart, and early detection of abnormalities such as atherosclerosis and myocardial infarction. Its non-invasive and rapid assessment of coronary artery calcification and vascular abnormality makes it an indispensable technology in clinical applications. Second, the combination of CT with theranostic nanomaterials is promising for simultaneous diagnosis and targeted therapy with improved patient benefit through the conjunction of imaging contrast and delivery of therapy in one modality (Wu *et. al.*, 2021). These developments are consistent with current clinical guidelines approving the use of CT in cardiovascular imaging and solidifying its utility in integrative disease management (Vahanian *et. al.*, 2021). Thus, CT remains a pillar of cardiovascular imaging, uniting advanced technology with practical clinical utility.

7.1.3. Magnetic Resonance Imaging (MRI)

Technological progress in cardiovascular diagnosis now largely depends upon advanced imaging modalities that provide precise anatomical and functional information without the need for invasive techniques. Of all these, MRI is most notable for its better characterization of tissues and usefulness in evaluating myocardial architecture and blood flow patterns. Particularly for conditions like arrhythmogenic cardiomyopathy, MRI's ability to non-invasively detect myocardial fibrotic replacement through late gadolinium enhancement has revolutionized diagnosis, risk stratification, and family screening efforts, highlighting its clinical importance beyond traditional imaging methods (Aleksandrova *et. al.*, 2024). Additionally, evolving techniques such as 4D

Flow MRI enable comprehensive quantification of blood flow throughout the cardiovascular system, albeit challenged by spatial resolution limitations. The integration of super-resolution approaches and ensemble learning models has demonstrated promising improvements in image quality and flow measurement accuracy, thereby augmenting MRI's diagnostic utility across diverse cardiovascular domains (Ericsson *et. al.*, 2024). Together, these innovations underscore MRI's pivotal role in advancing cardiovascular imaging and personalized patient management (Figure 7.5).

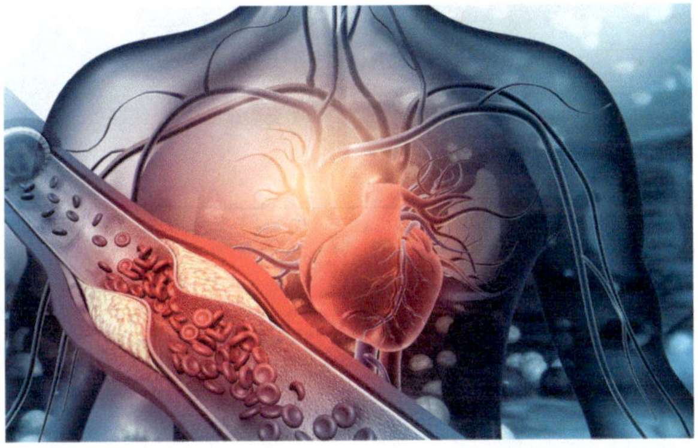

Figure 7.5. Magnetic Resonance Imaging (MRI) stands out for its superior tissue characterization and versatility in assessing myocardial structure and blood flow dynamics.

Source: https://greaterwaterburyimagingcenter.org/wp-content/uploads/2024/09/Cardiac-MRI-.jpg.

7.1.4. Ultrasound Imaging

Advances in imaging technology have had a significant effect on the diagnosis and treatment of CVD, especially through non-invasive approaches that improve safety for the patient and the accuracy of diagnosis. Among these, ultrasound imaging is particularly favored for its real-time nature and lack of ionizing radiation, making it ideal for repeated monitoring and functional evaluation. Recent progress has introduced more sophisticated ultrasound techniques that quantify hemodynamic parameters such as blood flow dispersion and wall shear stress, which are crucial to evaluating arterial stenosis and global vascular function. Though there are some limitations in their diagnostic value, they increase the utility of ultrasound as a tool by allowing multi-parametric measurement, which provides complementary information to other imaging techniques. The integration of ultrasound with complex fusion models further enhances coronary artery visualization and cardiac function analysis, highlighting its value in comprehensive cardiovascular diagnostics. This new role expounds on the value of ultrasound as a multifaceted and indispensable imaging tool for cardiovascular imaging (Du *et. al.*, 2024; Gargi, 2025).

7.1.5. Positron Emission Tomography (PET)

Improvements in cardiovascular imaging have served only to underscore the significance of molecular and metabolic assessment alongside anatomical visualization. Positron emission tomography (PET) plays a pivotal role within this endeavor by providing detailed information regarding myocardial viability and plaque biology not readily accessible by standard imaging modalities. PET's ability to use radiotracers such as [18F] FDG to identify metabolically viable myocardial tissue can even identify hibernating myocardium that would become functional following revascularization. PET viability imaging has been reported in new evidence, however, to have limited predictive value for recovery of left ventricular function and survival in patients with chronic ischemic heart failure, and must be interpreted cautiously in clinical decision-making (Kjærulff *et. al.*, 2025). Additionally, PET molecular imaging stands out in evaluating unstable atherosclerotic plaques by identifying inflammatory processes and macrophage activity, key indicators of adverse cardiac events. Though a hindrance for conditions like myocardial uptake interference,

PET is a prime candidate for early risk stratification and personalized therapeutic strategies (Tamaki *et. al.*, 2024) (Figure 7.6).

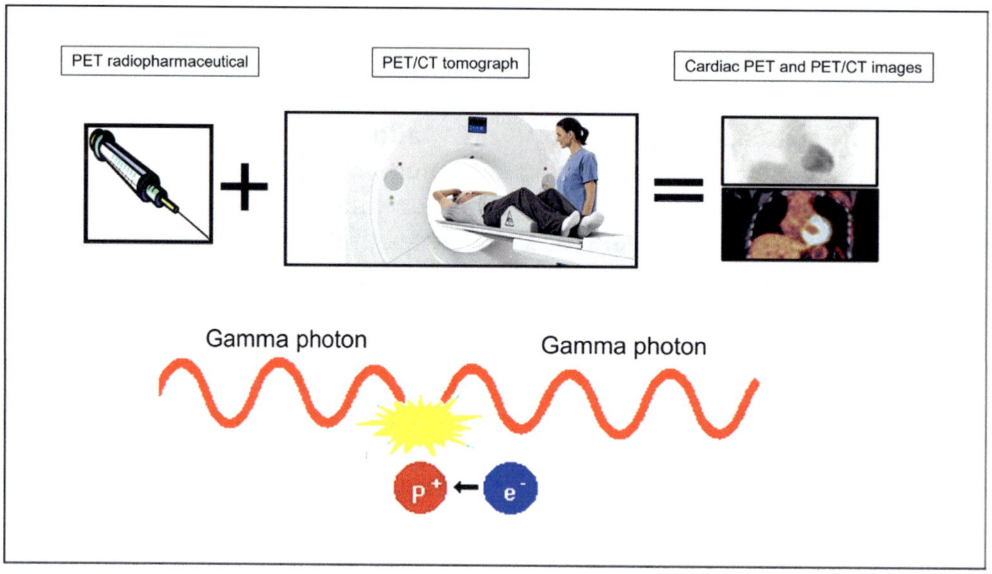

Figure 7.6. Positron emission tomography (PET) in cardiovascular imaging.

Source: https://www.mdpi.com/jcdd/jcdd-10-00220/article_deploy/html/images/jcdd-10-00220-g001.png.

7.1.6. Single Photon Emission Computed Tomography (SPECT)

Advances in technology in cardiovascular imaging have significantly enhanced the diagnostic accuracy, particularly in determining myocardial perfusion and viability. Single Photon Emission Computed Tomography (SPECT) is distinguished by its ability to provide precise functional information through the use of radiotracers that quantify blood flow and metabolic activity in the myocardium. This modality is beneficial in distinguishing ischemic from non-ischemic cardiomyopathies and in detecting viable but hypoperfused myocardium, and is beneficial in clinical decision-making in challenging cases like athletes with suspected cardiac abnormality or patients with multi-vessel coronary artery disease (Zorzi *et. al.*, 2024). Moreover, when combined with PET, SPECT offers exhaustive information, although its prognostic value for long-term functional recovery after revascularization is variable, indicating the heterogeneous nature of ischemic heart disease (Miia *et. al.*, 2015). Despite being underutilized, SPECT remains a cornerstone imaging modality in nuclear cardiology, preserving diagnostic specificity and tolerating acceptable radiation exposure, thus reaffirming its role in personalized cardiovascular management strategies.

7.1.7. Angiography

Technical advancements in cardiovascular imaging have maximally enhanced diagnostic and management potential for CVD, with angiography being a prime focus for these developments. By providing complete visualization of blood vessels, angiography facilitates precise identification of vascular pathologies, including obstructions and aneurysms. In the past, imaging modalities such as CT angiography and PET have been utilized to complement angiographic data in providing a comprehensive assessment of hemodynamics and coronary artery status. Existing approaches include image fusion and sophisticated analytical techniques like radiomics that distill weak quantitative features imperceptible to the human eye, thereby improving diagnostic precision and prognostic evaluation. Issues still exist, however, in imaging protocol heterogeneity and segmentation, thus necessitating standard acquisition and reporting paradigms in an effort to optimize angiographic value in clinical practice. They underscore the critical role of angiography in current cardiovascular diagnosis and management practice (Badesha *et. al.*, 2024; Gargi, 2025) (Figure 7.7).

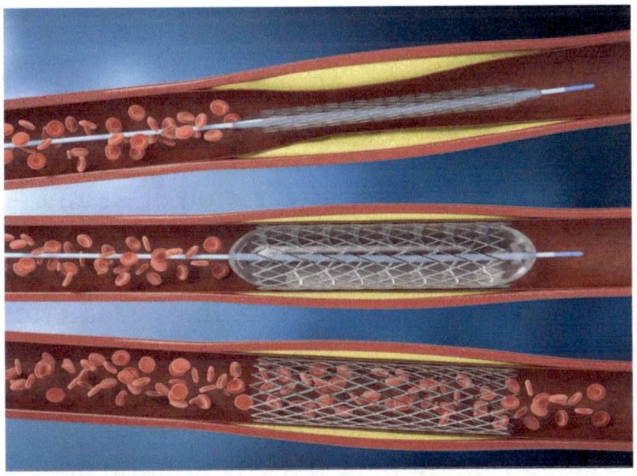

Figure 7.7. By providing detailed visualization of blood vessels, angiography allows for precise identification of vascular abnormalities, including blockages and aneurysms.

Source: https://ssbhealthcare.com/wp-content/uploads/2023/10/3d-rendering-balloon-angioplasty-procedure-with-stent-vein_1_1200x800-1200x900.webp.

7.1.8. Echocardiography

Advances in medical imaging technology have significantly enhanced diagnostic equipment for CVD, with echocardiography playing a significant role due to its capacity to image cardiac anatomy and function in real-time. Echocardiography plays a particularly significant role in cardio-oncology due to its critical role in the detection and management of cardiotoxicity induced by cancer therapy, such as anthracyclines and HER2-targeted agents. By providing baseline testing and ongoing monitoring, echocardiography minimizes cardiovascular morbidity in populations at high risk (Dobson *et. al.*, 2021). The dynamic nature of the beating heart also demands rapid acquisition of images and correct interpretation, and this is being overcome increasingly with the aid of AI. Applications of AI in echocardiography include the automated segmentation of cardiac chambers, functional analysis, and disease diagnosis, and not only enhance accuracy but also workflow efficiency (Zhou *et. al.*, 2021). In combination, these technologies emphasize echocardiography's central position in integrated cardiovascular imaging and patient management (Figure 7.8).

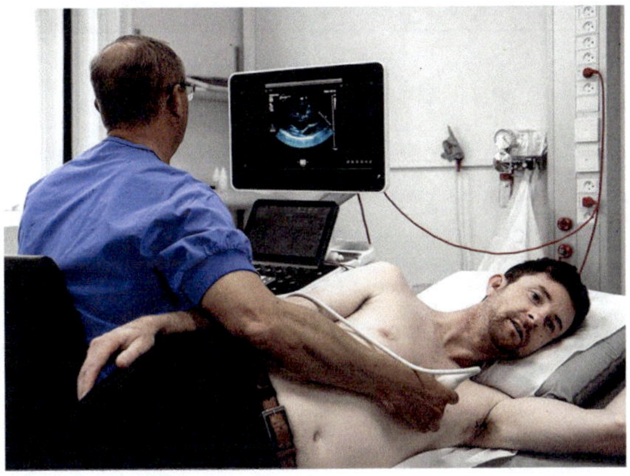

Figure 7.8. Echocardiography.

Source: https://media.post.rvohealth.io/wp-content/uploads/sites/3/2021/12/echocardiogram-doctor-patient-thumb.jpg.

7.1.9. Hybrid Imaging Techniques

Advances in cardiovascular imaging have put increased focus on the integration of more than one modality to enhance diagnostic effectiveness as well as patient management. Hybrid imaging techniques, where anatomical and functional information are blended together, represent a significant advance in this regard. For example, PET fusion with CT or MRI allows clinicians to assess myocardial perfusion and coronary anatomy simultaneously, leading to an increase in the identification and characterization of coronary artery disease. These hybrid approaches have strengths when compared to single modalities because they provide complementary information that is valuable to clinical decision-making. Additionally, the development of deep learning algorithms has enabled effective interpretation of the vast amounts of data generated with hybrid imaging, making possible enhanced risk stratification as well as customized treatment schemes (Bizopoulos *et. al.*, 2021). With their further development, ongoing research is necessary in order to make the best use of their potential in daily cardiovascular practice Glaudemans, A. W., Rouzet, F., Galli, F., Signore, A., *et. al.* (2015).

Test Your Knowledge

1. What are the main types of cardiovascular imaging modalities used in clinical practice?
2. What are the primary advantages and limitations of cardiac CT angiography?

7.2. Applications of Cardiovascular Imaging

Learning Outcome

1. Perform diagnosis of cardiovascular diseases
2. Learn assessment of heart function
3. Explain the evaluation of vascular diseases
4. Focus on preoperative planning
5. Describe postoperative monitoring
6. Identify risk stratification in patients
7. Understand research applications in cardiology
8. Know the role in emergency medicine
9. Focus on patient education and engagement

Advances in technology have enormously increased cardiovascular imaging applications and potential, making it possible to diagnose CVD earlier and more precisely. Traditional imaging techniques, although proficient at defining vessel anatomy, are found to be lacking in assessing the biochemical composition of plaques, a critical prerequisite for specific treatment. Emerging technologies, such as Raman spectroscopy, offer marker-free, high-resolution analysis of plaque composition, improving diagnostic sensitivity and real-time tracking of the progression of the disease (Xie *et. al.*, 2025). Besides, integration of AI and ML with cardiovascular imaging has revolutionized the clinical workflow by supporting image interpretation, patient outcome prediction, and optimization of resource allocation. AI models augment clinical decision-making with increased accuracy and reduced human error, thereby strengthening patient monitoring and treatment stratification (Mohammed *et. al.*, 2025). Combined, these advances in technology not only increase the diagnostic accuracy but also enable personalized therapy, underscoring the revolutionary promise of cardiovascular imaging in contemporary medicine.

7.2.1. Diagnosis of Cardiovascular Diseases (CVD)

Technological innovation in cardiovascular imaging has revolutionized the diagnosis of complex heart diseases, specifically congenital heart diseases (CHD) and structural defects like coarctation of the aorta (CoA). Early-stage diagnosis by innovative imaging modalities is a critical determinant in bringing about early intervention and maximizing patient outcomes. Genetic diagnosis has become a principal aid to the understanding of the etiology of CHD, adding to older clinical assessments the capability of making a more focused and detailed diagnosis and treatment. Further, imaging equipment such as MRI and CT scanning provides non-invasive, high-resolution visualization of cardiovascular anatomy, essential for initial diagnosis as well as for long-term surveillance of conditions like CoA. The technologies allow clinicians to track hemodynamic implications and detect complications after repair, thus enhancing patient care by continuous monitoring and maximally optimal therapeutic interventions (Leo *et. al.*, 2023). Genetic knowledge, combined with high-tech imaging, is a central approach in the diagnostic assessment of CVD (Figure 7.9).

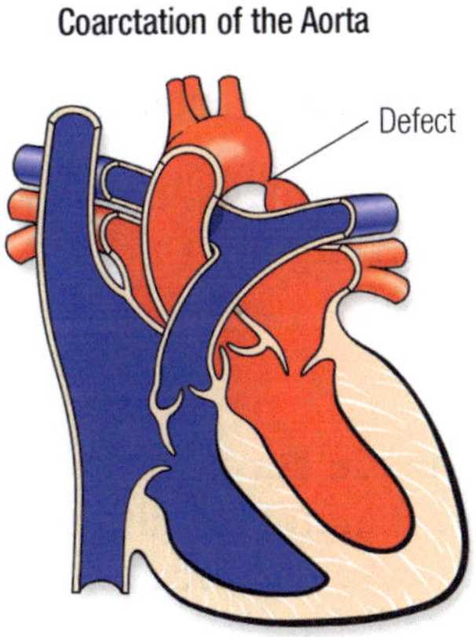

Figure 7.9. Coarctation of the aorta (CoA).

Source: https://www.heart.org/-/media/Images/Health-Topics/Congenital-Heart-Defects/50_1683_50a_CoA.jpg?sc_lang=en.

7.2.2. Assessment of Heart Function

Technological improvements in cardiovascular imaging have vastly enhanced the ability to evaluate heart function more accurately and with greater complexity. Imaging techniques such as CMR imaging can study myocardial structure and function in exquisite detail and provide quantitative information about ventricular volume, ejection fraction, and characterization of myocardial tissue. For instance, in experimental models of aortic coarctation, CMR demonstrates minimal adverse myocardial remodeling along with the concomitant capture of hemodynamic alterations with 4D flow MRI, including localized alterations in flow velocity and patterns, which are crucial in pathophysiology (Gober *et. al.*, 2024). Besides, the inclusion of more sophisticated modalities like 4D flow MRI and arterial spin labeling increases the assessment by imaging detailed intraventricular flow details and quantifying myocardial blood flow with early detection and risk stratification of heart failure patients (Alkhalifah, 2024). These imaging modalities together constitute an integrated approach to assessing cardiac function, ranging from anatomical, functional, and hemodynamic understanding, which is important in tailored clinical management.

7.2.3. Evaluation of Vascular Diseases

Understanding of the intricate pathophysiology of vascular diseases requires a whole-greatness approach that harmonizes biology with advanced diagnostic facilities. Existing research has delineated the manner in which systemic inflammation, metabolic derangements, and focal vascular changes contribute to disease occurrence, particularly in high-risk groups such as type 2 diabetes mellitus and chronic kidney disease. For instance, higher visceral adipose tissue correlates with heightened arterial inflammation, while markers like albuminuria suggest subclinical vascular abnormalities in the form of micro-calcification and arterial stiffness. All such pathophysiologic processes further underscore the employment of cardiovascular imaging modalities in parallel with laboratory investigations—like insulin resistance testing and tests of renal function—to offer precise risk stratification and individualized treatment algorithms. Imaging not only detects but also monitors the evolution of vascular abnormalities and is thus a critical resource in the evaluation of vascular diseases as well as the elaboration of respective preventive strategies (Kitsiou *et. al.*, 2013; Reijrink *et. al.*, 2022) (Figure 7.10).

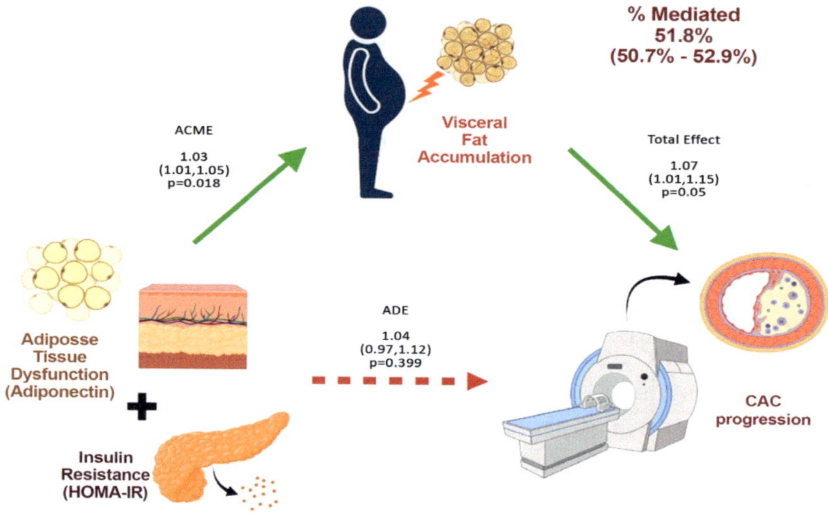

Figure 7.10. Increased visceral adipose tissue correlates with heightened arterial inflammation.

Source: https://media.springernature.com/lw1200/springer-static/image/art%3A10.1186%2Fs12933-023-01807-6/MediaObjects/12933_2023_1807_Fig4_HTML.png.

7.2.4. Preoperative Planning

The addition of newer cardiovascular imaging technologies has made surgical preparation more beneficial by enabling better and more individualized preoperative planning. Multidetector CT with high-resolution anatomic assessment, for instance, allows aortic valve calcification quantification and assessment of the suitability of various prosthetic devices, directly impacting estimation of risk of complications such as paravalvular leak following transcatheter aortic valve implantation. This advanced interpretation aids in selecting the optimal prosthesis size, which is a key determinant of minimizing postoperative complications and enhancing patient outcomes (Pollari *et. al.*, 2019). Moreover, the evolution of autonomous surgical technology, depending on real-time cardiovascular imaging data, has the prospect of advancing surgical proficiency by improving accuracy and velocity, especially in complex procedures challenging human capacity. This synergy of imaging modalities and robotic autonomy is a step ahead in preoperative planning, emphasizing the pivotal role of cardiovascular imaging in personalized treatment and improved surgical efficacy (Das *et. al.*, 2017).

7.2.5. Postoperative Monitoring

Effective postoperative care following cardiovascular surgery is critical in order to optimize patient outcomes and reduce complications. Postoperative monitoring, particularly through cardiovascular imaging, is an integral part of this process that enables early detection of functional abnormalities and potential complications such as graft failure or extension of aortic dissection. Tailored surveillance schemes integrating imaging modalities with clinical evaluation enhance risk stratification and steer intervention appropriately at the right time. Besides, systematic approaches with prognostic prediction models improve patient detection of higher risk for adverse events, hence steering individualized monitoring practices and therapy (Moons *et. al.*, 2019). Emerging technologies such as virtual wards enable remote and sustained monitoring of vital parameters like blood pressure, which is pivotal to minimizing postoperative dangers and improving survival rates in advanced cardiovascular disorders (Pruna-Guillen *et. al.*, 2024). Thus, the convergence of predictive analytics and advanced imaging technologies creates an integrated system for postoperative cardiovascular medicine care (Figure 7.11).

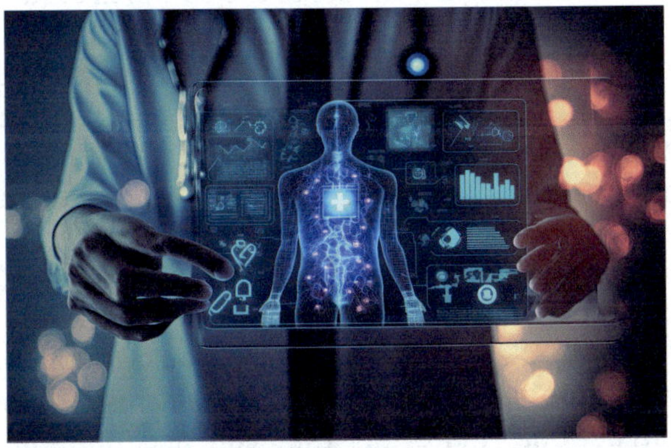

Figure 7.11. Personalized surveillance programs that integrate imaging techniques alongside clinical evaluations enhance risk stratification and guide timely interventions.

Source: https://healthsnap.io/wp-content/uploads/2023/09/ea27d8d0-dbbb-4c22-a505-bf61b98dd200.png.

7.2.6. Risk Stratification in Patients

Accurate quantification of the severity of disease and risk of adverse events is critical to the management of cardiovascular disease. Advances in cardiovascular imaging have facilitated significant risk stratification by precise elucidation of myocardial structure and function. For instance, cardiovascular magnetic resonance (CMR) is precise in the identification of myocardial fibrosis, a critical substrate for arrhythmias and sudden cardiac death in dilated cardiomyopathy, through techniques such as late gadolinium enhancement and T1 mapping, with the ability to differentiate replacement and interstitial fibrosis and inform prognosis (Feng *et. al.*, 2025). To this is contributed the novel modality of 4D flow MRI and arterial spin labeling, which allows measurement of complex cardiac blood flow patterns and myocardial perfusion with the ability to detect subtle functional impairments undetected by conventional methods (Alkhalifah, 2024). Integrating these imaging innovations, preclinical identification of high-risk patients is made possible through a multimodal combination of anatomical and hemodynamic data, thereby optimizing clinical decision-making and patient outcomes through tailoring interventions.

7.2.7. Research Applications in Cardiology

Technological innovation in cardiovascular imaging has expanded research opportunities in cardiology significantly by providing more accurate therapeutic and diagnostic tools. Intravascular optical coherence tomography (OCT) is one such technology that offers high-definition images, allowing for the precise characterization of plaques and aiding percutaneous coronary interventions with enhanced accuracy. Not only does this technology enhance visualization of coronary artery structure, but it is also likely to result in better clinical outcomes through the optimization of stent placement and real-time assessment during intervention, as evidenced by recent trials showing OCT over intravascular ultrasound and traditional angiography (Sacoto *et. al.*, 2024). With it, bringing AI and ML techniques into cardiovascular imaging has advanced the study by enabling automated data analysis and predictive modeling. These approaches improve diagnostic performance and prognostic estimates in interventional cardiology, although problems remain regarding interpretability, generalizability, and ethics. These developments collectively emphasize the transformative effect of advanced imaging and computer-based approaches on planning future cardiology trials (Ali *et. al.*, 2021) (Figure 7.12).

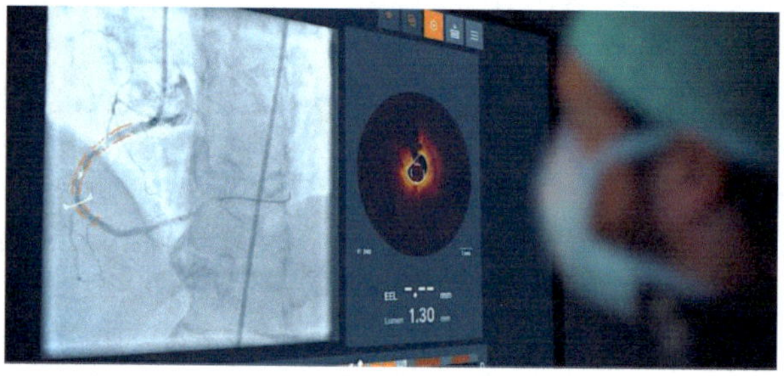

Figure 7.12. Intravascular optical coherence tomography (OCT).

Source: https://www.dicardiology.com/sites/default/files/styles/slider/public/Abbott_AI_OCT_Ultreon_1.0_Software_2.jpg?itok=MeV_ac4V.

7.2.8. Role in Emergency Medicine

In acute illness scenarios, timely and accurate diagnosis is important for effective patient management, particularly in cardiovascular emergencies. Imaging modalities are crucial in emergency medicine by offering rapid visualization of cardiac anatomy and integrity of vessels so that immediate clinical decision-making is possible. Imaging modalities assist the clinicians in the detection of life-threatening illnesses such as myocardial infarction, aortic dissection, or pulmonary embolism, which need urgent intervention. Incorporation of big patient data with ML also enhances diagnostic accuracy and prognostic assessment, guiding patient-specific care plans in critical care (Rajkomar *et. al.*, 2019). Additionally, adherence to established clinical guidelines ensures that responsible use of cardiovascular imaging is made to optimize resource utilization while upholding excellent levels of patient care (Kirchhof *et. al.*, 2016). Accordingly, the contribution of cardiovascular imaging to emergency medicine is inestimable, improving outcomes through simplified diagnosis and evidence-based therapeutic interventions that respond to the latest available knowledge.

7.2.9. Patient Education and Engagement

Cardiovascular imaging technology not only enhanced the accuracy of diagnosis but also redefined patient education and participation, allowing for a more patient-focused healthcare system. Three-dimensional printing, for example, produces a tangible model of the complex cardiac anatomy, allowing patients to better understand their disease and its treatment, thereby improving informed consent and adherence to care plans (Anwar *et. al.*, 2018). It facilitates more effective communication between multidisciplinary teams and patients, bridging knowledge gaps that would otherwise discourage active participation in one's own care. Online cardiovascular imaging-related platforms also allow for continuous education and empowerment through readily accessible instructional materials that can accommodate patient educational requirements (Copeland *et. al.*, 2020). Such engagement strategies result in enhanced clinical outcomes as they encourage active management of care and highlight the importance of follow-up treatment. In total, the merging of advanced imaging modalities with patient-centered educational approaches is a significant move towards optimizing cardiovascular disease control and fostering shared decision-making in clinical practice (Figure 7.13).

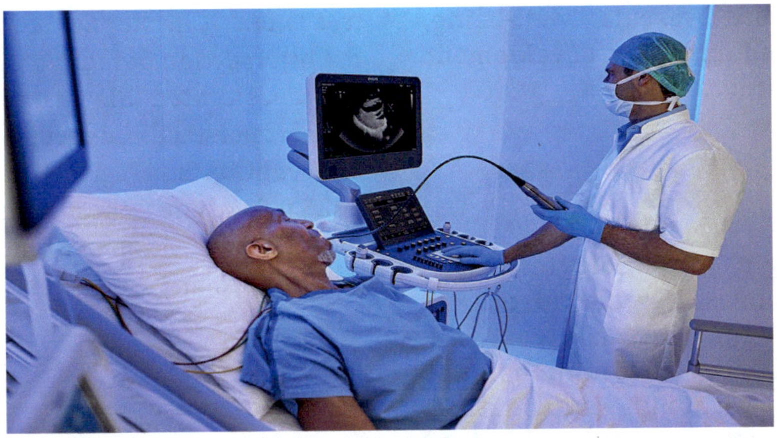

Figure 7.13. Advancements in cardiovascular imaging have not only enhanced diagnostic accuracy but also transformed patient education and engagement, fostering a more collaborative healthcare environment.

Source: https://www.philips.com/c-dam/corporate/innovation-and-you/global/sep-2024/cardiac-care-header.jpg.

Test Your Knowledge

1. What is the role of echocardiography in evaluating heart failure?
2. What are the applications of cardiovascular imaging in congenital heart disease?

7.3. Advances in Cardiovascular Imaging Technology

Learning Outcome

1. Explain development of 3D imaging techniques
2. Learn the integration of artificial intelligence
3. Focus on improvements in image resolution
4. Discuss innovations in contrast agents
5. Know real-time imaging capabilities
6. Identify portable imaging devices
7. Define telemedicine and remote imaging
8. Describe radiation dose reduction techniques
9. Understand future technological trends

Continuing innovation in medical technology has significantly enhanced the ability for diagnosis and treatment of CVD with increased precision. Newer technologies in cardiovascular imaging have enabled novel techniques such as high-resolution CT and MRI, enabling the clinician to visualize cardiac structures with unprecedented detail. Such advances enable early identification of pathology, facilitate interventional strategies, and improve patient outcomes. Precisely, the integration of three-dimensional imaging and functional assessment is achievable for complete assessment beyond normal anatomical imaging. Additionally, improvements in ultrasound technology have also improved capabilities in real-time imaging, which are very critical during surgery. This was achieved through increased image resolution as well as processing rate, as reflected through contemporary imaging devices providing detailed anatomical as well as dynamic functional information. Further, the creation of hybrid modalities combining multiple imaging modalities offers a more complete view of cardiovascular well-being, underscoring a groundbreaking development in diagnostic capabilities.

7.3.1. Development of 3D Imaging Techniques

Advances in imaging technologies have revolutionized cardiovascular diagnostics by allowing more precise anatomical and functional assessment. Traditional two-dimensional imaging methods, although informative, often lack spatial context, which hinders understanding of complex cardiovascular anatomy and diseases. Advances in three-dimensional imaging modalities have overcome such limitations by allowing greater depth perception and volumetric visualization.

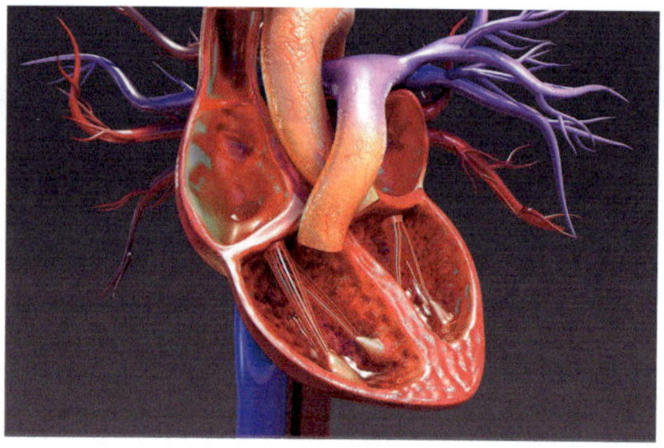

Figure 7.14. The evolution of imaging technologies has revolutionized the field of cardiovascular diagnostics by enabling more precise anatomical and functional assessments.

Source: https://eremedium.in/wp-content/uploads/2024/07/heart-images-in-human-body.jpg.

This development has been complemented by the integration of computational fluid dynamics (CFD) with patient-specific imaging information, allowing for dynamic hemodynamic factor analysis in cardiovascular disease. Stereoscopic display environments allow clinicians to interactively explore high-resolution, 3D-represented models, improving diagnostic accuracy and planning treatment (Christopher *et. al.*, 2015). Besides, the intersection of radiomics and AI in radiology has accelerated 3D imaging optimization to support personalized medicine and more efficient intervention strategies (Augustynowicz *et. al.*, 2023). Combined, these technologies emphasize the leading position of 3D imaging in optimizing cardiovascular care (Figure 7.14).

7.3.2. Integration of Artificial Intelligence

Technological progress in imaging has exponentially expanded the array of information to be found in cardiovascular diagnostics, challenging clinicians to interpret and integrate this information effectively. Synthesis of AI offers a revolutionary approach to this complexity through the enhancement of diagnostic insight and prognostication. ML algorithms like deep learning can enable the identification and examination of weak imaging markers that are not specific to humans, particularly in imaging modalities like nuclear cardiology imaging and coronary CT angiography. Although central AI models have potential in leveraging big data for speedy prototyping, their functionality is task-specific and data-dependent. End-to-end learning strategies explicitly designed for cardiovascular imaging have reported higher clinical-grade accuracy and lower diagnostic variation, mitigating the issue of high computational expense associated with generalized models. Therefore, a hybrid approach through the integration of foundation models with domain-specialized training has the highest potential to maximize the integration of AI into cardiovascular imaging practice (Mulliqi *et. al.*, 2025; Slart *et. al.*, 2021).

7.3.3. Improvements in Image Resolution

Advancements in imaging technology have significantly enhanced the visualization of the morphology of the cardiovascular system, making cardiac pathophysiology more measurable. Increased resolution in images permits precise examination of complex anatomical and functional traits, which is vital in the diagnosis and treatment of CVD. For example, the integration of high-resolution patient-specific imaging information with CFD within virtual reality visualization environments has improved the spatial and temporal recognition of hemodynamic patterns to aid in clinical interpretation as well as intervention planning (Christopher *et. al.*, 2015). Additionally, sophisticated techniques such as diffusion tensor imaging with late gadolinium enhancement cardiovascular magnetic resonance have yielded submillimeter resolution images that define microstructural remodeling of myocardial infarcts. This degree of resolution captures fine changes in fiber direction and scar tissue structure, thus giving an in-depth characterization of post-infarction remodeling processes in both animal models and human hearts (Bluemke *et. al.*, 2017). These advances not only promote diagnostic accuracy but also provide insight into myocardial pathophysiology and therapeutic targeting (Figure 7.15).

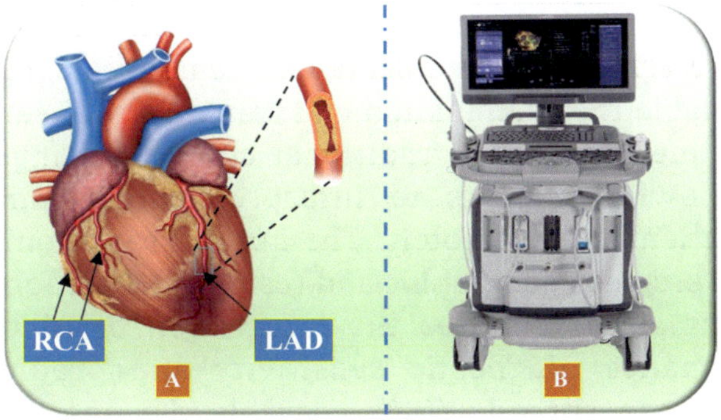

Figure 7.15. Advancements in imaging technology have profoundly enhanced the visualization of cardiovascular structures, allowing more precise assessment of cardiac pathophysiology.

Source: https://www.mdpi.com/diagnostics/diagnostics-15-00848/article_deploy/html/images/diagnostics-15-00848-g001.png.

7.3.4. Innovations in Contrast Agents

There are new imaging technologies that have greatly enhanced cardiovascular diagnostics' ability, particularly by way of novel contrast agents that improve tissue differentiation and molecular specificity. Spectral photon-counting computed tomography (SPCCT) is one recent innovation that leverages the features of photon-counting detectors with the capability to discriminate between energies in order to improve contrast resolution and lower artifacts typically linked to conventional imaging methods. The ability to image multiple contrast agents in parallel enables quantitative characterization of cardiovascular tissues with high precision for improved evaluation of myocardial perfusion and tissue characterization (Meloni *et. al.*, 2024). Similarly, targeted ultrasound molecular probes have revolutionized ultrasound imaging by chemical modification of microbubbles with site-specific antibodies or ligands that bind to cellular markers, providing real-time imaging of pathologic alterations at the molecular level. Not only does this technology enhance diagnostic accuracy but also allows for targeted drug delivery and therapy monitoring, constituting a tremendous milestone toward combined diagnostic and therapeutic approaches in cardiovascular medicine (Wen *et. al.*, 2023). All these breakthroughs herald a revolutionary era for contrast agent development for cardiovascular imaging.

7.3.5. Real-time Imaging Capabilities

Technological innovations in imaging have profoundly impacted many fields, such as cardiovascular diagnosis, where the ability to capture and process real-time information is critical for effective patient management. The ability to perform real-time imaging is critical since it allows practitioners to observe dynamic functions of the heart, such as blood flow and myocardial motion, so that heart wellness can be accurately assessed and intervention can be done if necessary. Such technology, fueled by innovation in other high-demand applications such as satellite imagery and aerial surveillance, employs high-performance onboard processing and rapid data acquisition methods to reduce latency while increasing resolution (Garcia *et. al.*, 2024). Furthermore, state-of-the-art detection models originally trained for real-time object detection in drone images further demonstrate the potential to advance cardiovascular imaging precision and speed with a focus on interdisciplinary breakthroughs that allow this technology (Muzammul *et. al.*, 2024). The ability to process complex cardiovascular images in real time not only facilitates improved diagnosis but also facilitates complex procedural guidance, thereby improving clinical outcomes (Figure 7.16).

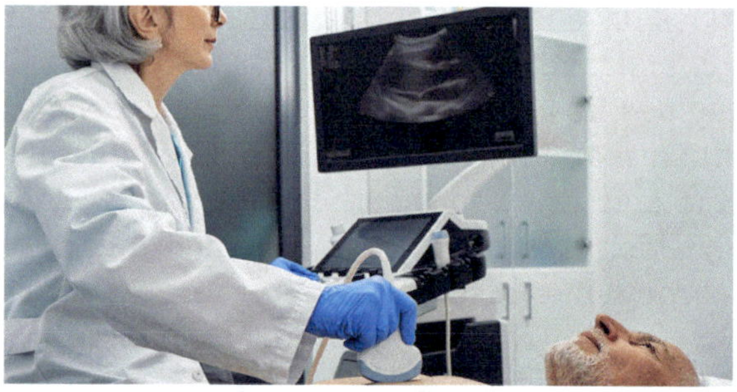

Figure 7.16. Real-time imaging capabilities allow clinicians to observe dynamic cardiac functions, such as blood flow and myocardial motion, enabling accurate assessment of heart health and immediate intervention if necessary.

Source: https://smithchason.edu/wp-content/uploads/2024/03/blog-10.jpg.

7.3.6. Portable Imaging Devices

Medical technology has made cardiovascular diagnostics more available and effective. Portable imaging equipment has been among the most significant advances , especially at the level of primary healthcare, where specialized personnel may not be readily available. These devices have been equipped with ultrasound facilities, allowing for non-invasive scanning of the carotid artery, the potential early identification of cardiovascular disease, and eventually the saving of lives. The addition of robotic aid in portable ultrasound systems has also increased their use with the ability of semi-automatic scanning and precise positioning of the probe, correcting for patient movement and cardiac phases, to improve image accuracy and reproducibility. The use of AI on these systems also makes possible detailed segmentation and analysis of vascular anatomy, assisting in the detection of significant pathologies such as carotid stenosis. Clinical studies confirm that the point-of-care systems are effective, simple to use, and receive great feedback from both patients and operators in testimony to their ability to revolutionize cardiovascular imaging and diagnosis (Tan *et. al.*, 2024).

7.3.7. Telemedicine and Remote Imaging

Technological innovation has significantly transformed the delivery of health care, particularly in cardiovascular imaging, where early diagnosis and continuous monitoring are critical. Telemedicine and remote imaging enable the examination and treatment of heart ailments beyond traditional clinical settings, allowing experts to interpret images and patient data remotely. The approach not only overcomes geographic and resource limitations but also facilitates the integration of AI to enhance diagnostic sensitivity and predict disease spread. With wearable devices and mobile applications, healthcare professionals can monitor vital signs and cardiac biomarkers in real-time to promote proactive intervention and personalized treatment. Studies indicate that telemonitoring patients have increased confidence in managing their disease on their own and are content with phone consultations, reflecting improved engagement in care (Marozzi *et. al.*, 2024). Furthermore, the combination of telemedicine with AI analytics for data analysis can potentially achieve rural healthcare equality, provide personalized care to practitioners, and improve overall cardiovascular disease management results (Nwankwo *et. al.*, 2024) (Figure 7.17).

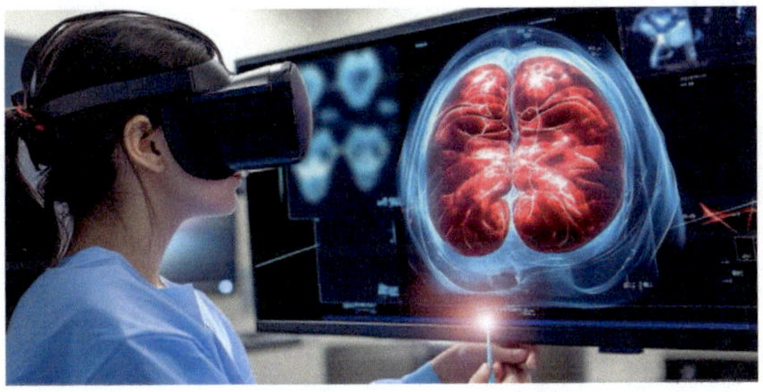

Figure 7.17. Telemedicine and remote imaging facilitate the assessment and management of cardiac conditions beyond traditional clinical settings, enabling specialists to interpret images and patient data remotely.

Source: https://tateeda.com/wp-content/uploads/2024/10/Top-8-Telemedicine-Trends-and-Technologies-in-2025-6-1024x597.jpg.

7.3.8. Radiation Dose Reduction Techniques

Developments in CT technology have significantly improved the safety profile of cardiovascular imaging by addressing concerns related to ionizing radiation exposure. Among such technologies, iterative image reconstruction algorithms have emerged as a game-changing approach by optimizing the quality of images through recursive computations that effectively reduce noise and artifacts without compromising diagnostic accuracy. This is especially helpful for challenging clinical situations such as imaging high body mass index patients or those with heavy coronary calcification, where traditional methods struggle to maintain clarity. Making ,more explicit images using less radiation, iterative reconstruction enables clinically relevant dose reductions in routine and follow-up cardiovascular CT scans to meet mounting calls for lower risk of imaging. Furthermore, modern coronary artery calcium scoring protocols incorporate technical developments that also constrain radiation exposure while preserving the prognostic value of the scans. These additive methods are a significant stride toward optimizing risk-benefit ratios in cardiovascular imaging (Cho *et. al.*, 2014; Kaitlin *et. al.*, 2016).

7.3.9. Future Technological Trends

Technological advances in cardiovascular imaging will likely be heavily influenced by upcoming trends that value integration, automation, and real-time monitoring. Integration with cutting-edge bioinformatics and nanotechnology in medical devices will likely contribute diagnostic precision and therapeutic efficacy, enabling more individualized patient treatment.

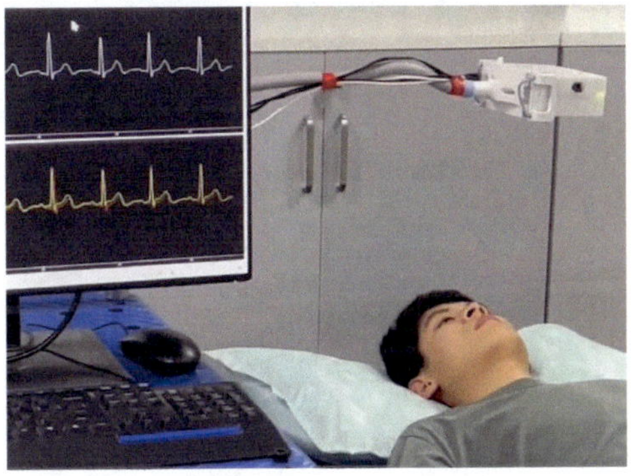

Figure 7.18. Continuous electrocardiogram (ECG).

Source: https://spectrum.ieee.org/media-library/less-than-p-greater-than-the-researchers-demonstrated-an-experimental-setup-for-contactless-ecg-monitoring-using-millimeter-wave-radar-less-than-p-greater-than.jpg?id=32121458.

Automatic systems with real-time electrocardiogram (ECG) and RR interval monitoring are increasingly prominent in order to identify diseases like atrial fibrillation more efficiently, thereby facilitating earlier intervention and reduction of morbidity and mortality rates. These technologies envision a future where cardiovascular imaging extends beyond hospital facilities but into usual patient care by wearable and implantable devices. Though highly promising, these advances face serious technological and regulatory challenges to overcome. Nonetheless, the drive to leverage big data and integrate AI in cardiovascular imaging is part of the overall health objectives of achieving improved outcomes at lower costs and staying competitive in the medical device industry (Acharya *et. al.*, 2020; Baio *et. al.*, 2025) (Figure 7.18).

Test Your Knowledge

1. What are the key recent advancements in cardiac MRI technology?
2. How has artificial intelligence (AI) improved the accuracy and efficiency of cardiovascular imaging interpretation?

7.4. Challenges and Limitations of Cardiovascular Imaging

Learning Outcome

1. Identify cost and accessibility issues
2. Know patient safety concerns
3. Discuss limitations of specific imaging modalities
4. Focus on interpretation challenges
5. Explain variability in imaging quality
6. Discuss ethical considerations in imaging
7. Understand training and expertise requirements
8. Learn integration into clinical practice
9. Identify future research needs

Even with vast improvements, cardiovascular imaging is confronted with many limitations that prevent it from reaching its ultimate clinical applications. Its limiting factor is the fast movement of the heart, which makes it difficult to obtain sharp and precise images, particularly in modalities such as echocardiography. Such fast motion requires advanced techniques and skilled interpretation to prevent diagnostic pitfalls. Despite the potential of AI to improve image recognition and functional measurements, practical application requires huge, standardized databases and precise image annotation, which are difficult to obtain on a routine basis (Zhou *et. al.*, 2021). In addition, multimodal imaging data integration, facilitated by medical image registration, is central to enhanced visualization but comes with limitations such as variability in imaging parameters and lack of reliable ground truth for verification. Despite the fact that ML has accelerated registration processes, reproducibility and accuracy are principal impediments (Liu *et. al.*, 2019). Such obstacles significantly limit diagnostic accuracy and the extensive use of cardiovascular imaging in practice.

7.4.1. Cost and Accessibility Issues

Advancements in cardiovascular imaging have dramatically improved treatment planning and diagnostic sensitivity, but their overall use remains constrained by cost and access factors. Sophisticated modalities such as MRI and CT scanning, while able to deliver higher degrees of detail in imaging, tend to be costly and specialized in equipment requirements, and therefore less accessible to resource-poor environments. Qualified personnel must also operate these devices and interpret results, adding to access problems. New technologies like generative AI have the promise to enhance patient education and even make imaging procedures more standardized, particularly in resource-poor settings. However, such technologies also present quality of data, infrastructure, and ethics that must be addressed to utilize them optimally (Marey *et. al.*, 2024). Balancing the need for novel imaging modalities with practical issues about affordability and availability is critical to ensure cardiovascular care is equitable, calling for tailor-made approaches that maximize cost-effectiveness without compromising on diagnostic efficacy (Lee, 2025) (Figure 7.19).

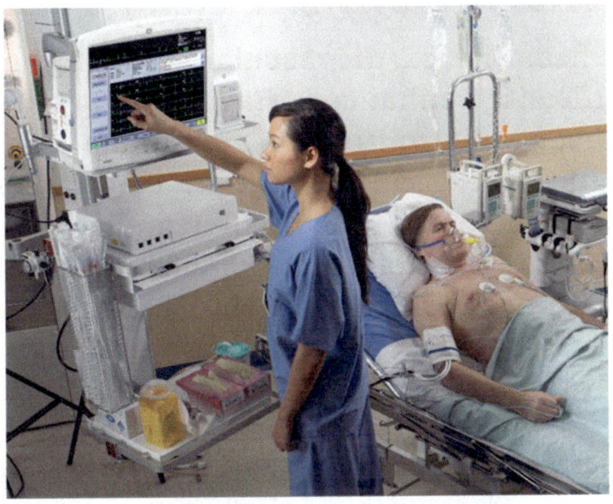

Figure 7.19. High-end modalities such as MRI and CT scans, while offering superior imaging detail, often require substantial financial investment and specialized infrastructure, limiting availability in resource-constrained settings.

Source: https://clinicalview.gehealthcare.com/sites/default/files/Clinician%20touching%20a%20monitor%20next%20to%20a%20male%20patient%20laying%20on%20a%20bed.png.

7.4.2. Patient Safety Concerns

Increased reliance on advanced cardiovascular imaging techniques underscores the crucial need to address patient safety concerns, particularly radiation exposure and contrast agent use. Pregnant patients represent a high-risk population whose imaging considerations go beyond short-term diagnostic benefits, with the necessity of stringent compliance with the ALARA principle to mitigate fetal hazards while providing proper assessment of cardiovascular disease. Such balance needs to be maintained in pregnancy-related CVD management without compromising the well-being of the mother and fetus (Lauriero *et. al.*, 2025). Concurrently, advances in medical care, such as adaptive learning algorithms employed in coronary artery angiography, offer hopeful means to reduce ionizing radiation doses safely. These algorithms optimize imaging protocols by adjusting dose parameters based on patient-specific variables, thereby enhancing imaging quality while minimizing radiological hazards. Despite the challenge in terms of variability and privacy of data, the union of these innovations is toward more secure, more personalized imaging methods that preserve diagnostic effectiveness and prioritize patient health (Tariq *et. al.*, 2024).

7.4.3. Limitations of Specific Imaging Modalities

Despite advances in cardiovascular imaging, other modalities pose intrinsic limitations that limit their diagnostic utility in specific clinical scenarios. For example, standard modalities such as MRI, CT, and ultrasound are prone to having problems of limited tissue penetration, acquisition time, and motion artifact susceptibility, which can complicate accurate assessment of dynamic blood flow or intracardiac disease (Marisa *et. al.*, 2024). Additionally, in patient subgroups, for example, left bundle branch block (LBBB), standard noninvasive techniques such as stress tests and nuclear scans are less successful in the diagnosis of ischemia on the basis of abnormal myocardial mechanics (Imamuddin *et. al.*, 2024). New technologies such as tissue Doppler imaging

(TDI) are more sensitive in these situations but are not yet universally accepted and require specialized expertise. This highlights the necessity for continued development and validation of novel imaging methodologies to overcome these constraints and improve cardiovascular diagnostic precision (Figure 7.20).

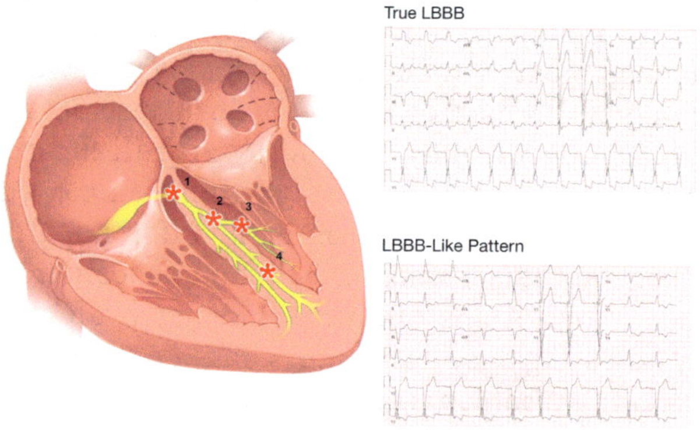

Figure 7.20. Left bundle branch block (LBBB).

Source: https://www.ahajournals.org/cms/10.1161/CIRCEP.119.008239/asset/7fc353d7-5348-44fc-abf3-1cad964c2829/assets/graphic/circep.119.008239.fig03.jpg.

7.4.4. Interpretation Challenges

Accurate interpretation of cardiovascular imaging data is critical for effective diagnosis and treatment planning, but it is commonly hindered by a number of interpretive challenges. Heterogeneous cardiac motion, inconsistency in patient anatomy, and artefacts in imaging are some of the challenges that contribute to the complexity of reliably identifying small structural and functional abnormalities.

Further, integration of multiple imaging planes often requires advanced computational techniques to reconstruct precise three-dimensional models because standard two-dimensional slices have the potential to limit diagnosis accuracy. Recent advances in automated image analysis and deep learning have shown potential in surmounting these challenges by enhancing image registration and enabling detailed 3D descriptions of cardiac anatomy (Banerjee *et. al.*, 2021).

The translation of ML techniques into the clinical setting, however, introduces novel challenges to study design, data quality, and algorithm reproducibility (Weikert *et. al.*, 2020). Subvention of these challenges of interpretation will need multidisciplinary alliances and robust testing of emerging technologies to yield appropriate and clinically relevant cardiovascular imaging measures.

7.4.5. Variability in Imaging Quality

Advances in cardiovascular imaging have significantly enhanced diagnostic precision; however, the uniformity of image quality remains a critical issue that could impact clinical outcomes. Inconsistent image quality results from variability in equipment calibration, operating expertise, patient characteristics, and institutional routine. Such variability can lead to diagnostic uncertainty, and that could lead to a delay in appropriate treatment or to inappropriate interpretation of pathologies. Moreover, standardization efforts are thwarted by the rapid rate of advancement of imaging modalities and the extensive variety of clinical settings for use.

The guidelines established by regulatory organizations emphasize the need to balance scientific data with clinical judgment in a bid to mitigate these differences, while encouraging professional responsibility for actual decision-making despite imaging performance variability (Cosentino *et. al.*, 2019; François *et. al.*, 2019). These discrepancies should be met with constant training, quality control measures, and technological advances to maximize the reliability and usefulness of cardiovascular imaging (Figure 7.21).

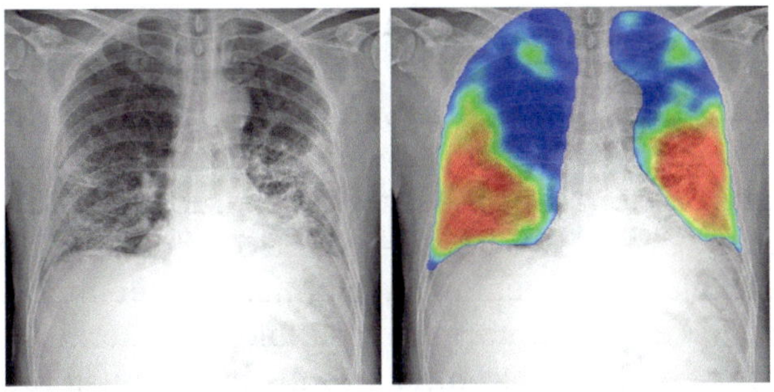

Figure 7.21. Variability in imaging performance.

Source: https://djq2z2zar5p7e.cloudfront.net/images/delft-imaging-cad4covid-xr.2e16d0ba.fill-800x400.png.

7.4.6. Ethical Considerations in Imaging

Technological advances in cardiovascular imaging have revolutionized diagnostic capability, but also bring with them complex ethical challenges that need careful thought. Maintenance of patient autonomy as informed consent is required, since patients must be informed of potential risks, benefits, and alternatives for testing and imaging. Also, concerns regarding equitable access are compromised in a market-driven healthcare environment where disparities limit access to vulnerable populations. The conflict between maximizing patient benefit and optimizing resource utilization forces practitioners to resolve these challenges cautiously. In addition, patient data confidentiality and privacy are still crucial as digital imaging databases expand, requesting strict guidelines for prevention against unauthorized posting or hacking (Copeland *et. al.*, 2019). Resolution of these ethical elements is crucial in ensuring trust and maintaining integrity in cardiovascular imaging practice in contemporary medical settings.

7.4.7. Training and Expertise Requirements

Growing demands for cardiovascular imaging, or echocardiography, underscore the necessity for advanced training and experience to deliver accurate diagnosis and patient care. As more patients are seen with fewer cardiologists available, boosting the skill level of physician assistants (PAs) has been a rational step in mitigating workforce shortages. Modern training for PAs typically does not involve formal postgraduate education in echocardiography, resulting in a lack of balance between clinical need and expertise. Recent efforts have aimed to produce systematic curricula that combine didactic modules online with supervised hands-on clinical training, with competency as assessed by Entrustable Professional Activities frameworks and simulation exams. These educational programs will work towards standardizing the gain of competence and ultimately create certification systems for non-physician providers, optimizing access and quality of cardiovascular imaging care. Continuous refinement and multi-center evaluation of these new curricula will be needed to demonstrate their effectiveness and integration within broader clinical practice (Kitsiou *et. al.*, 2013; Moon *et. al.*, 2017) (Figure 7.22).

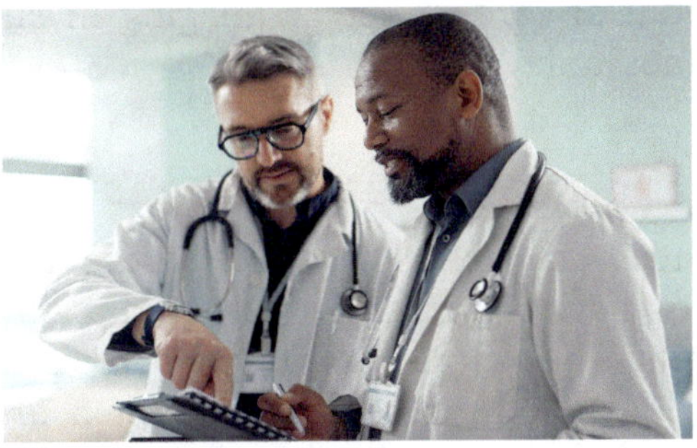

Figure 7.22. With a growing patient population and a simultaneous shortage of cardiologists, expanding the skill set of physician assistants (PAs) has emerged as a pragmatic strategy to alleviate workforce constraints.

Source: https://assets.isu.pub/document-structure/241114143629-97d78c64885bf745d4410105baf1cac8/v1/0050c85140baa95ec617e765ef733c75.jpeg.

7.4.8. Integration Into Clinical Practice

Technological advances in cardiovascular imaging have progressed well due to urgent advancements that improve precise diagnosis and treatment planning. The application of three-dimensional modeling and printing due to high-definition CT and MRI images is an ideal example of how advances in engineering benefit advances in interventional cardiology through facilitating clinicians to pre-procedure visualize patient-specific anatomy, improving outcome, and procedural efficacy (Celi *et. al.*, 2025). At the same time, clinical application of newer CMR technologies, such as T1/T2 mapping and automated segmentation, has been a persistent effort to integrate newer imaging modalities into routine use. These methods deliver quantitative data that support updating myocardial disease staging and risk stratification, progressing personalized medicine approaches (Julia *et. al.*, 2024). Despite limitations including validation, reproducibility, and availability of expertise staff, these technologies hold promise for substantial reductions in invasive testing and disease phenotyping, and demonstrate the revolutionary potential of cardiovascular imaging in clinical pipelines today.

7.4.9. Future Research Needs

Advances in technology for cardiovascular imaging have significantly increased diagnostic capability, but there remain great areas to be filled by ongoing research. One such area is further unraveling congenital heart defects (CHDs), which occur in a significant percentage of the population and have multifactorial causes involving genetic, epigenetic, and environmental factors. To optimize diagnostic precision and therapeutic intervention, it is crucial to integrate advanced genomic technology with comprehensive phenotypic characterization and create disease-specific models to establish molecular mechanisms (Reemtsen *et. al.*, 2017). Emerging technologies like mass spectrometry also offer promising avenues for the identification of biomarkers, for example, lipid profiles that can direct plaque morphology and cardiovascular risk stratification. However, further research is required to optimize the accuracy, reproducibility, and clinical relevance of such devices for cardiovascular imaging (Hassan *et. al.*, 2015). Addressing these areas of research will be essential to enabling personalized cardiovascular care, ultimately improving patient outcomes and reducing morbidity related to cardiac disease (Figure 7.23).

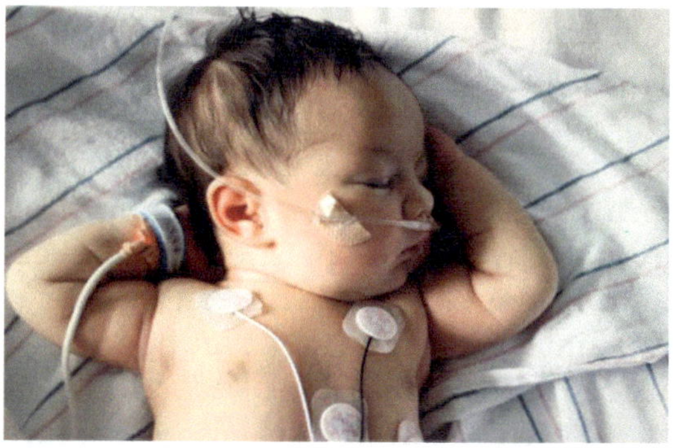

Figure 7.23. Understanding of congenital heart defects (CHDs).

Source: https://www.heart.org/-/media/Images/Health-Topics/Congenital-Heart-Defects/Survivor-photos/Sloan-in-hospital.jpg?h=533&w=800&sc_lang=en.

Test Your Knowledge

1. What are the major limitations of echocardiography in obese or critically ill patients?
2. How does patient motion affect the quality of cardiac MRI and CT images?

SUMMARY

The rapid development of cardiovascular imaging, driven by advances in AI technology, is a revolutionary era in cardiology. Greater incorporation of AI technologies into diagnosis pipelines holds the promise to introduce unprecedented advancements in accuracy, timeliness, and personalized patient care. The methods enhance image resolution, reduce processing time, and enable detection of subtle cardiac abnormalities that would otherwise go undetected. While these are optimistic benefits, they will depend on addressing issues of data standardization, regulatory compliance, and patient safety in order to realize the full potential of AI in clinical practice. It will be the joint effort of clinicians, researchers, and regulators to overcome the obstacles and ensure ethical application. Finally, the use of AI-based cardiovascular imaging has the potential to dramatically improve clinical decision-making and patient outcomes, representing a paradigm shift towards more precise and predictive cardiovascular care (Alotaibi *et. al.*, 2025; Tolu-Akinnawo *et. al.*, 2025).

Advances in technologies in cardiovascular imaging have led to significant improvements in diagnostic accuracy and clinical utility, which are mainly attributed to the introduction of new analytical techniques and technologies. Coupling patient-specific, high-resolution imaging with CFD enables the visualization of complicated hemodynamic patterns in detail, which improves spatial and temporal understanding beyond two-dimensional displays (Christopher *et. al.*, 2015). In addition, combinations of AI and ML algorithms have yielded promising results in differentiating cardiovascular disease, which typically has a similar clinical presentation, such as Takotsubo cardiomyopathy and myocardial infarction (Chew *et. al.*, 2024). These AI-based methods not only increase the specificity and sensitivity of diagnosis but also reduce human error, thus making them even more likely to enhance clinical decision-making. Together, these developments present a paradigm shift in cardiovascular imaging in which an elevated visualization capacity and intelligent data interpretation converge to facilitate better patient care and guide future scientific research in cardiovascular medicine.

KEY TERMS FROM THIS CHAPTER

- Cardiology
- Cardiovascular magnetic resonance (CMR)
- Coronary artery disease
- Heart failure
- Molecular levels
- Single-photon emission computed tomography
- Cardiovascular magnetic resonance
- Congenital heart defects
- Echocardiography
- Intracellular calcium signaling
- Nuclear imaging
- Systemic inflammation

CRITICAL THINKING QUESTIONS

1. Which imaging modality is considered the gold standard for assessing cardiac anatomy and function?

a. Chest X-ray
b. Echocardiography
c. Cardiac MRI
d. CT angiography

2. What is the primary use of stress echocardiography?

a. Evaluate valvular disease
b. Detect pericardial effusion
c. Assess myocardial ischemia
d. Visualize congenital defects

3. Which of the following is the best initial imaging study in a suspected aortic dissection in a hemodynamically stable patient?

a. Chest X-ray
b. Echocardiogram
c. CT angiography
d. Cardiac MRI

4. A coronary artery calcium (CAC) score of zero suggests:

a. High risk of coronary artery disease
b. Moderate plaque burden
c. No detectable atherosclerosis
d. Need for immediate angiography

5. Which of the following is true about cardiac CT with contrast?

a. It does not require heart rate control
b. It can accurately assess coronary plaque
c. It is preferred for myocardial perfusion
d. It is the gold standard for valve evaluation

Short Answer Questions

1. What imaging modality is considered the gold standard for evaluating cardiac anatomy and function?
2. How does echocardiography help in assessing valvular heart disease?
3. What is the role of CT angiography in the diagnosis of aortic dissection?
4. When is cardiac MRI preferred over echocardiography?
5. What does a coronary artery calcium score indicate about cardiovascular risk?
6. What is the most appropriate imaging technique for detecting a patent foramen ovale?
7. How is myocardial viability assessed in cardiovascular imaging?
8. In which scenarios is nuclear imaging used in cardiovascular evaluation?

Answers to Critical Thinking Questions

1. (c); 2. (c); 3. (c); 4. (c); 5. (b)

REFERENCES

1. Abubakar, M., Javed, I., Rasool, H. F., Raza, S., Basavaraju, D., Abdullah, R. M., Ahmed, F., *et. al.* (2023). Advancements in percutaneous coronary intervention techniques: A comprehensive literature review of mixed studies and practice guidelines. *Cureus, 15*. https://www.semanticscholar.org/paper/79f7c53c7bb7d51a7b8c7ad02bc6ca24eb55f8eb (accessed on 30 May 2025).
2. Acharya, U. R., Ciaccio, E. J., & Faust, O. (2020). A review of atrial fibrillation detection methods as a service. https://core.ac.uk/download/322489443.pdf (accessed on 30 May 2025).
3. Adertinto, N., David-Olawade, A. C., *et. al.* (2024). Advancements and applications of artificial intelligence in cardiology: Current trends and future prospects. https://core.ac.uk/download/603653360.pdf (accessed on 30 May 2025).
4. Aleksandrova, S., Glazkova, E. Y., & Golukhova, E. (2024). Cardiac magnetic resonance imaging in arrhythmogenic cardiomyopathy: Evolving diagnostic criteria and new capabilities. *Russian Journal of Cardiology*. https://www.semanticscholar.org/paper/1ec8dcb73f478e3325dab99306971ff7170b6fef (accessed on 30 May 2025).
5. Alkhalifah, B. (2024). Quantitative imaging for early detection and risk stratification of cardiovascular disease using 4D flow MRI and arterial spin labelling. *Bioinformation, 20*, 1769–1775. https://www.semanticscholar.org/paper/bf474985400da5a5792bea1d5368a62838101a20 (accessed on 30 May 2025).
6. Alotaibi, A., Contreras, R., Thakker, N., Mahapatro, A., Adla Jala, S. R., Mohanty, E., Devulapally, P., *et. al.* (2025). Bibliometric analysis of artificial intelligence applications in cardiovascular imaging: Trends, impact, and emerging research areas. *Annals of Medicine and Surgery, 87*, 1947–1968. https://www.semanticscholar.org/paper/ad69a66069ba6969622811c51bd90770146424c6 (accessed on 30 May 2025).
7. Anwar, A., Barach, B., Bhatla, Biglino, *et. al.* (2018). 3D printing is a transformative technology in congenital heart disease. https://core.ac.uk/download/212858839.pdf (accessed on 30 May 2025).
8. Augustynowicz, K., Morawski, P., Ostaszewska, S., Pactwa, *et. al.* (2023). Advancements in radiology and diagnostic imaging. https://core.ac.uk/download/587246519.pdf (accessed on 30 May 2025).
9. Badesha, A. S., Frood, R., Bailey, M. A., Coughlin, P., & Scarsbrook, A. (2024). A scoping review of machine-learning derived radiomic analysis of CT and PET imaging to investigate atherosclerotic cardiovascular disease. *Tomography, 10*, 1455–1487. https://www.semanticscholar.org/paper/ad44c35459c44bfd5ed11635c56787da532415b5 (accessed on 30 May 2025).
10. Baio, G., Magazzini, L., Oglialoro, C., *et. al.* (2025). Medical devices competitiveness and impact on public health expenditure. https://core.ac.uk/download/pdf/6464525.pdf (accessed on 30 May 2025).
11. Banerjee, A., Camps, J., Zacur, E., Andrews, C. M., Rudy, Y., Choudhury, R. P., Rodríguez, B., *et. al.* (2021). A completely automated pipeline for 3D reconstruction of human heart from 2D cine magnetic resonance slices. *Philosophical Transactions of the Royal Society A: Mathematical, Physical and Engineering Sciences, 379*. https://doi.org/10.1098/rsta.2020.0257.

12. Baron, K. B., Choi, A., & Chen, M. Y. (2016). Low radiation dose calcium scoring: Evidence and techniques. *Current Cardiovascular Imaging Reports, 9*. https://www.semanticscholar.org/paper/c31e547bae77e451f1c808f70fffc87540342c92 (accessed on 30 May 2025).

13. Ben Ali, W., Pesaranghader, A., Avram, R., Overtchouk, P., Perrin, N., Laffite, S., Cartier, R., *et. al.* (2021). Implementing machine learning in interventional cardiology: The benefits are worth the trouble. *Frontiers in Cardiovascular Medicine, 8*. https://www.semanticscholar.org/paper/7501d91e3f975dedc1e4e57e437525e5a6dd04a5 (accessed on 30 May 2025).

14. Bhogal, R. H., & Downing, R. (2011). The evolution of aortic aneurysm repair: Past lessons and future directions. https://cdn.intechopen.com/pdfs/22382/InTech-The_evolution_of_aortic_aneurysm_repair_past_lessons_and_future_directions.pdf

15. Bizopoulos, P., & Koutsouris, D. (2021). Deep learning in cardiology. http://arxiv.org/abs/1902.11122 (accessed on 30 May 2025).

16. Bluemke, D. A., Gai, N., Halperin, H., *et. al.* (2017). Submillimeter diffusion tensor imaging and late gadolinium enhancement cardiovascular magnetic resonance of chronic myocardial infarction. https://core.ac.uk/download/323064815.pdf (accessed on 30 May 2025).

17. Celi, S., Capellini, K., Fanni, B., Pizzuto, A., Santoro, G., & Gasparotti, E. (2025). 3D play: From bench to hybrid catheterization laboratory. *European Heart Journal. Imaging Methods and Practice, 3*. https://www.semanticscholar.org/paper/2f3dc3e8a999e0f1827b21abea073972dad79879 (accessed on 30 May 2025).

18. Chew, N., Chew, N., Huang, H., Huang, H., *et. al.* (2024). The utility of artificial intelligence and machine learning in the diagnosis of Takotsubo Cardiomyopathy: A systematic review. https://core.ac.uk/download/614960746.pdf (accessed on 30 May 2025).

19. Cho, Y. J., Schoepf, U., Silverman, J. R., Krazinski, A. W., Canstein, C., Deak, Z., Grimm, J., *et. al.* (2014). Iterative image reconstruction techniques: Cardiothoracic computed tomography applications. *Journal of Thoracic Imaging, 29*, 198–208. https://www.semanticscholar.org/paper/ee62b8bef30548ccb39c3074e8fdc7235f4748ba (accessed on 30 May 2025).

20. Chowdhury, M. A., Rizk, R., Chiu, C., Zhang, J. J., Scholl, J. L., Bosch, T. J., Singh, A., *et. al.* (2025). The heart of transformation: Exploring artificial intelligence in cardiovascular disease. *Biomedicines, 13*. https://www.semanticscholar.org/paper/5f96626de9d05f4fbf5a8c33bc0cfcd6b7fe2ec6 (accessed on 30 May 2025).

21. Copeland, L. I. B. T., James, Duinkerken, M. S. I., Kelsey, Gordon, *et. al.* (2020). Jefferson Digital Commons quarterly report: January-March 2020. https://core.ac.uk/download/299811518.pdf (accessed on 30 May 2025).

22. Cosentino, F., Grant, P. J., Aboyans, V., Bailey, C. J., Ceriello, A., Delgado, V., Federici, M., *et. al.* (2019). 2019 ESC Guidelines on diabetes, pre-diabetes, and cardiovascular diseases developed in collaboration with the EASD. *European Heart Journal, 41*, 255–323. https://doi.org/10.1093/eurheartj/ehz486.

23. Das, N., & Yip, M. (2017). Robot autonomy for surgery. *arXiv*. http://arxiv.org/abs/1707.03080 (accessed on 30 May 2025).

24. Dobson, R., Ghosh, A. K., Ky, B., Marwick, T. H., Stout, M., Harkness, A., Steeds, R. P., *et. al.* (2021). BSE and BCOS guideline for transthoracic echocardiographic assessment of adult cancer patients receiving anthracyclines and/or trastuzumab. *JACC Cardio Oncology, 3*, 1–16. https://doi.org/10.1016/j.jaccao.2021.01.011.

25. Du, Y., Wang, S., Lu, Z., Liu, Y., Guo, Y., An, X., Li, S., *et. al.* (2024). Research progress on medical imaging and new ultrasound techniques for assessing the degree of carotid artery stenosis. *Zhongguo Yi Liao Qi Xie Za Zhi = Chinese Journal of Medical Instrumentation, 48*(6), 624–630. https://www.semanticscholar.org/paper/3baaca7a785a0fe7e042f4ffd946535126da3032 (accessed on 30 May 2025).

26. Ericsson, L., Hjalmarsson, A., Akbar, M. U., Ferdian, E., Bonini, M., Hardy, B., Schollenberger, J., *et. al.* (2024). Generalized super-resolution 4D flow MRI – using ensemble learning to extend across the cardiovascular system. *IEEE Journal of Biomedical and Health Informatics, 28*, 7239–7250. https://www.semanticscholar.org/paper/d57885e8a9e13869076e2e7b864031d21bfd6141 (accessed on 30 May 2025).

27. Feng, X. Y., Zheng, Y. C., Yang, Y., He, W. F., Yang, F., Wang, L. L., Yang, H. F., *et. al.* (2025). Utilization of cardiac magnetic resonance imaging for assessing myocardial fibrosis in prognosis evaluation and risk stratification of patients with dilated cardiomyopathy. *Reviews in Cardiovascular Medicine, 26*. https://www.semanticscholar.org/paper/ec2336511c3626544e195c342968a55634995a40 (accessed on 30 May 2025).

28. Gargi, J. T. (2025). Survey of advanced image fusion techniques for enhanced visualization in cardiovascular diagnosis and treatment. *Journal of Clinical, Medical and Experimental Images*. https://www.semanticscholar.org/paper/121e90f887fa30b95c54f043dc5b52d874aace5c (accessed on 30 May 2025).

29. Glaudemans, A. W., Rouzet, F., Galli, F., Signore, A., *et. al.* (2015). Imaging infection and inflammation. https://core.ac.uk/download/54518572.pdf (accessed on 30 May 2025).

30. Gober, L., Stellon, M., Lamers, L. J., Frenkel, A., Irrer, D., & Alzate, A. R. (2024). Abstract 1089: Noninvasive assessment of aortic biomechanics using 4-D flow and cardiovascular magnetic resonance in a porcine model of aortic coarctation. *Arteriosclerosis, Thrombosis, and Vascular Biology*. https://www.semanticscholar.org/paper/5895267d917c335f5b12730007a813080cb7381c (accessed on 30 May 2025).

31. Carrillo Guerrero , D. (2024). Psoriasis: Definition and classification of a complex entity. *International Journal of Medical Science and Clinical Research Studies*. https://www.semanticscholar.org/paper/16c5be52f0e9c871134b401601650cf3f33d2535 (accessed on 30 May 2025).

32. Hassan, M., Jacob, S. S., & Yacoub, M. H. (2015). Utility of mass spectrometry for the diagnosis of the unstable coronary plaque. https://core.ac.uk/download/77008832.pdf (accessed on 30 May 2025).

33. Imamuddin, S., Srinivas, R., Parvathareddy, K., Nagula, P., Suneetha, K., & Ganesh, M. (2024). A study of the usefulness of tissue Doppler imaging for the diagnosis of coronary artery disease in patients with left bundle branch block. *Journal of The Indian Academy of Echocardiography & Cardiovascular Imaging*. https://www.semanticscholar.org/paper/c1ff3671a6fd82e0c15c11d5332751ddceee76ca (accessed on 30 May 2025).

34. Jo, J., Lee, S. Y., Kwon, W. D., Lee, S. J., Lee, J. Y., Lee, S. H., Shin, D., *et. al.* (2025). Intravascular imaging-guided versus angiography-guided complex PCI in patients with high bleeding risk: A secondary analysis of the RENOVATE-COMPLEX PCI trial. *Circulation: Cardiovascular Interventions, 18*(3), e014952. https://www.semanticscholar.org/paper/260f5c50fdd015b350f9fc9ad3cb0338fb0f8f83 (accessed on 30 May 2025).

35. Joshi, S., Geers, J., Gimelli, A., Hyafil, F., Habib, G., Erba, P., Gheysens, O., *et. al.* (2024). Current and emerging radiotracers in molecular cardiovascular imaging. *Circulation: Cardiovascular Imaging, 17*(10), e016323. https://www.semanticscholar.org/paper/1fece8a841d54a491ad17d23b0dd0f344abf2e32 (accessed on 30 May 2025).

36. Kirchhof, P., Benussi, S., Kotecha, D., Ahlsson, A., Atar, D., Casadei, B., Castellá, M., *et. al.* (2016). 2016 ESC guidelines for the management of atrial fibrillation developed in collaboration with EACTS. *European Heart Journal, 37*, 2893–2962. https://doi.org/10.1093/eurheartj/ehw210.

37. Kitsiou, A., Caforio, A. L. P., Porta-Sanchez, A., Vahanian, A., Iung, B., Carrera, C., Szymanski, C., *et. al.* (2013). ESC core curriculum for the general cardiologist (2013). https://core.ac.uk/download/55756305.pdf (accessed on 30 May 2025).

38. Kjærulff, M. L. B. G., Tolbod, L., Pryds, K., Nielsen, R., Madsen, S., Luong, T. V., & Gormsen, L. (2025). Clinical use of [15O]H_2O/[18F]FDG viability positron emission tomography does not reliably predict left ventricular ejection fraction improvement or survival after revascularization. *European Heart Journal. Cardiovascular Imaging*. https://www.semanticscholar.org/paper/03e22ce89bc027be881d1de46c3e4babec356b6e (accessed on 30 May 2025).

39. Larkee, C. E., Quam, D. J., Otake, H., Ladisa, J. F., Ladisa, J. F., Ellwein, L., Hayden, P., *et. al.* (2015). Immersive visualization for enhanced computational fluid dynamics analysis. https://core.ac.uk/download/213075191.pdf (accessed on 30 May 2025).

40. Lauriero, F., Mazza, G., Perazzolo, A., Ottoni, G., Cipriani, A., Castro Pereira, J. F., Marano, R., *et. al.* (2025). Pregnancy-related cardiovascular diseases: A radiological overview. *Journal of Cardiovascular Development and Disease, 12*. https://www.semanticscholar.org/paper/02f88ae18672c5a38fb2b44c7b3c3bccd3227a94 (accessed on 30 May 2025).

41. Lee, D. H. (2025). Recent advances and issues in imaging modalities for hepatocellular carcinoma surveillance. *Journal of Liver Cancer, 25*, 31–40. https://www.semanticscholar.org/paper/8186ab61545a4644ac410c2968902e4d88ef2284 (accessed on 30 May 2025).

42. Lehtinen, M. L., Schildt, J., Ahonen, A., Nikkinen, P., Lauerma, K., Sinisalo, J., Kankuri, E., *et. al.* (2015). Combining FDG-PET and 99mTc-SPECT to predict functional outcome after coronary artery bypass surgery. *European Heart Journal Cardiovascular Imaging, 16*(9), 1023–1030. https://www.semanticscholar.org/paper/67cb89b7a86c4ce8cf232e7f98c3831ea5c09ab7 (accessed on 30 May 2025).

43. Leo, I., Sabatino, J., Avesani, M., Moscatelli, S., Bianco, F., Borrelli, N., De Sarro, R., *et. al.* (2023). Non-invasive imaging assessment in patients with aortic coarctation: A contemporary review. *Journal of Clinical Medicine, 13*. https://www.semanticscholar.org/paper/9150d44df79de1caf79bfe24a35fa15985cb79d5 (accessed on 30 May 2025).

44. Liu, J., Singh, G., Al'Aref, S. J., Lee, B. C., Oleru, O., Min, J. K., Dunham, S., *et. al.* (2019). Image registration in medical robotics and intelligent systems: Fundamentals and applications. *Advanced Intelligent Systems, 1*. https://doi.org/10.1002/aisy.201900048.

45. Mach, F., Baigent, C., Catapano, A. L., Koskinas, K. C., Casula, M., Badimón, L., Chapman, M. J., *et. al.* (2019). 2019 ESC/EAS Guidelines for the management of dyslipidemias: Lipid modification to reduce cardiovascular risk. *European Heart Journal, 41*, 111–188. https://doi.org/10.1093/eurheartj/ehz455.

46. Marey, A., Saad, A. M., Killeen, B., Gomez, C., Tregubova, M., Unberath, M., & Umair, M. (2024). Generative artificial intelligence: Enhancing patient education in cardiovascular imaging. *BJR Open,*

6. https://www.semanticscholar.org/paper/dfccdb6b81b85329ccab8cf262b8e7408f89f074 (accessed on 30 May 2025).

47. Marozzi, M., Corvasce, F., Falcone, G., Desantis, V., Solimando, A., Ria, R., Vacca, A., *et. al.* (2024). Impact of remote monitoring on patients' quality of life: A single center study. *Journal of Hypertension, 42*, e154–e155. https://www.semanticscholar.org/paper/137e28b97f068b3453eae9397baff336d4307ec8 (accessed on 30 May 2025).

48. Meloni, A., Maffei, E., Clemente, A., De Gori, C., Occhipinti, M., Positano, V., Berti, S., *et. al.* (2024). Spectral photon-counting computed tomography: Technical principles and applications in the assessment of cardiovascular diseases. *Journal of Clinical Medicine, 13*. https://www.semanticscholar.org/paper/08877fb32b64f4d4671d71eb0935996f18f8ae17 (accessed on 30 May 2025).

49. Moccia, F., Fiorio Pla, A., Lim, D., Lodola, F., & Gerbino, A. (2023). Intracellular Ca2+ signaling: Unexpected new roles for the usual suspect. *Frontiers in Physiology, 14*. https://www.semanticscholar.org/paper/e3d7337cf46f3cc7e5e908054005468ba1373326 (accessed on 30 May 2025).

50. Moon, S. (2017). Echocardiography curriculum development for physician assistants using entrustable professional activities. https://core.ac.uk/download/215924737.pdf (accessed on 30 May 2025).

51. Moons, K., Wolff, R., Riley, R., Whiting, P., Westwood, M., Collins, G., Reitsma, J., *et. al.* (2019). PROBAST: A tool to assess risk of bias and applicability of prediction model studies: Explanation and elaboration. *Annals of Internal Medicine, 170*, W1–W33. https://www.semanticscholar.org/paper/2a5bed915f10e2467397f55d0fd0c7cbb51696e6 (accessed on 30 May 2025).

52. Mulliqi, N., Blilie, A., Ji, X., Szolnoky, K., Olsson, H., Boman, S. E., Titus, M., *et. al.* (2025). Foundation models–A panacea for artificial intelligence in pathology? https://www.semanticscholar.org/paper/516d76eb4547667ff9191853afc407fedb0564e4 (accessed on 30 May 2025).

53. Muthurangu, V., Puranik, R., & Taylor, A. M. (2017). The role of cardiovascular magnetic resonance in congenital heart disease. https://core.ac.uk/download/268426669.pdf (accessed on 30 May 2025).

54. Muzammul, M., Algarni, A., Ghadi, Y., & Assam, M. (2024). Enhancing UAV aerial image analysis: Integrating advanced SAHI techniques with real-time detection models on the VisDrone dataset. *IEEE Access, 12*, 21621–21633. https://www.semanticscholar.org/paper/16b9bd7b67e19d274c1c93267bac679f741b01eb (accessed on 30 May 2025).

55. Nwankwo, E. I., Emeihe, E. V., Ajegbile, M. D., Olaboye, J. A., & Maha, C. C. (2024). Integrating telemedicine and AI to improve healthcare access in rural settings. *International Journal of Life Science Research Archive*. https://www.semanticscholar.org/paper/a48d6d02742ddd4106ac2fb9d2e3aa9245c65e9c (accessed on 30 May 2025).

56. Pacheco, M. O., Gerzenshtein, I. K., Stoppel, W. L., & Rinaldi-Ramos, C. M. (2024). Advances in vascular diagnostics using magnetic particle imaging (MPI) for blood circulation assessment. *Advanced Healthcare Materials*. https://www.semanticscholar.org/paper/e18c46cbade707fb081eb8817666086e1acadd74 (accessed on 30 May 2025).

57. Garcia Parra , L., Furano, G., Ghiglione, M., Zancan, V., Imbembo, E., Ilioudis, C., Clemente, C., *et. al.* (2024). Advancements in onboard processing of synthetic aperture radar (SAR) data: Enhancing efficiency and real-time capabilities. *IEEE Journal of Selected Topics in Applied Earth Observations and Remote Sensing, 17,* 16625–16645. https://www.semanticscholar.org/paper/558a0f9946e32208fc185652ad01619f98b4b9c3 (accessed on 30 May 2025).

58. Patra, J. K., Das, G., Fernandes Fraceto, L., Campos, E. V. R., Rodriguez-Torres, M. P., Acosta-Torres, L. S., Díaz-Torres, L. A., *et. al.* (2018). Nano based drug delivery systems: Recent developments and future prospects. *Journal of Nanobiotechnology, 16.* https://doi.org/10.1186/s12951-018-0392-8.

59. Pollari, F. (2019). Risk factors for paravalvular leak after transcatheter aortic valve replacement. https://core.ac.uk/download/188825595.pdf (accessed on 30 May 2025).

60. Pruna-Guillen, R., Ghosh, L., Mastracci, T., Kapil, V., Lopez-Marco, A., & Oo, A. (2024). Challenges and innovations in postoperative care for acute type A aortic dissection: The role of structured surveillance and virtual wards. *Reviews in Cardiovascular Medicine, 25.* https://www.semanticscholar.org/paper/8b1fd06cf368abdbfaa7f7bc485811fd3176b244 (accessed on 30 May 2025).

61. Rajkomar, A., Dean, J. B., & Kohane, I. S. (2019). Machine learning in medicine. *New England Journal of Medicine, 380,* 1347–1358. https://doi.org/10.1056/nejmra1814259.

62. Ravi, R. S., Vanitha, K., & Anjana, T. K. (2024). A survey of cardiovascular disease identification and prediction using machine learning and deep learning methods. In *2024 International Conference on Emerging Research in Computational Science (ICERCS).* https://www.semanticscholar.org/paper/5035d8c3f8cb482fb0ffcc76cd89efb1ae682711 (accessed on 30 May 2025).

63. Reemtsen, B., Finn, J. P., Alejos, J., Touma, M., Halnon, N., Nelson, S. F., *et. al.* (2017). A path to implement precision child health cardiovascular medicine. https://doi.org/10.3389/fcvm.2017.00036.

64. Reijrink, M. (2022). *Cardiovascular disease in type 2 diabetes mellitus and chronic kidney disease: imaging modalities and pathogenetic mechanisms.* [Thesis fully internal (DIV), University of Groningen]. University of Groningen. https://doi.org/10.33612/diss.213637405

65. Roy, A., Mansour, M., Oxborough, D., Geberhiwot, T., & Steeds, R. (2022). Multi-modality cardiovascular imaging assessment in Fabry disease. *Applied Sciences.* https://www.semanticscholar.org/paper/3b49b0daf2ce600df49e040a51a96b57406d0479 (accessed on 30 May 2025).

66. Sacoto, V. M. A., Mite, A. P. C., Pilatasig, W. J. M., Mosquera-Ceprian, R. A., Muñoz Cunduri, E. V., Basantes Castillo, A. M., Polo Roldán, V. M., *et. al.* (2024). A systematic review of clinical applications and diagnostic efficacy of intravascular optical coherence tomography in cardiology. *International Journal of Research in Medical Sciences.* https://www.semanticscholar.org/paper/e75117f7831b9d54474cd8d711d1b22d6ed40979 (accessed on 30 May 2025).

67. Simkowski, J. M., Eck, B., Tang, W. H. W., Nguyen, C., & Kwon, D. (2024). Next-generation cardiac magnetic resonance imaging techniques for characterization of myocardial disease. *Current Treatment Options in Cardiovascular Medicine, 26,* 243–254. https://www.semanticscholar.org/paper/e6e4334cbe97393767418dff743ea2d474744d88 (accessed on 30 May 2025).

68. Situ, Y., Birch, S., Moreyra, C., & Holloway, C. J. (2020). Cardiovascular magnetic resonance

imaging for structural heart disease. *Cardiovascular Diagnosis and Therapy, 10*, 361–375. https://doi.org/10.21037/cdt.2019.06.02.

69. Slart, R., Williams, M., Juárez-Orozco, L., Rischpler, C., Dweck, M., Glaudemans, A., Gimelli, A., *et. al.* (2021). Position paper of the EACVI and EANM on artificial intelligence applications in multimodality cardiovascular imaging using SPECT/CT, PET/CT, and cardiac CT. *European Journal of Nuclear Medicine and Molecular Imaging, 48*, 1399–1413. https://www.semanticscholar.org/paper/40466aff2bca6b86070f2f329796710a131e3be4 (accessed on 30 May 2025).

70. Tamaki, N., Mititelu, R., Proaño-Bernal, L., Gilabert-Garcia, A., Sharma-Sharma, S., Mora-Barrera, C. M., Singer-De-la-Garza, J., *et. al.* (2024). Positron emission tomography and its role in the assessment of vulnerable plaques in comparison to other imaging modalities. *Frontiers in Medicine, 10*. https://www.semanticscholar.org/paper/d0bda09317ce2266c75d742e76bcedb17422058c (accessed on 30 May 2025).

71. Tan, L., Deng, Z., Hao, M., Zhang, P., Hou, X., Chen, C., Gu, X., *et. al.* (2024). 3D ultrasound image acquisition and diagnostic analysis of the common carotid artery with a portable robotic device. *2024 IEEE/RSJ International Conference on Intelligent Robots and Systems (IROS)*. https://www.semanticscholar.org/paper/150b296d706f28d3b5c711c5525572fb92dee6d3 (accessed on 30 May 2025).

72. Tariq, K., Munir, M. A., Aftab, H. T., Naveed, A., Yousaf, A., & Hassan, S. U. (2024). Adaptive learning algorithms for low dose optimization in coronary arteries angiography: A comprehensive review. *Journal of Rawalpindi Medical College*. https://www.semanticscholar.org/paper/a749575fb56289435fcb416937d7f5b8a41a1f09 (accessed on 30 May 2025).

73. Toktarbay, B., Zhankorazova, A., Khamitova, Z., Jumadilova, D., & Salustri, A. (2024). Ventricular-arterial coupling: Advances and current perspectives in cardiovascular research. *Journal of Clinical Medicine of Kazakhstan*. https://www.semanticscholar.org/paper/42a07b4202f0fae6631fad484a514ffac5860581 (accessed on 30 May 2025).

74. Tolu-Akinnawo, O., Ezekwueme, F., Omolayo, O., Batheja, S., & Awoyemi, T. (2025). Advancements in artificial intelligence in noninvasive cardiac imaging: A comprehensive review. *Clinical Cardiology, 48*. https://www.semanticscholar.org/paper/438993eec131848e01f335a9a3f30eebd875a809 (accessed on 30 May 2025).

75. Toma, M., Chong, L., Husain, G., Nasef, D., Vathappallil, P., & Matalia, M. (2024). Machine learning strategies for improved cardiovascular disease detection. *Medical Research Archives*. https://www.semanticscholar.org/paper/5c71f0b939e20c9b28fbac295075a7582fd40e84 (accessed on 30 May 2025).

76. Vahanian, A., Beyersdorf, F., Praz, F., Milojevic, M., Baldus, S., Bauersachs, J., Capodanno, D., *et. al.* (2021). 2021 ESC/EACTS guidelines for the management of valvular heart disease. *European Heart Journal, 43*, 561–632. https://doi.org/10.1093/eurheartj/ehab395.

77. Vishwakarma, K., Anish, P., Priyadarshi, R., Ranjan, R., Singh Rathore, *et. al.* (2024). Exploring the frontiers of unsupervised learning techniques for diagnosis of cardiovascular disorder: A systematic review. https://core.ac.uk/download/624275247.pdf (accessed on 30 May 2025).

78. Weikert, T., Francone, M., Abbara, S., Baeßler, B., Choi, B. W., Gutberlet, M., Hecht, E. M., *et. al.* (2020). Machine learning in cardiovascular radiology: ESCR position statement on design

requirements, quality assessment, current applications, opportunities, and challenges. *European Radiology, 31*, 3909–3922. https://doi.org/10.1007/s00330-020-07417-0.

79. Wen, Q., & Xu, S. (2023). Applications of ultrasound targeted micro/nano probes and intelligent ultrasound molecular imaging technology. *Journal of Biomedical Nanotechnology*. https://www.semanticscholar.org/paper/f7d4231ad018f9747f66ccf4e14666dece7b64d5 (accessed on 30 May 2025).

80. Wu, Y., Vazquez-Prada, K. X., Liu, Y., Whittaker, A. K., Zhang, R., & Ta, H. T. (2021). Recent advances in the development of theragnostic nanoparticles for cardiovascular diseases. *Nanotheranostics, 5*, 499–514. https://doi.org/10.7150/ntno.62730.

81. Xie, S., Zhu, X., Han, F., Wang, S., Cui, K., Xue, J., Xi, X., *et. al.* (2025). Discussion on the comparison of Raman spectroscopy and cardiovascular disease-related imaging techniques and the future applications of Raman technology: A systematic review. *Lasers in Medical Science, 40*. https://www.semanticscholar.org/paper/526a73ed51cd49cb5983a4407d52c03bd870d604 (accessed on 30 May 2025).

82. Zhang, H., Leng, S., Gao, F., Kovalik, J. P., Wee, H., Chua, K. V., Ching, J., *et. al.* (2024). Characteristics of pulmonary artery strain assessed by cardiovascular magnetic resonance imaging and associations with metabolomic pathways in human ageing. *Frontiers in Cardiovascular Medicine, 11*. https://www.semanticscholar.org/paper/ce04ca0279744f528ae73408b285a2e552f65bfd (accessed on 30 May 2025).

83. Zhou, J., Du, M., Chang, S., & Chen, Z. (2021). Artificial intelligence in echocardiography: Detection, functional evaluation, and disease diagnosis. *Cardiovascular Ultrasound, 19*. https://doi.org/10.1186/s12947-021-00261-2.

84. Zorzi, A., Bondarev, S., Graziano, F., Cecere, A., Giordani, A., Turk, L., Corrado, D., *et. al.* (2024). The role of nuclear medicine in the diagnostic work-up of athletes: An essential guide for the sports cardiologist. *Journal of Cardiovascular Development and Disease, 11*. https://www.semanticscholar.org/paper/9c8a39487f010ae7c4b94a6d08c140b39b7460ed (accessed on 30 May 2025).

ABDOMINAL IMAGING

8

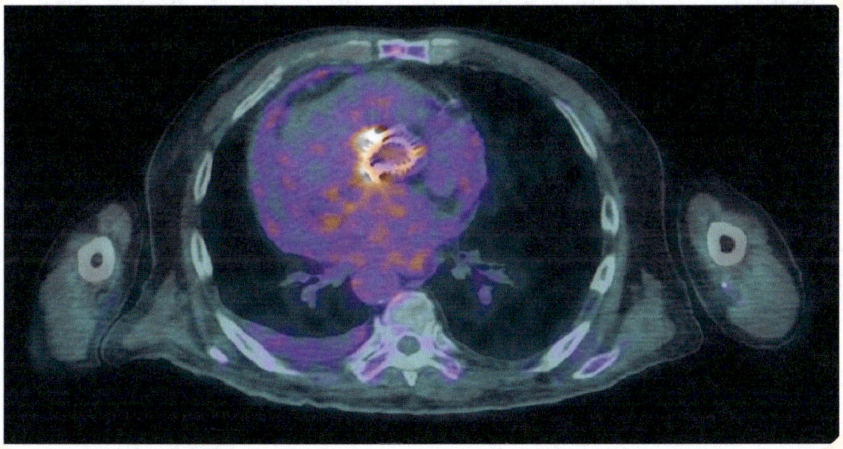

LEARNING OBJECTIVES

After studying this chapter, you will be able to:

1. Identify types of abdominal imaging techniques
2. Explain indications for abdominal imaging
3. Focus on safety and risks associated with abdominal imaging
4. Discuss the interpretation of abdominal imaging results

Introduction

Progress in medical technology has transformed diagnostic capability, especially for radiology, where imaging strategies are an integral part of detecting and monitoring abdominal illnesses. Since the abdomen houses a variety of critical organs and intricate structures, precise visualization is crucial in diagnosing illnesses, ranging from inflammatory conditions to cancerous ones. Technologies that are available now, for example, the use of AI, have revolutionized image interpretation through optimizing accuracy and efficiency, and therefore facilitating the clinician in making informed decisions. Regardless of increased reliance on sophisticated machines, the radiologist's contribution is still essential due to the fact that expert judgment together with clinical context is paramount in ensuring holistic patient care. Besides, management of recurrent abdominal diseases, such as primary sclerosing cholangitis, is a testament to the significance of reliable imaging modalities during diagnosis and monitoring (McGuigan *et. al.*, 2018; Pesapane *et. al.*, 2018). In this chapter, the fundamental techniques and new trends in abdominal imaging will be covered and their clinical relevance.

Definition of Abdominal Imaging

Medical technological advancements have greatly improved the diagnostic capabilities of equipment, particularly in imaging structures and organs inside the body. Abdominal imaging is a subspecialty of radiology that involves the use of a number of imaging modalities to image the abdominal cavity, including organs such as the liver, kidneys, intestines, and vascular organs. Imaging methods such as MRI, CT, and ultrasound produce detailed cross-sectional or real-time images, making detection of abnormalities ranging from tumors to inflammatory disease possible. New techniques, such as ferumoxytol-enhanced magnetic resonance angiography, for example, enable enhanced visualization of vascular anatomy without the nephrotoxicity of traditional contrast media in patients with renal disease, broadening the use of abdominal imaging (Hennessy *et. al.*, 2017).

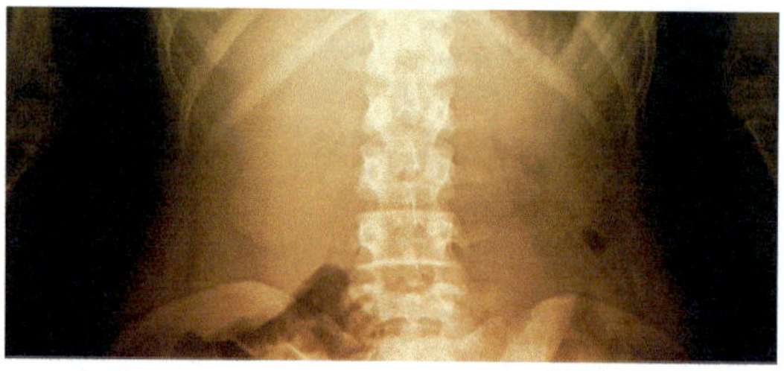

Figure 8.1. Abdominal imaging constitutes a specialized field within radiology that involves the use of various imaging modalities to examine the abdominal cavity, including organs such as the liver, kidneys, intestines, and vascular structures.

Source: https://s3-us-west-2.amazonaws.com/utsw-patientcare-web-production/original_images/abdominal-imaging-1600x732.jpg.

Furthermore, imaging is leading the way in the management of complex diseases like Crohn's disease through helping endoscopic techniques and facilitating diagnosis and monitoring therapy (Albert *et. al.*, 2011). Thus, abdominal imaging is an integral part of modern diagnostics, striking a balance between patient safety and accuracy (Figure 8.1).

Importance of Abdominal Imaging in Medical Diagnosis

Effective medical diagnosis often hinges on the ability to properly visualize internal anatomy, and abdominal imaging serves an essential function in that regard. Abdominal ultrasound, computerized tomography (CT), and other imaging procedures offer non-invasive methods to detect multifactorial conditions that are otherwise likely to be overlooked. For example, routine ultrasound screening enabled the early diagnosis of advanced hydatidosis in a patient occupationally exposed to it, and it enabled immediate surgical and pharmacological intervention, sufficiently lowering disease progression and complications (Bućan *et. al.*, 2025). Similarly, diagnosis of rare but life-threatening illnesses like diaphragmatic hernia with intestinal occlusion to a great extent relies on timely and correct imaging to facilitate effective treatment protocols and prevent detrimental effects (Mahir *et. al.*, 2024). These instances present how abdominal imaging not only serves to assist in the confirmation of disease impressions but also enhances patient prognosis through the provision of early, targeted therapeutic intervention, thus establishing its crucial position in comprehensive medical diagnosis.

Historical Development of Abdominal Imaging

The evolution of abdominal imaging follows a broader trend of technological and methodological progress in medical diagnosis. The beginning was originally set by the discovery of X-rays, which enabled visualization of abdominal anatomy without invasion and revolutionized clinical practice. This early advance led to subsequent developments such as EUS and CT, which dramatically enhanced image resolution and diagnostic specificity. Over time, MRI further expanded the scope and specificity of abdominal investigations to enable detailed characterization of soft tissues without resorting to ionizing radiation. Over recent years, the development of abdominal imaging has increasingly been influenced by applying AI and ML algorithms, permitting improved image segmentation, predictive modeling, and workflow optimization, a paradigm shift for radiologic interpretation and efficiency (Najjar, 2023). These technologies, in addition to the expanded deployment of networked biomedical devices via the Internet of Medical Things (IoMT), have transformed diagnostic capability and personalized treatment in abdominal imaging (Manickam *et. al.*, 2022).

Current Trends in Abdominal Imaging

Technical advances in imaging have transformed abdominal pathology diagnosis with enhanced accuracy and better patient outcomes. Multidetector computed tomography (MDCT) is one such technology, the gold standard for precise staging and evaluation of pancreatic cancer due to its high spatial resolution and rapid scanning speed. Supplementing MDCT, modalities such as endoscopic ultrasonography (EUS), contrast-enhanced EUS, and MRI with magnetic resonance cholangiopancreatography (MRCP) have enhanced the potential for accurate tumor characterization and the identification of faint lesions.

More recent techniques, such as elastography, provide non-invasive tissue stiffness measurements of paramount significance in fibrosis and malignancy assessment, while fine needle aspiration (FNA) continues to be a high-diagnostic-yield minimally invasive tissue sampling modality (Florina *et. al.*, 2024). In vascular imaging, advances in technology that combine biomechanical parameters as derived by ultrasound elastography and newer CT and MRI techniques facilitate patient-specific risk estimation of AAA. The advances, supplemented with AI and novel drug delivery systems, represent a leaning towards precision medicine in abdominal imaging (Alsabbagh *et. al.*, 2024) (Figure 8.2).

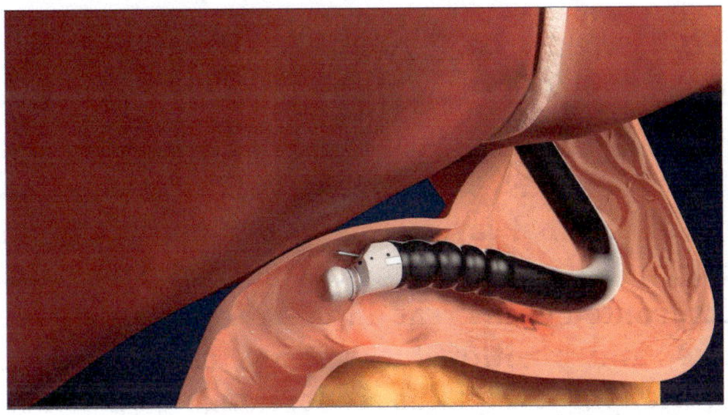

Figure 8.2. Endoscopic ultrasonography (EUS).

Source: https://drsukrit.com/assets/img/blogs/Understanding-EUS.jpeg.

Target Audience for Abdominal Imaging

Technological progress in abdominal imaging has increased its application, with the need for a correct understanding of the target group to maximize clinical gain. The ultimate users are adult and pediatric gastroenterologists who act as the central group that is to diagnose and treat abdominal disorders such as inflammatory bowel disease (IBD). However, disparities in education and application, as identified by reports of vast differences between formal ultrasound training and actual use, especially in nations like Turkey, highlight the need for improved educational materials and national guidelines to enhance capability and uptake among specialists (Bilican *et. al.*, 2025). Additionally, the integration of ML and deep learning models into longitudinal electronic health records presents a new clientele of clinicians and healthcare professionals who can benefit from predictive analytics for abdominal disease identification and surveillance. The timely diagnosis and individualized therapy facilitated by these tools increase the remit of abdominal imaging from radiologists to multidisciplinary teams with prevention and treatment optimization goals (Swinckels *et. al.*, 2023).

Challenges in Abdominal Imaging

Accurate diagnosis in abdominal imaging is often fraught with complex anatomy and heterogeneous pathological conditions within the abdominal cavity, and both radiologists and computer-based imaging diagnostic systems are confronted with great difficulties. Organ shape, size, and positional variations coupled with overlapping symptoms render imaging outcomes hard to interpret, which often necessitates complex preprocessing and feature extraction methods for improving detection accuracy.

Further, the emergence of neuropathic and gynecologic pain syndromes mimicking abdominal diseases increases diagnostic uncertainty, requiring thorough clinical evaluation over imaging to distinguish overlapping disorders effectively (Vijayan *et. al.*, 2025). New advancements in deep learning models like YOLOv9 have the potential to overcome the aforementioned challenges by enhancing the detection of disease using better algorithms and data augmentation techniques, but with limitations based on the need for high-resolution databases and the inability to classify small pathological changes effectively (Emre, 2025). These conditions underscore the ongoing necessity of multidisciplinary approaches combining imaging advances with meticulous clinical assessment to overcome present limitations in abdominal imaging (Figure 8.3).

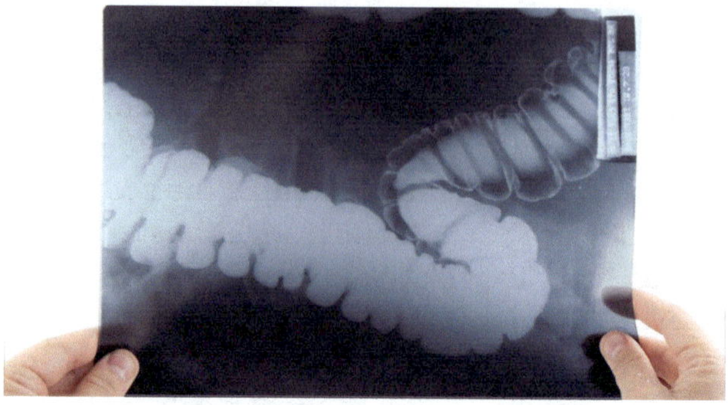

Figure 8.3. Variability in organ shape, size, and position coupled with overlapping symptoms complicates the interpretation of imaging results, often necessitating advanced preprocessing and feature extraction methods to improve detection accuracy.

Source: https://www.nps.org.au/assets/_1080x596_crop_center-center_80_none/c89ac3db2c072c8e-872d54b56811-abdomen-xray-shutterstock_707870.jpg.

Future Directions in Abdominal Imaging

There are emerging technologies that will revolutionize the landscape of abdominal imaging by enhancing diagnostic precision and surgical planning. The application of AI, particularly ML and deep learning algorithms, holds the promise of game-changing enhancement in image segmentation, computer-aided diagnosis, and predictive analytics, ultimately translating into improved clinical workflows and personalized patient care (Najjar, 2023). To this end, three-dimensional imaging modalities, augmented with advancements such as augmented reality and 3D-printing, have begun revolutionizing preoperative planning by providing surgeons with precise anatomical reconstructions and interactive environments in which to plan procedures (Cevik *et. al.*, 2023). The technology not only enhances the visualization of delicate abdominal structures but also facilitates personalized surgical interventions, reducing risk and improving outcomes. Ethical issues and infrastructure challenges remain significant roadblocks; however, even more transdisciplinary involvement and continued research are required to fulfill the full promise of these technologies. Combined, these breakthroughs portend a future of abdominal imaging with improved accuracy, efficiency, and patient-centeredness.

8.1. Types of Abdominal Imaging Techniques

Learning Outcome

1. Explain x-ray Imaging
2. Know ultrasound imaging
3. Focus on computed tomography (CT)
4. Describe magnetic resonance imaging (MRI)
5. Define positron emission tomography (PET)
6. Discuss fluoroscopy
7. Understand endoscopic ultrasound
8. Learn contrast studies
9. Identify interventional radiology techniques

Abdominal medical imaging has significantly enhanced the diagnostic evaluation of abdominal disease and, as an indirect result, patient outcomes. Among all the various techniques, ultrasound is a ubiquitous, non-invasive modality that is ideally suited for the initial assessment of abdominal organs and to guide biopsies since it is a real-time imaging method. Computed tomography (CT) offers high-resolution cross-sectional images with precise lesion localization and characterization, which is critical in cancer staging of cancers such as hepatocellular carcinoma (HCC) and renal masses (Steven et al., 2017; Vogel *et. al.*, 2018). MRI offers superior soft tissue contrast without ionizing radiation and is therefore very valuable in the characterization of complex cystic masses and tumor subtypes in liver and kidney pathology. Contrast-enhanced imaging also increases the diagnostic sensitivity of CT and MRI by highlighting vascular information and lesion perfusion. Contrast-enhanced ultrasound has also emerged to complement standard imaging, particularly in the evaluation of liver nodules. A combination of these modalities allows for full examination of the abdomen with patient-specific clinical considerations.

8.1.1. X-Ray Imaging

The technological progress in imaging has significantly enhanced diagnostic equipment in abdominal pathologies, in which X-ray imaging remains a fundamental component in clinical practice. While the traditional abdominal radiograph enables rapid, immediately available evaluation of conditions such as bowel obstruction or perforation, the employment of contrast media has facilitated visualization of vascular and gastrointestinal structures, increasing the diagnostic accuracy level.

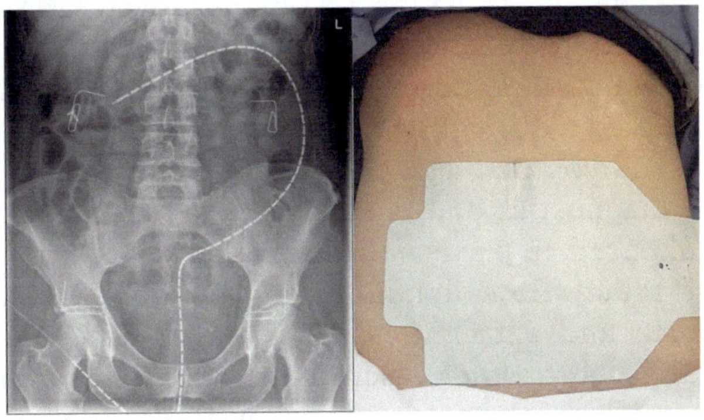

Figure 8.4. High-quality focal spot imaging also plays a vital role in enhancing detail resolution in X-ray abdominal studies, thereby facilitating precise clinical evaluation.

Source: https://media.springernature.com/lw1200/springer-static/image/art%3A10.1038%2Fs41598-024-54429-7/MediaObjects/41598_2024_54429_Fig1_HTML.jpg.

The use of iodinated contrast media with higher tube voltage settings allows for optimal image quality with decreased radiation exposure, which is a concern because of the cumulative risk associated with multiple imaging exams (Albrecht *et. al.*, 2017). Also contributing to better images with lower doses are technologies such as automated dose modulation and iterative reconstruction (IR) algorithms. The need to manage contrast volume and iodine concentration is highlighted in these guidelines, striking a balance between patient safety and diagnostic return. High-fidelity focal spot X-ray imaging also plays a significant role in optimizing detail resolution for abdominal X-ray examinations, thereby providing accurate clinical evaluation (Figure 8.4).

8.1.2. Ultrasound Imaging

Imaging diagnostic advances have profoundly impacted the treatment of abdominal diseases. Among them, ultrasound imaging stands out due to its versatility, real-time, and ionization-free characteristics, promoting improved safety and utility, particularly for the assessment of abdominal organs and vascular routes. Coupled with other new developments, like AI and contrast agent technology, its accuracy in diagnostics and clinical use has also been enhanced. In particular, ultrasound registration of blood flow dynamics of the abdominal aorta and extremities has brought hope for early detection of vascular insufficiencies and circulatory alterations of aging. In correlation and spectral analysis of rheographic curves, doctors may observe abnormal blood flow patterns, which can indicate arterial constriction or degenerative vessel changes. These data, with access and affordability enabled by existing ultrasound technology, hold broad potential for enhancing tailored patient care as well as systemwide health gains (Muhanna *et. al.*, 2022).

8.1.3. Computed Tomography (CT)

Technical developments in imaging have significantly enhanced abdominal diagnostic testing safety and accuracy, with CT as a central focus. CT provides high-resolution cross-sectional images, enabling accurate imaging of abdominal structures, allowing clear detection and characterization of pathology. While very useful for diagnosis, CT entails exposure to ionizing radiation, raising concerns over long-term risks, especially in vulnerable groups such as children. Consequently, optimization of radiation doses is a necessary requirement. Techniques like changing tube voltage and current, automatic exposure control, and the use of IR algorithms have been shown to reduce radiation dose considerably without compromising image quality. Diagnostic reference levels (DRLs) also add to dose reduction through measurement of allowable levels of radiation based on geographic location and patient population. For instance, Indian studies report higher abdominal CT doses compared to international standards, emphasizing the need for targeted optimization efforts (Malik *et. al.*, 2024). Pediatric imaging requires the application of multidimensional dose reduction techniques, including prefiltering and advanced post-processing methods, to enhance patient safety without compromising diagnostic performance (Sayed *et. al.*, 2024) (Figure 8.5).

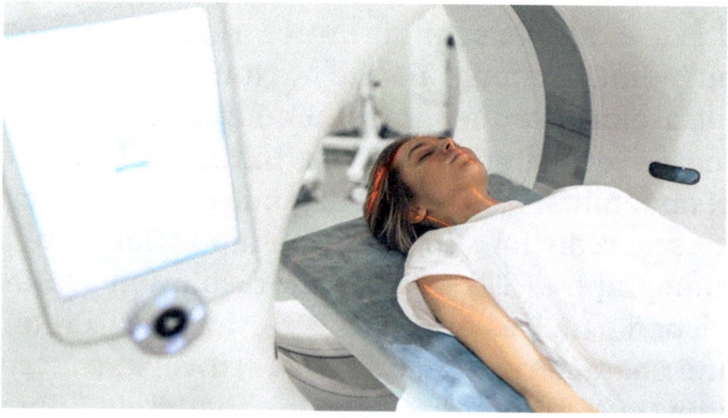

Figure 8.5. CT provides detailed cross-sectional images that enable precise visualization of abdominal structures, facilitating the detection and characterization of various pathologies.

Source: https://sjra.com/wp-content/uploads/2023/10/Woman-Lying-Down-During-CT-Scan.webp.

8.1.4. Magnetic Resonance Imaging (MRI)

Advances in imaging technology have significantly enhanced diagnostic possibilities in abdominal medicine, particularly with the use of MRI. Unlike ionizing radiation modalities, MRI is capable of delivering an improved soft tissue contrast, and therefore it is invaluable in defining complex pathologies in the abdominal cavity, such as hepatic tumors, pancreatic masses, and IBD. The multiplanar imaging capability of MRI provides excellent anatomical visualization, which assists in the precise localization and characterization of abnormalities. Furthermore, MRI's functional imaging sequences, such as diffusion-weighted imaging and magnetic resonance cholangiopancreatography (MRCP), provide additional insights into tissue composition and biliary tract anatomy, respectively. These advantages contribute to more accurate diagnoses without the risks associated with radiation exposure. The incorporation of MRI into emergency abdominal imaging guidelines also emphasizes its growing contribution to acute care settings where rapid, noninvasive evaluation is imperative for patient management (Muhmmed *et. al.*, 2024). Further, emerging techniques maximizing the sensitivity of MRI to fluid motion will likely improve intra-abdominal process assessment (Adam *et. al.*, 2024).

8.1.5. Positron Emission Tomography (PET)

Technological advancements have given unprecedented improvement to the diagnostic accuracy of abdominal pathologies, particularly with hybrid techniques combining functional and anatomical data. PET has been a valuable modality for this purpose, allowing metabolic information that is critical to diagnose and define abdominal cancers. When integrated with MRI or CT, PET allows morpho-metabolic evaluation on an integral scale, improving staging and follow-up of therapy response. This feature is most evident in complex cases such as pediatric musculoskeletal sarcomas and abdominal soft tissue sarcomas, where PET/MRI reduces radiation doses but offers excellent soft-tissue contrast in addition to metabolic data (Plaza *et. al.*, 2024). PET/CT has also been useful in veterinary oncology for the detection of gastric tumors and evaluation of metastasis, supporting surgical planning and post-operative follow-up with greater precision (Kim *et. al.*, 2024). In combination, PET's functional imaging capability complements structural modalities and offers a powerful tool for clinical and research abdominal imaging (Figure 8.6).

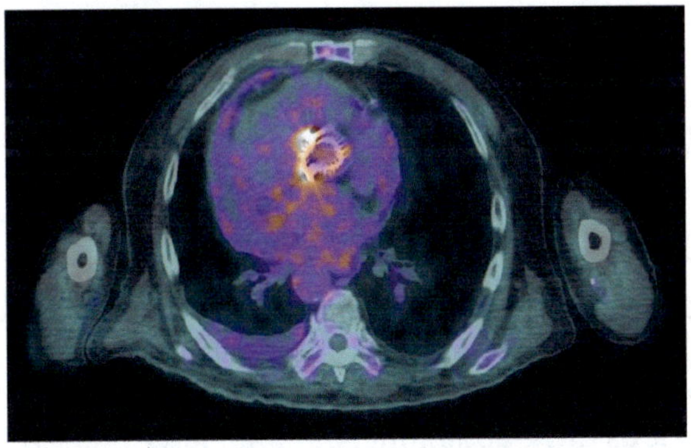

Figure 8.6. Positron Emission Tomography (PET) has emerged as a valuable modality in this context, offering metabolic insights that are crucial for detecting and characterizing abdominal tumors.

Source: https://pub.mdpi-res.com/jcm/jcm-13-04124/article_deploy/html/images/jcm-13-04124-g002.png?1721034627.

8.1.6. Fluoroscopy

In diagnostic imaging, visualization of dynamic physiological functions in real time provides certain advantages, particularly for abdominal examination. Fluoroscopy is a technique employing continuous X-ray beams to produce images in motion and enables doctors to evaluate functional dysfunction of hollow viscera such as the gastrointestinal tract and biliary system. Its value in the diagnosis of disorders like Mirizzi syndrome is priceless, where fluoroscopy-guided procedures like ERCP not only facilitate visualization of bile duct obstruction caused by impacted gallstones but also therapeutic procedures, proving its duality in diagnosis as well as intervention in abdominal imaging (Moosa *et. al.*, 2025). Furthermore, fluoroscopy complements other imaging modalities in delivering information on transient events that static imaging cannot possibly capture. While predominantly used in gastrointestinal and hepatobiliary imaging, its use also encompasses the guidance of surgical intervention in complex cases, underlining the significance of expertise in fluoroscopic techniques in achieving maximum patient success and minimizing complications in abdominal imaging protocols (Paramita *et. al.*, 2025).

8.1.7. Endoscopic Ultrasound (EUS)

Technological advancements in imaging of the abdomen have significantly enhanced the therapeutic and diagnostic approaches towards various intra-abdominal pathologies. Endoscopic ultrasound (EUS), with the combination of endoscopy and high-frequency ultrasound, is one such foundation modality that provides good visualization of the gastrointestinal wall as well as perigastrointestinal structures. Its capacity to yield real-time imaging assists in precise assessment of vascular anatomy, lymph nodes, and pancreatic lesions, which are typically hard to assess by conventional imaging modalities. EUS is an essential part of malignancy staging and fine-needle aspiration biopsy guidance, improving diagnostic yield with less invasiveness. EUS-guided interventions have also expanded the scope of therapeutic intervention, for example, being a flawless combination of imaging and therapy. This technique complements other imaging modalities by providing accurate anatomic information that informs clinical decision-making, particularly in complex presentation of vascular or neoplastic abdominal disease (Maeseneer *et. al.*, 2022; Patrick *et. al.*, 2020) (Figure 8.7).

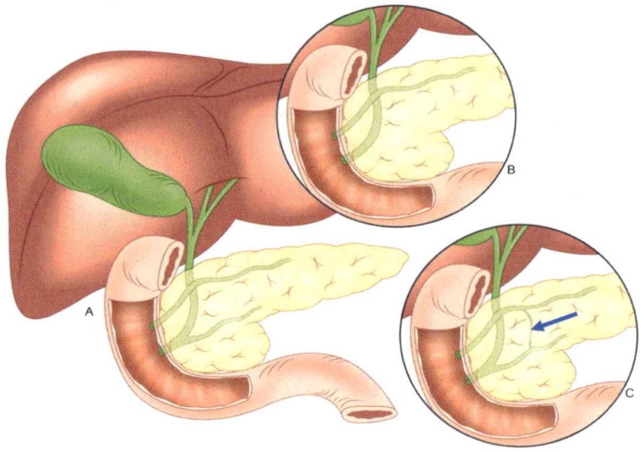

Figure 8.7. Endoscopic ultrasound (EUS) has emerged as a pivotal modality, combining endoscopy with high-frequency ultrasound to provide detailed visualization of the gastrointestinal wall and adjacent structures.

Source: https://www.mdpi.com/applsci/applsci-15-02948/article_deploy/html/images/applsci-15-02948-g001.png.

8.1.8. Contrast Studies

In imaging of abdominal pathology, the use of contrast agents is a deciding factor in obtaining vascular structure and soft tissue visualization. Contrast studies, traditionally reserved for CT scanning, significantly improve the discrimination of normal and abnormal tissues by recognizing perfusion and vascular defects. Such greater imaging ability is particularly valuable in postoperative surveillance, as in liver transplantation, where an early detection of complications is critical. Ultrasound is a first-line imaging modality with contrast-enhanced adjunctive techniques reserved for selectively defining indeterminate findings. Contrast-enhanced computed tomography (CECT) abdomen is also commonly applied due to its high-resolution cross-sectional images, despite the risks of ionizing radiation that require strict dose monitoring and optimization for patient protection (Aryal *et. al.*, 2025; Dammann *et. al.*, 2024). Therefore, contrast studies form an essential component of abdominal imaging, offering improved diagnostic accuracy at the expense of having a balanced risk and benefit.

8.1.9. Interventional Radiology Techniques

Imaging technologies have transformed the efficacy and precision of minimally invasive treatments in the abdominal cavity. Amongst these, interventional radiology treatments use real-time imaging technologies such as contrast-enhanced ultrasound (CEUS) to allow therapeutic intervention with enhanced safety and precision. CEUS is particularly valuable for the identification of complications such as endoleaks from endovascular AAA repair, allowing early diagnosis and tailored treatment. In addition, it also serves a critical function in the periprocedural thermal ablation by delineating target lesions and showing perfusion changes, thereby optimizing treatment and minimizing residual tumor burden. In HCC treatment, CEUS not only serves as intraoperative guidance and postoperative assessment but is of special significance for patients who cannot undergo standard contrast-enhanced CT or MRI. Such new directions emphasize interventional radiology's role in optimizing patient care in abdominal imaging, reducing reliance on more invasive diagnostic modalities, and improving procedural accuracy (Davis *et. al.*, 2024; HonShideler *et. al.*, 2024) (Figure 8.8).

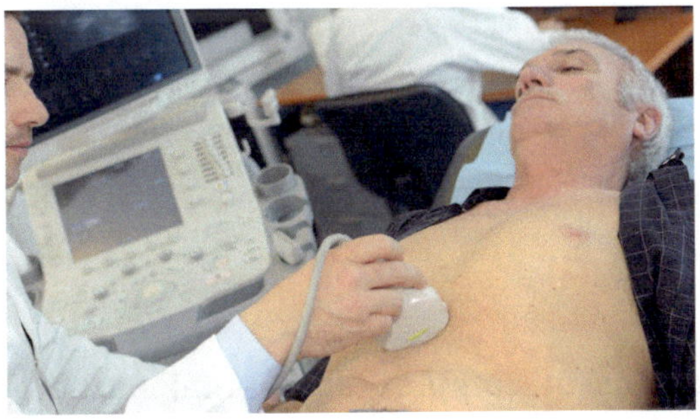

Figure 8.8. Contrast-enhanced ultrasound (CEUS).

Source: https://www.emedicalacademy.com/wp-content/uploads/2020/05/lung-ultrasound.jpg.

Test Your Knowledge

1. What are the main types of imaging techniques used for evaluating abdominal conditions?
2. What is the difference between contrast-enhanced and non-contrast CT in abdominal imaging?

8.2. Indications for Abdominal Imaging

Learning Outcome

1. Explain the evaluation of abdominal pain
2. Discuss the diagnosis of tumors and masses
3. Perform assessment of gastrointestinal disorders
4. Learn investigation of vascular conditions
5. Monitoring chronic diseases
6. Discuss preoperative planning
7. Understand postoperative evaluation
8. Explain trauma assessment
9. Focus on screening for abdominal diseases

Diagnosis of complex abdominal pathologies often mandates imaging to guide diagnosis and treatment plans. For instance, in patients with AAA, imaging is important for initial detection as well as follow-up surveillance after EVAR. Contrast-enhanced routine imaging is essential to assess sac exclusion and detect complications such as endoleaks, which can have an important impact on patient outcomes (Túlio *et. al.*, 2025). The same abdominal imaging is also indicated in chronic intestinal ischemic syndrome (CIIS), where circulatory insufficiency in the mesenteric arteries compromises visceral perfusion. Duplex ultrasound is a first-line diagnostic tool, with new imaging modalities, including angioplasty-guided radiologic intervention, playing a central role in therapy planning and evaluation (Zaitsev *et. al.*, 2024). These figures emphasize that the indications for abdominal imaging are broad, both for diagnostic clarification and for follow-up assessment in visceral and vascular disease to improve clinical care.

8.2.1. Evaluation of Abdominal Pain

Accurate diagnosis of acutely painful abdomen remains challenging with the widespread variety of potential etiologies ranging from self-resolving to potentially life-threatening conditions. Imaging plays an important role in narrowing differential diagnosis and guiding management by providing meticulous delineation of intra-abdominal anatomy. CT is generally the initial method of choice in indeterminate cases due to its high sensitivity and specificity in inflammation, obstruction, or ischemia.

For instance, epiploic appendagitis, which is a self-limiting and rare inflammation of the epiploic appendages, can closely mimic acute diverticulitis or appendicitis clinically but is demarcated by typical fat-attenuation lesions with hyperattenuating rings and central dots on CT (Giambelluca *et. al.*, 2019). Similarly, in the chronic conditions of Crohn's disease, cross-sectional imaging—MRI—is required to evaluate fibrotic strictures, which are wall thickening and narrowing of the lumen, and therapeutic response follow-up to prevent nontherapeutic surgery (Rieder *et. al.*, 2018) (Figure 8.9).

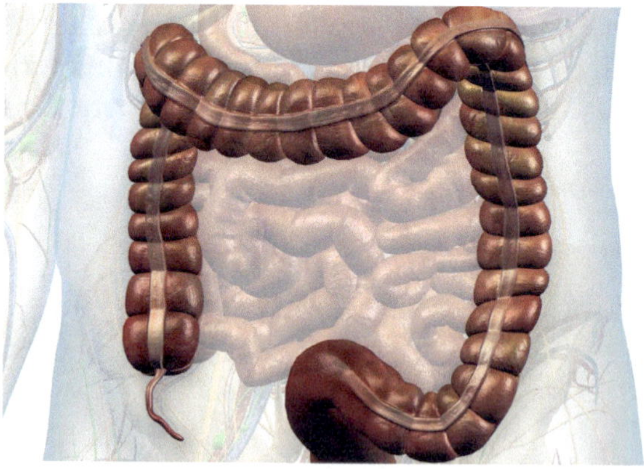

Figure 8.9. Accurate diagnosis in patients presenting with acute abdominal pain remains challenging due to the broad spectrum of potential causes, ranging from benign conditions to life-threatening emergencies.

Source: https://cdn-prod.medicalnewstoday.com/content/images/articles/320/320321/image-of-intestines-with-appendix.jpg.

8.2.2. Diagnosis of Tumors and Masses

Abdominal imaging plays a crucial role in the incidental detection and subsequent diagnosis of tumors and masses within the abdominal cavity, often identifying clinically occult neoplasms at early stages. For instance, renal cell carcinoma is frequently detected incidentally during imaging tests such as CT or ultrasound, and an estimated 70% of patients are diagnosed at stage I, highlighting the role of imaging modalities in early detection and improved survival outcomes (Tracy *et. al.*, 2024). In a similar manner, appendix neoplasms, while infrequent, are typically incidentally found during surgery or histopathologic examination during uncomplicated appendectomy, emphasizing the necessity of sound imaging and clinical assessment in patients with nonspecific abdominal pain (Sean *et. al.*, 2019). Cross-sectional imaging by CT or MRI is crucial for assessing tumor features, staging, and determining management. Integration of imaging information with clinical, histologic, and biochemical data ensures proper diagnosis, supports proper surgery planning, and ensures maximal patient prognoses in abdominal oncology.

8.2.3. Assessment of Gastrointestinal Disorders

Evaluation of gastrointestinal disease is challenging and needs a multidimensional process that pairs clinical history, symptom questionnaire, and high-tech imaging to arrive at a conclusive diagnosis. Functional gastrointestinal disease, such as irritable bowel syndrome (IBS), is highly burdensome for the healthcare system due to its indeterminate symptoms and absence of absolute biomarkers, thus requiring special approaches to diagnosis (Alexander *et. al.*, 2018). Imaging modalities, like cross-sectional studies, have a key role to play in the identification of structural abnormalities, therapeutic decision making, and ruling out organic causes. Supplementing these methods, novel nanomedicine technologies promise enhanced diagnostic precision with drug delivery and molecular imaging, potentially revolutionizing the model for assessment by enabling early detection and individualized treatment strategies (Patra *et. al.*, 2018). This wide-ranging diagnostic framework not only supports symptom classification and subclassification but also optimizes treatment outcomes through therapy individualization in relation to imaging findings and biochemical parameters, thereby overcoming the heterogeneity of gastrointestinal disease (Figure 8.10).

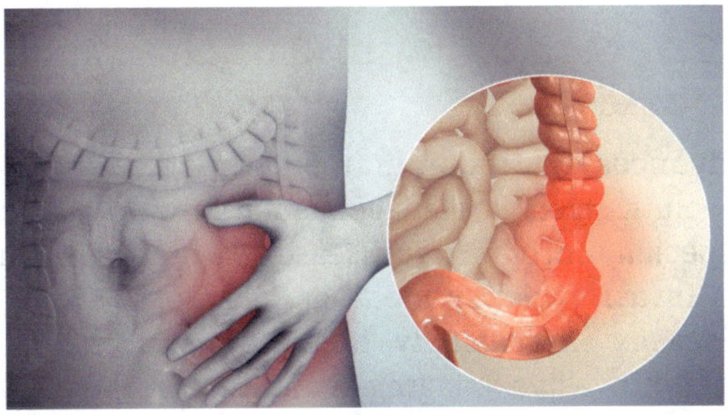

Figure 8.10. Irritable bowel syndrome (IBS).

Source: https://upload.wikimedia.org/wikipedia/commons/1/1a/Irritable_bowel_syndrome.jpg.

8.2.4. Investigation of Vascular Conditions

Advances in imaging modalities have revolutionized the assessment of complex anatomical regions, enabling accurate diagnosis and treatment planning. In abdominal imaging, assessment of vascular disease needs a strong method to assess blood flow patterns, vessel integrity, and pathologic conditions such as aneurysms, stenosis, or thrombosis. Modalities such as Doppler ultrasound, CT angiography, and MR angiography provide critical information about vascular pathophysiology, enabling early treatment and improved outcomes. Moreover, new imaging techniques are also assisting in the explanation of the relationship between vascular organs and adipose tissue, a new area of interest for its usefulness in cardiovascular disease and advancement of cardiovascular health (Agra *et. al.*, 2017). Although current imaging technology offers high-resolution, detailed anatomical data, functional abnormalities, as well as morphological changes, are still hard to differentiate. The integration of various imaging data, as illustrated in recent visual summations, enhances diagnostic accuracy and spotlights multimodal methods in vascular assessment in abdominal imaging standards.

8.2.5. Monitoring of Chronic Diseases

Advances in abdominal imaging have truly revolutionized the management of chronic disease, especially chronic liver disease. Previously reliant on invasive biopsy methods, diagnosis of such diseases increasingly benefits from the use of noninvasive imaging techniques that allow detailed anatomical and functional information. Techniques such as ultrasound, CT, and MRI enable physicians to assess critical factors, including fat deposition, iron loading, and fibrosis, with greater patient safety and comfort, facilitating earlier diagnosis and treatment (Narayanasamy *et. al.*, 2025). As adjuncts to imaging, noninvasive imaging studies, including elastography and serum biomarker panels, enhanced diagnosis by providing dynamic quantifications of disease severity and progression (Boon-Yasidhi *et. al.*, 2024). Cumulatively, these developments allow for adapted and individualized management strategies, less reliant on biopsies, to improve outcomes in patients. In spite of challenges related to standardization and cost, the addition of advanced imaging modalities represents a milestone towards more accessible and effective monitoring of abdominal chronic disease in daily practice (Figure 8.11).

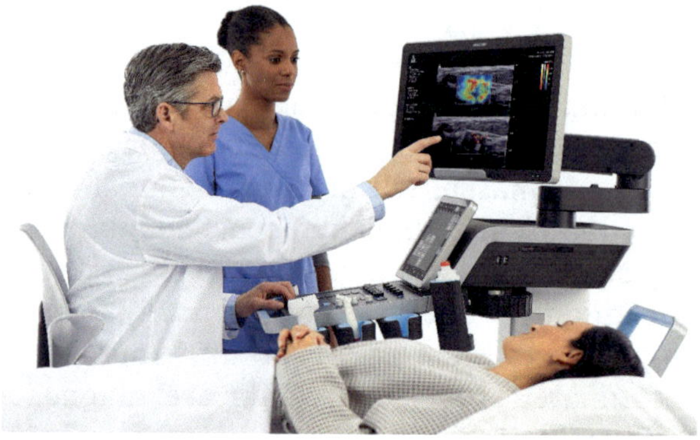

Figure 8.11. Elastography.

Source: https://www.itnonline.com/sites/default/files/field/image/Mach40_LS_0502_TriVu_sm.jpg.

8.2.6. Preoperative Planning

Imaging modality advancements have transformed dramatically surgical preparation, particularly in abdominal surgery, where anatomical complexity dictates precise preoperative planning. Three-dimensional reconstruction using MRI or CT enables surgeons to see complex vascular anatomy and tumor margins, thus permitting them to plan individualized approaches aimed at tissue preservation and minimizing operative risk. This computer modeling assists in defining solid masses and outlining major vessels, which is especially necessary in the surgery of pediatric tumors or complex retroperitoneal masses, thereby optimizing surgical results through improved spatial awareness (Lopez *et. al.*, 2024). Furthermore, computational surgery integrates mathematical models and simulations to further optimize these plans by predicting patient-specific responses and surgical results. Such approaches have intraoperative monitoring and postoperative monitoring potential, especially in diseases such as AAA, for which there is a need for precision for safety as well as long-term results (D'Oria *et. al.*, 2024). With advancements in technology, there comes enhanced precision and efficacy of abdominal surgery procedures.

8.2.7. Postoperative Evaluation

Optimal postoperative evaluation is a crucial factor in optimizing patient results following abdominal surgery by ensuring total resolution of the etiology and early detection of complications. Specialized imaging modalities, e.g., non-contrast CT scans and plain abdominal X-rays, are utilized routinely to define stone-free status after procedures such as percutaneous nephrolithotomy, providing objective information that guides subsequent care decisions (Bryan *et. al.*, 2025). Moreover, the use of intraoperative imaging modalities, including hyperspectral imaging and indocyanine green fluorescence, has been demonstrated to possess enhanced precision in outlining tumor margins and vascular pathologies, thereby augmenting surgical precision and decreasing residual disease (Wagner *et. al.*, 2023). Not only do these imaging modalities allow for early postoperative complication detection, such as arteriovenous malformations or residual tumors, but they also individualize patient management by directing customized follow-up regimens. With advancing technology, postoperative evaluation during abdominal imaging becomes increasingly focal to successful recovery and reduction of risk for re-intervention, pointing to its very important position within the continuum of perioperative care (Figure 8.12).

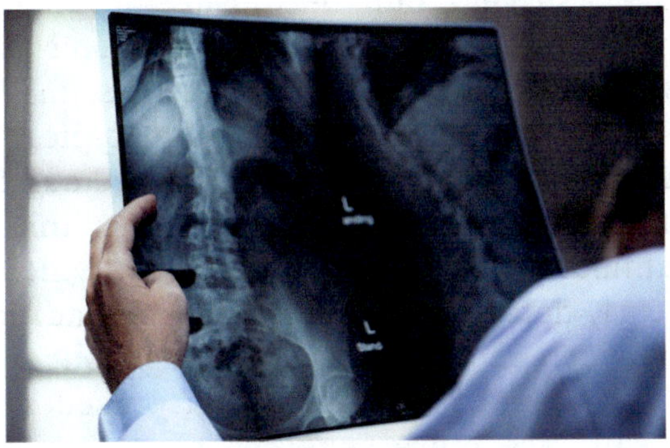

Figure 8.12. Plain abdominal X-rays.

Source: https://healthinfo.healthengine.com.au/assets/photo-1512615199361-5c7a110a8d11.jpeg.

8.2.8. Trauma Assessment

Effective treatment of abdominal trauma relies heavily on proper initial evaluation and effective imaging techniques to establish the extent and nature of internal injury. Due to the complex anatomy and critical vascular organs in the abdomen, trauma evaluation must focus on timely and precise diagnosis to guide appropriate intervention. CT has become the workhorse imaging modality, with high-resolution visualization of organ damage and vascular compromise, such as kidney and large vein injuries. Renal injury, for instance, typically occurs after blunt trauma and requires multiphasic CT protocols to characterize the severity of injury and stage interventional radiology procedures when nonoperative therapy is contemplated (Gorsi *et. al.*, 2025). Similarly, traumatic injuries of large abdominal veins such as the inferior vena cava mandate extensive imaging assessment for determining hemorrhage or thrombosis and contemporaneous implications for surgical or endovascular treatment (Abad-Santos *et. al.*, 2025). Abdominal imaging is, therefore, a crucial platform in reducing morbidity and enhancing outcomes in comprehensive trauma evaluation.

8.2.9. Screening for Abdominal Diseases

Effective screening for abdominal diseases is a critical component of early diagnosis and improved patient outcomes, particularly in conditions such as HCC, where early detection may significantly influence prognosis. Abdominal imaging modalities, including ultrasound, CT, and MRI, are the initial tests in surveillance protocols for risk populations, such as those with liver disease. Ultrasound remains the cornerstone for routine screening due to its availability and non-invasive nature, but is operator-dependent and stage-dependent for sensitivity, prompting an adjunctive use of advanced imaging modalities as necessary. A combination of imaging with clinical risk factors and biomarkers enhances diagnostic accuracy and thereby guides appropriate therapeutic interventions. Furthermore, strict preoperative medical assessment and infection prevention measures have become part of standard abdominal imaging protocols, especially in the context of an increased number of infectious threats, in order to ensure diagnostic efficacy while ensuring safety (Zheng *et. al.*, 2020). The changes in abdominal cancer patterns underscore the ongoing need for enhanced screening modalities predicated upon demographic and etiologic trends (Vogel *et. al.*, 2018) (Figure 8.13).

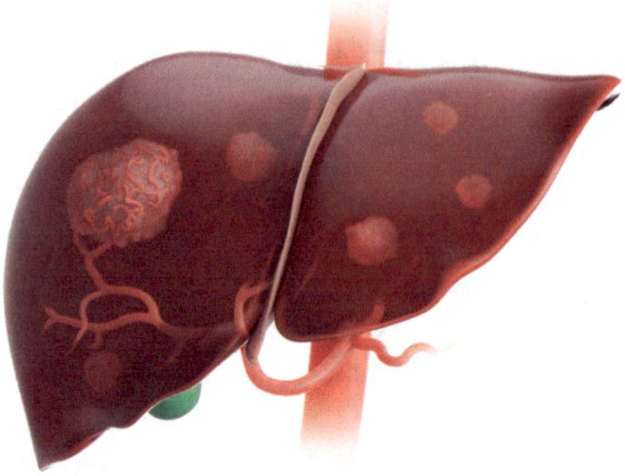

Figure 8.13. Hepatocellular carcinoma (HCC) is the most common form of primary liver cancer.

Source: https://trisaluslifesci.com/wp-content/uploads/2022/05/TriSalus_Pipeline_HCC-1024x785.png.

Test Your Knowledge

1. What are the most common clinical indications for ordering an abdominal ultrasound?
2. In what scenarios is a contrast-enhanced CT of the abdomen preferred?

8.3. Safety and Risks Associated with Abdominal Imaging

Learning Outcome

1. Focus on radiation exposure in X-rays and CT scans
2. Explain contrast agent reactions
3. Describe MRI safety concerns
4. Identify risks of invasive procedures
5. Learn guidelines for minimizing risks
6. Focus on patient education on imaging safety
7. Give special considerations for vulnerable populations
8. Identify long-term effects of imaging
9. Understand regulatory standards for imaging safety

Abdominal imaging has improved vastly, adding significantly to diagnostic accuracy, but safety cannot be overlooked. Modalities such as CT scans are of tremendous value in detecting complications such as internal hernias following bariatric surgery, but re-exposure to radiation carries a cumulative risk that has to be judiciously utilized (Romulo *et. al.*, 2024). Besides, imaging is a requirement in the detection of atypical but severe complications such as retained surgical sponges, or gossypibomas, that can initiate inflammatory or fibrotic reactions, which, if not early detected, can lead to lethal conditions (Al-Wageeh *et. al.*, 2024). The diagnostic yield heavily depends on the modality used since CT scans are more sensitive than X-rays or ultrasound in complex post-surgical conditions (Al-Wageeh *et. al.*, 2024). To ensure they optimize patient safety, the clinicians must balance diagnostic benefits against radiation exposure hazards and ensure they adequately account for deep communication between radiological and surgical staff in reducing negligence cases and ensuring timely and accurate diagnoses (Al-Wageeh *et. al.*, 2024; Romulo *et. al.*, 2024).

8.3.1. Radiation Exposure in X-rays and CT Scans

Diagnostic imaging technologies have advanced abdominal assessments profoundly, but radiation exposure problems are central to clinical decision-making. Abdominal imaging widely uses X-rays and CT scans, which are based on ionizing radiation, which transfers energy to tissues and can cause potential harm to health depending on the dose absorbed. Effective dose in millisieverts (mSv) is the amount of radiation needed to attain diagnostic images to restrict damage.

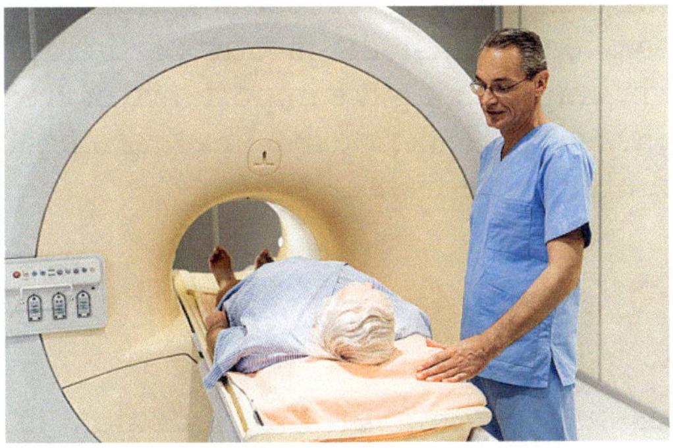

Figure 8.14. X-rays and CT scans, widely used in abdominal imaging, utilize ionizing radiation, which deposits energy in tissues and carries potential health risks depending on the dose absorbed.

Source: https://domf5oio6qrcr.cloudfront.net/medialibrary/2043/conversions/w1010c16207233089387-thumb.jpg.

Research has demonstrated that CT is the predominant artificial source of per capita effective dose, with variations in patient body composition, such as weight and body mass index, influencing image quality and amount of radiation exposure (Lin *et. al.*, 2023). While CT scans do have greater specificity for abdominal pathology, radiation exposure from them must be applied cautiously . Other modalities, like MRI, which are non-ionizing, expand the options between diagnostic utility and patient safety in abdominal imaging (Yaseen, 2022). Thus, optimization of imaging protocols to find a compromise between image quality and radiation dose is important for minimizing radiation hazards during abdominal examination (Figure 8.14).

8.3.2. Contrast Agent Reactions

In the imaging of the abdomen, intravenous use of contrast media is one aspect of the technique to help raise diagnostic specificity, but with the risk of causing adverse effects. These range from minor discomfort, such as rash or nausea, to rare but potentially fatal allergic reactions. Emerging advances in imaging technology, such as low-dose CT and low-concentration contrast media, have shown a promising decrease in the occurrence and severity of such reactions without compromising image quality and diagnostic performance. For instance, studies have shown that patients exposed to lower contrast during lower extremity CTA experienced fewer mild adverse reactions compared to traditional protocols, hypothesizing a lower risk profile for vulnerable populations (Gao *et. al.*, 2024). Besides, the level of endotoxin is directly related to contrast agent safety, as contamination would cause pyrogenic immune reactions. Current reviews affirm that strict endotoxin limits are required to minimize such risks so that contrast media are less likely to induce harmful effects in abdominal imaging procedures (Aziz *et. al.*, 2024).

8.3.3. MRI Safety Concerns

Development in medical imaging has significantly enhanced diagnostic capability, but safety issues still remain paramount, especially involving

MRI. While MRI can offer the best spatial and contrast resolution without subjecting patients to ionizing radiation, application of MRI in sensitive populations, such as pregnant women, has pertinent issues of safety related mainly to the use of gadolinium-based contrast media. Gadolinium-based contrast agents can cross the placental barrier and potentially harm the fetus during development. There is little published data on the long-term effects of exposure to gadolinium during pregnancy, and this has been a stimulus to develop alternative contrast agents that have limited placental transfer, such as nanoparticle-based preparations designed to minimize fetal exposure. This conservative approach points out the equilibrium clinicians must maintain between diagnostic accuracy and the potential for harm, in this case that of imaging the abdomen during pregnancy, where both fetal and maternal health are overriding concerns (Gatta *et. al.*, 2021). Unlike ultrasound, whose greater safety record in prenatal imaging presents fewer technical disadvantages, MRIs' greater cost and technical disadvantages further complicate its routine use in such a circumstance (Heling *et. al.*, 2020) (Figure 8.15).

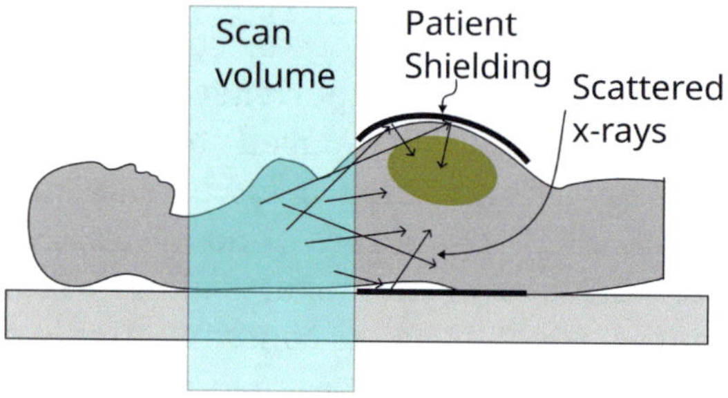

Figure 8.15. While MRI offers excellent spatial and contrast resolution without ionizing radiation exposure, its use in sensitive populations, such as pregnant women, raises important safety questions chiefly related to the administration of gadolinium-based contrast agents.

Source: https://media.springernature.com/lw1200/springer-static/image/art%3A10.1007%2Fs00261-023-03861-w/MediaObjects/261_2023_3861_Fig5_HTML.png.

8.3.4. Risks of Invasive Procedures

Despite advances in imaging technology to enhance diagnostic specificity, invasive procedures remain a component of abdominal imaging but are inherently dangerous and must be balanced with caution. They entail penetration of tissues or manipulation of organs and can lead to complications such as bleeding, infection, and tissue damage. For example, with prostate cancer diagnosis, while standard image-guided biopsies work well, they are painful for patients and lead to potential procedural complications, which may deter some from obtaining necessary evaluation (Hnumber *et. al.*, 2025). Similarly, minimally invasive surgery methods in diseases like cervical cancer, though associated with less perioperative complication than with traditional open surgeries, still remain issues for procedural difficulty and potential adverse consequences (Ferrari *et. al.*, 2024). Thus, in selecting an invasive procedure, risks have to be weighed against diagnostic or therapeutic benefit, emphasizing the importance of creating non-invasive or less invasive imaging modalities to counter these risks.

8.3.5. Guidelines for Minimizing Risks

Successful imaging of the abdomen is not only based on technical effectiveness but also on adherence to guidelines established to minimize patient risks, particularly procedural complications. Adequate pre-procedure assessment, e.g., careful hemostatic status evaluation and suspicion of vascular diseases, is of great significance in averting bleeding-related complications during imaging-guided procedures. Current evidence emphasizes that routine coagulation tests are often inadequate alone to predict bleeding risk, especially among patients with more than one disease, such as liver disease; hence, clinical practice should entail integrated assessment of the comorbidities of patients and procedure risks

(Patrick *et. al.*, 2020). In addition, ultrasound guidelines accommodate reducing exposure time and employing the minimum power levels necessary, respecting the ALARA principle to avoid bioeffects during imaging (Caterina *et. al.*, 2023). Importantly, operator technical skills and incorporation of real-time guidance technologies also reduce the risk of adverse events. These formal guidelines ensure diagnostic efficacy and prioritize patient safety during abdominal imaging exams (Figure 8.16).

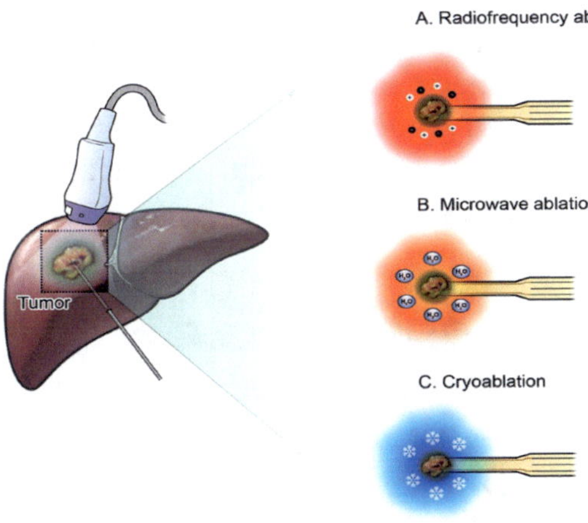

Figure 8.16. Careful pre-procedural evaluation, including a thorough assessment of hemostatic status and potential vascular abnormalities, is crucial to avoid bleeding complications during imaging-guided interventions.

Source: https://www.e-jlc.org/upload//thumbnails/jlc-2024-08-04f1.jpg.

8.3.6. Patient Education on Imaging Safety

Effective communication between healthcare professionals and patients is imperative to ensure safe and well-informed use of imaging techniques in abdominal imaging. Patients are typically apprehensive due to inadequate information regarding the radiation risks involved, mirroring the importance of effective education on imaging safety. Health professionals must establish the standards of justification and optimization in such a way that imaging tests are justified and conducted with the minimum radiation exposure to balance the diagnostic benefits against potential harms. In an open process, informed consent is supported, and patients are empowered to be active participants in their health care. The inclusion of explicit, understandable information on radiation doses, potential late effects such as stochastic risks, and shielding helps build patient trust and compliance. Furthermore, regulation-standardized educational materials and discussion items created collaboratively with regulatory bodies can reduce misinformation and harmonize clinical practice against mutually agreed-upon guidelines. This maintains both patient safety and ethical standards compliance in abdominal imaging practice (François *et. al.*, 2019; Modarai *et. al.*, 2022).

8.3.7. Special Considerations for Vulnerable Populations

In abdominal imaging in vulnerable groups, there are certain challenges that require the skill and expertise of specialized approaches to perform and optimize diagnostic capability and patient safety. Patients with chronic illness, the elderly, or pediatric patients often require repeated imaging, causing concern regarding cumulative ionizing radiation. Advances in technology with AI have shown to be promising in rendering low-dose imaging regimens viable without causing compromises in diagnostic quality and reducing radiation risks, thus enhancing safety in such vulnerable populations (David-Olawade *et. al.*, 2025). Other pathologies like stercoral colitis, which primarily present in immobilized or older patients, but can also occur in young patients similarly underscore the necessity of personalized diagnostic vigilance. Imaging modalities such as CT scans play a key role in the detection of complications early on, guiding timely interventions that mitigate fatal morbidity and mortality risks (Max *et. al.*,

2024). In accordance, a patient-driven approach integrating contemporary imaging technology and clinical acumen is required to maximize outcomes for vulnerable populations exposed to abdominal imaging (Figure 8.17).

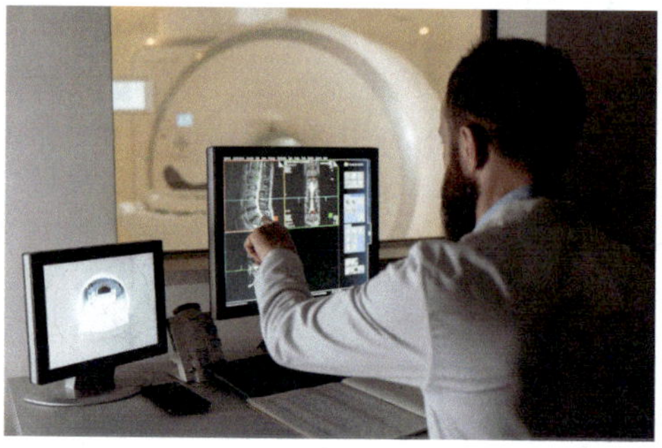

Figure 8.17. When addressing abdominal imaging in vulnerable populations, unique challenges arise that necessitate specialized approaches to balance diagnostic efficacy and patient safety.

Source: https://nam.edu/wp-content/uploads/2022/09/stock-photo.png.

8.3.8. Long-Term Effects of Imaging

Advances in abdominal imaging techniques have facilitated increased precision in diagnosis and follow-up, but their long-term effect is still vital. Imaging techniques such as MRI not only aid in preliminary assessments but are also important in tracking tissue changes in the longer term, as evidenced by stable muscle growth and fat reduction after non-surgical treatments by High-Intensity Focused Electromagnetic technology after six months (Brian *et. al.*, 2018). These chronic anatomical alterations highlight the potential of imaging to guide and assess the results of therapy with no acute impairing effect. However, repeated imaging, especially with ionizing radiation, is under suspicion for cumulative exposure and resultant risk, particularly in vulnerable populations, including chronic abdominal disease like pancreatitis, where ongoing monitoring needs to be performed in order not to have repeated complications (Szatmary *et. al.*, 2022). Hence, balancing the therapeutic and diagnostic utility of the abdominal imaging against potential long-term risks calls for precaution to optimize care for the patient and minimize harm in the long run.

8.3.9. Regulatory Standards for Imaging Safety

The development of imaging modalities for abdominal diagnosis necessitates stringent regulatory requirements to ensure patient protection and image quality. The regulatory frameworks need strict testing protocols and quality control guidelines governing the design, manufacturing, and clinical application of imaging devices.

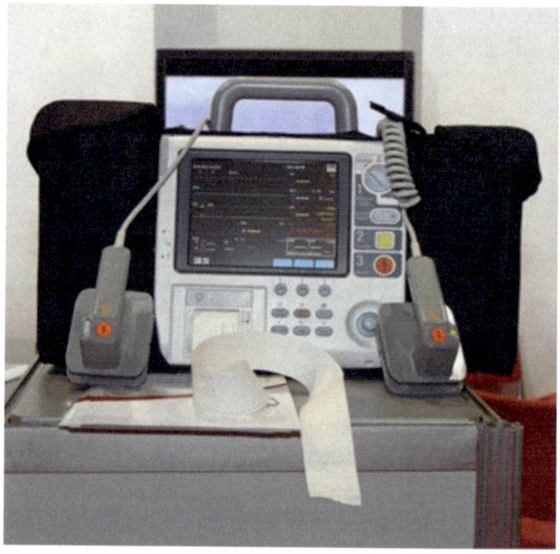

Figure 8.18. Regulatory frameworks mandate rigorous testing protocols and quality assurance measures that govern the design, manufacturing, and clinical application of imaging devices.

Source: https://pannam.com/wp-content/uploads/2017/03/stockfresh_2788594_defibrillator-and-monitor_sizeXS.jpg.

Standards aim to minimize risks like radiation overexposure and equipment malfunction, which could tamper with diagnostic integrity or patient safety. The integration of sophisticated evaluation methods, including non-destructive testing and nanometrology, becomes imperative to ensure device integrity and compliance with safety standards throughout the imaging device life cycle (Igunma *et. al.*, 2025). Regulatory compliance further extends beyond the licensure of devices to encompass procedures of constant monitoring and innovation, providing safer therapeutic regimens and imaging modalities (Kaistha *et. al.*, 2025). This whole-brain approach is of highest priority in abdominal imaging, where good visualization and low risk are the best in successful diagnosis and treatment (Figure 8.18).

Test Your Knowledge

1. What are the primary risks associated with repeated CT scans of the abdomen?
2. How does radiation exposure from abdominal imaging vary between X-ray, CT, and MRI?

8.4. Interpretation of Abdominal Imaging Results

Learning Outcome

1. Identify the role of radiologists in interpretation
2. Explain common findings in abdominal imaging
3. Know differential diagnosis based on imaging
4. Discuss the importance of clinical correlation
5. Know limitations of imaging techniques
6. Explain the use of imaging in treatment planning
7. Describe case studies illustrating interpretation
8. Understand advances in imaging technology and interpretation
9. Discuss future trends in imaging analysis

Interpretation of abdominal imaging results demands an advanced understanding of imaging techniques and pathological conditions for which they are diagnostic. Variability in contrast of image quality, anatomical complexity, and presence of overlapping structures may hamper diagnosis, necessitating the use of advanced analytical techniques. Advanced understanding of AI, particularly deep learning algorithms, has revolutionized diagnostic accuracy through the avoidance of human mistakes and the acceleration of image analysis. These technologies have been very sensitive and specific for all imaging modalities, including CT and ultrasound, to further improve workflow efficiency and clinical decision-making in the assessment of abdominal pathology (Al-Awfi, 2024). Additionally, simulation software generating synthetic but realistic-looking imaging datasets holds the promise of augmenting interpretation expertise by providing extensive ground-truth data, enabling improved algorithm training for computerized analysis (Daniek *et. al.*, 2024). Overall, these developments point to the evolving panorama of abdominal imaging in which integrating traditional radiologic understanding with AI-driven methods is central to improving diagnostic yields.

8.4.1. Role of Radiologists in Interpretation

Accurate diagnosis in abdominal imaging often depends upon the radiologist's ability to understand complex and sometimes dubious results. Radiologists are central to interpreting imaging tests such as CT scans, MRI, and ultrasound, where subtle variations can mean benign disease versus deadly tumors or critical vascular problems. For example, radiologic interpretation of polymorphous and non-diagnostic imaging information in atypical lesions, such as inflammatory myofibroblastic tumors, requires specialized expertise to guide ensuing clinical decision-making, emphasizing the importance of correlation of radiologic data with histopathologic correlation (Fagkrezos *et. al.*, 2024). Radiologists are also directly involved in opportunistic detection of asymptomatic conditions such as AAA through imaging for unrelated indications. Such subtle screening, particularly in lumbar spine MRIs, expands the role of radiologists from diagnosis to preventive medicine, and the emphasis lies in being vigilant in capturing risk factors and early warnings in many patient groups (Mashhood *et. al.*, 2024). Their interpreting skills thus also play a critical role in patient outcomes in abdominal imaging (Figure 8.19).

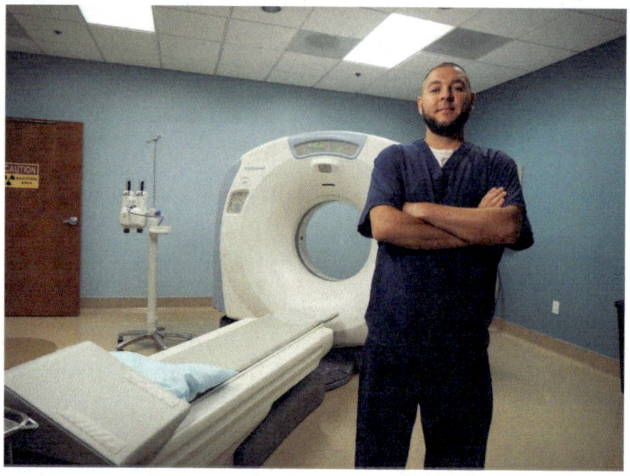

Figure 8.19. Role of radiologists in interpretation in critical vascular abnormalities.

Source: https://www.eroftexas.com/ct-vs-mri-what-s-difference/images/ct-vs-mri-what-s-difference.jpg.

8.4.2. Common Findings in Abdominal Imaging

Advances in abdominal imaging have expanded early detection of most pathologies, particularly with modalities like EUS and MRI. Recurrent findings that are frequently met include structural lesions such as ectopic ureters, typically identified by MRI, which may have symptoms ranging from urinary incontinence to abdominal pain and are associated with complicated anomalies such as duplex collecting systems or syndromes such as Zinner syndrome (Rani *et. al.*, 2024). Additionally, imaging plays a crucial role in multisystem disorder detection; for instance, neonatal screening accompanied by skeletal radiography and abdominal EUS has revealed early onset of mucopolysaccharidosis manifesting as vertebral features and impairment of abdominal organs that correlate with biochemical indices (Lee *et. al.*, 2025). This form of imaging not only facilitates early diagnosis but also affects clinical management by enabling critical evaluation at presymptomatic stages. Therefore, appreciating these common patterns on abdominal imaging is imperative for optimizing patient outcomes by early detection and tailored treatment regimens.

8.4.3. Differential Diagnosis Based on Imaging

Accurate diagnosis on abdominal imaging relies heavily on an orderly method that distinguishes between several pathological processes, allowing for clinical decision-making. Modalities such as ultrasound, CT, and MRI provide critical information about organ size, morphology, and tissue composition, which aid in distinguishing between benign and malignant processes and structural abnormalities. For instance, in the evaluation of lower urinary tract symptoms, imaging can reveal prostate shape and size, and intravesical protrusions, which all influence benign prostatic hyperplasia treatment plans (Lori *et. al.*, 2021). Moreover, attention to possible infectious risks and technique-related difficulties of imaging-guided interventions has been emphasized during the COVID-19 outbreak, emphasizing the application of rigorous safety protocols to protect patients and healthcare professionals (Zheng *et. al.*, 2020). Thus, differential diagnosis with imaging not only guides therapeutic interventions but also minimizes dangers from invasive diagnostic interventions, making it an essential component of abdominal pathophysiology assessment (Figure 8.20).

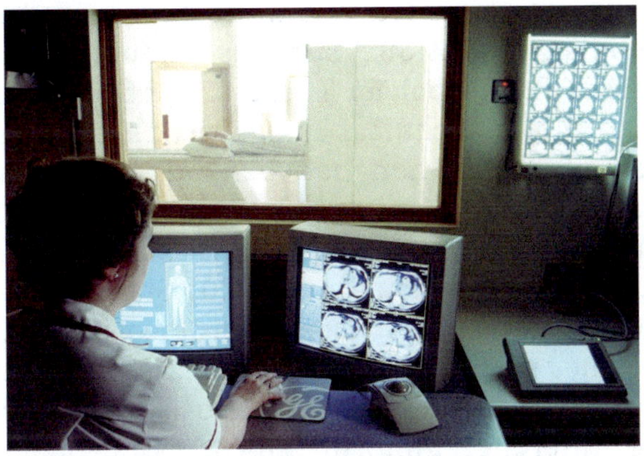

Figure 8.20. Accurate diagnosis in abdominal imaging relies heavily on a systematic approach that distinguishes between various pathological conditions, enhancing clinical decision-making.

Source: https://cdn.britannica.com/78/80578-050-BF193014/Magnetic-resonance-imaging-organs-structures-X-rays-radiation.jpg.

8.4.4. Importance of Clinical Correlation

The interpretation of abdominal imaging findings is greatly enhanced when integrated with comprehensive clinical correlation to enhance diagnostic accuracy and patient management. The imaging abnormalities alone are often nonspecific, independent of the underlying cardiovascular, metabolic, or gastrointestinal disease processes influencing organ function and form. For instance, the study of aortic wall motion in patients with a history of repair operations illustrates the effect of diabetes and hypertension on aortic distensibility over and above structural changes to scans, the value of imaging correlation with risk factors and patient history to enable prediction of vascular integrity (Croccia *et. al.*, 2012). Similarly, noninvasive techniques like electrogastrography show the value of combining imaging data with functional assessments in the evaluation of gastrointestinal motility disorders and filling the gap between morphologic appearance and physiological relevance (Coleman *et. al.*, 2018). Thus, clinical correlation moves beyond abdominal imaging as an exclusively anatomical science to become a varied diagnostic approach that harmonizes radiologic results with the clinical context of the patient and ultimately guides targeted interventions.

8.4.5. Limitations of Imaging Techniques

Despite the tremendous advances in abdominal imaging modalities, several limitations exist that restrict their diagnostic precision and clinical relevance. For instance, modalities like CT find it difficult to accurately assess injury to hollow organs following blunt abdominal trauma at least in part due to the absence of widely standardized diagnostic criteria and the subtle nature of radiographic findings. This doubt can lead to false positives and unwarranted surgeries, as highlighted in clinical series demonstrating that the simple occurrence of free air does not necessarily call for laparotomy, favoring a more conservative approach (Aljiffry *et. al.*, 2024). Additionally, image registration techniques critical for abdominal CT scan longitudinal imaging have proven challenging with the multi-organ, complicated anatomy of the abdomen, with available techniques being organ-specific and less effective across dissimilar structures. Breakthroughs with multi-layer decomposition of deformation fields have been promising in addressing such challenges with better alignment precision across several organs and better potential for general abdominal evaluation (Pham *et. al.*, 2025).

8.4.6. Use of Imaging in Treatment Planning

Effectively treated abdominal illness depends to a great extent on precise imaging modalities that inform clinical choice and yield the optimal patient result. The use of CT and MRI imaging modalities is worthwhile in depicting tumor morphology and metastatic spread, the data required for surgical and therapeutic care optimization. For example, in adrenal malignancies like adrenocortical carcinoma and pheochromocytoma, CT and MRI are not only necessary for differential diagnosis but also for staging and metastasis detection, and hence directly influencing treatment strategy (Faßnacht *et. al.*, 2020). Additionally, in conditions like diverticulitis, CT scanning is the cornerstone for assessing severity, distinguishing between uncomplicated and complicated disease, and guiding nonoperative versus surgical management (Hall *et. al.*, 2020). These applications illustrate how advanced imaging techniques integrate anatomical and functional information so that treatment planning can be optimized and prognosis better predicted in abdominal pathology (Figure 8.21).

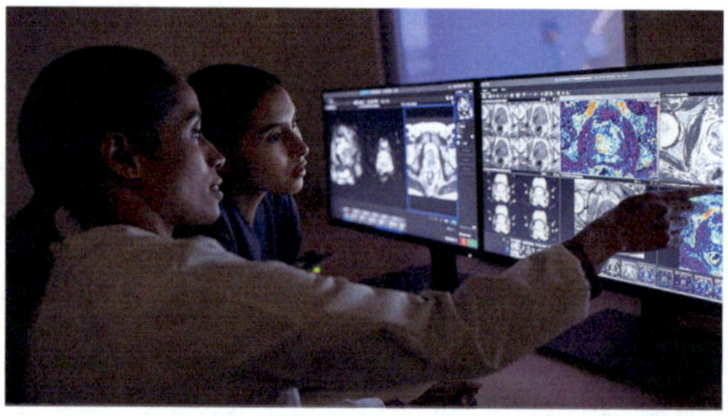

Figure 8.21. Effective treatment of abdominal conditions relies heavily on precise imaging techniques that inform clinical decision-making and ensure optimal patient outcomes.

Source: https://www.philips.com/c-dam/corporate/newscenter/global/standard/resources/healthcare/2023/philips-quibim/header-philips-mr-workspace-radiologist-technologist-image-review.jpg.

8.4.7. Case Studies Illustrating Interpretation

Clinical cases are very helpful in refining the skill of interpretation for abdominal imaging. With the careful consideration of individual patient presentations, clinicians are presented with a broad range of presentations, from trauma-associated hemopericardium to complex conditions such as endometriotic lesions in the pelvis. These case reports not only depict technical image acquisition but also discrimination between false positives and negatives, enhanced understanding of pathological appearance on sonographic inspection (Brandon *et. al.*, 2020). Standardized nomenclature and consensus protocols, such as the ones proposed for sonographic appearance of deep infiltrating endometriosis, also show the difference uniform interpretation makes to diagnosis accuracy and enable multicenter research collaboration (Guerriero *et. al.*, 2016). By embracing these exemplars, the practitioners develop a critical mindset towards site-specific deviance so that better mapping of disease extent is possible and, ultimately, improved outcomes in patient management are achieved. It highlights the interaction between hands-on case practice and theoretical models in becoming skilled at interpreting abdominal images.

8.4.8. Advances in Imaging Technology and Interpretation

The evolution of imaging modalities has greatly enhanced accuracy and the scope of abdominal diagnosis, providing better insight into complex pathologies. Improvements in time-resolved x-ray crystallography and advanced scattering techniques now enable the visualization of molecular dynamics at the atomic scale to provide insight into biological macromolecules crucial for disease description and drug development (Henning *et. al.*, 2024). In parallel, the evolution of interventional photoacoustic imaging offers unmatched soft tissue contrast and real-time feedback for minimally invasive therapies without the limitations inherent in traditional ultrasound or fluoroscopy (van Soest *et. al.*, 2019). Not only does this integration of optical and acoustic imaging improve instrument guidance and tissue differentiation, but it also facilitates targeted therapies with enhanced specificity and reduced side effects. These developments necessitate sophisticated interpretation methods, integrating structural and functional data to optimally organize clinical decision-making in abdominal imaging and intervention, thus facilitating better and individualized patient care.

8.4.9. Future Trends in Imaging Analysis

Advances in imaging technology have the potential to turn abdominal imaging into a more precise diagnostic tool and allow for more individualized treatment plans. Novel techniques, such as hyperspectral imaging, hold the potential for quick, noninvasive, multidimensional analysis capable of recording tissue composition with greater precision than current technology, crucial to the comprehension of nutritional and disease status within abdominal organs (Zuo *et. al.*, 2024). Moreover, the union of functional magnetic resonance imaging (fMRI) with sophisticated computational software is expanding capacity for imaging intricate physiological processes and subtle disease manifestations in real time. Bibliometric publications show growing research interest in further developing the modalities to refine spatial resolution and functional mapping, potentially significantly enhancing intervention strategies (Wang *et. al.*, 2025). As ML and AI continue to integrate with these imaging technologies, abdominal imaging interpretation in the future will be all about automated pattern recognition and predictive analytics, facilitating earlier diagnosis and targeted treatments further.

Test Your Knowledge

1. What are the radiologic signs of small bowel obstruction on CT and X-ray?
2. What are the key CT findings in acute pancreatitis?

SUMMARY

Advances in abdominal imaging have significantly improved diagnostic accuracy and patient management, particularly with new techniques that allow for functional and anatomical evaluation. The field is promising much in oncology, with such methods as intravoxel incoherent motion MRI offering a fine technique of measuring tissue perfusion and diffusion, enabling improved lesion characterization outside the confines of conventional imaging (Aleksandra *et. al.*, 2020). Also, quantitative metrics like CT histogram analysis offer useful diagnostic insights, for example, the potential to discriminate between metastatic bone disease and multiple myeloma involvement of the abdominal and thoracic cavities (Yıldırım *et. al.*, 2020). Despite these advances, problems persist, and standardization of imaging techniques and analysis to allow for reproducibility and clinical significance continues to be required. In conclusion, abdominal imaging is still a pillar of diagnostic medicine that continues to develop with ongoing research critical to the optimization of methods for delivering clinicians more innovative tools for exact diagnosis and enhanced patient outcomes.

Advances in abdominal imaging have significantly influenced clinical decision-making, particularly the management of liver tumors and the application of AI in diagnostic workup. Recent evidence highlights that percutaneous thermal ablation is preferable to liver resection for central tumors since it is associated with a lower rate of complications and shorter hospitalization, while liver resection is the preferred method for subcapsular tumors or tumors near important structures in order to have an adequate margin (Tombesi *et. al.*, 2025). Along with this, the rapid growth of AI-enhanced abdominal CT has brought revolutionary developments, with deep learning and radiomics being the leading methods that maximize image reconstruction, segmentation, and quantitative measurement. These developments are supported by robust international and industry-academic collaborations, evidencing the increasing reliance on AI for maximizing clinical effectiveness and streamlining radiology workflows (Gülay, 2025). Together, these advances illustrate the evolving times of abdominal imaging, balancing accurate treatment with emerging diagnostic technologies.

KEY TERMS FROM THIS CHAPTER

- Informed decisions
- Abdominal imaging
- Kidneys
- Vascular organs
- Abdominal ultrasound
- Primary sclerosing cholangitis
- Liver
- Intestines
- Crohn's disease
- Hydatidosis

CRITICAL THINKING QUESTIONS

1. **What is the first-line imaging modality for evaluating right upper quadrant abdominal pain?**
   a. CT scan
   b. MRI
   c. Ultrasound
   d. X-ray
2. **Which imaging modality is most sensitive for detecting liver metastases?**
   a. X-ray
   b. Ultrasound
   c. CT with contrast
   d. MRI with contrast
3. **In a patient with suspected acute appendicitis, what is the preferred imaging modality in adults?**
   a. X-ray
   b. Ultrasound
   c. CT scan
   d. MRI
4. **Which of the following findings on ultrasound is most suggestive of acute cholecystitis?**
   a. Gallbladder wall calcification
   b. Gallstones without pain
   c. Gallbladder wall thickening and positive Murphy's sign
   d. Biliary duct dilation
5. **What is the most appropriate imaging study for evaluating a suspected abdominal aortic aneurysm in the emergency setting?**
   a. Abdominal X-ray
   b. Ultrasound
   c. Non-contrast MRI
   d. CT angiography

Short Answer Questions

1. What are the common imaging modalities used for abdominal evaluation?
2. When is ultrasound preferred over CT in abdominal imaging?
3. What are the typical CT findings in acute appendicitis?
4. How does MRI help differentiate benign from malignant liver lesions?
5. What is the role of contrast in abdominal CT scans?
6. How is abdominal imaging used to diagnose bowel obstruction?
7. What are the limitations of plain abdominal X-rays in diagnosing abdominal conditions?
8. What is the imaging modality of choice for evaluating suspected gallstones?
9. What are the imaging features of acute pancreatitis on CT?

Answers to Critical Thinking Questions

1.(c); 2. (d); 3. (c); 4. (c); 5. (d)

REFERENCES

1. Ab Aziz, A., Mappiare, S., Nam, H. Y., Devi, D., Johan, M. R., & Kamarul, T. (2024). Endotoxin detection in magnetic resonance imaging contrast agent using optimizing chromogenic Limulus Amebocyte Lysate assay. *The Malaysian Journal of Medical Sciences: MJMS, 31*, 284–291. https://www.semanticscholar.org/paper/3484c55dfbc7e214b6fa24f1897178c0120378bf (accessed on 30 May 2025).
2. Abad-Santos, M., Jeffries, J. C., Hua, C., & Johnson, G. E. (2025). Traumatic abdominal venous injury: Diagnosis and management. *Digestive Disease Interventions*. https://www.semanticscholar.org/paper/bfe1a44b479d3348be61bdfa5b8caa1362a57630 (accessed on 30 May 2025).
3. Agra, A., Alexander, A., Alexopoulos, A., *et. al.* (2017). Investigating interactions between epicardial adipose tissue and cardiac myocytes: What can we learn from different approaches? https://core.ac.uk/download/82983603.pdf (accessed on 30 May 2025).
4. AL Muhanna, S. S., AL Khamis, W. A. S., AL Anazi, M. A., *et. al.* (2022). Exploring the multifaceted applications of ultrasound imaging in medical diagnostics. *International Journal of Bio-Medical Informatics and e-Health*. https://www.semanticscholar.org/paper/3556650545d70cdc9f83c41003978776778f241e (accessed on 30 May 2025).
5. Al-Awfi, A. M. S. (2024). The role of deep learning in revolutionizing radiological imaging and interpretation. *Power System Technology*. https://www.semanticscholar.org/paper/7bbffbdf134278d9c436224873f21d99aa006a1a (accessed on 30 May 2025).
6. Albert, J. G., & Hausmann, J. (2011). Detecting and managing small bowel Crohn's disease–Capsule endoscopy becoming a first line diagnostic method? https://core.ac.uk/download/14524212.pdf (accessed on 30 May 2025).
7. Albrecht, T., Aschoff, A. J., Catalano, C., *et. al.* (2017). Low radiation dose in computed tomography: The role of iodine. https://core.ac.uk/download/98341308.pdf (accessed on 30 May 2025).
8. Aljiffry, M., & Bawazeer, M. A. (2024). A comparative analysis of conservative management and laparotomy in cases of free air after blunt abdominal trauma: A comprehensive case series investigation. *Saudi Surgical Journal*. https://www.semanticscholar.org/paper/c79c031274e69d82adf9b9a212d320d8ba555450 (accessed on 30 May 2025).
9. Alsabbagh, Y., Erben, Y., Vandenberg, J., & Farres, H. (2024). New trends of personalized medicine in the management of abdominal aortic aneurysm: A review. *Journal of Personalized Medicine, 14*. https://www.semanticscholar.org/paper/c3b949a7ffcd0cdc65aeca849671ba4d2880c72d (accessed on 30 May 2025).
10. Al-wageeh, S., Alshoaibi, I., Abdo, B., Ahmed, F., Ghabisha, S. A., Badheeb, M., & Ameen, M. (2024). Unraveling the enigma of gossypiboma: A series of 14 cases highlighting the prevalence, root causes, and outcomes in resource-limited settings. *Cureus, 16*. https://www.semanticscholar.org/paper/8e9f4601d5ecff45fb52d275527d57076787ea3c (accessed on 30 May 2025).
11. Aryal, B., Bhat, M. R., Wani, A. A., & Islam, J. U. (2025). Assessment of radiation exposure: An in-depth analysis of dose evaluation in contrast-enhanced computed tomography abdomen imaging. *Annals of the National Academy of Medical Sciences (India)*. https://www.

semanticscholar.org/paper/f0b7f1ca5fdb0fdf9af7eac1f50918f54123d5e4 (accessed on 30 May 2025).

12. Bilardo, C. M., Chaoui, R., Hyett, J., Kagan, K. O., Karim, J., Papageorghiou, A. T., Poon, L. C., *et. al.* (2023). ISUOG practice guidelines (updated): Performance of 11–14-week ultrasound scan. *Ultrasound in Obstetrics and Gynecology, 61*, 127–143. https://doi.org/10.1002/uog.26106.

13. Bilican, G., Karakan, T., Eğritaş Gürkan, Ö., Sabhan, H., Hedin, C., Forss, A., Petrousis, G., *et. al.* (2025). P0376 Advancing intestinal ultrasound for IBD in Turkey: Results of a national survey. *Journal of Crohn's and Colitis*. https://www.semanticscholar.org/paper/30611e47cd0b36def50c23f1da2c6676be6ab456 (accessed on 30 May 2025).

14. Boon-Yasidhi, P., & Karnsakul, W. (2024). Non-invasive biomarkers and breath tests for diagnosis and monitoring of chronic liver diseases. *Diagnostics, 15*. https://www.semanticscholar.org/paper/06a70e0cd37e96aef828bba8438de5ff3f08ec03 (accessed on 30 May 2025).

15. Brandon, C., Moran, J., Sajed, D., & Kang, T. L. (2020). Focused assessment with sonography in trauma (FAST). *Oxford University Press eBooks*. https://doi.org/10.1093/med/9780190696825.003.0001.

16. Bućan, D., Neveščanin, M., & Bućan, I. (2025). Multiple cystic echinococcosis: The importance of preventive examination and collaborative treatment. *Archives of Industrial Hygiene and Toxicology, 76*, 67–70. https://www.semanticscholar.org/paper/a1a673976f1a9420b48e87ffe2d7fc385b66842a (accessed on 30 May 2025).

17. Campbell, S. C., Uzzo, R. G., Allaf, M. E., Bass, E. B., Cadeddu, J. A., Chang, A., Clark, P. E., *et. al.* (2017). Renal mass and localized renal cancer: AUA guideline. *The Journal of Urology, 198*(3), 520–529. https://doi.org/10.1016/j.juro.2017.04.100.

18. Cevik, J., Seth, I., Hunter-Smith, D. J., & Rozen, W. M. (2023). A history of innovation: Tracing the evolution of imaging modalities for the preoperative planning of microsurgical breast reconstruction. *Journal of Clinical Medicine, 12*, 5246. https://doi.org/10.3390/jcm12165246.

19. Gharibans, A.A., Smarr, B.L., Kunkel, D.C. *et. al.* Artifact Rejection Methodology Enables Continuous, Noninvasive Measurement of Gastric Myoelectric Activity in Ambulatory Subjects. *Sci Rep* **8**, 5019 (2018). https://doi.org/10.1038/s41598-018-23302-9

20. Croccia M, Levantino M, Marraccini P, Franchi F, Bortolotti U. Influence of Cardiovascular Risk Factors on Aortic Wall Motion After Repair of Type A Aortic Dissection: An Electrocardiography-Gated Computed Tomography Study. Aorta (Stamford). 2013 Oct 1;1(5):235-43. doi: 10.12945/j.aorta.2013.13-034. PMID: 26798700; PMCID: PMC4682767.

21. D'Oria, M., Raffort, J., Condino, S., Cutolo, F., Bertagna, G., Berchiolli, R., Scali, S., *et. al.* (2024). Computational surgery in the management of patients with abdominal aortic aneurysms: Opportunities, challenges, and future directions. *Seminars in Vascular Surgery, 37*(3), 298–305. https://www.semanticscholar.org/paper/4e04864834703478738c7bcf2e75f82b79513ab6 (accessed on 30 May 2025).

22. Dammann, E., Ording-Müller, L., Franchi-Abella, S., Verhagen, M. V., Mcguirk, S., Bokkers, R., Clapuyt, P. R. M., *et. al.* (2024). European Society of Pediatric Radiology survey of perioperative imaging in pediatric liver transplantation: (3) Postoperative imaging. *Pediatric Radiology, 54*, 276–284. https://www.semanticscholar.org/paper/b0a57e9756c5b2d6b54763e35e2edd1ed73df6f7 (accessed on 30 May 2025).

23. David-Olawade, A. C., Olawade, D., Vanderbloemen, L., Rotifa, O. B., Fidelis, S. C., Egbon, E., Akpan, A. O., *et. al.* (2025). AI-driven advances in low-dose imaging and enhancement—A review. *Diagnostics, 15.* https://www.semanticscholar.org/paper/44051b152f1c9fdf0599bfc6f3bf4a45b07ac104 (accessed on 30 May 2025).

24. Davis, L. M., Martinez-Correa, S., Freeman, C., Adams, C., Sultan, L. R., Le, D. Q., Lemessa, N. F., *et. al.* (2024). Ultrasound innovations in abdominal radiology: Techniques and clinical applications in pediatric imaging. *Abdominal Radiology (New York), 50*, 1744–1762. https://www.semanticscholar.org/paper/384926c5227775a5ff44582cb2924f7566a01039 (accessed on 30 May 2025).

25. De Maeseneer, M., Kakkos, S. K., Aherne, T., Bækgaard, N., Black, S., Blomgren, L., Giannoukas, A., *et. al.* (2022). Editor's choice–European Society for Vascular Surgery (ESVS) 2022 clinical practice guidelines on the management of chronic venous disease of the lower limbs. *European Journal of Vascular and Endovascular Surgery, 63*, 184–267. https://doi.org/10.1016/j.ejvs.2021.12.024.

26. Fagkrezos, D., Kakavelou, M., Charitaki, E., Delis, S., Papaparaskeva, K., Triantopoulou, C., Maniatis, P., *et. al.* (2024). A rare inflammatory myofibroblastic tumor of the spleen: A case report. *Cancer Diagnosis & Prognosis, 4*(3), 379–383. https://www.semanticscholar.org/paper/cbd4b332fe87950dfcb2467b374fc271e32973a3 (accessed on 30 May 2025).

27. Faßnacht, M., Assié, G., Baudin, E., Eisenhofer, G., de la Fouchardière, C., Haak, H. R., de Krijger, R. R., *et. al.* (2020). Adrenocortical carcinomas and malignant phaeochromocytomas: ESMO–EURACAN clinical practice guidelines for diagnosis, treatment and follow-up. *Annals of Oncology, 31*, 1476–1490. https://doi.org/10.1016/j.annonc.2020.08.2099.

28. Ferrari, F., Giannini, A., Pecorino, B., Cuccu, I., Gozzini, E., Majd, H. S., Barra, F., *et. al.* (2024). Minimally invasive vs. open surgery: Comparison of surgical complications in radical hysterectomy for cervical cancer. *Mini-invasive Surgery*. https://www.semanticscholar.org/paper/6a823248889ccd2da2c5689d4ad2b7adf67ee223 (accessed on 30 May 2025).

29. Ford, A. C., Moayyedi, P., Chey, W. D., Harris, L. A., Lacy, B. E., Saito, Y. A., & Quigley, E. M. M. (2018). American College of Gastroenterology monograph on management of irritable bowel syndrome. *The American Journal of Gastroenterology, 113*, 1–18. https://doi.org/10.1038/s41395-018-0084-x.

30. Gao, Y., Ma, J., Lu, T., & Qi, J. (2024). Efficacy and safety of 128 slice CT low-dose scanning technique combined with low-density contrast agent in computed tomography angiography of diabetic foot and lower limb. *American Journal of Translational Research, 16*(11), 7136–7144. https://www.semanticscholar.org/paper/48fbb3322fcfdbca11ac3b255e65e99d0777e567 (accessed on 30 May 2025).

31. Gatta, G., Di Grezia, G., Cuccurullo, V., Sardu, C., Iovino, F., Comune, R., Ruggiero, A., *et. al.* (2021). MRI in pregnancy and precision medicine: A review from literature. *Journal of Personalized Medicine, 12.* https://www.semanticscholar.org/paper/0603da4b27da542195eed2b94f097eed16acc7e5 (accessed on 30 May 2025).

32. Giambelluca, D., Cannella, R., Caruana, G., Salvaggio, L., Grassedonio, E., Galia, M., Midiri, M., *et. al.* (2019). CT imaging findings of epiploic appendagitis: An unusual cause of abdominal pain. *Insights into Imaging, 10.* https://doi.org/10.1186/s13244-019-0715-9.

33. Glasgow, S. C., Gaertner, W. B., Stewart, D. A., Davids, J. S., Alavi, K., Paquette, I. M., Steele, S. R., *et. al.* (2019). The American Society of Colon and Rectal Surgeons, clinical practice guidelines for the management of appendiceal neoplasms. *Diseases of the Colon & Rectum, 62*(12), 1425–1438. https://doi.org/10.1097/dcr.0000000000001530.

34. Gorsi, U., & Shivaji, S. C. (2025). Interventional radiology in renal trauma. *Digestive Disease Interventions.* https://www.semanticscholar.org/paper/accb9bbbdd780ef6f72ba89e26d6869e266206c5 (accessed on 30 May 2025).

35. Guerriero, S., Condous, G., Van den Bosch, T., Valentin, L., Leone, F., Van Schoubroeck, D., Exacoustòs, C., *et. al.* (2016). Systematic approach to sonographic evaluation of the pelvis in women with suspected endometriosis, including terms, definitions and measurements: A consensus opinion from the International Deep Endometriosis Analysis (IDEA) group. *Ultrasound in Obstetrics and Gynecology, 48*, 318–332. https://doi.org/10.1002/uog.15955.

36. Güngör, G. (2025). Bibliographic analysis of artificial intelligence-assisted publications used in abdominal CT imaging in the last 10 years. *Turkish Journal of Clinics and Laboratory.* https://www.semanticscholar.org/paper/6e9dad2f85827649366fe2331accf0f0f0b6587c (accessed on 30 May 2025).

37. Hall, J., Hardiman, K. M., Lee, S. H., Lightner, A. L., Stocchi, L., Paquette, I. M., Steele, S. R., *et. al.* (2020). The American Society of Colon and Rectal Surgeons clinical practice guidelines for the treatment of left-sided colonic diverticulitis. *Diseases of the Colon & Rectum, 63*, 728–747. https://doi.org/10.1097/dcr.0000000000001679.

38. Heling, K., & Kozlowski, P. (2020). Safety aspects of ultrasound in prenatal diagnosis. *Ultra Schall in der Medizin–European Journal of Ultrasound, 41*, 116–119. https://www.semanticscholar.org/paper/91edb67c6d94ff49662ea9357bfc0247a6d6d1f0 (accessed on 30 May 2025).

39. Hennessy, M., Kasthuri, R., Kingsmore, D. B., *et. al.* (2017). Ferumoxytol-enhanced magnetic resonance angiography for the assessment of potential kidney transplant recipients. DOI: 10.1007/s00330-017-4934-5

40. Henning, R., Kosheleva, I., Šrajer, V., Kim, I., Zoellner, E., & Ranganathan, R. (2024). BioCARS: Synchrotron facility for probing structural dynamics of biological macromolecules. *Structural Dynamics, 11*. https://www.semanticscholar.org/paper/894f5e506764602fd93945fb6544dd3987faad24 (accessed on 30 May 2025).

41. HonShideler, C., Coffin, B., & Guez, D. (2024). Imaging in interventional radiology: Applications of contrast-enhanced ultrasound. *Seminars in Interventional Radiology, 41*(3), 241–245. https://www.semanticscholar.org/paper/7fd7be350529c4f837058c89ea11c3b5f6a768b5 (accessed on 30 May 2025).

42. Huang, X., Ye, H., Hu, Y., Lei, Y., Tian, Y., Huang, X., Zhang, J., *et. al.* (2025). Ultrasound super-resolution imaging for non-invasive assessment of micro vessel in prostate lesion. *Cancer Imaging, 25*. https://www.semanticscholar.org/paper/f63bf5de32d8c28a1f2384443512c3833ee9fc8e (accessed on 30 May 2025).

43. Igunma, T. O., Adeleke, A. K., & Nwokediegwu, Z. S. (2025). Developing nanometrology and non-destructive testing methods to ensure medical device manufacturing accuracy and safety. *Gulf Journal of Advance Business Research.* https://www.semanticscholar.org/paper/28158738ec88631052f4e0817a528a54445874cb (accessed on 30 May 2025).

44. Jones, M. J., Adeyemi, E., & Kouyoumjian, S. (2024). Stercoral colitis: An unexpected presentation in a young adolescent. *Cureus, 16*. https://www.semanticscholar.org/paper/1aadc4dfcf8a3187d17667f42f9c2b5070914c81 (accessed on 30 May 2025).

45. Kaistha, S., Devi, P., Sharma, N., & Sagar, S. (2025). Navigating regulatory frameworks and compliances for bacteriophages as therapeutic agents. *Current Pharmaceutical Biotechnology*. https://www.semanticscholar.org/paper/4b3e0b52e4938931e87f7628accc8fbcebcfd474 (accessed on 30 May 2025).

46. Kim, S., Chae, Y., Kang, B. T., & Lee, S. (2024). Use of 18-fluorodeoxyglucose positron emission tomography and near-infrared fluorescence-guided imaging surgery in the treatment of a gastric tumor in a dog. *Animals, 14*. https://www.semanticscholar.org/paper/3906e27e01fa9f1a0a16e472e3bf5b274d52a575 (accessed on 30 May 2025).

47. Kinney, B. M., & Lozanova, P. (2018). High intensity focused electromagnetic therapy evaluated by magnetic resonance imaging: Safety and efficacy study of a dual tissue effect based non-invasive abdominal body shaping. *Lasers in Surgery and Medicine*, *51*, 40–46. https://doi.org/10.1002/lsm.23024.

48. Kıran, H. E. (2025). Deep learning-based detection of abdominal diseases using YOLOv9 models and advanced preprocessing techniques. *Computers and Electronics in Medicine*. https://www.semanticscholar.org/paper/a027bc40b774975a59910bd50897ae66a541d9e9 (accessed on 30 May 2025).

49. Lee, C. L., Chang, S. W., Fang, H. H., Chuang, C., Chiu, H. C., Chang, Y. H., Tu, Y. R., *et. al.* (2025). Systematic analysis of multiple imaging modalities in infants diagnosed with mucopolysaccharidosis by newborn screening. *Diagnostics, 15*. https://www.semanticscholar.org/paper/ccd53ea9490fe2cd8f5eade2bf1ac9594f3cffa2 (accessed on 30 May 2025).

50. Leite, T. F. de O., Silva, E. R. da, Evelyn, K., Tirapelli, D., & Joviliano, E. (2025). Expression of plasma levels of miRNA-181b and miRNA-21 in patients with abdominal aortic aneurysms and their effect on clinical outcome after endovascular treatment. *Journal of Endovascular Therapy*. https://www.semanticscholar.org/paper/7334232cdfb330d7cb50529f0d2c547a63f0c864 (accessed on 30 May 2025).

51. Lerner, L. B., McVary, K. T., Barry, M. J., Bixler, B. R., Dahm, P., Das, A. K., Gandhi, M. C., *et. al.* (2021). Management of lower urinary tract symptoms attributed to benign prostatic hyperplasia: AUA guideline part II—Surgical evaluation and treatment. *The Journal of Urology, 206*, 818–826. https://doi.org/10.1097/ju.0000000000002184.

52. Lin, C., Shen, X., Gu, Y., Qiao, Z., & Peng, W. (2023). A cross-sectional study on the correlation of image quality, effective dose, and body composition with thyroid, chest, and abdominal computed tomography scans. *Quantitative Imaging in Medicine and Surgery, 14*, 4031–4040. https://www.semanticscholar.org/paper/b850e72af8221602840e6040eac69ae3af573c24 (accessed on 30 May 2025).

53. Lind, R. P., Goncalves, G. R., Belluzzi, A., Hage, K., Antunes, J., Ghanem, M., Jawad, M. A., *et. al.* (2024). Internal hernia in patients after duodenal switch: A multi-centered comparative analysis. *Clinical Obesity*. https://www.semanticscholar.org/paper/a57abc95cf54e4cf29c3df1139d78700f6a193ea (accessed on 30 May 2025).

54. Lopez, P., Belgacem, A., Sarnacki, S., Arnaud, A., Houari, J., Piguet, C., Baudouin, M., *et. al.* (2024). Enhancing surgical planning for abdominal tumors in children through advanced

3D visualization techniques: A systematic review of future prospects. *Frontiers in Pediatrics, 12.* https://www.semanticscholar.org/paper/1d718d79efe83635ecfa8b17a9940571ea8b68e0 (accessed on 30 May 2025).

55. Mach, F., Baigent, C., Catapano, A. L., Koskinas, K. C., Casula, M., Badimón, L., Chapman, M. J., *et. al.* (2019). 2019 ESC/EAS guidelines for the management of dyslipidemias: Lipid modification to reduce cardiovascular risk. *European Heart Journal, 41*, 111–188. https://doi.org/10.1093/eurheartj/ehz455.

56. Mahir, M., Zidani, A., Slioui, B., Belasri, S., Hammoune, N., & Mouhsine, A. (2024). The role of imaging in diagnosis and management of diaphragmatic hernia with intestinal occlusion: A case report. *Journal of Innovations in Medical Research.* https://www.semanticscholar.org/paper/39571b8ed615a21c015891b92d3228bc4ca04315 (accessed on 30 May 2025).

57. Malik, M. M., Alqahtani, M. M., Hadadi, I., AlQhtani, A. G. M., & Alqarni, A. (2024). An analysis of computed tomography diagnostic reference levels in India compared to other countries. *Diagnostics, 14.* https://www.semanticscholar.org/paper/dda368edfa44698b613b4b935cbde8677d12a2cb (accessed on 30 May 2025).

58. Manickam, P., Mariappan, S. A., Murugesan, S. M., Hansda, S., Kaushik, A., Shinde, R. B., & Thipperudraswamy, S. P. (2022). Artificial intelligence (AI) and Internet of Medical Things (IoMT) assisted biomedical systems for intelligent healthcare. *Biosensors, 12*, 562. https://doi.org/10.3390/bios12080562.

59. Mashhood, A., Malik, S., & Yoon, B. C. (2024). Implicit screening of abdominal aortic aneurysms among veterans using lumbar spine MRI. *Current Problems in Diagnostic Radiology.* https://www.semanticscholar.org/paper/24c9818ecab2f17468d3d60d594d798f72c7ead7 (accessed on 30 May 2025).

60. McGuigan, A., Kelly, P., Turkington, R., Jones, C., Coleman, H. G., & McCain, R. S. (2018). Pancreatic cancer: A review of clinical diagnosis, epidemiology, treatment and outcomes. *World Journal of Gastroenterology, 24*, 4846–4861. https://doi.org/10.3748/wjg.v24.i43.4846.

61. Modarai, B., Haulon, S., Ainsbury, E. A., Böckler, D., Vañó-Carruana, E., Dawson, J., Farber, M. A., *et. al.* (2022). Editor's choice–European Society for Vascular Surgery (ESVS) 2023 clinical practice guidelines on radiation safety. *European Journal of Vascular and Endovascular Surgery, 65*, 171–222. https://doi.org/10.1016/j.ejvs.2022.09.005.

62. Moosa, H., Jaffer, S., Khan, M. N., Aftab, A., Hussain, R., Mirza, A., Zuberi, M. A. W., *et. al.* (2025). Mirizzi syndrome: Clinical insights, diagnostic challenges, and surgical outcomes–A 5-year experience from a tertiary care hospital in Pakistan. *Qatar Medical Journal.* https://www.semanticscholar.org/paper/e09bd838f82e4ad5810ffbfd76b530a83f294e18 (accessed on 30 May 2025).

63. Muhmmed, B., Muhmmed, A., Mohammed, D., Alsaeedi, S., Salem, A., Mohammed, Y., Alotibi, F. O., *et. al.* (2024). Radiology in emergency medicine: Life-saving imaging. *Power System Technology.* https://www.semanticscholar.org/paper/64f1ceaad160e745a4b22e0bb715d7cee391faa6 (accessed on 30 May 2025).

64. Najjar, R. (2023). Redefining radiology: A review of artificial intelligence integration in medical imaging. *Diagnostics, 13*, 2760. https://doi.org/10.3390/diagnostics13172760.

65. Narayanasamy, S., Franca, M., Idilman, I., Yin, M., & Venkatesh, S. (2025). Advanced imaging techniques for assessing fat, iron, and fibrosis in chronic liver disease. *Gut and Liver, 19,*

31–42. https://www.semanticscholar.org/paper/9e04cc994c5cda72f5d74e780a906e76ee7fd243 (accessed on 30 May 2025).

66. Northup, P. G., García-Pagán, J. C., García-Tsao, G., Intagliata, N. M., Superina, R., Roberts, L. N., Lisman, T., *et. al.* (2020). Vascular liver disorders, portal vein thrombosis, and procedural bleeding in patients with liver disease: 2020 practice guidance by the American Association for the Study of Liver Diseases. *Hepatology, 73*, 366–413. https://doi.org/10.1002/hep.31646.

67. Panelewen, B. P., Arianto, E., Astram, A., Toreh, C., & Wihono, F. (2025). Validation of Guy's Stone Score, RUSS, S-RESC SCORE, and S.T.O.N.E score for predicting stone free rate in percutaneous nephrolithotomy in a residency teaching hospital. *Medical Scope Journal*. https://www.semanticscholar.org/paper/4c343af0f19e66fff67c3ae4a5a8ef0450880ca7 (accessed on 30 May 2025).

68. Paramita, B. D., Suhartomo, D. M., Sukarsa, M. R. A., Rinaldi, A., Ma'soem, A., & Adriansyah, P. N. A. (2025). Imaging and diagnostic challenges in an 11-year-old girl with vaginal agenesis: A case report. *The American Journal of Case Reports, 26*. https://www.semanticscholar.org/paper/71a76e560ba1d6ef9c0ed185a0d613ff4c617b5f (accessed on 30 May 2025).

69. Patra, J. K., Das, G., Fraceto, L. F., Campos, E. V. R., Rodriguez-Torres, M. del P., Acosta-Torres, L. S., Díaz-Torres, L. A., *et. al.* (2018). Nano based drug delivery systems: Recent developments and future prospects. *Journal of Nanobiotechnology, 16*. https://doi.org/10.1186/s12951-018-0392-8.

70. Pesapane, F., Codari, M., & Sardanelli, F. (2018). Artificial intelligence in medical imaging: Threat or opportunity? Radiologists again at the forefront of innovation in medicine. *European Radiology Experimental, 2*. https://doi.org/10.1186/s41747-018-0061-6.

71. Pham, X. L., Prokop, M., Ginneken, B., & Hering, A. (2025). Divide to conquer: A field decomposition approach for multi-organ whole-body CT image registration. *ArXiv*. https://www.semanticscholar.org/paper/3a1597a9fa8fd98e97a7acc9f144e1678f3e3e3f (accessed on 30 May 2025).

72. Plaza de Las Heras, I. S., García Cañamaque, L., Quílez Caballero, E., Camacho-Arias, M., Cárdenas Soriano, M. del P., & Martel Villagrán, J. (2024). Positron emission tomography-magnetic resonance imaging applications in pediatric musculoskeletal tumors. *Quantitative Imaging in Medicine and Surgery, 14*, 7825–7838. https://www.semanticscholar.org/paper/d06e80758b9d186811bf041afc9c05bdd421b528 (accessed on 30 May 2025).

73. Rani, K., Surolia, P., Jaipal, U., & Mannan, N. (2024). Ectopic ureter: Spectrum of magnetic resonance imaging findings. *Cureus, 16*. https://www.semanticscholar.org/paper/ba290dc8145e485a3b7fa576dc88b6c56b06c031 (accessed on 30 May 2025).

74. Rieder, F., Bettenworth, D., Ma, C., Parker, C. E., Williamson, L. A., Nelson, S., Van Assche, G., *et. al.* (2018). An expert consensus to standardize definitions, diagnosis and treatment targets for anti-fibrotic stricture therapies in Crohn's disease. *Alimentary Pharmacology & Therapeutics, 48*, 347–357. https://doi.org/10.1111/apt.14853.

75. Rose, T. L., & Kim, W. Y. (2024). Renal cell carcinoma. *JAMA, 332*(10), 1001. https://doi.org/10.1001/jama.2024.12848.

76. Sayed, I. S., & Yusof, M. I. M. (2024). Techniques and strategies to minimize radiation exposure in pediatric computed tomography (CT) abdominal examinations: A review. *Cureus, 16*. https://www.semanticscholar.org/paper/938562bde5aaf50e9dd81b58f28093ff7676f34a (accessed on 30 May 2025).

77. Şolea, S. F., Brisc, M. C., Orăşeanu, A., Venter, F. C., Brisc, C., Şolea, R., Davidescu, L., *et. al.* (2024). Revolutionizing the pancreatic tumor diagnosis: Emerging trends in imaging technologies: A systematic review. *Medicina, 60*. https://www.semanticscholar.org/paper/314685a654aec8a57355ec0923cff6061c779e96 (accessed on 30 May 2025).

78. Swinckels, L., Bennis, F., Ziesemer, K. A., Scheerman, J., Bijwaard, H., de Keijzer, A., & Bruers, J. (2023). The use of deep learning and machine learning on longitudinal electronic health records for the early detection and prevention of diseases: Scoping review. *Journal of Medical Internet Research, 26*. https://www.semanticscholar.org/paper/bbb3bd1ff203e5707eb29234cb5666cb68c0a264 (accessed on 30 May 2025).

79. Szatmary, P., Grammatikopoulos, T., Cai, W., Huang, W., Mukherjee, R., Halloran, C., Beyer, G., *et. al.* (2022). Acute pancreatitis: Diagnosis and treatment. *Drugs, 82*, 1251–1276. https://doi.org/10.1007/s40265-022-01766-4.

80. Szubert-Franczak, A. E., Naduk-Ostrowska, M., Pasicz, K., Podgórska, J., Skrzyński, W., & Cieszanowski, A. (2020). Intravoxel incoherent motion magnetic resonance imaging: Basic principles and clinical applications. *Polish Journal of Radiology, 85*, e624–e635. https://www.semanticscholar.org/paper/d0ce42943ee2ce97a266f6d5976bb361e58480cb (accessed on 30 May 2025).

81. Tombesi, P., Cutini, A., Di Vece, F., Grasso, V., Politti, U., Capatti, E., & Sartori, S. (2025). Surgery or percutaneous ablation for liver tumors? The key points are: When, where, and how large. *Cancers, 17*. https://www.semanticscholar.org/paper/214bb196b3569fd963a995208a2652d9b2a83b41 (accessed on 30 May 2025).

82. Van Aarle, D. A. C., Fasen, F., Schmeitz, H. A. W., de Bruijn, F. J., van Sambeek, M. V., Schwab, H. M., & Lopata, R. G. P. (2024). Numerical simulation of intravascular ultrasound images based on patient-specific computed tomography. *IEEE Transactions on Ultrasonics, Ferroelectrics, and Frequency Control, 72*, 215–225. https://www.semanticscholar.org/paper/a098966f0d2af0ad27d3207df7a1cf8030100178 (accessed on 30 May 2025).

83. van Soest, G., & Desjardins, A. (2019). Interventional photoacoustic: Using light to sound out the path to safe, effective interventions. *Physics in Medicine & Biology, 64*. https://www.semanticscholar.org/paper/3b4cccbe863c199c9e4af720685ee78181c7fee8 (accessed on 30 May 2025).

84. Vijayan, V., Savira, M., Vasanthi, R., Emmanuel, C. E. S., Prasanna, M., & Bagchi, S. (2025). Revolutionizing gynecologic pain management: Exploring modern trends and innovations. *Hellenic Journal of Obstetrics and Gynecology*. https://www.semanticscholar.org/paper/b08a5752e234eb50b8dbcef41d2ee7566582a0f8 (accessed on 30 May 2025).

85. Vogel, A., Cervantes, A., Chau, I., Daniele, B., Llovet, J. M., Meyer, T., Nault, J. C., *et. al.* (2018). Hepatocellular carcinoma: ESMO clinical practice guidelines for diagnosis, treatment and follow-up. *Annals of Oncology, 29*, iv238–iv255. https://doi.org/10.1093/annonc/mdy308.

86. Wagner, T., Mustafov, O., Hummels, M., Grabenkamp, A., Thomas, M. N., Schiffmann, L., Bruns, C. J., *et. al.* (2023). Image guided surgery during arteriovenous malformation of gastrointestinal stromal tumor using hyperspectral and indocyanine green visualization techniques: A case report. *World Journal of Clinical Cases, 11*(22), 5530–5537. https://www.semanticscholar.org/paper/21ac22c7981ef593a9abf95ea34207e1e95d66b5 (accessed on 30 May 2025).

87. Wang, Z., Chen, L., Jiang, T., Zhang, Q., Zhao, J., & Wang, F. (2025). Research status and trends of functional magnetic resonance imaging technology in the field of acupuncture: A bibliometric analysis over the past two decades. *Frontiers in Neuroscience, 19*. https://www.semanticscholar.org/paper/0083e3b42579e7ed2e05d40412217274aa8bacf7 (accessed on 30 May 2025).

88. Wright, A. M., Wu, Y. C., Feng, L., & Wen, Q. (2024). Diffusion magnetic resonance imaging of cerebrospinal fluid dynamics: Current techniques and future advancements. *NMR in Biomedicine, 37*, e5162. https://www.semanticscholar.org/paper/86531a4d1484b56def142398dbe891307f6c58a2 (accessed on 30 May 2025).

89. Yaseen, H. F. (2022). Study the difference between the measurement of the radiation dose of MRI and CT scan. *EUREKA: Health Sciences*. https://www.semanticscholar.org/paper/013a9105df96aa7ab465e03402205bff3e61a2d4 (accessed on 30 May 2025).

90. Yıldırım, M., & Baykara, M. (2020). Differentiation of multiple myeloma and lytic bone metastases: Histogram analysis. *Journal of Computer Assisted Tomography*. https://www.semanticscholar.org/paper/f6fa28cc3aa52a695c8c9a1a58521322148450a8 (accessed on 30 May 2025).

91. Zaitsev, O. V., Kopeykin, A. A., Surov, D. E., Surov, I. Y., Yudin, V. A., Koshkina, A. V., & Kochetkov, F. D. (2024). Balloon angioplasty and stenting of superior mesenteric artery in chronic intestinal ischemia associated with decompensated chronic heart failure (clinical case report). *I.P. Pavlov Russian Medical Biological Herald*. https://www.semanticscholar.org/paper/2f066f4f2343974c1125d14aa55baba08757f5c3 (accessed on 30 May 2025).

92. Zheng, M., Boni, L., & Fingerhut, A. (2020). Minimally invasive surgery and the novel coronavirus outbreak: Lessons learned in China and Italy. *Annals of Surgery, 272*, e5–e6. https://doi.org/10.1097/sla.0000000000003924.

93. Zuo, J., Peng, Y., Li, Y., Chen, Y., & Yin, T. (2024). Advancements in hyperspectral imaging for assessing nutritional parameters in muscle food: Current research and future trends. *Journal of Agricultural and Food Chemistry*. https://www.semanticscholar.org/paper/f0fcb5ca6b7d6bf77868cfbb4a58505001451bf7 (accessed on 30 May 2025).

HEPATOBILIARY AND PANCREATIC IMAGING

9

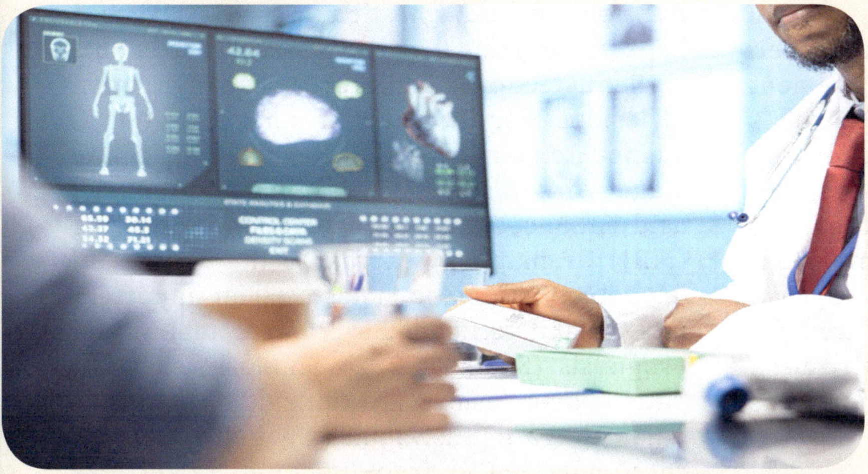

LEARNING OBJECTIVES

After studying this chapter, you will be able to:

1. Explain imaging modalities
2. Identify common hepatobiliary conditions
3. Explain pancreatic disorder
4. Focus on interventional imaging techniques

Introduction

Advances in imaging have completely transformed the diagnosis and management strategies of complex organ systems. Among them, the hepatobiliary and pancreatic regions pose unique challenges in the context of their complex anatomy and prevalence of diverse pathologies, i.e., malignancies and inflammatory conditions. Accurate imaging is key to successful characterization, staging, and treatment planning, which thereafter determines outcomes in patients. Recent technological innovations, such as increased contrast agents and multimodal imaging techniques, have improved visualization and diagnosis sensitivity in the field. Also, the new field of nanomedicine offers exciting possibilities for targeted imaging agents and improved resolution at the molecular level, which may transform early disease detection and monitoring (Pelaz *et. al.*, 2017). Proficiency in the internal understanding of common imaging modalities like ultrasound, computed tomography (CT), and MRI, and their specific functions is mandatory to optimize clinical management strategies for hepatobiliary and pancreatic disease (Dow-Koh *et. al.*, 2016).

Definition of Hepatobiliary and Pancreatic Imaging

Medical imaging plays a very significant role in the diagnosis of diseases of complex anatomical organs, where proper visualization will significantly aid treatment planning. Of these, hepatobiliary and pancreatic imaging is specifically devoted to acquiring precise images of the liver, bile ducts, gallbladder, and pancreas, which form an important component of the excretory and digestive systems. This advanced imaging allows clinicians to identify such abnormalities as tumors, blockages, and inflammation, allowing early intervention. For instance, hepatobiliary imaging is important in assessing cholangiocarcinoma, a neoplasm arising at various levels of the biliary tree, for which precise localization and characterization are necessary because of its variable pathogenesis and behavior (Alvaro *et. al.*, 2018).

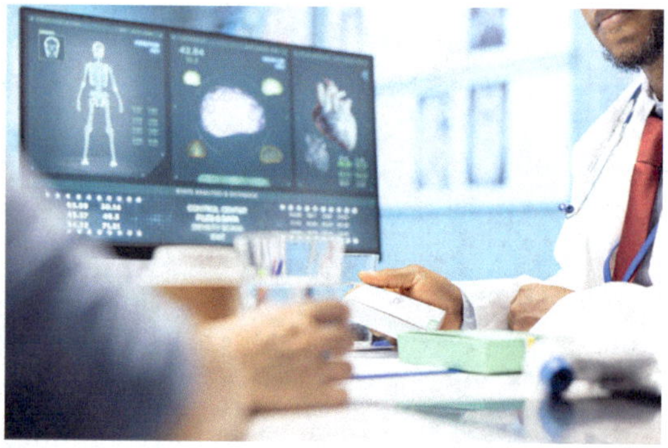

Figure 9.1. Medical imaging plays a critical role in diagnosing diseases involving complex anatomical structures, where accurate visualization is essential for effective treatment planning.

Source: https://www.ominext.com/storage/files/1/100693.webp.

Similarly, pancreatic imaging provides critical information on trauma or injury to this organ, and there is a great impact on treatment outcomes (Ndongo *et. al.*, 2010). In conclusion, hepatobiliary and pancreatic imaging integrates new modalities to enhance the accuracy of diagnosis in the evaluation of diseases of these interconnected organ systems (Figure 9.1).

Importance of Imaging in Diagnosing Liver and Pancreatic Diseases

Technological advances in imaging have transformed the diagnostic approach to advanced hepatobiliary and pancreatic diseases to enable earlier detection and improved characterization of lesions. For instance, in pancreatic ductal adenocarcinoma, usually diagnosed at a late stage with a guarded prognosis, gadoxetic acid-enhanced magnetic resonance imaging (MRI) dramatically increases the sensitivity for detecting hepatic metastasis, an important factor that determines surgical resectability and prognosis (Shaikh, 2022). Similarly, cirrhotic patient liver lesions are difficult to diagnose, particularly in distinguishing hepatocellular carcinoma (HCC) from its mimics, such as neuroendocrine or prostate cancer metastases. The liver imaging-reporting and data system (LI-RADS) schema assists radiologists in classifying such lesions; however, indeterminate findings sometimes require a multidisciplinary framework with the risks of biopsy balanced against potential misdiagnosis (Gazelakis *et. al.*, 2021). Together, these advances underscore the pivotal role of sophisticated imaging modalities in the attainment of early and precise diagnosis as well as in liver and pancreatic disease management planning.

Historical Context of Hepatobiliary and Pancreatic Imaging

Technical advancement in imaging has revolutionized the diagnosis and management of hepatobiliary and pancreatic disease on the basis of a rich heritage of technological development and clinical acumen. Early methods were predominantly radiographic but were restricted by resolution and specificity, and additions of EUS, CT, and MRI added greater visualization of pancreatic and liver anatomy, permitting earlier and more accurate detection of pathology. The simultaneous evolution of genetic and molecular sciences, with studies utilizing model organisms like the zebrafish, has enlightened understanding of liver pathology, which forms the basis of imaging modalities aimed at specifically targeting disease mechanisms and regenerative schemes (Shimizu *et. al.*, 2023). Besides, the tactical use of multimodal imaging methods emerged as a resolution to the difficulties in differentiating between benign and malignant lesions in the hepatobiliary tree, improving the diagnosis of cancer and therapy monitoring, especially in pediatric patients (Donald *et. al.*, 2023). The above background showcases the synergy of technological innovation and clinical acumen in hepatobiliary and pancreatic imaging.

Current Trends in Imaging Technology

Technological developments in imaging have had a transformative impact on the diagnostic strategy for hepatic, biliary, and pancreatic disease, allowing earlier discovery and more precise characterization of lesions. Advances such as contrast-enhanced ultrasound, multiphase CT, and MRI with hepatocyte-specific agents have enhanced tissue discrimination and vascular assessment, central to the detection of malignancies like HCC. These developments align with updated clinical recommendations that focus more on the integration of imaging modalities to enable all-encompassing evaluation and personalized planning of treatment (Association *et. al.*, 2019). The greater understanding of obesity as a risk factor impacting the occurrence of cancer has also necessitated the need for imaging techniques capable of accommodating diverse body habitus, improving diagnostic sensitivity, and surveillance (Pati *et. al.*, 2023). These precision medicine approaches, founded on advanced imaging modalities, allow clinicians to stratify risk in patients, tailor interventions, and ultimately improve outcomes in hepatobiliary and pancreatic oncology (Figure 9.2).

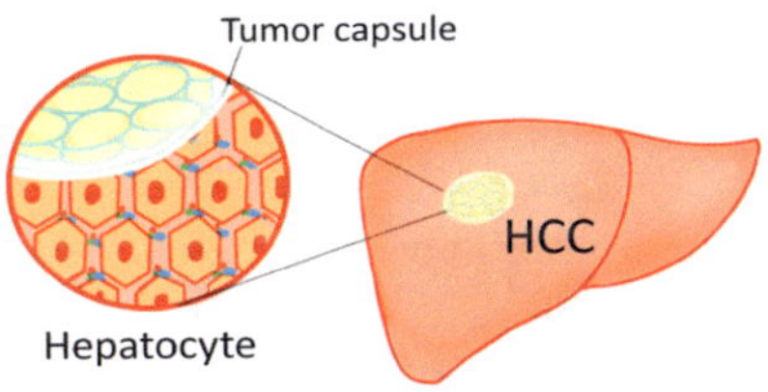

Figure 9.2. Hepatocellular carcinoma (HCC).

Source: https://www.researchgate.net/publication/348989255/figure/fig3/AS:987024307789824@1612336341579/Hepatocellular-carcinoma-HCC-often-possesses-a-fibrous-capsule-with-a-clear-cut-margin.jpg.

Relevance to Clinical Practice

Accurate diagnosis and effective management of hepatobiliary diseases are largely reliant on advances in imaging techniques, highlighting the prime role these play in clinical practice. In disorders such as primary sclerosing cholangitis (PSC), imaging techniques such as magnetic resonance imaging with cholangiopancreatography (MRCP) provide noninvasive visualization of biliary strictures, enabling early detection and follow-up without subjecting patients to invasive procedures like ERCP, which is risky. This imaging-driven paradigm has established diagnostic protocols, allowing for differentiation among PSC variants and identification of clinically important strictures that are linked with obstructive cholestasis and cholangitis (Christopher *et. al.*, 2022). Furthermore, the integration of imaging findings along with clinical and biochemical data enhances risk stratification. It directs treatment, such as surveillance for complications, including cholangiocarcinoma, which remains a leading cause of mortality in PSC. Thus, hepatobiliary imaging plays a critical role not only in diagnosis but also in patient stratification and personalized management, addressing unmet clinical needs and improving prognosis (Tom *et. al.*, 2017).

9.1. Imaging Modalities

Learning Outcome

1. Understand ultrasound in hepatobiliary and pancreatic imaging
2. Know computed tomography (CT) applications
3. Explain magnetic resonance imaging (MRI) techniques
4. Focus on endoscopic ultrasound (EUS) advantages
5. Discuss positron emission tomography (PET) in oncology
6. Give a comparison of imaging modalities
7. Identify limitations of each imaging technique
8 Focus on future advancements in imaging technology
9. Describe the role of artificial intelligence in imaging

Advances in technology for the diagnosis of hepatobiliary and pancreatic disease have illustrated intrinsic limitations of traditional imaging methods, such as poor specificity and sensitivity for precise diagnosis and treatment. Routine modalities such as CT and MRI provide good anatomical detail but frequently cannot differentiate between malignant and benign lesions, thereby complicating clinical decision-making.

Recent comparative reviews highlight the growing worth of functional imaging modalities, most importantly 18F-FDG PET, with higher positive predictive value and overall accuracy to distinguish malignant pancreatic cystic lesions from CT or MRI. This suggests a critical role for PET in preoperative assessment, with greater diagnostic confidence and potential for customized management plans. Moreover, innovative approaches like radiomics, which extract quantitative characteristics from imaging data, have the potential to maximize tumor characterization and prognostication, and possibly overcome shortcomings inherent to traditional imaging while improving long-term patient outcomes in hepatobiliary and pancreatic oncology (Grewal *et. al.*, 2023; Lee *et. al.*, 2022).

9.1.1. Ultrasound in Hepatobiliary and Pancreatic Imaging

Technical developments in imaging have significantly enhanced diagnostic accuracy for complex abdominal disease, particularly that of the liver, biliary system, and pancreas. Ultrasound is employed as an initial non-invasive test due to availability, real-time imaging capability, and lack of ionizing radiation. It is employed in the diagnosis of hepatobiliary derangement, such as gallstones, bile duct obstruction, and liver lesions, and is valuable in primary diagnosis as well as follow-up. Moreover, ultrasound allows for the guidance of interventional therapy, thereby improving therapeutic outcomes. Despite its advantages, its efficacy is compromised by patient habitus and operator dependence and needs adjunct imaging modalities in some cases. Its evolving role includes the integration of contrast-enhanced techniques that improve sensitivity and specificity in tumor characterization, in keeping with multidisciplinary management planning of malignant biliary neoplasms (Cannavale *et. al.*, 2016). This is in line with greater endeavors in clinical care to maximize imaging for greater diagnostic specificity in differing clinical presentations (Ndongo *et. al.*, 2010) (Figure 9.3).

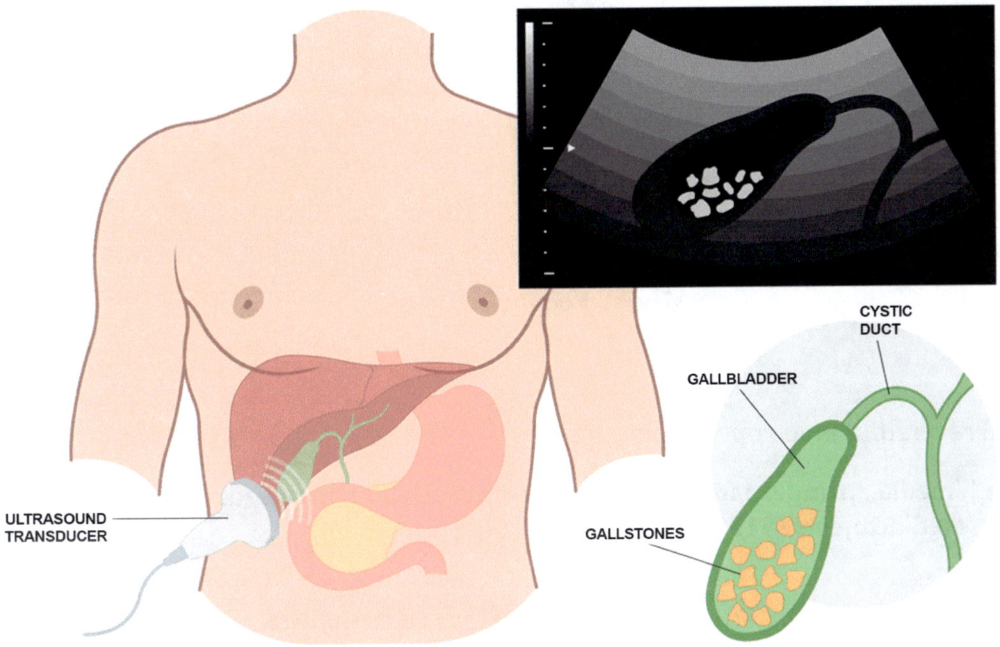

Figure 9.3. Ultrasound in hepatobiliary and pancreatic imaging.

Source: https://gastroclinic.com.sg/wp-content/uploads/2023/07/Illustration-of-what-to-expect-from-US-Hepatobiliary-System.png.

9.1.2. Computed Tomography (CT) Applications

Improved technology in imaging has significantly enhanced the preoperative planning and treatment plans of hepatobiliary and pancreatic disease to a high degree of accuracy. Among these, computed tomography (CT) leads with very detailed cross-sectional images that improve tumor detection and vascular mapping. For instance, three-dimensional reconstruction based on enhanced CT data allows for meticulous preoperative planning of complex procedures like pancreatoduodenectomy, with accurate volumetric measurements and revealing significant vascular anomalies that inform operative planning and patient outcome (Zhang *et. al.*, 2022). CT imaging is also an integral part in guiding novel interventional therapies like irreversible electroporation (IRE), with image guidance allowing accurate placement of the needle electrode for ablation of tumors. In addition, CT and functional imaging modalities combined facilitate real-time assessment of metastatic pancreatic ductal adenocarcinoma treatment response, grounding novel methods involving ablation and immunotherapy integration (Geboers *et. al.*, 2021). Overall, the multi-faceted applications of CT continue evolving diagnostic and therapeutic efficacy in hepatobiliary and pancreatic imaging (Figure 9.4).

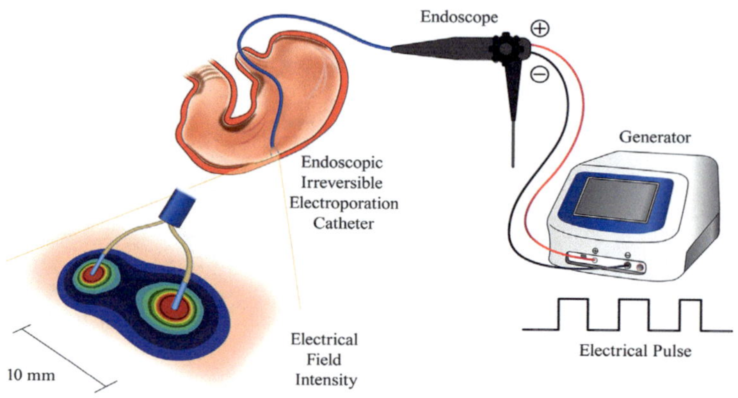

Figure 9.4. Irreversible electroporation (IRE).

Source: https://media.springernature.com/full/springer-static/image/art%3A10.1038%2Fs41598-021-94583-w/MediaObjects/41598_2021_94583_Fig1_HTML.png.

9.1.3. Magnetic Resonance Imaging (MRI) Techniques

Imaging has made a remarkable impact on the diagnosis of hepatobiliary and pancreatic disease, with MRI playing the pivotal role in the diagnostic and management scheme. Of all the MRI modalities, magnetic resonance cholangiopancreatography (MRCP) is an imaging technique that is noninvasive in nature and, to a great extent, has supplanted endoscopic techniques in outlining the pancreatic and biliary ducts. Although MRCP is done with standard hardware, there is a requirement for technical special knowledge to overcome image quality and artifact reduction problems that are openly related to diagnostic precision. There is a need for developed protocols and operator experience to maximize image quality and comprehensive assessment of ductal anatomy and pathology. Furthermore, MRI provides priceless information concerning postoperative complications, for instance, biliary strictures following liver transplantation, where subtle information may be overwhelmed by surgical artifacts and tissue edema. Early and precise interpretation of MRI data thus enables early therapeutic intervention and improved patient outcomes in hepatobiliary imaging (Al-Ruzzeh *et. al.*, 2008; Cillo *et. al.*, 2023).

9.1.4. Endoscopic Ultrasound (EUS) Advantages

Advancements in imaging devices have significantly contributed to improved diagnosis and treatment of pancreatic disease, with EUS as a prime tool. EUS has a very high spatial resolution that enables careful visualization of pancreatic tissues and lesions that are classically hard to image with conventional imaging methods. Its ability to guide fine needle aspiration facilitates direct cystic fluid or tissue sampling, allowing precise pathological diagnosis and differential evaluation of cystic tumors. Such dual diagnostic and interventional capability enhances clinical decision-making, for instance, in challenging examples such as intraductal papillary mucinous neoplasms, where differential identification of malignant versus benign characteristics is desired. Despite concerns of operator dependency, recent information proves EUS sensitivity greater than 90% for mural nodule detection comparable or superior to MRCP and CT. Thus, EUS is a valuable adjunct tool in hepatobiliary and pancreatic imaging with the capability of providing detailed morphological and pathological data that improves accuracy and patient outcomes (Ghaffar *et. al.*, 2025; Ohno *et. al.*, 2024) (Figure 9.5).

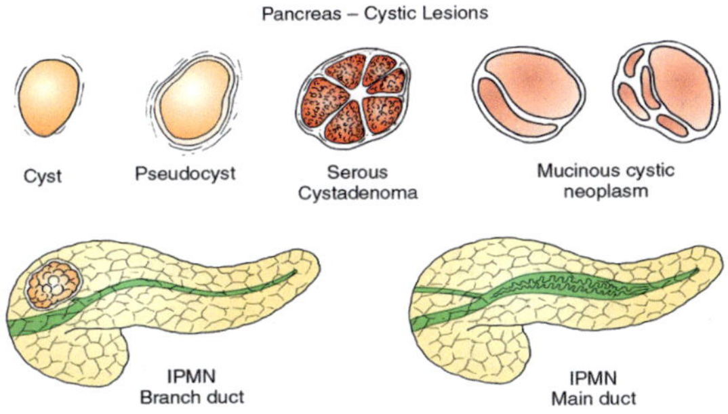

Figure 9.5. Cystic tumors.

Source: https://radiologykey.com/wp-content/uploads/2021/06/f14-01-9780323680615.jpg.

9.1.5. Positron Emission Tomography (PET) in Oncology

Imaging modality innovation has significantly altered the diagnostic and therapeutic approach to hepatobiliary and pancreatic cancer. PET is one such important modality, particularly in the field of oncology, which enhances tumor detection, staging, and monitoring of treatment response. PET scanning utilizes radiotracers such as 18F-FDG, which detects the metabolic activity of cancer cells, allowing for the precise localization and characterization of HCC and neuroendocrine tumors. Other newer studies have also discussed new tracers like 18F-DOPA and 11C-Choline that are used to improve detection rates, especially in cases where the general 68Ga-labeled somatostatin analog PET imaging may be inadequate. Furthermore, the application of PET in clinical medicine allows for the selection and monitoring of targeted therapies, such as the selective internal radiation therapy (SIRT) that targets yttrium-90 microspheres directly into the liver tumors, improving outcomes of therapy (Cannavale *et. al.*, 2016). This PET integration highlights the importance of PET in improving preoperative staging and also personalized treatment planning for complex biliary and pancreatic cancers (Cannavale *et. al.*, 2016).

9.1.6. Comparison of Imaging Modalities

Accurate diagnosis and staging of hepatobiliary and pancreatic disease are highly reliant on making the optimum imaging selections, each with its advantages and disadvantages. CT and MRI remain the gold standards for evaluating the extent of tumor and vascular invasion due to their superior spatial resolution and multiplanar capahty.

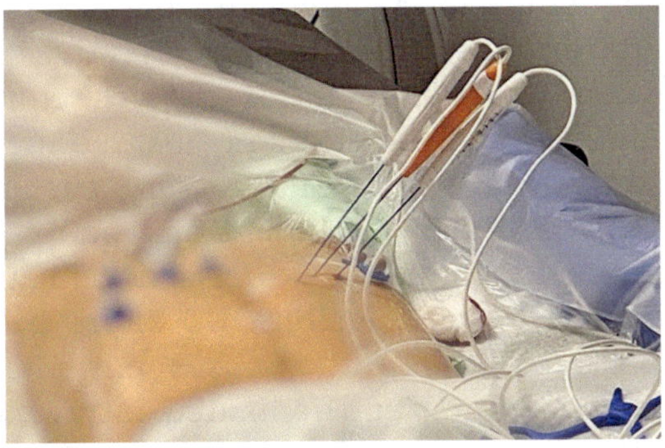

Figure 9.6. Emerging techniques such as irreversible electroporation (IRE) have introduced imaging-guided therapeutic interventions that complement traditional modalities, particularly for tumors adjacent to critical structures where thermal ablation poses risks.

Source: https://www.surgnova.com/upload/image/202103/02/0645070080.jpg.

Ultrasound, endoscopic, and conventional imaging allow real-time imaging but are compromised by operator and patient variability. Emerging techniques such as IRE have introduced imaging-guided therapy procedures that complement traditional modalities, particularly for lesions adjacent to sensitive structures where thermal ablation is risky. The application of IRE underscores the evolving synergy among diagnostic imaging and site-specific treatment in hepatobiliary oncology, indicating the necessity of proper imaging in planning and follow-up (Astras *et. al.*, 2017; Cannavale *et. al.*, 2016). This comparative information facilitates individualized clinical management to improve outcomes through the coordination of advanced imaging and interventional devices in complex hepatobiliary and pancreatic disease (Figure 9.6).

9.1.7. Limitations of Each Imaging Technique

Despite tremendous advances, all imaging techniques used in hepatobiliary and pancreatic evaluation are intrinsically defective and influence diagnostic accuracy and clinical management. Even though ultrasound is available everywhere and is very cheap, it is highly operator-dependent and limited by patient body habitus and bowel gas attenuation, which can obscure lesions. CT offers better spatial resolution but exposes patients to ionizing radiation and iodinated intravenous contrast material, which are hazards for patients with compromised renal function. MRI provides improved soft tissue contrast without radiation exposure but is more costly, time-consuming, and contraindicated in certain patients with implants or claustrophobia. Endoscopic ultrasonography (EUS) combines imaging with biopsy but is invasive and operator-dependent, with less use applicable to widespread practice. No single technique addresses all the diagnostic challenges, and multimodal approaches are needed to optimize the detection and characterization of pathology. These limitations underscore the significance of continual technological enhancement and contextual use in clinical practice (Addiss *et. al.*, 2018; Ndongo *et. al.*, 2010).

9.1.8. Future Advancements in Imaging Technology

Technical innovations in surgical imaging and patient-customized medical devices are poised to transform hepatobiliary and pancreatic imaging. Fluorescence-guided surgery, as indocyanine green application, is fast becoming the leading innovation, with surgeons now being able to visualize tumors and crucial biliary anatomy in real time intraoperatively, enhancing the safety and precision of resections. This technique can potentially maximize outcomes by detecting lesions undetectable through conventional imaging methods, enabling directed therapy (Coco *et. al.*, 2023). Additionally, new developments in three-dimensional printing technology have enabled the production of patient-specific biliary stents that include living cells, tailored to individual anatomy and pathophysiology. These bio-integrated stents are not just improving device function and biocompatibility but also have the potential to reduce complications such as obstruction and biofilm formation (Alexander *et. al.*, 2019). All these technological advances point towards an era of greater convergence of imaging and intervention, leading to more minimally invasive and personalized pancreatic and hepatobiliary disease management.

9.1.9. Role of Artificial Intelligence in Imaging

The incorporation of artificial intelligence (AI) in hepatobiliary and pancreatic imaging has brought a new level of diagnostic accuracy and efficiency. Deep learning algorithms and ML, with convolutional neural networks especially, have shown excellent ability in the detection and segmentation of pancreatic tissues, differentiation between benign and malignant lesions, and the prediction of patient outcomes, including survival and recurrence risk (Podină *et. al.*, 2025). These advances transcend pancreatic diseases to facilitate improved diagnosis and characterization of hepatobiliary pathologies through quantitative imaging approaches and radiomics that extract rich tissue information from modalities like CT and MRI (Mark *et. al.*, 2024). AI-powered approaches not only enhance clinical decision-making but also optimize radiology workflows, boosting the productivity and precision of imaging interpretation. In spite of these tremendous advantages, hurdles such as algorithm explainability, data protection, and ethics need to be overcome to achieve the full potential of AI's revolutionary impact on hepatobiliary and pancreatic imaging (Mark *et. al.*, 2024; Podină *et. al.*, 2025) (Figure 9.7).

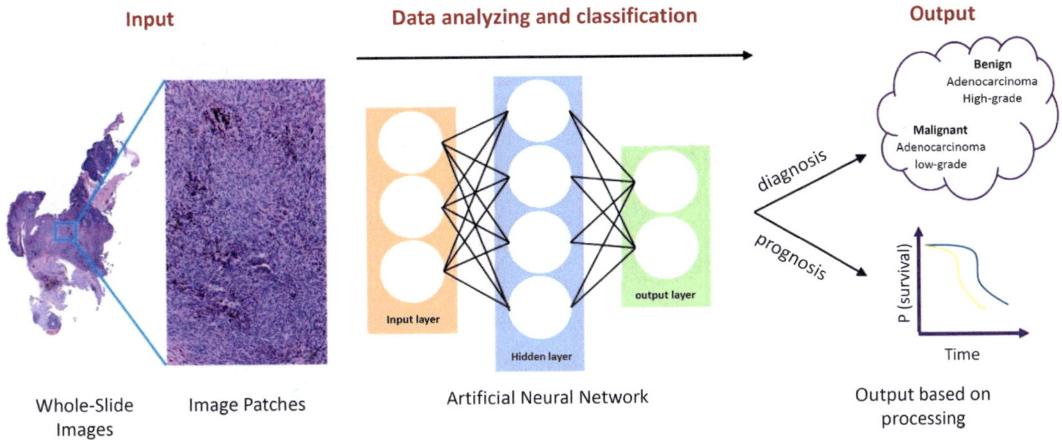

Figure 9.7. Machine learning and deep learning algorithms, particularly convolutional neural networks, have demonstrated remarkable capability in detecting and segmenting pancreatic tissues, distinguishing benign from malignant lesions, and predicting patient outcomes such as survival and recurrence risk.

Source: https://www.mdpi.com/cancers/cancers-14-05264/article_deploy/html/images/cancers-14-05264-g001.png.

Test Your Knowledge

1. What is the imaging modality of choice for detecting gallstones?
2. When is MRCP preferred over ERCP for evaluating the biliary tree?

9.2. Common Hepatobiliary Conditions

Learning Outcome

1. Understand hepatitis and its imaging characteristics
2. Explain cirrhosis and its complications
3. Focus on liver tumors
4. Describe biliary obstruction and imaging findings
5. Define cholangiocarcinoma imaging features
6. Focus on fatty liver disease and its diagnosis
7. Identify liver abscesses and their imaging appearance
8. Discuss hemangiomas and focal nodular hyperplasia
9. Know the role of imaging in liver transplantation

Technological advances in imaging modalities have significantly improved the diagnosis and management of hepatobiliary pathologies, which most commonly present as HCC, cholangitis, gallstones, and biliary strictures. Of these, HCC remains the most common primary liver cancer and requires precise non-invasive diagnostic tools. MRI, especially with hepatobiliary-specific contrast media, is more sensitive and more specific than CT and ultrasound and enables precise evaluation of tumor characteristics such as vascular supply, cellular metabolism, and tissue elasticity. Techniques like magnetic resonance elastography and diffusion-weighted imaging provide another dimension of malignant behavior assessment, enabling a multi-dimensional perspective on disease development and treatment response (Jiang *et. al.*, 2024). Simultaneously, novel deep learning methodologies like the Anisotropic Hybrid Network also augment hepatobiliary imaging through the addition of uncertainty quantification and three-dimensional data analysis for enhanced diagnostic accuracy and clinical decision-making purposes (Singh *et. al.*, 2025). They further emphasize the evolving nature of hepatobiliary imaging in the management of widespread yet complex liver diseases.

9.2.1. Hepatitis and its Imaging Characteristics

Awareness of the imaging characteristics of hepatobiliary diseases is crucial to accurate diagnosis and effective management of the patient. Of these diseases, hepatitis poses unique challenges since it has so many causes and possesses overlapping imaging characteristics with other liver diseases. Ultrasound, CT, and MRI are significant imaging tools for the detection of hepatic inflammation, cellular injury, and fibrosis.

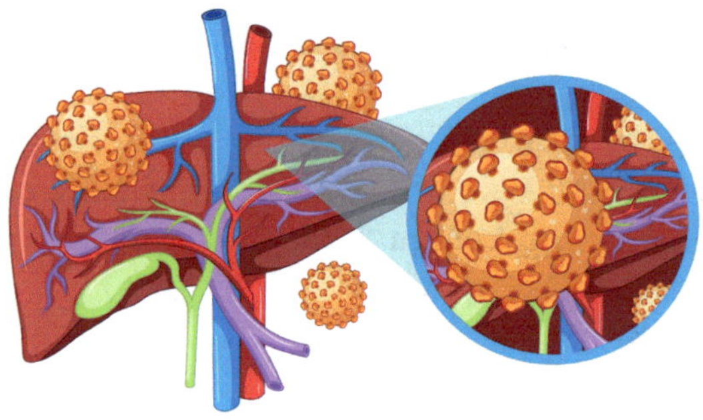

Figure 9.8. Hepatitis.

Source: https://drramchandrasoni.in/wp-content/uploads/2023/10/Best-Hepatologist-in-Faridabad-Hepatitis-A-Dr-RC-Soni-scaled-e1697342185203.jpg.

Hepatitis typically presents as hepatomegaly with diffuse or focal alteration in liver parenchymal signal intensity or echotexture and periportal edema on T2-weighted MRI images. Furthermore, drug-induced hepatitis also presents specific imaging characteristics that, if observed, can direct clinicians to the right diagnosis, especially in complex hepatobiliary examinations (Ichikawa *et. al.*, 2023). Whereas imaging is primarily useful for the exclusion of other causations and assessment of complications, newer guidelines emphasize its use in conjunction with biochemical and histological data for the management of related hepatic disease in a comprehensive manner (Christopher *et. al.*, 2022). Multimodal imaging helps better appreciate hepatitis in the broader context of hepatobiliary and pancreatic disease (Figure 9.8).

9.2.2. Cirrhosis and its Complications

Cirrhosis represents the advanced stage of chronic liver disease with widespread fibrosis and alteration of the architecture of the liver parenchyma, often resulting in severe hepatobiliary dysfunction. This chronic scarring results from continued liver injury from a wide range of etiologies, such as chronic cholestatic disorders like PSC. The following cirrhotic complications are portal hypertension, which can result in variceal hemorrhage and ascites, as well as impaired hepatic synthetic function manifested as coagulopathy and hypoalbuminemia. In addition, cirrhotic patients risk developing HCC and cholangiocarcinoma, where the occurrence of the latter is most closely linked with chronic biliary inflammation and strictures typical of cholangiopathies (Christopher *et. al.*, 2022; Paul *et. al.*, 2021). Accurate imaging with modalities like MRI with cholangiopancreatography is central to both the diagnosis of cirrhotic change and surveillance for malignant transformation within the hepatobiliary tree. Through integration of imaging information with clinical and biochemical data, immediate intervention is facilitated, which is vital to optimizing prognostic outcomes within this multifactorial disease.

9.2.3. Liver Tumors: Benign vs Malignant

Differential diagnosis between malignant and benign liver tumors is significant in management and prognosis. Benign liver lesions, whether of epithelial or mesenchymal origin, are often discrete masses on imaging and are usually asymptomatic. On the other hand, malignant tumors like primary HCC and metastases are more aggressive in nature and more complex in imaging characteristics. Sophisticated MRI techniques, such as diffusion-weighted imaging and hepatobiliary contrast agents, enable accurate tissue characterization and differentiation of malignant from benign lesions without the use of invasive procedures. The diagnostic enhancement on the basis of noninvasive evaluation leads to enhanced precision and guides treatment planning, which is especially useful because of the complexity of hepatobiliary cancers and associated comorbidities. Optimal management of malignant tumors like HCC includes a multidisciplinary approach synthesizing imaging findings with clinical and pathologic findings to inform surgical, transplant, and systemic therapy decisions (Al B Benson *et. al.*, 2021; Gatti *et. al.*, 2022) (Figure 9.9).

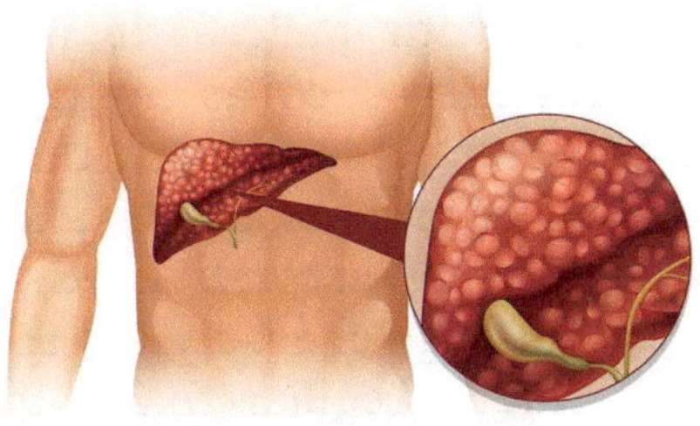

Figure 9.9. Liver tumors.

Source: https://max-website20-images.s3.ap-south-1.amazonaws.com/liver_cancer_a221cfc41d.jpg.

9.2.4. Biliary Obstruction and Imaging Findings

Imaging plays a central role in diagnosing and treating biliary obstruction by demarcating the anatomical location and causative etiology of the blockade. Recent modalities such as ultrasound and

CT provide valuable information concerning bile duct dilatation and intraluminal or extraluminal obstructions. For instance, in a case of extrahepatic biliary obstruction in a potbelly pig, both ultrasound and CT identified gross dilatation of the common bile duct with obstruction by inspissated biliary content, as surgically confirmed (Sannajust *et. al.*, 2024). In addition, rare conditions like mucinous cystadenoma of the gallbladder that can extend to the cystic and common bile ducts and cause obstruction have been reported on the basis of descriptive imaging features. This contributes to greater preoperative clarification and differentiation from more common obstructive etiologies (Liu *et. al.*, 2023). Imaging, thus, not only facilitates timely diagnosis but also guides specific therapeutic interventions in biliary obstruction.

9.2.5. Cholangiocarcinoma Imaging Features

Accurate imaging is crucial in the diagnosis and treatment planning of cholangiocarcinoma, a biliary epithelial malignancy that shares several pathophysiological and morphological characteristics with pancreatic neoplasms. Imaging modalities such as multiphasic CT and MRI are essential in defining the location, size, and vascular invasion of the tumor, which determines staging as well as therapeutic planning. Imaging characteristics in the character include irregular thickening of the bile duct wall, luminal narrowing, and delayed enhancement patterns consistent with the fibrous stroma of the tumor. MRCP also provides valuable noninvasive visualization of biliary ductal obstruction and secondary intrahepatic dilatation. These imaging techniques not only discriminate cholangiocarcinoma from benign biliary disease but also provide preoperative staging within a multidisciplinary plan. The complexity of management confirms the importance of ongoing imaging advancements for prognostication and monitoring of therapy (Alvaro *et. al.*, 2019; Cannavale *et. al.*, 2016).

9.2.6. Fatty Liver Disease and its Diagnosis

Advances in hepatobiliary imaging have significantly enhanced the detection and characterization of fatty liver disease, a condition increasingly causing liver morbidity worldwide. Prompt recognition is crucial because fatty liver disease can progress to steatohepatitis, fibrosis, and ultimately cirrhosis if not diagnosed.

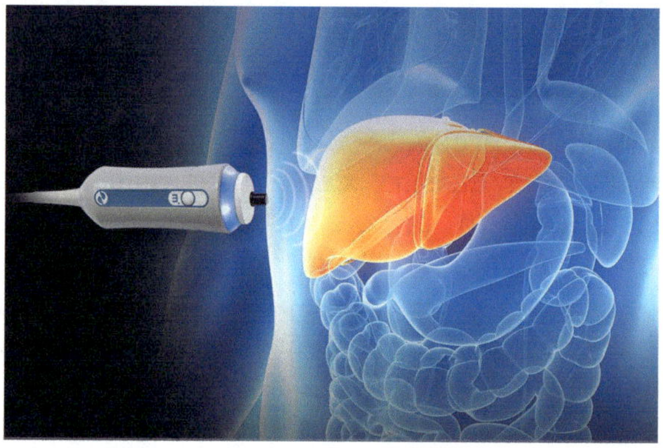

Figure 9.10. Fatty liver disease.

Source: https://precisiondigestivecare.com/wp-content/uploads/2023/04/FibroScanimage-PDC-1024x693.jpg.

The imaging agents used are mostly ultrasound, CT, and MRI to evaluate hepatic steatosis on a noninvasive scale. Ultrasound is commonly used as an initial screening tool due to its convenience, low cost, and ability to show increased echogenicity secondary to fat deposition. MRI, specifically proton density fat fraction imaging, offers greater quantitation of the amount of hepatic fat and stages of fibrosis. Elastography also offers complementary measurements through assessment of liver stiffness to aid in detecting fibrosis. As the nonspecific laboratory findings of fatty liver disease, an imaging combined modality is still required to provide an accurate diagnosis and follow-up. This is most crucial for early treatment and management to prevent progression towards HCC, within the overall hepatobiliary imaging paradigms (Al B Benson *et. al.*, 2021; Hilscher *et. al.*, 2022) (Figure 9.10).

9.2.7. Liver Abscesses and Their Imaging Appearance

Imaging plays a crucial role in the differentiation of liver abscesses from other hepatic lesions, especially when clinical presentation is not definitive. Early abscesses are visualized as heterogeneous solid masses on CT, and differentiation from tumors may be challenging. With maturation of the abscess, an expected hypoattenuating necrotic center with rim enhancement can typically be identified, which aids in diagnosis. MRI gives additional diagnostic clues; e.g., the double target sign, with layered wall enhancement, is more typically associated with abscesses than malignancy. Overlap in imaging features some-times necessitates biopsy to establish a diagnosis. Clinical presentation and signs such as fever and leukocytosis, together with elevated alkaline phosphatase, add to imaging findings in establishing the diagnosis. According to these complexities, multiphasic CT and hepatobiliary-specific MRI contrast agents enable lesion characterization by differential enhancement patterns between liver parenchyma and lesions (Khaled *et. al.*, 2021). Accurate identification of liver abscesses plays an important role in guiding timely and effective treatment plans under the overall scenario of hepatobiliary imaging (Jean-Dumonceau *et. al.*, 2018).

9.2.8. Hemangiomas and Focal Nodular Hyperplasia (FNH)

Benign lesions of the liver have a tendency to present diagnostic challenges in hepatobiliary imaging due to their varied vascular signatures and overlap of imaging features with malignant tumors. Hemangiomas and focal nodular hyperplasia (FNH) are the most frequent among them. Hemangiomas have a typical peripheral nodular enhancement pattern with centripetal fill-in at increasingly advanced phases on contrast-enhanced studies, which allows for easy recognition. In contrast, FNH usually demonstrates intense arterial phase enhancement with a central scar visible on delayed imaging, which reflects its characteristic vascular supply and fibrous stroma. Accurate differentiation between these lesions is necessary to avoid unnecessary interventions and appropriately guide patient management. Progress in imaging modalities, i.e., contrast-enhanced ultrasound, CT, and MRI, contributes to improved characterization by standardized protocol and lexicon such as the Liver Imaging Reporting and Data System (LI-RADS), particularly useful in the absence of cirrhosis but incidental liver lesions (Agostini *et. al.*, 2023; Berzigotti *et. al.*, 2023) (Figure 9.11).

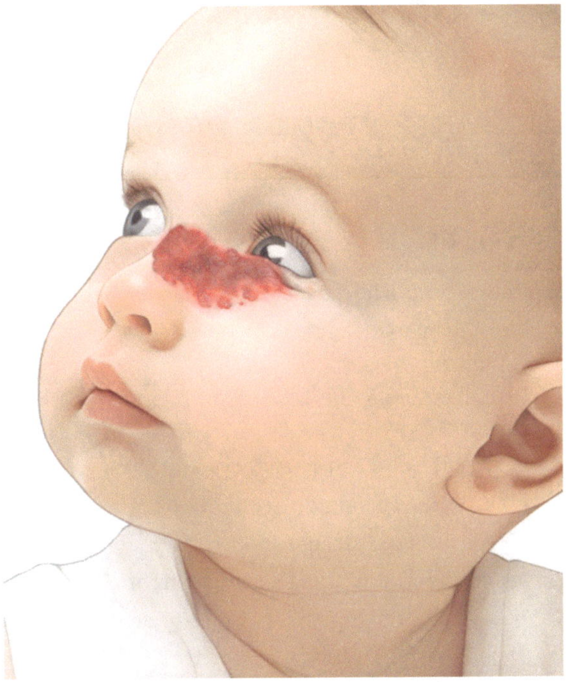

Figure 9.11. Hemangiomas (infantile).

Source: https://www.informedhealth.org/grafiken/en_haemangiom_saeugling-in-augennaehe_replacement_image.png.

9.2.9. Role of Imaging in Liver Transplantation

Accurate assessment and surveillance of the liver's vascular and biliary anatomy are crucial factors in liver transplantation success. Imaging modalities, such as ultrasound, CT, and MRI, play crucial roles pre- and post-transplant by evaluating donor liver anatomy, detecting potential complications, and guiding interventional treatments. For instance, percutaneous transhepatic biliary drainage, as a rule, image-guided, has been shown to have excellent technical and clinical success rates in the management of postoperative biliary leakages, with great benefit to patients. Additionally, early diagnosis of vascular complications such as hepatic artery bleeding, while rare but potentially lethal, relies heavily on accurate imaging, such that intervention can be early with stent-graft placement or surgery (Ndongo *et. al.*, 2010). The use of advanced imaging modalities ensures comprehensive evaluation, which enhances transplant planning and postoperative care, and ultimately reduces morbidity and mortality of liver transplant patients in complex clinical situations (Ndongo *et. al.*, 2010).

Test Your Knowledge

1. What is the typical ultrasound appearance of a gallbladder polyp?
2. How is liver cirrhosis identified on imaging?

9.3. Pancreatic Disorders

Learning Outcome

1. Understand acute pancreatitis imaging findings
2. Define chronic pancreatitis and its complications
3. Explain staging and imaging of pancreatic cancer
4. Focus on cysts and pseudocysts of the pancreas
5. Identify neuroendocrine tumors of the pancreas
6. Discuss imaging in pancreatic trauma
7. Learn the role of imaging in pancreatic surgery
8. Describe endoscopic techniques for pancreatic imaging
9. Explain emerging imaging techniques for pancreatic disorders

Advances in imaging techniques have facilitated greatly the diagnosis and management of pancreatic disease, which traditionally presents complex challenges due to the position of the pancreas and its close relationship with adjacent structures. Pancreatic injury, though relatively rare, is frequently compounded by duodenal and biliary injury, making clinical management difficult and necessitating prompt, precise imaging to facilitate treatment planning. The hemodynamic stability was normally the deciding factor for the treatment plan to be followed, with non-operative care getting increasingly popular when evidence-based and with proper imaging modalities. Endoscopic and radiological interventions have enhanced multimodal treatment for pancreatic trauma and its complications without surgery, but major injuries typically necessitate operative intervention to counteract the high morbidity risk (Hecker *et. al.*, 2019). Furthermore, MRCP has been a non-invasive, reliable modality that complements conventional ones like cholangiopancreatography (ERCP), offering high diagnostic yield in detecting pancreaticobiliary disorders and thus avoiding unnecessary invasive procedures (Gondal *et. al.*, 2018).

9.3.1. Acute Pancreatitis Imaging Findings

Accurate imaging plays an important role in the diagnosis and management of acute pancreatitis, with the capability of diagnosing complications and guiding therapeutic planning. Early in the course of the illness, contrast-enhanced CT is the preferred modality to assess pancreatic inflammation, necrosis, and peripancreatic fluid collections. Imaging typically shows pancreatic hypertrophy, heterogeneous enhancement, and non-enhancing regions compatible with necrosis. MRI can provide improved soft tissue differentiation and detect biliary etiologies or subtle ductal changes, while ultrasound is only suited for the detection of gallstones as a causative agent.

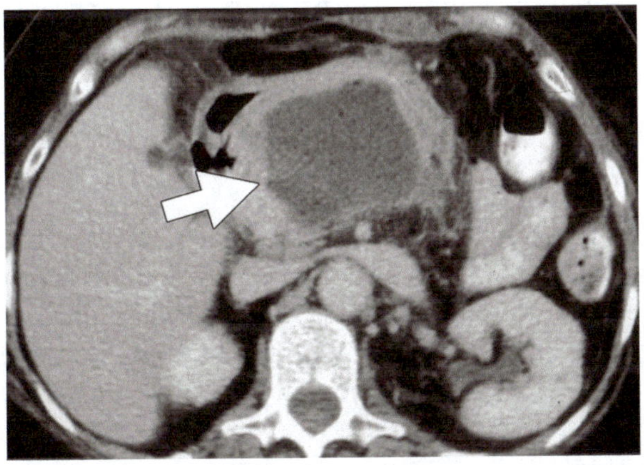

Figure 9.12. Acute pancreatitis imaging.

Source: https://www.ajronline.org/cms/10.2214/AJR.10.4338/asset/images/08_10_4338_07.jpeg.

Common findings are diffuse or focal pancreatic hypertrophy, fat stranding in the peripancreatic tissues, and fluid collections that mature into pseudocysts or abscesses. Prompt detection of these radiographic findings ensures appropriate clinical management and hence prevents morbidity. Although imaging findings in drug-induced pancreatitis are rare, expertise in differentiating such presentations from alternative etiologies is essential to a correct diagnosis (Ichikawa *et. al.*, 2023). Further, advanced imaging techniques are recommended to describe the severity of inflammation and biliary tract extension in complicated cases (Christopher *et. al.*, 2022) (Figure 9.12).

9.3.2. Chronic Pancreatitis and its Complications

Advances in imaging have significantly enhanced the diagnosis and management of idiopathic complex pancreatic illness, particularly chronic pancreatitis, with its definition of chronic inflammation resulting in irreversible pancreatic damage. It tends to cause complications such as ductal strictures, calcification, and exocrine and endocrine insufficiency, and thus necessitates precise imaging modalities to assess structural and functional alterations. Moreover, chronic inflammation also makes the patients susceptible to secondary complications like pseudocyst formation and biliary obstruction, which are crucial for therapeutic approaches. The overlapping effect of chronic pancreatitis with immune-mediated disease, i.e., IgG4-related disease, emphasizes the necessity of a comprehensive diagnostic approach by serology, histology, and imaging to guide appropriate glucocorticoid treatment regimens effectively (Matthias *et. al.*, 2020). Additionally, new evidence suggests a potential role of microbial biofilms in sustaining chronic pancreatic inflammation, supporting refractory disease, and complicating intervention strategies. Detection of involvement of biofilm through advanced imaging can help in the early detection of stable foci of infection that are crucial for successful management (Lene *et. al.*, 2020).

9.3.3. Pancreatic Cancer: Staging and Imaging

Accurate staging of pancreatic cancer is necessary to determine appropriate treatment plans and improve patient outcomes. Cross-sectional imaging, particularly CECT and MRI, plays an important role in the assessment of tumor size, vascular invasion, and the occurrence of metastasis. Advanced new modalities such as PET/MRI combine metabolic and anatomic data to enhance diagnostic accuracy by better lesion characterization and correct localization than with PET/CT (Samuel *et. al.*, 2021). Moreover, EUS-guided fine-needle aspiration or biopsy offers complementary tissue diagnosis and locoregional staging that connects imaging findings to histopathologic diagnosis. Despite international guidelines, the most suitable diagnostic strategy remains heterogeneous, reflecting clinical practice and patient variability (Sahai *et. al.*, 2020). Therefore, multimodal imaging and endoscopic therapies together form extensive staging that is crucial for surgical planning, neoadjuvant therapy decision, and palliation in patients with pancreatic cancer (Figure 9.13).

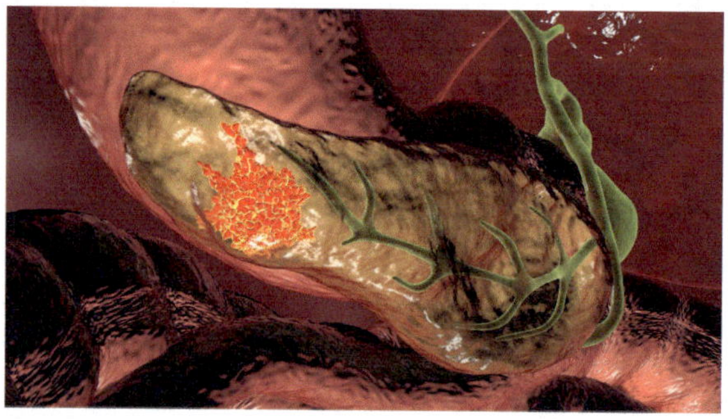

Figure 9.13. Pancreatic cancer.

Source: https://www.genengnews.com/wp-content/uploads/2022/06/Aug21_2020_Getty_1215121154_PancreaticCancer-scaled.jpg.

9.3.4. Cysts and Pseudocysts of the Pancreas

Accurate diagnosis and treatment of pancreatic cystic lesions remain a challenging clinical dilemma due to their diverse etiologies and variable malignant potential. The capacity for differentiation between benign cysts, cystic neoplasms, and pseudocysts is necessary for the establishment of treatment regimens, yet routine cytology and biomarkers in cyst fluid often fail to provide definitive diagnoses. Recent advancements highlight the value of proteomic analysis to identify specific protein biomarkers in pancreatic cystic neoplasms, enhancing diagnostic accuracy and enabling detection of the risk of malignancy (Kwon *et. al.*, 2011). Pancreatic pseudocysts can also, in certain cases, extend to extrapancreatic sites such as gastrohepatic or hepatoduodenal ligaments, complicating clinical presentation and imaging diagnoses. These extensions show that there is a great need for high clinical suspicion and extensive imaging assessment to avoid epigastric mass misdiagnosis (Goyal *et. al.*, 2012). Thus, the integration of advanced biomarker diagnosis and accurate imaging techniques is highly essential in the improvement of patients with pancreatic pseudocysts and cysts.

9.3.5. Neuroendocrine Tumors of the Pancreas

Effective imaging approaches play a critical role in the diagnosis and treatment of advanced hepatic and pancreatic disease, particularly in the management of metastatic disease. Pancreatic neuroendocrine tumors (PNETs), although rare, frequently present with liver metastases, strongly influencing prognosis and treatment planning (Aurello *et. al.*, 2018). Accurate estimation of liver tumor burden is important, considering that metastatic involvement occurs in 40–80% and significantly affects patient outcomes. More recent advances in imaging, specifically gadoxetic acid-enhanced magnetic resonance imaging (Gd-EOB MRI), have demonstrated unmatched sensitivity for the detection and measurement of neuroendocrine liver metastases. Moreover, integration with AI-based segmentation models allows for three-dimensional volumetry assessment, improving accuracy and efficiency in clinical use. These developments not only maximize treatment response evaluation but also have a strong association with multidisciplinary board review evaluations, which promote their potential for enhancing individualized patient care for liver-involving neuroendocrine pancreatic cancer (Figure 9.14).

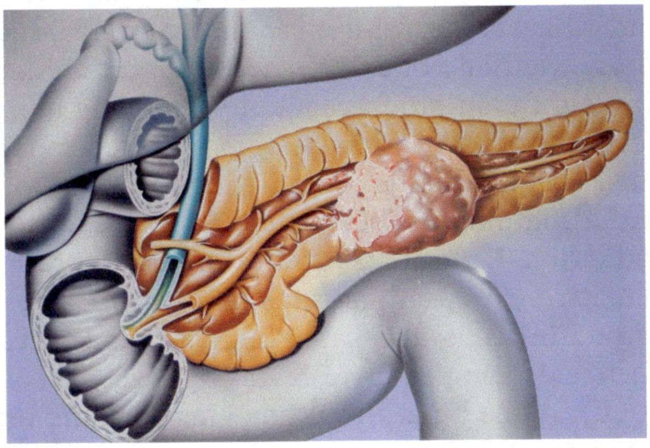

Figure 9.14. Neuroendocrine tumors of the pancreas.

Source: https://www.endocrinologyadvisor.com/wp-content/uploads/sites/9/2020/03/Pancreatic-cancer_SS_SS21222423.jpg.

9.3.6. Imaging in Pancreatic Trauma

Proper assessment of pancreatic injury is the key to guiding appropriate clinical management and improving patient outcomes. Imaging plays a pivotal role in establishing the scope of injury, particularly in light of the retroperitoneal location of the pancreas and intimate association with adjacent vascular and biliary structures. CT remains the first-line modality due to its widespread availability and ability to provide high-resolution imaging of parenchymal disruption and associated complications such as hematomas or ductal injury. More advanced imaging modalities, such as CT angiography, turn out to be greatly useful in identifying vascular anomalies or pseudoaneurysms that can add to the risk of bleeding, especially in complicated cases or congenital anomalies such as situs inversus totalis (Christopher *et. al.*, 2019). Concomitant modalities such as MRI and EUS may offer enhanced soft-tissue differentiation and ductal evaluation to aid in planning and intervention during surgery. End-to-end integration of entire imaging results ensures a multidisciplinary approach tailored to the intricate anatomy and pathology of pancreatic trauma (Dennison *et. al.*, 2010).

9.3.7. Role of Imaging in Pancreatic Surgery

The evolution of medical imaging has transformed preoperative assessment and intraoperative surgery of pancreatic diseases.

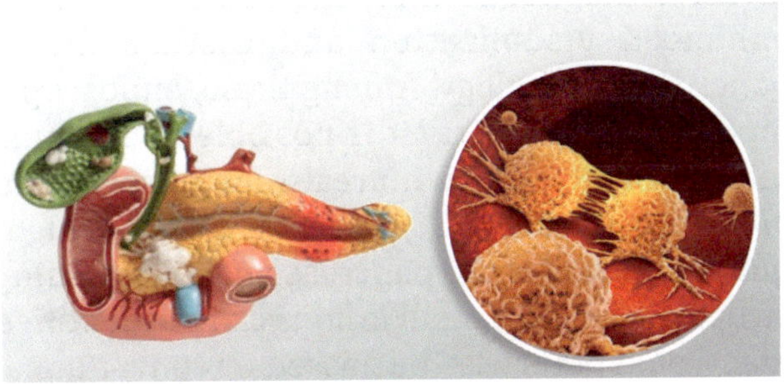

Figure 9.15. Imaging in pancreatic surgery.

Source: https://gemhospitals.com/frontend/assets/images/team/grid/pancreaticcancer.webp.

Accurate imaging procedures are essential to establish tumor size, vascular spread, and metastatic spread, which directly influence the surgery plan and prognosis. Imaging modalities such as contrast-enhanced CT, MRI, and EUS provide panoramic views of the pancreas and surrounding structures and enable individualized treatment and reduced operative risk. These imaging modalities are accurate for staging and are now key to multidisciplinary treatment, optimizing patient outcomes. Furthermore, ongoing technological refinements promise enhanced resolution and functional evaluation, with potential advantages for early detection and monitoring response. Although most famous for evaluating malignant biliary tumors, imaging's expanding role in pancreatic surgery serves to underscore its integral contribution to therapeutic choice and postoperative follow-up in hepatobiliary care (Cannavale *et. al.*, 2016). Although trauma imaging is heterogeneous by environment, understanding pancreatic trauma injury patterns remains useful to emergent surgical intervention across environments (Ndongo *et. al.*, 2010) (Figure 9.15).

9.3.8. Endoscopic Techniques for Pancreatic Imaging

Technological advancement in minimally invasive diagnostic methods has significantly enhanced visualization and assessment of pancreatic pathology. Among these, endoscopic methods stand out as it is possible to combine direct visualization with real-time imaging and biopsy acquisition. EUS, for instance, yields high-quality images of the pancreas and surrounding structures, so that small lesions can be identified that would otherwise be missed by conventional imaging modalities. In addition, ERCP not only facilitates careful imaging of pancreatic ducts but also provides therapeutic options such as stenting in the obstructive scenario. The techniques have assumed a central role in the diagnostic workup for pancreatic cancers, where precise staging is synonymous with appropriate management. These techniques are integrated to complement cross-sectional imaging and enhance a multidisciplinary approach to both improve the diagnostic yield and outcome of the patient in pancreatic disease (Cannavale *et. al.*, 2016). The evolving role of endoscopy in pancreatic and hepatobiliary imaging is an expression of the trend toward more focused, less invasive therapies (Ndongo *et. al.*, 2010).

9.3.9. Emerging Imaging Techniques for Pancreatic Disorders

Current advances in imaging have significantly enhanced pancreatic disorder diagnosis and treatment, overcoming the limitations embedded in their heterogeneity. Traditional modalities such as ultrasound, CT, and MRI remain the cornerstone; however, newer modalities such as contrast-enhanced ultrasound, diffusion-weighted MRI, and EUS-guided elastography are finding growing application in early detection and characterization of pancreatic lesions. These methods offer enhanced resolution and tissue differentiation capability, enabling more accurate staging and malignant assessment, such as pancreatic ductal adenocarcinoma, and inflammatory disease. Of interest, the reduction in ionizing radiation exposure in sensitive groups illustrates the growing role of non-invasive and safer imaging modalities, particularly in pediatric cases (Nydegger *et. al.*, 2010). While biliary tract imaging remains the primary focus, improvement in modality-related advances in pancreatic pathology highlights the importance of interdisciplinary coordination to optimize patient outcomes for care, as with the multifactorial pathogenesis determined for associated hepatobiliary diseases (Alvaro *et. al.*, 2018) (Figure 9.16).

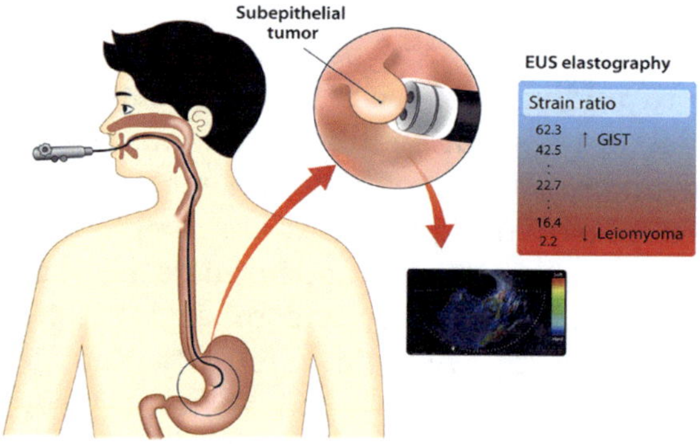

Figure 9.16. Endoscopic ultrasound-guided elastography.

Source: https://www.giejournal.org/cms/10.1016/j.gie.2019.09.012/asset/8031cae9-8b03-4964-ae73-2483cdfed208/main.assets/fx1_lrg.jpg.

Test Your Knowledge

1. How can imaging help detect complications of pancreatitis, such as necrosis or abscess formation?
2. How is autoimmune pancreatitis diagnosed using imaging?

9.4. Interventional Imaging Techniques

Learning Outcome

1. Explain the role of imaging in guided biopsies
2. Learn drainage procedures for abscesses
3. Discuss radiofrequency ablation in liver tumors
4. Define transarterial chemoembolization (TACE)
5. Focus on stereotactic body radiation therapy (SBRT)
6. Describe endoscopic retrograde cholangiopancreatography (ERCP)
7. Focus on imaging-guided interventions in pancreatitis
8. Describe the future of interventional imaging
9. Understand ethical considerations in interventional procedures

Medical imaging technology improvements have revolutionized the accurate diagnosis and management of pancreatic and hepatobiliary disease, particularly with the use of interventional imaging techniques that enable minimally invasive therapy. Such techniques combine real-time imaging guidance with targeted interventions, allowing clinicians to accurately map out complex anatomy in a way that minimizes patient morbidity. Therapeutic modalities such as ultrasound-guided biopsy, fluoroscopy-guided drainage, and CT–guided tumor ablation are currently the standard in the management of hepatic and pancreatic diseases, with improved therapeutic outcomes and reduced recovery time. Moreover, nanotechnology at the nanoscale, which has been explored by recent nanomedicine advances, promises superior imaging resolution and site-specific delivery within these organs and, subsequently, enhances interventional accuracy and efficacy (Pelaz *et. al.*, 2017). Despite these advances, there are still challenges in optimizing vector-based therapies using safe and effective delivery systems for therapy, which is congruent with the challenges in integrating viral vector designs into clinical practice (Bulcha *et. al.*, 2021). Overall, these interventional imaging advances are an important piece in the new age of hepatobiliary and pancreatic imaging.

9.4.1. Role of Imaging in Guided Biopsies

Accurate tissue sampling is critical to hepatobiliary and pancreatic disease diagnosis, and therefore imaging-guided biopsies form an integral component of clinical practice. Advanced imaging technologies such as real-time three-dimensional ultrasound enhance localization accuracy through dynamic visualization of the target anatomy, which maximizes the accuracy of needle positioning compared with traditional two-dimensional approaches. This augmented targeting maximizes the minimization of sampling errors and procedural complexity with a guarantee of representative tissue retrieval, depicted in experimental models demonstrating significant improvement of accuracy in targeting areas for biopsy (Moreau-Gaudry *et. al.*, 2007). In pancreatic cancer, where therapeutic planning is guided by early and precise diagnosis, integration of multimodal imaging with endoscopic EUS and CT maximizes biopsy guidance through delineation of tumor location and vascular involvement, thus enhancing staging and treatment planning. These imaging-guided biopsies support clinician decision-making that maximizes surgical treatment, neoadjuvant treatment, or palliative care and ultimately maximizes patient benefit in this challenging disease environment (Caputo *et. al.*, 2023) (Figure 9.17).

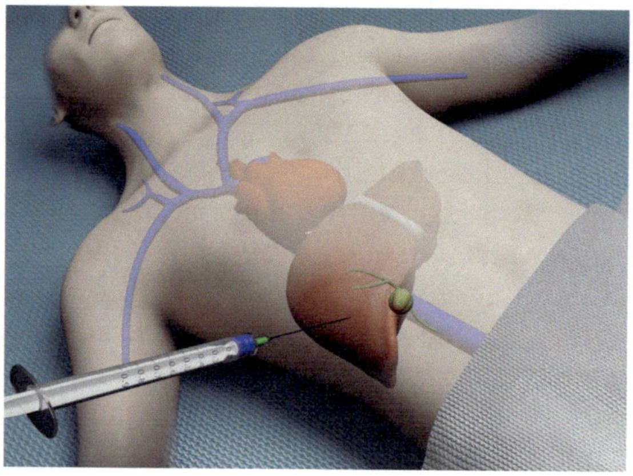

Figure 9.17. Accurate tissue sampling is crucial for diagnosing hepatobiliary and pancreatic diseases, making imaging-guided biopsies an indispensable component of clinical practice.

Source: https://www.mdpi.com/diagnostics/diagnostics-13-00784/article_deploy/html/images/diagnostics-13-00784-g001.png.

9.4.2. Drainage Procedures for Abscesses

Effective treatment of abscesses within the hepatobiliary and pancreatic systems relies on timely and precise drainage. Therapy guided by imaging has become pivotal, with the facility for targeted drainage with fewer complications. Percutaneous catheter drainage, preferably under ultrasound or CT guidance, is preferred because of its minimally invasive nature and high success rate, particularly when surgical access is less than ideal. Endoscopic drainage, either via stents or nasobiliary drains, is also significant, especially if abscesses are biliary obstruction or malignancy related. The choice of drainage procedure depends on the abscess size, location, and causation. For example, preoperative biliary drainage employing self-expandable metal stents is applicable in some malignant obstructions for symptom palliation and in a bid to optimize surgical outcome (Jean-Dumonceau *et. al.*, 2018). Advances in imaging not only enable accurate localization of abscesses but also provide therapy guidance, enhancing prognosis in widespread hepatobiliary infection and malignancies such as cholangiocarcinoma (Blechacz, 2016).

9.4.3. Radiofrequency Ablation in Liver Tumors

Technical advancements have significantly enhanced the efficacy of minimally invasive treatments for liver tumors, offering improved therapeutic outcomes. Among these treatments, radiofrequency ablation (RFA) has become a routine modality for the treatment of HCC and metastatic liver tumors. RFA delivers thermal energy to induce coagulative necrosis in tumors, so it is especially suitable for those patients who are not candidates for surgical resection. Intraoperative ultrasound plays a significant role in RFA guidance by clearly defining tumor margins and assessing vascular involvement, thereby maximizing ablation margins and minimizing complications (Bartoş *et. al.*, 2018).

RFA is also as effective as traditional surgery methods but with minimal postoperative pain and hospital stays. However, emerging alternatives such as IRE are promising by avoiding collateral thermal damage to essential hepatic and biliary anatomy, with growing evidence for complementary roles in hepatic oncology (Astras *et. al.*, 2017). Such advancements emphasize the value of integrating imaging modalities with ablation devices in hepatobiliary oncology (Figure 9.18).

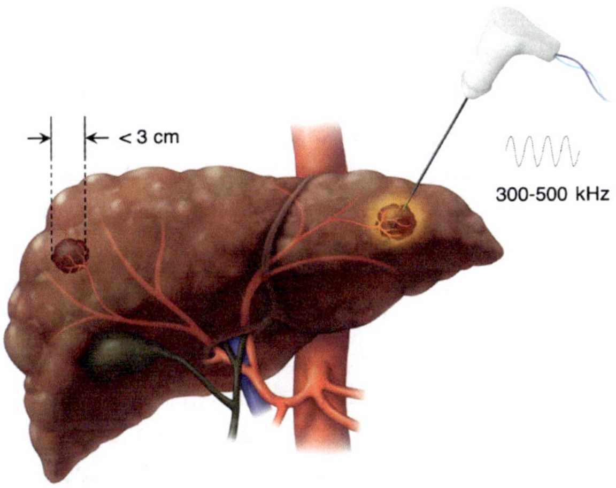

Figure 9.18. Radiofrequency ablation (RFA) has emerged as a widely accepted modality for managing hepatocellular carcinoma and metastatic liver lesions.

Source: https://www.researchgate.net/publication/338026987/figure/fig4/AS:837642967085058@1576721054984/Radiofrequency-ablation-RFA-Treatment-is-typically-used-to-treat-hepatocellular.jpg.

9.4.4. Transarterial Chemoembolization (TACE)

Locoregional therapies have contributed enormously to the therapeutic armamentarium of patients with unresectable liver cancer, particularly those who are not suitable candidates for systemic chemotherapy. TACE, among others, has been a valuable intervention by providing targeted drug delivery to hepatic tumors and simultaneously causing ischemia through embolization. The two modalities enhance tumor necrosis and maintain systemic toxicity under control. The method is very reliant on precise imaging techniques to achieve correct catheter placement as well as assess tumor vascularity, underlining the importance of hepatobiliary imaging for successful application. The role of TACE is particularly pertinent in metastatic liver disease management where curative measures are unfeasible and systemic treatments fail with resistance. In addition, its complementarity with advanced technologies, such as MR-guided interventions, has the potential to improve targeting and adaptive treatment planning, leading potentially to higher-quality outcomes with fewer side effects (Boldrini *et. al.*, 2021; Kylie *et. al.*, 2021).

9.4.5. Stereotactic Body Radiation Therapy (SBRT)

Advances in imaging technology have significantly enhanced the precision and effectiveness of oncologic treatments, particularly in complex regions such as the hepatobiliary and pancreas systems. Among the developments is the introduction of SBRT that offers a non-surgical approach for the delivery of tumor destruction with less damage to surrounding tissue.

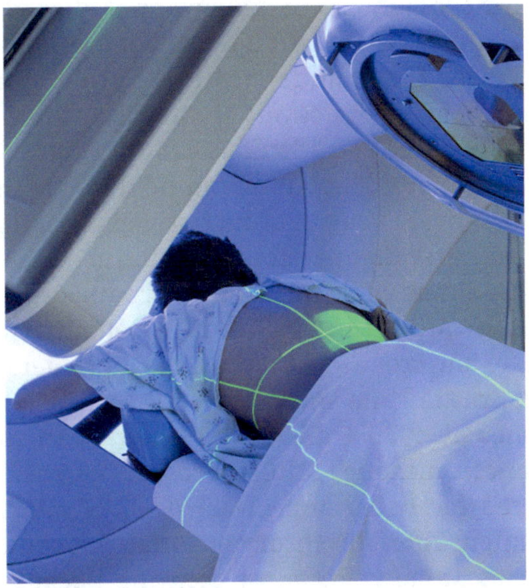

Figure 9.19. Stereotactic body radiation therapy (SBRT).

Source: https://kentuckianacancer.com/wp-content/uploads/2023/11/sbrtsmall.png.

With the use of sophisticated imaging modalities, clinicians can achieve accurate tumor localization and organ motion correction with a resultant maximization of radiation delivery. This accuracy is especially critical for liver tumors, for which MR-guided radiotherapy has improved volume visualization and enabled adaptive treatment planning, leading to better clinical outcomes and reduced toxicity (Boldrini *et. al.*, 2021). Similarly, in locally advanced pancreatic cancer, SBRT has emerged as a useful adjuvant by providing high-dose localized radiation resulting in increased local tumor control and also possibly enabling increased systemic immune responses, and therefore potential for prolonging overall survival in a disease hitherto and historically associated with poor prognosis (Bolli *et. al.*, 2024) (Figure 9.19).

9.4.6. Endoscopic Retrograde Cholangiopancreatography (ERCP)

Accurate diagnosis of biliary tract disease is precariously dependent upon advanced imaging modalities that can delineate the etiology and location of obstruction or disease. Of these modalities, ERCP stands alone as both a diagnostic and therapeutic modality and holds its highest value in evaluating bile duct stones, strictures, and tumors. Comparison with ultrasound has revealed that while ultrasound produces a non-invasive initial survey with high sensitivity for tumors and stones, ERCP provides more detailed visualization and interventional facilities and reaches over 90% diagnostic accuracy in some instances. Although MRCP becomes increasingly favored for being non-invasive, ERCP remains indispensable for interventional procedures such as stone removal or stenting because of its diagnostic acuity with therapy (Gondal *et. al.*, 2018). ERCP therefore remains a cornerstone in pancreatic and hepatobiliary imaging, balancing risk against clinical benefit.

9.4.7. Imaging-guided Interventions in Pancreatitis

Effective management of pancreatitis often requires individualized therapy that prevents complications such as fluid collections, necrosis, and fibro-obliterative fibrosis of bile ducts. Imaging-directed interventions, and particularly ones that employ EUS and CT, have become central to diagnosis as well as therapeutic strategies. These imaging modalities allow drainage of pancreatic pseudocysts or walled-off necrosis with minimally invasive modalities, which is achieved with much less morbidity compared to surgical approaches. Besides, imaging plays a critical role in the diagnosis of biliary strictures and obstructions secondary to pancreatitis to enable targeted stent placement to regain patency of the ducts. For example, endoscopic placement of self-expandable metal stents is employed in malignant biliary obstruction while plastic stents treat benign strictures or leaks, which optimizes the patient's outcome (Jean-Dumonceau *et. al.*, 2018). MRCP also maximizes pancreatic and biliary ductal pathology characterization, guiding intervention planning by distinguishing benign from malignant stricture etiology, which is central to prevention of inappropriate invasive therapies (Venkata *et. al.*, 2014). Imaging-guided interventions thus form a cornerstone of contemporary pancreatitis management in hepatobiliary and pancreatic imaging (Figure 9.20).

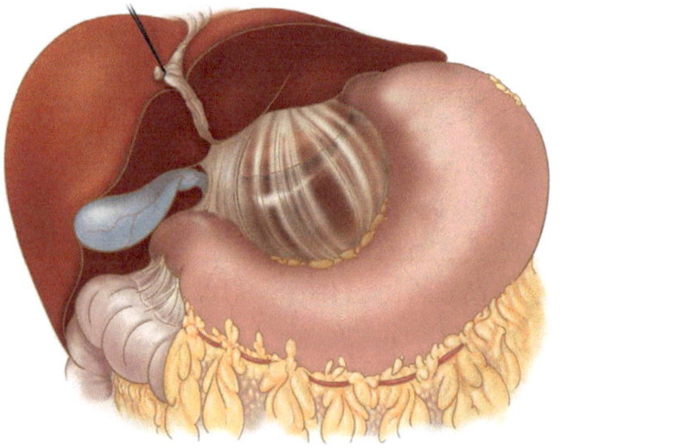

Figure 9.20. Invasive drainage of pancreatic pseudocysts.

Source: https://www.laparoscopicexperts.com/wp-content/uploads/2016/09/laparoscopic-drainage-pancreatic-pseudocyst-b.jpg.

9.4.8. Future of Interventional Imaging

Innovations in technology continue to re-shape the domain of hepatobiliary and pancreatic interventions with the potential for augmented diagnostic accuracy and therapeutic efficacy. Motorized spiral enteroscopy with device-assisted enteroscopy is one illustration of how technology surpasses anatomical constraints in patients with altered surgical anatomy, thereby simplifying and rendering advanced procedures such as ERCP easier and safer. These devices enhance maneuverability, reduce procedural time, and maximize therapeutic potential, ultimately contributing to improved patient care. Moreover, the synergism of molecular imaging with targeted therapies directed at preselected genetic abnormalities, such as fibroblast growth factor receptor fusions or isocitrate dehydrogenase mutations in cholangiocarcinoma, has potential for tailored interventional imaging approaches that not only target tumors but also guide individualized therapy (Paul *et. al.*, 2021). Combined, these technological and molecular advances herald a future where interventional imaging will be increasingly specific, less invasive, and integrated into multidisciplinary models of hepatobiliary and pancreatic care.

9.4.9. Ethical Considerations in Interventional Procedures

Advances in hepatobiliary and pancreatic imaging have significantly enhanced the accuracy of interventionist procedures, facilitating greater therapeutic and diagnostic value. However, these advances also call for rigorous ethical examination to ensure patient safety, informed consent, and fairness of access. Physicians must carefully balance the potential benefits of novel approaches, such as nanoscale targeting for cancer treatment, with unidentified long-term risks and the possibility of unforeseen complications upon clinical translation (Chehelgerdi *et. al.*, 2023). Moreover, therapy decisions, particularly in complex cases such as neuroendocrine liver metastasis, must be candid regarding risks versus benefits of surgery versus other treatments, with emphasis on patient autonomy and individualized planning for treatment (Jordan *et. al.*, 2020). Ethical issues are also implicated in resource allocation and justification of expensive or innovative treatment. Finally, professional clinical practice entails multidisciplinary collaboration, proper education of patients, and adherence to ethical standards that balance efficacy and patients' general welfare who are undergoing hepatobiliary and pancreatic interventions.

Test Your Knowledge

1. When is ultrasound-guided biopsy preferred over CT-guided biopsy?
2. What are the key advantages of image-guided biopsy compared to surgical biopsy?

SUMMARY

Advancements in pancreatic and hepatobiliary imaging have greatly improved the early detection and characterization of diseases and, as such, improved clinical outcomes. Precise imaging methods are critical to diagnose complex conditions like immunoglobulin G4-related disease, where early identification is necessary in order to avoid irreversible organ damage through timely intervention (Katz *et. al.*, 2021). Imaging is also critical in the diagnosis and management of cholangiocarcinoma, which has multifactorial pathogenesis and unpredictable presentation and needs precise anatomical and pathological assessment for optimal treatment planning (Paul *et. al.*, 2021). Still, challenges lie ahead, though, in differentiating disease mimickers and correlating imaging findings with clinical and pathological data for successful treatment. Future research in the optimization of imaging modalities and their integration with molecular and genetic markers holds the promise of improving diagnostic performance and patient prognosis in hepatobiliary and pancreatic diseases. Imaging is therefore a cornerstone of multidisciplinary management in this context.

Advances in hepatobiliary and pancreatic imaging have significantly enhanced diagnostic accuracy and patient management. Recent research indicates that MRCP is a valuable non-invasive imaging agent for detecting pancreatic and biliary pathologies, particularly in resource-poor areas. Retrospective analysis showed that MRCP effectively diagnosed obstructive cholelithiasis and pancreatic head tumors with obstructive jaundice as the primary imaging indication, highlighting its clinical use in hepatobiliary disease (Rabiu *et. al.*, 2025). At the same time, research on the biological effect of static magnetic fields employed for MRI shows therapeutic potential in models of pancreatic trauma. Specifically, moderate-intensity static magnetic fields reduced alcohol-induced pancreatic damage and inflammation and oxidative stress in acute pancreatitis and were proposed to be secondarily useful aside from imaging for clinical use (Wang *et. al.*, 2025). Globally, these findings reflect on the double role of magnetic resonance technologies as applied in diagnosis and emerging treatment options for hepatobiliary and pancreatic diseases.

KEY TERMS FROM THIS CHAPTER

- Nanomedicine
- Bile ducts
- Tumors
- Inflammation
- Hepatocellular carcinoma (HCC)
- Molecular level
- Gallbladder
- Blockages
- Liver lesions

CRITICAL THINKING QUESTIONS

1. **What is the imaging modality of choice for initial evaluation of suspected gallstones?**
   a. CT scan
   b. MRI
   c. Ultrasound
   d. Plain X-ray
2. **Which of the following is most sensitive for detecting liver hemangiomas?**
   a. Non-contrast CT
   b. Ultrasound
   c. MRI with contrast
   d. Plain abdominal X-ray
3. **What imaging finding is most indicative of chronic pancreatitis?**
   a. Homogenous pancreatic enhancement
   b. Dilated pancreatic duct with calcifications
   c. Pancreatic mass with cystic components
   d. Biliary dilatation only
4. **What is the best imaging modality for detecting acute pancreatitis and its complications?**
   a. Abdominal X-ray
   b. CT scan with contrast
   c. MRI without contrast
   d. Endoscopy
5. **Which imaging technique is best for evaluating bile duct obstruction non-invasively?**
   a. MRCP (Magnetic Resonance Cholangiopancreatography)
   b. ERCP
   c. Ultrasound
   d. Plain radiograph

Short Answer Questions

1. What are the first-line imaging modalities for evaluating right upper quadrant pain?
2. How is ultrasound used to assess gallbladder inflammation?
3. What imaging features help differentiate a hepatic cyst from a liver abscess?
4. When is MRI preferred over CT in evaluating liver lesions?
5. What is the role of MRCP in the assessment of biliary tract obstruction?
6. What are the characteristic imaging findings of hepatocellular carcinoma on contrast-enhanced CT?
7. In which clinical scenarios is ERCP used diagnostically and therapeutically?
8. How can pancreatic pseudocysts be identified and monitored on imaging?

Answers to Critical Thinking Questions

1. (c); 2. (c); 3. (b); 4. (b); 5. (a)

REFERENCES

1. Jourdan PM, Lamberton PHL, Fenwick A, Addiss DG. Soil-transmitted helminth infections. Lancet. 2018 Jan 20;391(10117):252-265. doi: 10.1016/S0140-6736(17)31930-X. Epub 2017 Sep 4. PMID: 28882382.
2. Agostini, A., Barile, A., Borgheresi, A., Brunese, P., *et. al.* (2023). Diagnostic approach to focal liver lesions at cross-sectional imaging: A primer for beginners. https://core.ac.uk/download/616533102.pdf (accessed on 30 May 2025).
3. Alexander, J. S., Ballard, D., Boktor, M., Boktor, M., *et. al.* (2019). 3D printing for bio-synthetic biliary stents. https://core.ac.uk/download/212867687.pdf (accessed on 30 May 2025).
4. Mandarano, G., & Sim, J. (2008). The diagnostic MRCP examination: Overcoming technical challenges to ensure clinical success. *Biomedical Imaging and Intervention Journal, 4*(4), Article e28. https://doi.org/10.2349/biij.4.2.e28
5. Alvaro, D., Arcidiacono, P. G., Capurso, G., Cardinale, V., *et. al.* (2019). Common features between neoplastic and preneoplastic lesions of the biliary tract and the pancreas. https://core.ac.uk/download/231748248.pdf (accessed on 30 May 2025).
6. Alvaro, D., Bragazzi, M. C., Cardinale, V., Carpino, G., *et. al.* (2018). Intrahepatic cholangiocarcinoma: Review and update. https://core.ac.uk/download/159269704.pdf (accessed on 30 May 2025).
7. Kourounis G, Paul Tabet P, Moris D, Papalambros A, Felekouras E, Georgiades F, Astras G, Petrou A. Irreversible electroporation (Nanoknife® treatment) in the field of hepatobiliary surgery: Current status and future perspectives. J BUON. 2017 Jan-Feb;22(1):141-149. PMID: 28365947.
8. Aurello, P., Crovetto, A., Debs, T., Mangogna, A., *et. al.* (2018). Treatment options for PNET liver metastases: A systematic review. https://core.ac.uk/download/159636090.pdf (accessed on 30 May 2025).
9. Bartoș, A., Bartoș, D., Breazu, C., Iancu, D., *et. al.* (2018). Intraoperative ultrasound of the liver: Actual status and indications. https://core.ac.uk/download/322435138.pdf (accessed on 30 May 2025).
10. Benson, A. B., D'Angelica, M. I., Abbott, D. E., Anaya, D. A., Anders, R. A., Are, C., Bachini, M., *et. al.* (2021). Hepatobiliary cancers, version 2.2021, NCCN clinical practice guidelines in oncology. *Journal of the National Comprehensive Cancer Network, 19*, 541–565. https://doi.org/10.6004/jnccn.2021.0022.
11. Berzigotti, A., Cui, X., Dietrich, C. F., Dong, Y., Faiss, S., Gorg, C., Lim, A., *et. al.* (2023). Focal liver lesions other than hepatocellular carcinoma in cirrhosis: Diagnostic challenges. https://core.ac.uk/download/611917193.pdf (accessed on 30 May 2025).
12. Juillard, C., Etoundi Mballa, G.A., Bilounga Ndongo, C. *et. al.* Patterns of Injury and Violence in Yaoundé Cameroon: An Analysis of Hospital Data. *World J Surg* **35**, 1–8 (2011). https://doi.org/10.1007/s00268-010-0825-5
13. Blechacz, B. (2016). Cholangiocarcinoma: Current knowledge and new developments. *Gut and Liver, 11*, 13–26. https://doi.org/10.5009/gnl15568.
14. Boldrini, L., Corradini, S., Dawson, L., Gani, C., *et. al.* (2021). MR-guided radiotherapy for liver malignancies. https://core.ac.uk/download/427547140.pdf (accessed on 30 May 2025).

15. Boldrini, L., Corradini, S., Gani, C., Henke, L. E., Hosni, A., Romano, A., & Dawson, L. A. (2021). MR-guided radiotherapy for liver malignancies. *Frontiers in Oncology, 11*. https://doi.org/10.3389/fonc.2021.616027.

16. Bolli, M., Erdem, S., Narayanan, J. S., White, S., *et. al.* (2024). Local ablative therapies and the effect on antitumor immune responses in pancreatic cancer–A review. https://core.ac.uk/download/631293057.pdf (accessed on 30 May 2025).

17. Bowlus, C. L., Arrivé, L., Bergquist, A., Deneau, M., Forman, L., Ilyas, S. I., Lunsford, K. E., *et. al.* (2022). AASLD practice guidance on primary sclerosing cholangitis and cholangiocarcinoma. *Hepatology, 77*, 659–702. https://doi.org/10.1002/hep.32771.

18. Brindley, P. J., Bachini, M., Ilyas, S. I., Khan, S. A., Loukas, A., Sirica, A. E., Teh, B. T., *et. al.* (2021). Cholangiocarcinoma. *Nature Reviews Disease Primers, 7*. https://doi.org/10.1038/s41572-021-00300-2.

19. Bulcha, J., Wang, Y., Ma, H., Tai, P. W. L., & Gao, G. (2021). Viral vector platforms within the gene therapy landscape. *Signal Transduction and Targeted Therapy, 6*(1). https://doi.org/10.1038/s41392-021-00487-6.

20. Cannavale, A., Catalano, C., Fanelli, F., Fiocca, R., *et. al.* (2016). Updated management of malignant biliary tract tumors: An illustrative review. https://core.ac.uk/download/98341455.pdf (accessed on 30 May 2025).

21. Caputo, D., Cimini, P., Coppola, A., Coppola, M., *et. al.* (2023). Advances in pre-treatment evaluation of pancreatic ductal adenocarcinoma: A narrative review. https://core.ac.uk/download/577160691.pdf (accessed on 30 May 2025).

22. Chehelgerdi, M., Chehelgerdi, M., Allela, O. Q. B., Pecho, R. D. C., Narayanan, J., Rao, D. P., Thamaraikani, T., *et. al.* (2023). Progressing nanotechnology to improve targeted cancer treatment: Overcoming hurdles in its clinical implementation. *Molecular Cancer, 22*. https://doi.org/10.1186/s12943-023-01865-0.

23. Cillo, U., Crimi, F., Mercante, I., Quaia, E., Tong, X. X., & Vernuccio, F. (2023). Biliary complications after liver transplantation: A computed tomography and magnetic resonance imaging pictorial review. https://core.ac.uk/download/614221091.pdf (accessed on 30 May 2025).

24. Cloyd, J. M., Ejaz, A., Konda, B., Makary, M. S., & Pawlik, T. M. (2020). Neuroendocrine liver metastases: A contemporary review of treatment strategies. *HepatoBiliary Surgery and Nutrition, 9*(4), 440–451. https://doi.org/10.21037/hbsn.2020.04.02.

25. Coco, D., & Leanza, S. (2023). IndoCyanine Green fluorescence guided resections in hepatobiliary surgery. https://core.ac.uk/download/613693828.pdf (accessed on 30 May 2025).

26. Deniz, S. (2024). Percutaneous transhepatic biliary drainage (PTBD) in patients with nondilated biliary system: Technical success, clinical outcomes and overall success. https://core.ac.uk/download/636730040.pdf (accessed on 30 May 2025).

27. Dennison, A., & Maddern, G. (2010). *Operative Solutions in Hepatobiliary and Pancreatic Surgery*. https://www.semanticscholar.org/paper/7757251f1fe1856c20006f8e0c1234ed838cd6cd (accessed on 30 May 2025).

28. Dumonceau, J. M., Tringali, A., Papanikolaou, I. S., Bléro, D., Mangiavillano, B., Schmidt, A., Vanbiervliet, G., *et. al.* (2018). Endoscopic biliary stenting: Indications, choice of stents, and results: European Society of Gastrointestinal Endoscopy (ESGE) Clinical Guideline–Updated October 2017. *Endoscopy, 50*(9), 910–930. https://doi.org/10.1055/a-0659-9864.

29. Elbanna, K. Y., & Kielar, A. Z. (2021). Computed tomography versus magnetic resonance imaging for hepatic lesion characterization/diagnosis. *Clinical Liver Disease, 17*(4), 159–164. https://doi.org/10.1002/cld.1089.

30. Frush, D. P., Callahan, M. J., Coley, B. D., Nadel, H., & Guillerman, R. P. (2023). Comparison of the different imaging modalities used to image pediatric oncology patients: A COG diagnostic imaging committee/SPR oncology committee white paper. *Pediatric Blood & Cancer, 70*(e30298). https://doi.org/10.1002/pbc.30298.

31. Galgano, S. J., Calderone, C., Xie, C. L., Smith, E. N., Porter, K. K., & McConathy, J. (2021). Applications of PET/MRI in abdominopelvic oncology. *Radiographic, 41*(6), 1750–1765. https://doi.org/10.1148/rg.2021210035.

32. Gatti, M., Maino, C., Tore, D., Carisio, A., Darvizeh, F., Tricarico, E., Inchingolo, R., *et. al.* (2022). Benign focal liver lesions: The role of magnetic resonance imaging. *World Journal of Hepatology, 14*(5), 923–943. https://doi.org/10.4254/wjh.v14.i5.923.

33. Gazelakis, K., Mendis, S., Wang, S., Wong, S., Lovett, G., & Valaydon, Z. (2021). Hepatobiliary and pancreatic: Liver lesions in cirrhosis: When to biopsy? *Journal of Gastroenterology and Hepatology, 37*(2), 283. https://www.semanticscholar.org/paper/146b003f5ae34cdc71d19abff7fad5f1b819551b (accessed on 30 May 2025).

34. Geboers, B., Timmer, F., Ruarus, A., Pouw, J. E. E., Schouten, E., Bakker, J., Puijk, R., *et. al.* (2021). Irreversible electroporation and nivolumab combined with intratumoral administration of a toll-like receptor ligand, as a means of *in vivo* vaccination for metastatic pancreatic ductal adenocarcinoma (PANFIRE-III): A phase-I study protocol. *Cancers, 13.* https://www.semanticscholar.org/paper/f315580c204d52f02ba8a75315567bba9898740e (accessed on 30 May 2025).

35. Ghaffar, W., & Batool, T. (2025). Comparison between magnetic resonance cholangiopancreatography and ultrasound for diagnosing patients with pancreatic tumor. *Insights-Journal of Health and Rehabilitation*. https://www.semanticscholar.org/paper/6a20735fe896a0fd7b45972a13d713a9831d5289 (accessed on 30 May 2025).

36. Gondal, M., Mushtaq Ch, S., Ahmad, I., Hussain, T., Awan, S., Fatima, K., Gondal, M., *et. al.* (2018). Accuracy of MRCP in comparison with ERCP for diagnosing hepato-pancreatic-biliary pathologies. https://core.ac.uk/download/553166222.pdf (accessed on 30 May 2025).

37. Goyal, S., Raju, R., & Yadav, S. (2012). Pancreatic pseudocyst of gastrohepatic ligament: A case report and review of management. https://core.ac.uk/download/619642468.pdf (accessed on 30 May 2025).

38. Grewal, M., Ahmed, T., & Javed, A. (2023). Current state of radiomics in hepatobiliary and pancreatic malignancies. *Artificial Intelligence Surgery*. https://www.semanticscholar.org/paper/7316b83056095f5f4b3ef3dc0e4ecb29ac521c08 (accessed on 30 May 2025).

39. Hecker, A., Kirkpatrick, A., Leppaniemi, A., Pikoulis, A., Mefire, A. C., De Simone, B., Sakakushev, B., *et. al.* (2019). Duodeno-pancreatic and extrahepatic biliary tree trauma: WSES-AAST guidelines. https://core.ac.uk/download/288798568.pdf (accessed on 30 May 2025).

40. Hilscher, M., Wells, M., Venkatesh, S. K., Cetta, F., & Kamath, P. S. (2022). Fontan-associated liver disease. *Hepatology, 75*(4), 1300–1321. https://doi.org/10.1002/hep.32406.

41. Ichikawa, S., & Goshima, S. (2023). Key CT and MRI findings of drug-associated hepatobiliary and

pancreatic disorders. *Japanese Journal of Radiology, 42*(3), 235–245. https://doi.org/10.1007/s11604-023-01505-z.

42. Jiang, J. H., Yang, D. W., Wang, Y. X., Dong, X., & Yang, Z. H. (2024). Application and prospects of magnetic resonance imaging techniques in the diagnosis and evaluation of hepatocellular carcinoma. *Zhonghua Gan Zang Bing Za Zhi = Zhonghua Ganzangbing Zazhi = Chinese Journal of Hepatology, 32*(8), 695–701. https://www.semanticscholar.org/paper/68ba02b90ed70deeac88a00e04985849752c6bd2 (accessed on 30 May 2025).

43. Kalmar, C. L., Gilmore, R. C., Taylor, J., & Makary, M. (2019). Frey procedure for chronic pancreatitis with situs inversus totals. *The American Surgeon, 85*(3), 392–393. https://www.semanticscholar.org/paper/199681aa27727a50b57978d8ce85bb0eeb256af3 (accessed on 30 May 2025).

44. Karlsen, T. H., Folseraas, T., Thorburn, D., & Vesterhus, M. (2017). Primary sclerosing cholangitis–a comprehensive review. *Journal of Hepatology, 67*(6), 1298–1323. https://doi.org/10.1016/j.jhep.2017.07.022.

45. Katabathina, V. S., Dasyam, A. K., Dasyam, N., & Hosseinzadeh, K. (2014). Adult bile duct strictures: Role of MR imaging and MR cholangiopancreatography in characterization. *Radiographic, 34*(3), 565–586. https://doi.org/10.1148/rg.343125211.

46. Katz, G., & Stone, J. H. (2021). Clinical perspectives on IgG4-related disease and its classification. *Annual Review of Medicine, 73*, 545–562. https://doi.org/10.1146/annurev-med-050219-034449.

47. KLCA Korean Liver Cancer Association, & NCC National Cancer Center. (2019). 2018 Korean Liver Cancer Association–National Cancer Center Korea practice guidelines for the management of hepatocellular carcinoma. *Gut and Liver, 13*(3), 227–299. https://doi.org/10.5009/gnl19024.

48. Koh, D. M., Kaste, S. C., Vinnicombe, S., Morana, G., Rossi, A., Herold, C., McLoud, T. C., *et. al.* (2016). Proceedings of the International Cancer Imaging Society (ICIS) 16th Annual Teaching Course. *Cancer Imaging, 16*(1). https://doi.org/10.1186/s40644-016-0079-z.

49. Kwon, R. S., & Simeone, D. M. (2011). The use of protein-based biomarkers for the diagnosis of cystic tumors of the pancreas. doi: 10.1155/2011/413646.

50. Lee, S. W., Shim, S., Jeong, S., & Kim, S. J. (2022). Comparison of preoperative imaging modalities for the assessment of malignant potential of pancreatic cystic lesions. *Clinical Nuclear Medicine, 47*(9), 849–855. https://www.semanticscholar.org/paper/6b14beb7768d3d038abbc244d7d5b52f8240bb38 (accessed on 30 May 2025).

51. Liu, J., & Mao, Z. (2023). Imaging findings of mucinous cystadenoma of cystic duct with biliary obstruction: A case report. *Radiology & Imaging Journal*. https://www.semanticscholar.org/paper/0435cff5118e8b9b37f1e8f4572f7bcda62e4f43 (accessed on 30 May 2025).

52. Löhr, M., Beuers, U., Vujasinović, M., Alvaro, D., Frøkjær, J. B., Buttgereit, F., Capurso, G., *et. al.* (2020). European guideline on IgG4-related digestive disease–UEG and SGF evidence-based recommendations. *United European Gastroenterology Journal, 8*(6), 637–666. https://doi.org/10.1177/2050640620934911.

53. Loper, M. R., & Makary, M. S. (2024). Evolving and novel applications of artificial intelligence in abdominal imaging. *Tomography, 10*, 1814–1831. https://www.semanticscholar.org/paper/aa7fa9ac802bd09be609b16171f0c97fa797a001 (accessed on 30 May 2025).

54. Moreau-Gaudry, A., Aus, C., Djavan, B., Epstein, H., Hodge, E., *et. al.* (2007). Prostate biopsies guided by three-dimensional real-time (4-D) transrectal ultrasonography on a phantom: Comparative study versus two-dimensional transrectal ultrasound-guided biopsies. *arXiv.* http://arxiv.org/abs/0712.0531 (accessed on 30 May 2025).

55. Nievelstein RA, Robben SG, Blickman JG. Hepatobiliary and pancreatic imaging in children-techniques and an overview of non-neoplastic disease entities. Pediatr Radiol. 2011 Jan;41(1):55-75. doi: 10.1007/s00247-010-1858-5.

56. Ohno, E., Kuzuya, T., Kawabe, N., Nakaoka, K., Tanaka, H., Nakano, T., Funasaka, K., *et. al.* (2024). Current status of endoscopic ultrasound in the diagnosis of intraductal papillary mucinous neoplasms. *DEN Open, 5*(1). https://www.semanticscholar.org/paper/f2d2b8fd3b6a302341a4f54af733e924cb3d661e (accessed on 30 May 2025).

57. Pati, S., Irfan, W., Jameel, A. T., Ahmed, S., & Shahid, R. (2023). Obesity and cancer: A current overview of epidemiology, pathogenesis, outcomes, and management. *Cancers, 15*(2), 485. https://doi.org/10.3390/cancers15020485.

58. Pelaz, B., Alexiou, C., Álvarez-Puebla, R. A., Alves, F., Andrews, A. M., Ashraf, S., Balogh, L., *et. al.* (2017). Diverse applications of nanomedicine. *ACS Nano, 11*, 2313–2381. https://doi.org/10.1021/acsnano.6b06040.

59. Podină, N., Gheorghe, E. C., Constantin, A., Cazacu, I., Croitoru, V., Gheorghe, C., Balaban, D., *et. al.* (2025). Artificial intelligence in pancreatic imaging: A systematic review. *United European Gastroenterology Journal, 13*, 55–77. https://www.semanticscholar.org/paper/ba90db863b28e1bb6b1b9576c8eaba98bbe0cf51 (accessed on 30 May 2025).

60. Rabiu, N. M., Muhammad, A. R., Umar, A. B., Donzomga, S. D., Garzali, I., Abba, S. M., & Ismail, A. (2025). Evaluation of hepatobiliary disorders using magnetic resonance cholangiopancreatography in a low-resource setting in Kano, Nigeria: A retrospective study. *BMC Gastroenterology, 25*. https://www.semanticscholar.org/paper/4b6edd8f644a49231822b633f9c0c211a55bc6e0 (accessed on 30 May 2025).

61. Sahai, A. V., Arya, N., Wyse, J. M., Jayaraman, S., Ball, C. G., Lam, E., Paquin, S. C., *et. al.* (2020). A proposal for the ideal algorithm for the diagnosis, staging, and treatment of pancreas masses suspicious for pancreatic adenocarcinoma: Results of a working group of the Canadian Society for Endoscopic Ultrasound. *Endoscopic Ultrasound, 9*, 154–154. https://doi.org/10.4103/eus.eus_28_20.

62. Sannajust, K., Palmisano, M. G., Whisenant, K., Slack, J., Holt, D., Woodrow, J. S., & Manzi, T. J. (2024). Computed tomographic diagnosis of a common bile duct abscess and secondary extrahepatic biliary duct obstruction in a potbelly pig. *Veterinary Radiology & Ultrasound.* https://www.semanticscholar.org/paper/1903fe268e9f7a7f6544757d23b09e76d8480966 (accessed on 30 May 2025).

63. Shaikh, S. (2022). Editorial for "Abbreviated Gadoxetic Acid-Enhanced MRI for the detection of liver metastases in patients with potentially respectable pancreatic ductal adenocarcinoma." *Journal of Magnetic Resonance Imaging, 56*. https://www.semanticscholar.org/paper/afcbf36b2246461e8c9ef829b7b03a6900b22581 (accessed on 30 May 2025).

64. Shimizu, N., Shiraishi, H., & Hanada, T. (2023). Zebrafish as a useful model system for human liver disease. *Cells, 12*(18), 2246. https://doi.org/10.3390/cells12182246.

65. Singh, Y., Andersen, J. B., Hathaway, Q. A., Venkatesh, S. K., Gores, G. J., & Erickson, B. J. (2025). Deep learning-based uncertainty quantification for quality assurance in hepatobiliary imaging-based techniques. *Oncotarget, 16*, 249–255. https://www.semanticscholar.org/paper/955b3f29c30d707e3f539fd427e2471b8c25782d (accessed on 30 May 2025).

66. Veenstra, E. (2023). Nuclear imaging and therapy: Towards a personalized approach in HCC and NET. https://core.ac.uk/download/581197670.pdf (accessed on 30 May 2025).

67. Vestby, L. K., Grønseth, T., Simm, R., & Nesse, L. L. (2020). Bacterial biofilm and its role in the pathogenesis of disease. *Antibiotics, 9*(2), 59. https://doi.org/10.3390/antibiotics9020059.

68. Wang, Y., Chen, W., Wang, J., Song, C., Zhang, L., & Zhang, X. (2025). The effects of moderate to high static magnetic fields on pancreatic damage. *Journal of Magnetic Resonance Imaging: JMRI*. https://www.semanticscholar.org/paper/fe9dd31fc0a76f24c614bdee761a2ec1c7324714 (accessed on 30 May 2025).

69. Zane, K. E., Cloyd, J. M., Mumtaz, K., Wadhwa, V., & Makary, M. S. (2021). Metastatic disease to the liver: Locoregional therapy strategies and outcomes. *World Journal of Clinical Oncology, 12*(9), 725–745. https://doi.org/10.5306/wjco.v12.i9.725.

70. Zhang, Y., Yang, G., Lei, P., & Zhang, D. (2022). Clinical application of 3D visualization technology in pancreatoduodenectomy. *Surgical Techniques Development*. https://www.semanticscholar.org/paper/aa2839d8b7b427072a9565204b231ebfefe5ef1e (accessed on 30 May 2025).

GENITOURINARY IMAGING

10

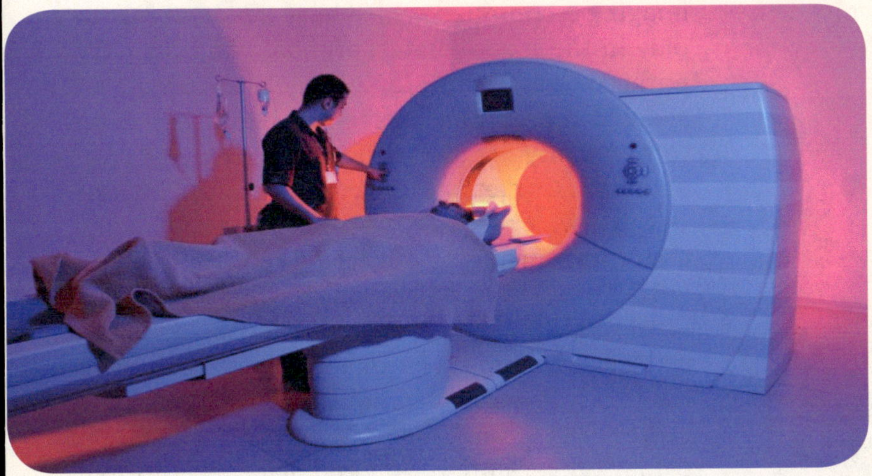

LEARNING OBJECTIVES

After studying this chapter, you will be able to:

1. Identify imaging modalities in genitourinary imaging
2. Explain clinical applications of genitourinary imaging
3. Focus on advances in genitourinary imaging technology
4. Describe challenges and limitations in genitourinary imaging

Introduction

Imaging technologies in medicine have greatly influenced therapeutic and diagnostic management across all major specialties, allowing high-resolution visualization of complex anatomical details and early detection of diseases. In particular, genitourinary imaging is significant in kidney, bladder, prostate, and reproductive organ diseases, where precision and image quality are key factors in determining patient outcomes. The combination of newer imaging techniques has enhanced the ability to noninvasively image physiological and pathologic changes in these systems and to gain significant information about conditions ranging from benign anomalies to malignancies. Continuing advances in technology and the integration of functional and structural information hold out significant promise for better diagnosis and targeted treatment planning. This chapter explores the state of genitourinary imaging, emphasizing new modalities and their clinical applications with a focus on the broader implications noted in the other areas of medical imaging research (Naranjo *et. al.*, 2024; Sarker *et. al.*, 2024).

Definition of Genitourinary Imaging

Advances in medical imaging have significantly enhanced diagnostic effectiveness in most specialties by making accurate visualization of anatomical features and pathologies. Genitourinary imaging in this context may be termed as specialized use of imaging modalities to assess the organs and systems involved in urinary and reproductive activity.

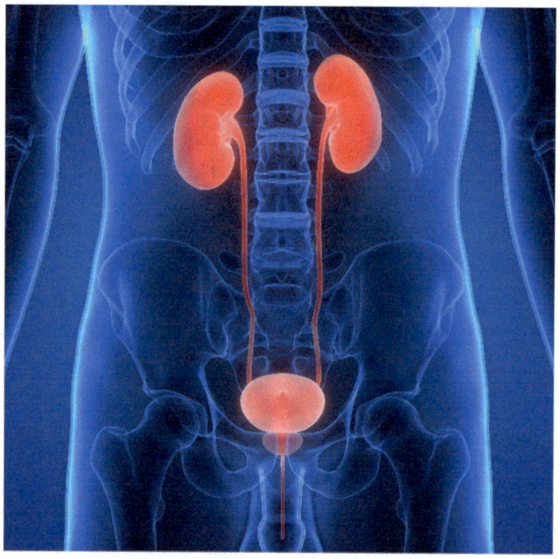

Figure 10.1. Genitourinary imaging.

Source: https://fonteva-customer-media.s3.amazonaws.com/00D20000000o6nVEAQ%2FosLMEqxB_GU+image.jpg.

It encompasses several modalities, including molecular imaging techniques like fluciclovine (18F) PET/CT, that have been more sensitive for the detection of recurrence of prostate cancer and the guidance of targeted therapies after prostatectomy (Jani *et. al.*, 2021). Other angiographic procedures also play a significant role in elucidating vascular abnormalities within the genitourinary tract, offering morphologic information required for diagnosis and treatment planning (Rösch, 1999). Thus, genitourinary imaging integrates various advanced techniques to provide thorough evaluation, which allows for informed therapeutic decision and maximization of patient outcomes in urologic oncology and related fields (Figure 10.1).

Importance of Imaging in Urology

Urological diagnosis and treatment planning have been significantly enhanced by advances in imaging techniques, which have a pivotal role to play in the management of most genitourinary pathologies. Technologies such as prostate-specific membrane antigen positron emission tomography (PSMA PET) have improved detection of metastatic prostate cancer lesions with low prostate-specific antigen levels, enabling earlier and more accurate staging with direct therapeutic implications (William *et. al.*, 2023). Furthermore, advancements in the conversion from traditional open techniques to minimally invasive techniques like robot-assisted radical cystectomy, facilitated by intracorporeal urinary diversion, have been achieved through the provision of meticulous preoperative imaging that reduces perioperative morbidity and improves patient outcomes (Mastroianni *et. al.*, 2022). These imaging modalities not only enhance the visualization of anatomical and pathological information but also allow for the integration of targeted therapies and customized treatment plans, demonstrating their essential role in urological practice today in the world of genitourinary imaging.

Historical Context of Genitourinary Imaging

Medical diagnosis has always widened the understanding and control of complex organ systems, and genitourinary imaging has been the foundation of this revolution. Early methods relied mainly on basic radiographic techniques that, while revolutionary for the time, were quite limited in detail and typically needed invasive processes to obtain acceptable information. Over time, the use of a greater depth of imaging technologies, including ultrasound, computed tomography (CT), and magnetic resonance imaging (MRI), maximized visualization of genitourinary anatomy, maximizing diagnostic sensitivity and patient outcomes. This expansion of technology was paralleled with the greater appreciation for the importance of precise infectious disease diagnosis in the genitourinary tract and the need for a reliable and accessible laboratory backup alongside imaging (Jm *et. al.*, 2024). More recently, the amalgamation of AI with imaging analysis is meant to further optimize treatment and diagnosis plans, testament to continued commitment to innovation in genitourinary care, combined with the necessity for careful consideration of ethical and legal implications (Karalis, 2024).

Current Trends in Imaging Technology

Advanced technology in imaging has significantly influenced genitourinary imaging, optimizing diagnosis and treatment planning. New technologies such as multiparametric MRI and emerging ultrasound methodologies allow physicians to see anatomical and functional details better, optimizing the detection of abnormalities at an earlier point. This is very applicable in prostate cancer, where tumor extent delineation plays a crucial role in therapeutic decision-making. Moreover, the union of AI and ML algorithms is beginning to revolutionize predictive modeling, especially in radiotherapy dosimetry. By analyzing complex datasets, these technologies permit more personalized treatment protocols, minimizing toxic side effects and maximizing clinical endpoints in patients (Ali *et. al.*, 2024). Although these advances have immense clinical potential, research and cross-disciplinary collaboration must continue to pursue ongoing to maximize their potential utility. Imaging modality development continues to propel genitourinary care in the future, an extension of a broader precision medicine movement (Burity *et. al.*, 2014) (Figure 10.2).

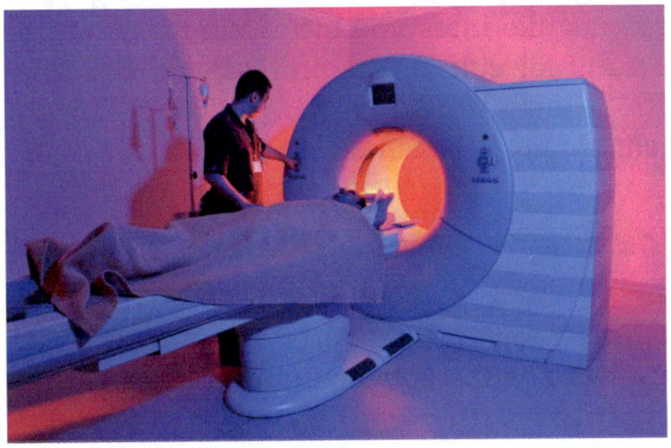

Figure 10.2. Multiparametric prostate MRI.

Source: https://thepelvicspecialists.co.uk/wp-content/uploads/2023/04/mri-scan-1024x680.jpg.

Target Audience for Genitourinary Imaging

Medical imaging technologies demand a clear understanding of the specific populations that are to be benefited most by the various means of diagnosis. Genitourinary imaging is primarily targeted towards those patients who come with symptoms of urinary and reproductive tract abnormalities, i.e., patients with hematuria, pelvic pain, or with suspected cancers. This is a wide clinical spectrum of audience ranging from young adults to elderly patients, including the patient with chronic diseases like inflammatory bowel disease that can potentially involve the adjacent genitourinary organs. Further, the healthcare professionals—urologists, radiologists, and general physicians—are another essential aspect of the target audience, requiring proper imaging protocols to enable maximum diagnosis and treatment. The incorporation of culturally tailored, individualized strategies into imaging practice has the possibility of enhancing patient engagement and diagnostic yield, commensurate with results highlighting the importance of culturally tailored content in promoting response and meaning for diverse groups (St Aöckl *et. al.*, 2025). Alongside this, shifting adoption patterns and learning needs in areas like intestinal ultrasound indicate the demand for continuous professional education to maximize the use of genitourinary imaging technologies (Bilican *et. al.*, 2025).

Challenges in Genitourinary Imaging

Diagnosis and appropriate treatment of genitourinary disease rely significantly on advanced imaging technologies, but these modalities suffer from challenges, rendering clinical decision-making increasingly complicated.

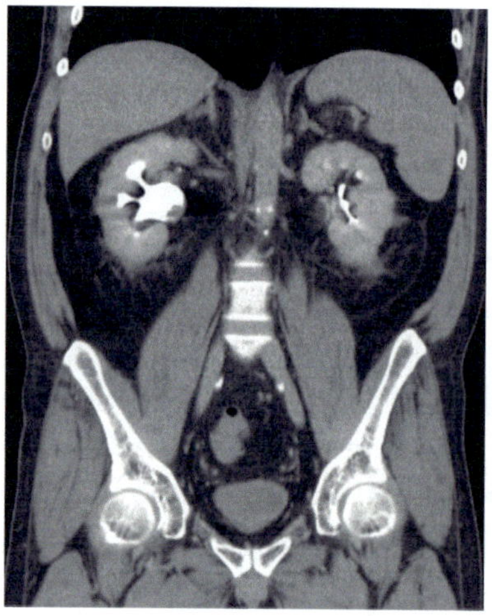

Figure 10.3. Neoplastic processes in the genitourinary tract.

Source: https://media.springernature.com/full/springer-static/image/art%3A10.1038%2Fnrurol.2016.252/MediaObjects/41585_2017_Article_BFnrurol2016252_Fig1_HTML.jpg.

It is frequently difficult to distinguish between infectious, inflammatory, and neoplastic genitourinary tract conditions since atypical presentations—such as rare parasitic infections mimicking common bacterial epididymo-orchitis—may be overlooked in the first diagnosis and need multidisciplinary processes to confirm and treat (Donoso *et. al.*, 2025). Apart from this, radiation therapy for prostate cancer is also faced with significant imaging analysis challenges and toxicity prediction because of dose parameters variability that requires precise measurement to avoid detrimental effects on surrounding structures such as the bladder and rectum (Ali *et. al.*, 2024). Integration of new technologies, such as AI, is possible in enhancing predictive power and individualizing treatment planning. Nevertheless, overcoming the inherent anatomical heterogeneity and complexity of pathological appearances is a major challenge to optimizing genitourinary imaging performance and promoting improved patient outcomes (Figure 10.3).

Future Directions in the Field

Technological innovations and interdisciplinary cooperative efforts are poised to revolutionize genitourinary imaging in the next few years. Emerging imaging modalities, such as molecular and functional imaging, are poised to provide more accurate diagnosis and focused treatment planning, particularly in oncology. Integration with artificial intelligence algorithms may also facilitate faster image interpretation and predictive analysis, leading to improved patient outcomes. The growth in research activity worldwide, as seen in other medical specialties facing urgent health challenges, underscores the need for targeted investment and innovation in genitourinary imaging to address unmet clinical needs (Ahmed *et. al.*, 2018). Similarly, of critical importance will be knowledge transfer across specialties like radiology, urology, and pathology to maximize imaging protocols and develop novel contrast agents targeted to genitourinary disease. Although the research scholarship of experienced investigators from a range of disciplines has enriched adjacent fields (Burity *et. al.*, 2014), targeted research programs are still essential to advance genitourinary imaging to a novel future of precision medicine.

10.1. Imaging Modalities in Genitourinary Imaging

Learning Outcome

1. Understand ultrasound in genitourinary imaging
2. Explain computed tomography (CT) scans
3. Define magnetic resonance imaging (MRI)
4. Discuss x-rays and their applications
5. Focus on nuclear medicine techniques
6. Identify fluoroscopy in urological procedures
7. Give comparison of imaging modalities
8. Know advantages and disadvantages of each modality
9. Explain role of imaging in diagnosis and treatment planning

Advances in imaging technology have significantly enhanced diagnostic accuracy and clinical management of genitourinary conditions. Among these, hybrid technologies such as positron emission tomography and magnetic resonance imaging (PET/MR) yield multi-modal insights by integrating metabolic and anatomical information. This integration is particularly valuable in the detection of pelvic nodal metastases, evaluation of prostate, endometrial, and cervical cancers, and radiation therapy planning. PET/MR excels over conventional single-modality imaging due to increased resolution and functional data, allowing for precise metastasis identification and response to treatment. Furthermore, the development of ML techniques, such as Vision Transformers augmented by new patching methods, has the promise of extending biomedical image analysis by acquiring complex spatial relationships beyond conventional convolutional neural networks. All of these technological developments contribute to enhanced, personalized patient care in genitourinary imaging part of a trend toward multimodal and AI-driven diagnostic approaches that enhance sensitivity and specificity in clinical practice (Habib *et. al.*, 2025; Kohan *et. al.*, 2024).

10.1.1. Ultrasound in Genitourinary Imaging

Advances in medical imaging have significantly improved diagnosis and treatment of genitourinary disease, and ultrasound has been an extremely valuable tool among them. It is non-invasive, does not involve ionizing radiation, and produces real-time images; hence, it is ideal for evaluating the kidneys, bladder, prostate, and reproductive organs. Ultrasound has excellent ability to detect abnormalities such as cysts, tumors, stones, and obstructions in the urinary tract, which are critical for making clinical decisions.

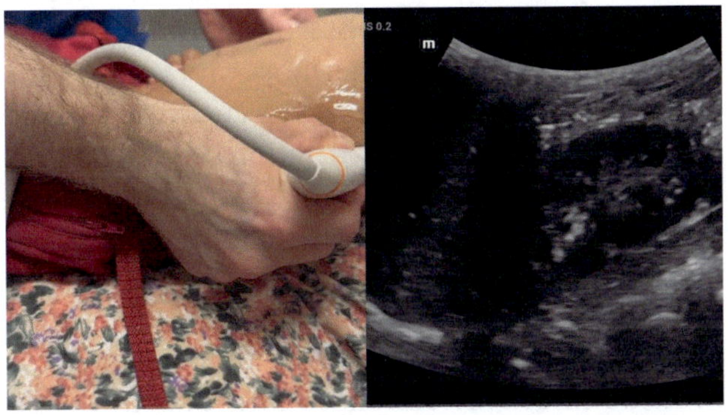

Figure 10.4. Ultrasound in genitourinary imaging.

Source: https://i.ytimg.com/vi/q4JaObHVkLk/maxresdefault.jpg.

In addition, Doppler ultrasound improves assessment by visualizing blood flow, which is vital in the identification of vascular issues or tumor vascularity. Despite its operator variability and less penetration in the obese, ultrasound remains a first-line modality for most genitourinary pathology due to its availability and cost-effectiveness. Subsequent research emphasizes its evolving function, such as adding enhanced contrast methods to more clearly delineate lesions and function, emphasizing its expanding use in this field (Burity *et. al.*, 2014). This merging of improved ultrasound techniques further maximizes the precision of genitourinary imaging (Figure 10.4).

10.1.2. Computed Tomography (CT) Scans

Advances in medical imaging have significantly enhanced the diagnosis and management of genitourinary conditions, and one of the key tools in this field has become the CT scan. CT scans produce high-resolution cross-sectional images that allow for detailed visualization of the kidneys, bladder, ureters, and surrounding structures, which are indispensable for accurate disease characterization and treatment planning. Its ability to separate tissue densities makes tumor, infection, and obstructive pathologies readily identifiable. Furthermore, the application of sophisticated algebraic reconstruction techniques such as total variation regularization and compressed sensing has improved the quality of images and speeded up scans, overcoming noise and artifacts problems that have been long-standing obstacles to diagnostic accuracy (Jessica, 2024). This technological evolution not only enhances clinical confidence but also broadens access in resource-limited settings. Additionally, the combination of CT imaging with novel deep learning methods holds the promise of refining tumor detection and staging and thereby optimizing treatment within genitourinary oncology (Sundar *et. al.*, 2024).

10.1.3. Magnetic Resonance Imaging (MRI)

Advances in imaging technology have significantly enhanced prenatal diagnosis, and by extension, the detection of congenital genitourinary system anomalies. MRI has become a valuable complement to ultrasonography (US), particularly in cases where oligohydramnios compromises the effectiveness of ultrasound. It's improved contrast for soft tissue makes fetal anatomy easier to view in detail, yielding significant information that boosts diagnostic accuracy and aids clinical decision-making for postnatal care. For example, MRI has been highly accurate in the diagnosis of conditions like ventriculomegaly but may be less so for cerebral hemorrhage and cortical malformations, thus depicting both its use and limitation in prenatal evaluation (Oudah *et. al.*, 2023). Besides, novel noninvasive MRI techniques promise wider uses by adding data on fluid dynamics and tissue properties, potentially extending diagnostic capabilities to functional testing rather than structural imaging, eventually enhancing understanding of developmental pathologies in the genitourinary and adjacent systems (Kamagata *et. al.*, 2023) (Figure 10.5).

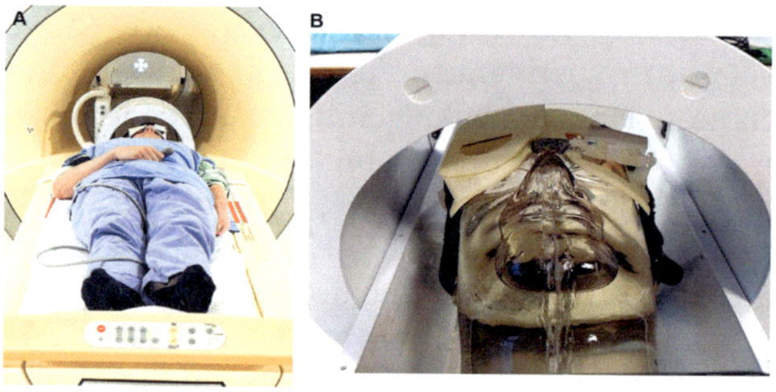

Figure 10.5. Magnetic Resonance Imaging (MRI) has emerged as a vital complement to ultrasonography, especially when factors such as oligohydramnios limit ultrasound effectiveness.

Source: https://www.researchgate.net/publication/340960526/figure/fig1/AS:11431281256584379@1719547713738/A-Setup-for-high-resolution-ocular-magnetic-resonance-MR-imaging-consisting-of-a.jpg.

10.1.4. X-Rays and Their Applications

Medical imaging technologies have revolutionized diagnostic practice in urology, particularly with the applications of X-rays, which remain a cornerstone technology in genitourinary imaging.

The unique ability of X-rays to penetrate body tissues and generate detailed images of internal structures makes it simple to evaluate renal calculi, urinary obstructions, and anatomical abnormalities. Techniques such as intravenous urography and retrograde pyelography utilize contrast-enhanced X-rays to accurately visualize the urinary tract, allowing for early diagnosis and treatment planning. Continuing innovation has also improved image resolution and reduced exposure to radiation, ensuring maximum patient safety and diagnostic performance. Moreover, the integration of digital radiography systems has improved image acquisition and storage speed, making clinical workflow more efficient. These developments underscore the ongoing importance of X-ray technology in genitourinary imaging and attest to its critical role in the diagnosis and treatment of a variety of urinary maladies.

10.1.5. Nuclear Medicine Techniques

Advances in imaging modalities have considerably expanded the scope of the potential for diagnosis of genitourinary disorders, and nuclear medicine techniques are at the forefront. Nuclear medicine techniques, such as renal scintigraphy and positron emission tomography (PET), provide functional and physiological data that complement structural imaging. Through the use of radiotracers selectively targeted to renal function or genitourinary cancer, nuclear medicine provides for the precise assessment of renal perfusion, glomerular filtration, and malignancy detection at the earliest stage. Such functional data is crucial in treatment planning and follow-up of therapeutic response, particularly in complex scenarios where conventional imaging is inadequate. In addition, integration of hypofractionated radiotherapy schedules according to evidence from nuclear imaging is also being tested, a sign of ongoing clinical refinement to maximize therapeutic benefit while minimizing toxicity in the treatment of prostate cancer (Chen *et al.*, 2019). Recent improvements in imaging resolution and tracer specificity also promise further enhancements to the application of nuclear medicine in genitourinary imaging, as illustrated by recent studies and novel strategies (Figure 10.6).

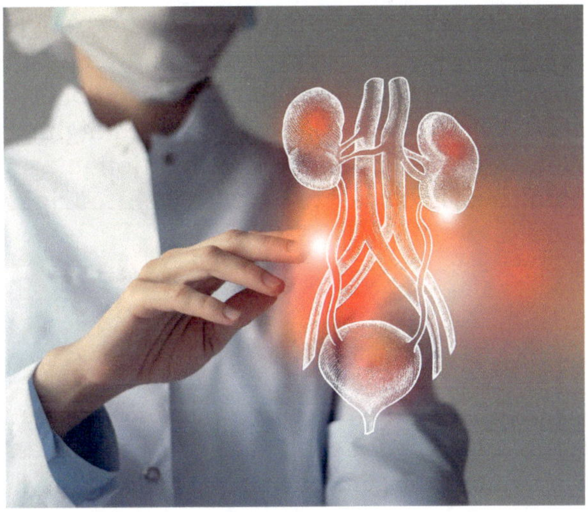

Figure 10.6. Genitourinary tumors.

Source: https://www.clevelandclinicabudhabi.ae/cancercenter/-/media/images/oncology/about-img/gu-cancer-program.jpg?h=1100&w=1260&la=en&hash=0F519903AF0F0F601C59203759281A79

10.1.6. Fluoroscopy in Urological Procedures

Innovations in imaging techniques have revolutionized urological therapeutics and diagnosis, greatly benefiting patients. Among these, fluoroscopy plays a critical role in real-time imaging for numerous urological procedures, such as retrograde pyelography, ureteral stenting, and percutaneous nephrolithotomy. Fluoroscopy's dynamic imaging capability facilitates accurate tool guidance and real-time assessment of anatomical structures, thereby enhancing the accuracy of procedures. But, fluoroscopy does expose patients to ionizing radiation, the precise management of which requires control in terms of dose and patient protection. Current practice emphasizes balancing the clinical benefits of fluoroscopy against minimizing radiation exposure, in line with principles of justification and optimization of medical imaging (Ferrero *et. al.*, 2019). Moreover, recent advances such as nanotechnology also promise greater imaging specificity and better therapeutic targeting in urology, which may serve as a complement to fluoroscopic procedures in the future (Bhat *et. al.*, 2016). Collectively, these advances highlight the need for integrating new generation imaging modalities in order to further genitourinary care.

10.1.7. Comparison of Imaging Modalities

Advancements in imaging technologies have significantly enhanced the diagnosis and management of genitourinary cancers, but the modality selection typically depends on certain clinical scenarios. In prostate cancer treatment, for instance, external beam radiation therapy (EBRT) based on conventional or moderately hypofractionated schedules is controversial among experts regarding whether to use traditional or moderately hypofractionated external beam radiation therapy, depending on different interpretations of efficacy and toxicity trials (Chen *et. al.*, 2019). Additionally, bladder cancer diagnosis is usually initiated with cystoscopy, even though the technique is restricted in its ability to find carcinoma in situ along with differentiating benign from malignant masses. Both CT and MRI serve complementary roles in the staging process, where CT urography contributes to diagnosis, and MRI differentiates between muscle-invasive and non-muscle-invasive disease, despite their sensitivity for nodal disease being less than ideal (Halpern *et. al.*, 2018). PET with CT or MRI offers better nodal staging and tissue characterization, yet no imaging modality alone thoroughly addresses all the staging and diagnostic problems, so there is a requirement for future development of targeted and multimodal methodologies (Halpern *et. al.*, 2018) (Figure 10.7).

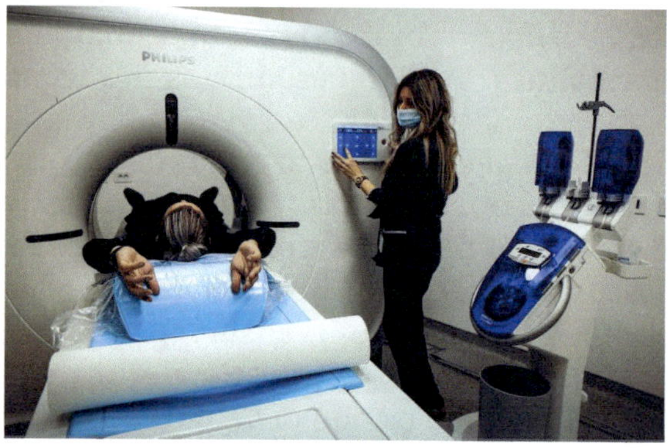

Figure 10.7. CT urography.

Source: https://pulskardioloskicentar.rs/wp-content/uploads/2021/04/Sta-je-CT-urografija-i-kako-vam-moze-pomoci.jpg.

10.1.8. Advantages and Disadvantages of Each Modality

In the imaging of genitourinary disease, each imaging modality has inherent strengths and limitations that influence diagnostic accuracy and clinical management. Ultrasound offers non-invasive, radiation-free imaging with excellent initial evaluation capability but lacks precise tissue characterization. CT is excellent in anatomical detail and most commonly applied for primary staging and diagnosis, but it exposes patients to ionizing radiation and often cannot distinguish between the earliest stages of the tumor, such as T1 and T2 bladder cancer (Halpern *et. al.*, 2018). MRI offers better soft tissue contrast and differentiation of muscle-invasive bladder carcinoma, but costliness and limited availability restrict widespread use. PET in combination with CT or MRI, boosts nodal staging and metabolism but adds complexity and additional expenses (Halpern *et. al.*, 2018). In addition, the incorporation of smoothing filters in the processing of image data, such as median and Savitzky-Golay filters, allows for improved image clarity in diagnosis but is yet to be optimized to effectively reduce artifacts.

10.1.9. Role of Imaging in Diagnosis and Treatment Planning

Medical technology progress has revolutionized the potential for accurate detection and assessment of genitourinary disease, for decisively improved outcomes. Imaging technologies such as ultrasound, CT, and MRI offer high-resolution visualization of anatomy and pathologic changes, allowing precise diagnosis. These technologies enable the early identification of malignancies, urinary tract obstructions, and inflammatory disorders, which are crucial in developing individualized treatments. Moreover, imaging aids treatment planning by guiding minimally invasive surgery and therapy, enhancing therapeutic precision and preventing complications. It also enables real-time assessment of disease progression and treatment response. Integration of recent imaging technologies into clinical practice is therefore indispensable for maximizing patient care in genitourinary medicine, necessitating continued technological innovation and multilogical cooperation (Burity *et. al.*, 2014).

Test Your Knowledge

1. What is the primary imaging modality for the initial evaluation of renal stones?
2. How does ultrasound help in assessing renal function and detecting structural abnormalities in the kidneys?

10.2. Clinical Applications of Genitourinary Imaging

Learning Outcome

1. Explain imaging for kidney diseases
2. Identify prostate imaging techniques
3. Discuss bladder imaging and assessment
4. Focus on imaging in urinary tract infections (UTIs)
5. Perform evaluation of testicular conditions
6. Discuss imaging for renal tumors
7 Describe role of imaging in trauma cases
8. Learn imaging in congenital anomalies
9. Understand follow-up imaging protocols

Advances in imaging technology have significantly enhanced the diagnostic and management approaches in genitourinary medicine. Imaging modalities such as ultrasound, CT, and MRI enable precise visualization of the kidneys, bladder, prostate, and surrounding structures, enabling early detection of pathology and precise characterization of lesions. For example, multiparametric MRI has become a standard tool in the evaluation of prostate cancer, improving the precision of tumor localization and staging, an issue with direct implication in treatment planning. In addition, imaging plays an important role in the management of urinary tract infections (UTIs), congenital anomalies, and trauma by allowing noninvasive measurement and monitoring. These uses not only allow interventions to be initiated early, but also reduce the need for exploratory studies, hence minimizing patient risk. The use of genitourinary imaging is a demonstration of how technology leads to improved patient outcomes as well as personalized approaches to care (Burity *et. al.*, 2014).

10.2.1. Imaging for Kidney Diseases

Advanced imaging techniques have revolutionized the diagnostic pathway for kidney disorders. Among them, convolutional neural networks (CNNs) have been found to possess remarkable potential in differentiating kidney pathologies such as cysts, tumors, and stones, by scanning CTs with remarkable accuracy. EfficientNetB3, in particular, demonstrated greater than 90% accuracy over other CNN architectures and indicated the power of deep learning in substantiating diagnostic certainty and patient outcomes (Kaushik *et. al.*, 2024). Augmenting this, new techniques based on a combination of residual networks and LSTM models have been utilized in iris image analysis, a new non-invasive biomarker for kidney disease detection. This method achieved an incredible 95% classification accuracy, pointing to a convergence of image processing and ML in facilitating painless, real-time early diagnoses (Priya *et. al.*, 2024). Each of these steps in combination points to growing impetus from advanced imaging modalities in facilitating better clinical management of kidney disorders (Figure 10.8).

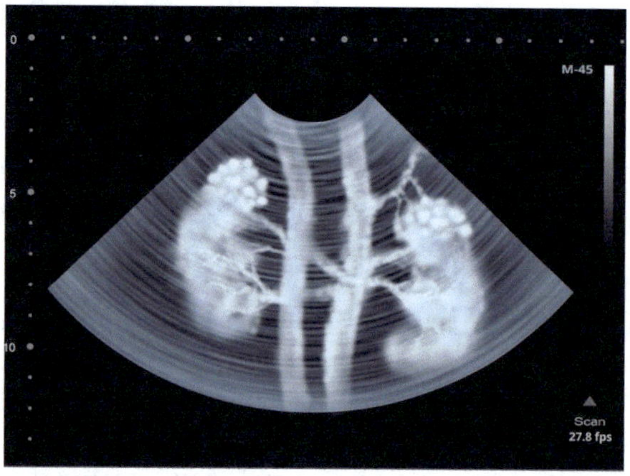

Figure 10.8. Imaging for kidney diseases.

Source: https://media.post.rvohealth.io/wp-content/uploads/2020/08/renal-scan_thumb.jpg.

10.2.2. Prostate Imaging Techniques

Technological advances in imaging modalities have revolutionized the diagnostic landscape of prostate cancer, offering improved accuracy and efficacy in detection and characterization. Among the newer modalities, positron emission tomography/magnetic resonance imaging (PET/MR) stands out in that it has the potential to provide metabolic as well as anatomical information simultaneously, enabling improved detection of pelvic nodal metastases and improved planning of radiation therapy with greater accuracy (Kohan *et. al.*, 2024). To this end, nonlinear microscopy (NLM) is a new fluorescence-based technology that has the ability to perform rapid, high-resolution imaging of newly biopsied prostate samples with near-histopathology-matching resolution at a fraction of the evaluation time of conventional histopathology. NLM not only provides real-time evaluation during biopsies but also high diagnostic sensitivity and specificity in carcinoma detection and identification, with the potential for improved patient management and reduced anxiety (Lucas *et. al.*, 2021). Together, these advances mark a shift toward more complete and faster prostate imaging modalities in genitourinary oncology that promise enhanced diagnostic pathways and customized treatments.

10.2.3. Bladder Imaging and Assessment

Medical imaging has significantly enhanced the evaluation of organ function, and less invasive alternatives are now available for traditional diagnostic methods. For bladder imaging and assessment, ultrasound has been shown to be a valuable adjunct to invasive urodynamics—traditionally the diagnostic gold standard for functional bladder disease. Ultrasound techniques, such as 2D and 3D modalities, allow real-time evaluation of bladder volume, wall thickness, compliance, and biomechanical properties during filling. These imaging modalities bypass patient discomfort and procedural distortions inherent to catheterization, providing a better physiologic examination milieu. While promising results are present, further investigation is required to validate these ultrasound uses prior to their incorporation in daily practice. This shift is an indication of trends throughout other imaging practices where noninvasive modalities augment gold-standard tests with greater frequency, indicating the evolving nature of diagnostic practice in genitourinary therapy (McCormack *et. al.*, 2024). Although the quoted cardiac imaging survey focuses on modality selection and its integration in clinical practice (Soliman-Aboumarie *et. al.*, 2022), its applicability to future development of imaging technology remains pertinent (Figure 10.9).

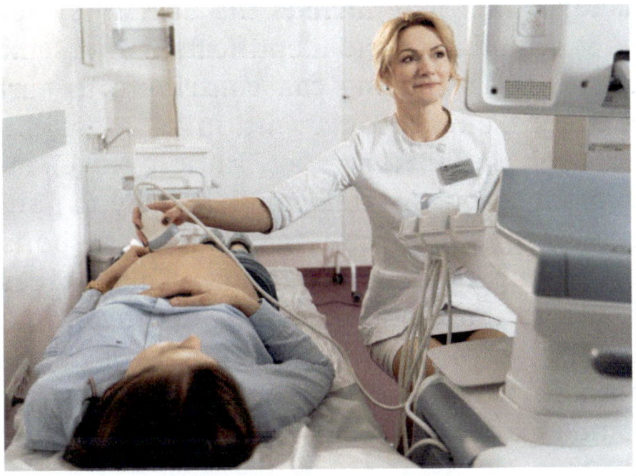

Figure 10.9. Bladder imaging and assessment.

Source: https://phoenix-ultrasound.co.uk/wp-content/uploads/2023/06/A-Comprehensive-Guide-to-Kidneys-Ureters-and-Bladder-KUB-Imaging2-1024x768.png.

10.2.4. Imaging in Urinary Tract Infections (UTIs)

Accurate diagnosis of UTIs often entails imaging to assess complications or atypical presentation. While uncomplicated UTIs can typically be diagnosed clinically, imaging is important in the diagnosis of underlying pathology such as obstruction, abscess, or renal infection. Ultrasound is frequently employed due to its accessibility and safety profile, and it allows visualization of renal size, parenchymal changes, or foreign bodies that predispose to infection, such as intravesical objects, where bedside ultrasound played an important role in differential diagnosis (Hajiran *et. al.*, 2013). In complex or chronic infections, particularly those with suspected tuberculosis (TB) involvement, high-end imaging modalities like CT provide accurate information regarding anatomical distortion and functional compromise, leading to early intervention to prevent irreversible renal damage (Aguirre-Avalos *et. al.*, 2018). Imaging, therefore, serves not only as an adjunct to diagnosis but also as a therapeutic management guide in UTIs within the broader context of genitourinary imaging.

10.2.5. Evaluation of Testicular Conditions

Accurate diagnosis of testicular pathology is crucial for proper management and improved patient outcomes, making genitourinary imaging an important component of the assessment. Imaging techniques such as ultrasound with its high resolution and real-time capability are the initial imaging modality of choice for detecting abnormalities such as tumors, torsion, and infection. In addition to morphological assessment, advanced molecular awareness has pushed the adoption of targeted treatments with a focus on the significance of complete characterization of tumors to guide treatment strategies (Anand *et. al.*, 2022).

Furthermore, evaluation is conducted at the functional level, including sperm DNA integrity necessary for fertility assessment. Although sperm DNA fragmentation testing remains controversial and not within the routine clinical practice, it provides informative data on testicular pathology-associated sperm quality, particularly in the case of idiopathic infertility (Agarwal *et. al.*, 2020). Therefore, an integrated approach with structural and molecular assessment by genitourinary imaging and ancillary tests enhances diagnostic accuracy and treatment planning in testicular pathologies (Figure 10.10).

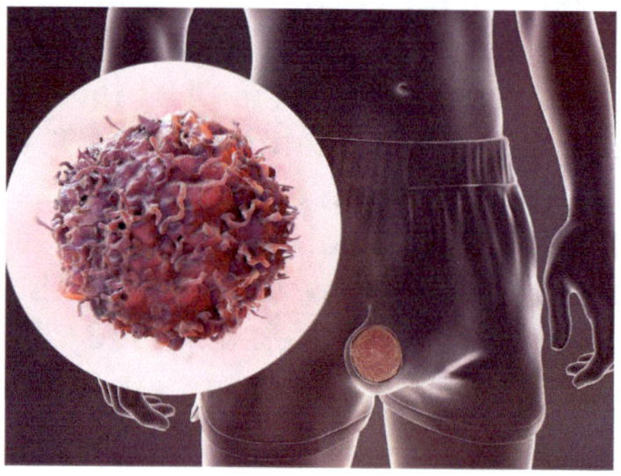

Figure 10.10. Evaluating testicular cancer.

Source: https://urodoc.sg/wp-content/uploads/2023/10/testicular-cancer-1.jpg.

10.2.6. Imaging for Renal Tumors

Technologic innovations have played a significant role in the diagnostic accuracy and management of renal tumors within the broader genitourinary imaging framework. New modalities such as CT and MRI provide accurate anatomical and functional information to enable accurate tumor localization, characterization, and staging. Contrast-enhanced imaging is critically important in distinguishing benign from malignant lesions, assessing tumor vascularity, and determining involvement of adjacent structures. Furthermore, new techniques that include molecular diagnostics and next-generation sequencing (NGS) enable a more personalized approach for cancer detection and prognosis, signifying the move towards personalized medicine in uro-oncology (Cimadamore *et. al.*, 2020). Although traditional imaging remains the cornerstone of initial evaluation, research goes on to highlight the role of advanced imaging biomarkers to maximize results. These advancements point toward an age where renal tumor imaging is more predictive and precise, underlining its pivotal role in ideal clinical decision-making (Burity *et. al.*, 2014).

10.2.7. Role of Imaging in Trauma Cases

In genitourinary trauma, early and accurate evaluation is of prime importance in prevention of long-term sequelae such as erectile dysfunction and organ loss. Imaging modalities are of pivotal significance in defining the extent of injury, both as a guide to management and diagnosis. Penile duplex Doppler EUS, for example, is critical to differentiate ischemic from non-ischemic priapism following trauma, the differentiation having dramatic implications for management schemes (Trinity *et. al.*, 2021). CT scanning is also beneficial in assessing intricate pelvic fractures that may include the urinary system and vasculature. Rapid identification of vascular injuries with imaging can contribute to early treatment and the prevention of morbidity. Although laboratory and radiologic exams augment diagnosis, imaging is the key to guide surgical planning and therapeutic response monitoring in urologic injury. This process of integration emphasizes the significant role imaging plays in the optimization of patient care and prognostication among genitourinary trauma patients (Nigel *et. al.*, 2019) (Figure 10.11).

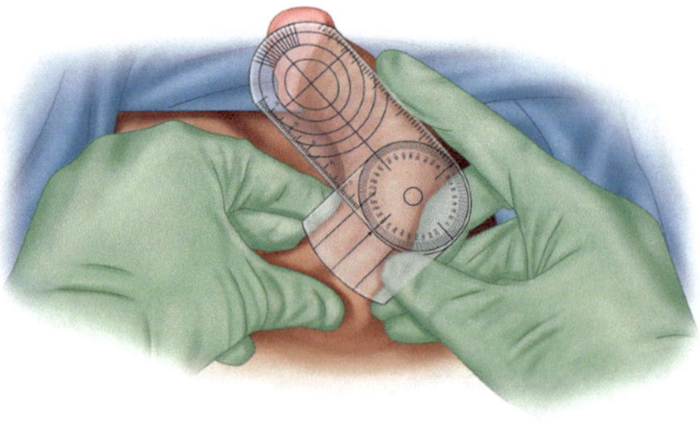

Figure 10.11. Penile duplex doppler ultrasonography.

Source: https://media.springernature.com/lw685/springer-static/image/chp%3A10.1007%2F978-3-030-52309-1_7/MediaObjects/145750_3_En_7_Fig23_HTML.png.

10.2.8. Imaging in Congenital Anomalies

Advances in technology have significantly transformed the diagnostic image of congenital malformations in the genitourinary system to provide earlier and more precise detection, ultimately to direct better management. Fetal MRI is among the new technologies, functioning as a valuable adjunct to routine ultrasound, since it provides better visualization of complex malformations that otherwise would be difficult to delineate. This non-invasive imaging method complements sonography with enhanced soft tissue contrast and multi-planar imaging, to facilitate more accurate assessment of abnormalities such as urinary tract obstruction, renal dysplasia, and extrarenal malformations. Of note, fetal MRI also increases the ability of clinicians to offer informed counseling to parents regarding prognosis and treatment options, which equates to more informed decision-making. Also, the integration of imaging findings with clinical information encourages comprehensive prenatal care, resonating with the critical necessity for interprofessional collaboration in the care of congenital genitourinary anomalies (Baldacchino *et. al.*, 2016). Such evolution is consonant with broader intellectual undertakings within the medical fraternity, with much emphasis on the necessity of further research and education (Burity *et. al.*, 2014).

10.2.9. Follow-up Imaging Protocols

Careful follow-through of standardized protocols is required to ensure repeatable and reproducible imaging results during follow-up exams so as not to overlook subtle morphologic changes, which may happen in genitourinary imaging. Morphologic changes may be subtle, but they can be clinically significant. Image acquisition parameters and reconstruction algorithms may vary between scanners and can restrict diagnostic performance and longitudinal correlation. Therefore, audits and protocol reviews become essential at regular intervals to maintain image quality without compromising radiation safety principles like ALARA. Incorporation of novel technologies like iterative reconstruction and deep learning has seemed to enhance image clarity and reduce the amount of radiation dose, thereby maximizing patient safety in serial follow-up (Mikkelsen *et. al.*, 2025). Further, use of AI in follow-up imaging also holds promise for disease progression assessment automation, reduction of inter-reader variability, and speeding up analysis—albeit with further refinement being needed before its widespread use in clinical practice (Nagy *et. al.*, 2024). Thus, well-defined and systematically evaluated follow-up imaging protocols are crucial to successful management of genitourinary disorders (Figure 10.12).

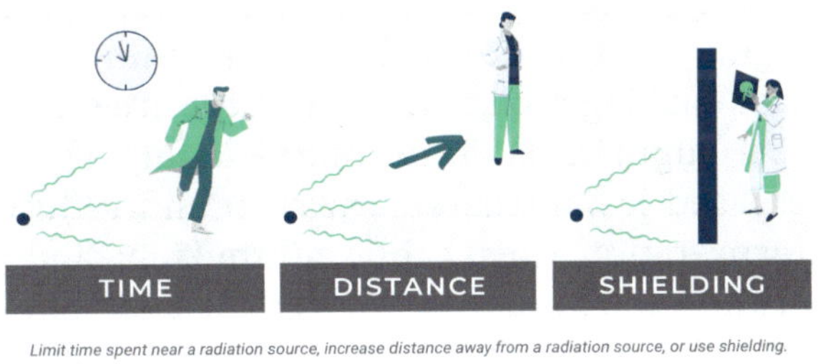

Figure 10.12. Routine audits and protocol reviews are essential to maintain image quality while adhering to radiation safety principles such as ALARA.

Source: https://versantphysics.com/wp-content/uploads/2021/03/Time-Distance-Shielding7.png.

Test Your Knowledge

1. In what cases is CT urography used in the work-up of hematuria, and what findings are indicative of malignancy?
2. What role does Doppler ultrasound play in assessing renal artery stenosis and hypertension?

10.3. Advances in Genitourinary Imaging Technology

Learning Outcome

1. Learn innovations in ultrasound technology
2. Discuss developments in CT imaging
3. Focus on MRI advancements and their implications
4. Describe artificial intelligence in imaging
5. Identify 3D imaging techniques
6. Learn contrast agents and their evolution
7. Define telemedicine and remote imaging
8. Discuss integration of imaging with other diagnostic tools
9. Explain future technologies on the horizon

Advancements in technology in recent years have greatly enhanced the diagnostic yield and accuracy of genitourinary imaging, with earlier detection and improved management of urological diseases. Of these advancements, multiparametric MRI has emerged as a critical modality, offering high-resolution soft tissue imaging and functional assessment without the use of ionizing radiation. Conversely, integration of AI algorithms into image analysis has increased lesion characterization and reduced interpretation times, thus optimizing clinical workflows. The advent of contrast-enhanced ultrasound also enhances traditional modalities in the sense that it offers dynamic evaluation of vascularity of renal and bladder pathologies. The technology not only allows individualized treatment of patients but also contributes to less invasive diagnostic techniques. Additionally, research on hybrid imaging techniques that combine anatomical and molecular information is still promising a revolution through optimal specificity and sensitivity in tumor detection. This development is a revolutionary era in genitourinary imaging that is both technologically sophisticated and clinically relevant (Burity *et. al.*, 2014).

10.3.1. Innovations in Ultrasound Technology

Technological advances in medical imaging have significantly enhanced the diagnosis of genitourinary diseases, particularly with ultrasound imaging. New technology has been accompanied by higher resolution imaging and three-dimensional reconstructions that allow improved visualization of anatomical structures and pathologic changes in the kidneys, bladder, and reproductive organs. The inclusion of contrast-enhanced ultrasound techniques has also allowed for improved differentiation between benign and malignant lesions; therefore, there is minimal need for invasive intervention.

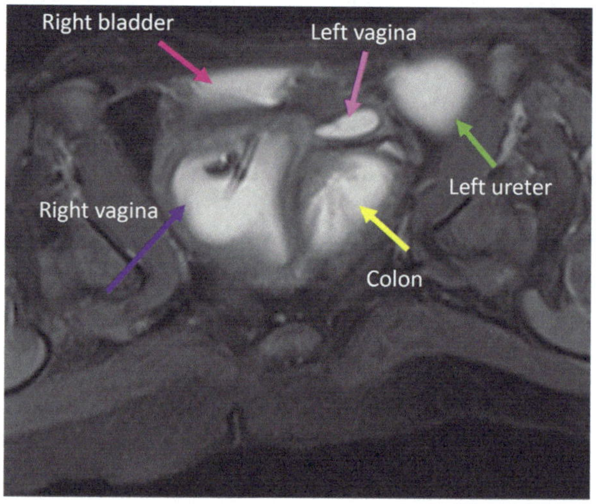

Figure 10.13. Recent innovations have introduced higher-resolution imaging and three-dimensional reconstructions, allowing for more precise visualization of anatomical structures and pathological changes within the kidneys, bladder, and reproductive organs.

Source: https://www.goldjournal.net/cms/10.1016/j.urology.2022.12.024/asset/f390edca-2b96-44bc-beb9-c66d56442ee4/main.assets/gr1_lrg.jpg.

These developments also include the addition of elastography, which measures tissue stiffness to more precisely delineate tumors or fibrosis. Portability and real-time imaging capabilities of modern ultrasound machines facilitate point-of-care testing, allowing for earlier diagnosis and pre-treatment planning. Furthermore, AI algorithms are beginning to assist image interpretation, allowing further gains in accuracy and efficiency. Such technological progress not only improves clinical outcomes but also demonstrates the dynamic evolution of genitourinary imaging modalities (Burity *et. al.*, 2014) (Figure 10.13).

10.3.2. Developments in CT Imaging

Technical advancements in imaging have significantly enhanced diagnostic capability in genitourinary medicine, particularly through the optimization of CT scanning. Technical advancements, such as increased detector sensitivity and faster gantry rotation times, have improved scan resolution and decreased acquisition times, allowing visualization of complex anatomical structures with greater precision. This is crucial in evaluating pathologies such as renal masses, urinary tract obstruction, and vascular anomalies. Further, technological advances in dose reduction have minimized radiation exposure risks and enabled safer repeated imaging if required. Post-processing tools, like multiplanar reconstructions and three-dimensional volume rendering, now permit more accurate assessments, aiding surgical planning and intervention. All these technical upgrades have led to improved staging and characterization of genitourinary cancers with greater accuracy, resulting in improved patient outcomes. Though still an evolving process, the incorporation of AI and ML into CT imaging will continue to improve diagnostic accuracy and workflow efficiency in this field (Burity *et. al.*, 2014).

10.3.3. MRI Advancements and Their Implications

Recent technical advances have significantly enhanced the role of MRI in genitourinary diagnosis, with improved visualization of soft tissue anatomy and disease. These include advances in field strength as well as coil design, providing improved spatial resolution and contrast differentiation to facilitate early detection and characterization of malignancies in organs like prostate and kidneys. In parallel, functional MRI techniques like diffusion-weighted imaging and dynamic contrast enhancement are helpful in evaluating tissue physiology and vascularity to aid treatment planning and prognostication. Further, AI and ML algorithms play a significant role in elevating diagnostic accuracy by capitalizing on lesion segmentation and classification with automated approaches. These developments in aggregate reduce the need for invasive procedures and optimize patient care while ushering in an era of a paradigm shift in genitourinary imaging. Aggregate impact emphasizes the importance of ongoing research and interdisciplinarity collaboration to further MRI's clinical potential (Burity *et. al.*, 2014) (Figure 10.14).

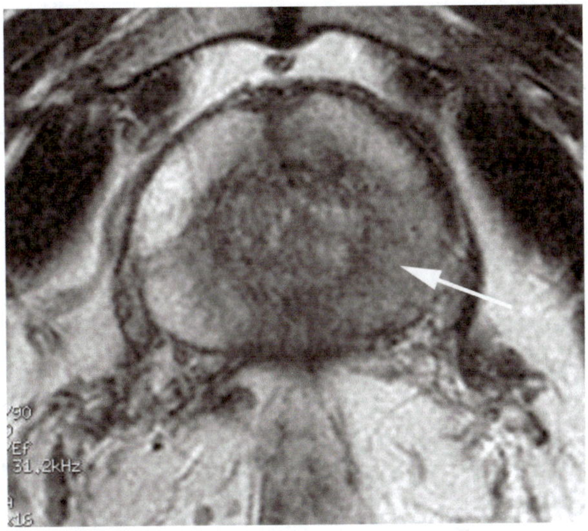

Figure 10.14. Diffusion-weighted imaging.

Source: https://www.ajronline.org/cms/10.2214/AJR.04.1584/asset/images/00_04_1584_01a.jpeg.

10.3.4. Artificial Intelligence in Imaging

Technological advancements have significantly reconfigured genitourinary imaging, introducing novel instruments to enhance therapeutic outcomes and diagnostic yield. Amongst these, AI has emerged as a revolutionizing force, particularly in radiotherapy optimization for prostate cancer patients. Doctors can accurately predict radiation-induced toxicities using predictive AI-based models, thus being able to design more personalized treatment plans with fewer side effects and greater therapeutic gain. They often incorporate fundamental dosimetric parameters, like Vdose, Dmax, and Dmean, to predict genitourinary and gastrointestinal toxicity risk accurately (Ali *et. al.*, 2024). Additionally, ML models in conjunction with process optimization models, for instance, Lean Six Sigma, facilitate plan quality evaluation and optimization in volumetric modulated arc therapy. Such AI-driven systems identify high-risk plans in advance, thereby enhancing patient safety while reducing avoidable workload through targeted quality assurance (Bresolin *et. al.*, 2024). Cumulatively, such technologies bring with them a new era of precision and efficiency in genitourinary imaging and treatment.

10.3.5. 3D Imaging Techniques

Advances in medical imaging have significantly transformed diagnostic and treatment strategies, particularly in the field of genitourinary imaging. Among these advances, three-dimensional imaging techniques have emerged as essential tools, providing full spatial visualization of anatomy and disease. Compared with conventional two-dimensional imaging, 3D modalities enable clinicians to better analyze the intricate relationships between organs and tissues and facilitate diagnosis and treatment planning. For instance, in prostate cancer radiotherapy, 3D imaging allows precise delineation of tumors and nearby critical structures, which are crucial for radiotherapy target optimization and avoidance of collateral damage. Recent studies aim at the integration of predictive models with data from 3D imaging to assess dosimetric parameters more accurately, ultimately reducing treatment toxicity and enhancing patient outcomes (Ali *et. al.*, 2024). With advancing technical capabilities of these imaging methods, their utilization in genitourinary environments is the best demonstration of the intersection of cutting-edge visualization and tailored medicine, concordant with more general theoretical frameworks highlighted in recent sociological accounts of healthcare technologies (Burity *et. al.*, 2014) (Figure 10.15).

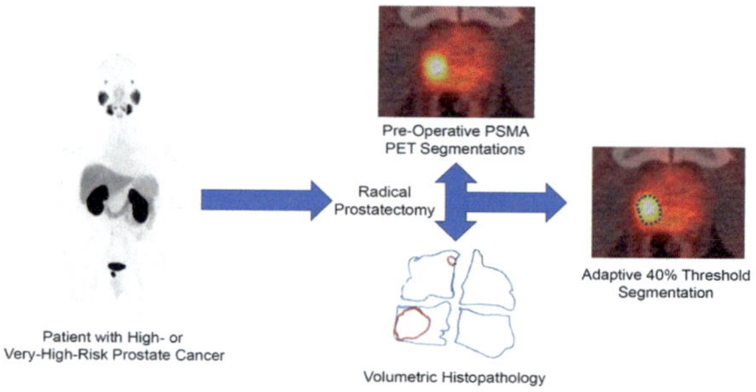

Figure 10.15. In prostate cancer management, 3D imaging facilitates precise delineation of tumors and surrounding critical structures.

Source: https://jnm.snmjournals.org/content/jnumed/65/1/87/F1.large.jpg.

10.3.6. Contrast Agents and Their Evolution

It has been closely linked with the progressive development of contrast agents enhancing tissue distinction and vascular characterization. It initially primarily amplified urinary tract anatomy visualization but had a tendency to reveal toxic as well as allergy-related hazards. Over time, sophistication with respect to agents developed, particularly in MRI, where gadolinium-based agents became the standard due to their better safety profile and enhanced soft tissue contrast. This advancement has allowed more precise definitions of pathologic changes, such as the non-perfused volume that represents necrotic tissue following interventions like MRI-guided transurethral ultrasound ablation (TULSA) for prostate treatment. Contrast-enhanced MRI can trace tissue response following ablation with distinct visualization of dynamic changes in necrosis resolution up to a year after treatment (Mäkelä *et. al.*, 2024). Also, the development of agents that minimize artifact interference further recommends accurate imaging in complex conditions near implants, as demonstrated in the advanced treatment of prostate cancer, with the significant role of innovative contrast agents in maximizing diagnostic accuracy and therapy assessment within genitourinary imaging.

10.3.7. Telemedicine and Remote Imaging

The advancement in digital technology has revolutionized diagnostic practice to a large extent, particularly in the area of genitourinary imaging. The combination of telemedicine with distant imaging modalities is a revolutionary pattern of patient care by circumventing geographical barriers and enhancing access to specialist expertise. Employing systems with high-definition medical image transmission in addition to genetic screening capacity permits clinicians to offer more accurate and timely diagnostics and facilitate customized treatment plans even from distant sites (Song *et. al.*, 2024). The employment of AI, in addition to convolutional neural networks, also facilitates advanced image analysis as well as pattern detection, thereby improving diagnostic efficiency as well as functionality in remote settings (Wang *et. al.*, 2024). These innovations collectively allow a more efficient, accessible, and informed clinical process, demonstrating the critical role of telemedicine and distant imaging in the expansion of genitourinary diagnostic reach and effect. As such, these technologies promise to usher in revolutionary improvements in patient outcomes and healthcare modalities.

10.3.8. Integration of Imaging with Other Diagnostic Tools

Technological progress in genitourinary imaging has advanced by leaps and bounds in diagnostic accuracy, yet there is even more potential for enhancing clinical decision-making with the merging of imaging modalities with ancillary diagnostic methods. Molecular imaging technologies such as fibroblast activation protein inhibitor (FAPI) PET/CT have been a hope in the diagnosis of genitourinary malignancies, particularly in situations where conventional imaging may not succeed, for instance, PSMA-negative prostate cancer.

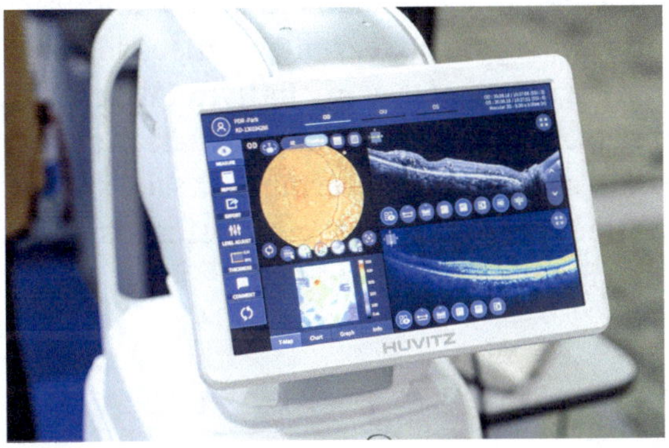

Figure 10.16. Optical coherence tomography (OCT).

Source: https://www.edmundoptics.com/media/fn0mpicr/oct-fig4.png?rmode=max.

This emphasizes the value of integrating functional imaging with routine anatomical assessments to improve lesion localization and staging (Hagens *et. al.*, 2024). In addition, the integration of techniques like optical coherence tomography (OCT), when combined with artificial intelligence (AI), shows how non-invasive methods can improve early cancer detection and surgical precision, again improving patient outcomes (Jerjes *et. al.*, 2024). These multimodal methods enable clinicians to better understand tumor biology and extent of disease, and to design treatment on an individualized basis, better manage genitourinary disease. Additional work is required to determine these integrated strategies and prove their usefulness in the clinic (Figure 10.16).

This emphasizes the value of integrating functional imaging with routine anatomical assessments to improve lesion localization and staging (Hagens *et. al.*, 2024). In addition, the integration of techniques like optical coherence tomography (OCT), when combined with artificial intelligence (AI), shows how non-invasive methods can improve early cancer detection and surgical precision, again improving patient outcomes (Jerjes *et. al.*, 2024). These multimodal methods enable clinicians to better understand tumor biology and extent of disease, and to design treatment on an individualized basis, better manage genitourinary disease. Additional work is required to determine these integrated strategies and prove their usefulness in the clinic (Figure 10.16).

10.3.9. Future Technologies on the Horizon

Technological advances in imaging have remained at the forefront of diagnosis and management, and genitourinary imaging stands poised on the cusp of revolution with the development of new imaging modalities. The intersection of AI and ML holds particular promise, enabling unprecedented accuracy in the detection and characterization of genitourinary pathology. These technologies are revolutionizing predictive modeling, most notably in prostate radiotherapy for cancer, where dosimetric factors like Vdose, Dmax, and Dmean can be studied more accurately to minimize toxic side effects and maximize therapeutic outcomes (Ali *et. al.*, 2024). Moreover, improved image acquisition and processing techniques are expected to improve real-time monitoring and personalized treatment planning, which will directly benefit patient quality of life. While some groundwork has been laid to invest in such advances, ongoing multidisciplinary research is required to further actualize such potential and integrate these into standard practice, catapulting genitourinary imaging into a new era of diagnostic and therapeutic differentiation (Burity *et. al.*, 2014).

Test Your Knowledge

1. How does contrast-enhanced ultrasound (CEUS) enhance the evaluation of renal tumors over traditional ultrasound?
2. How has artificial intelligence (AI) and machine learning been integrated into genitourinary imaging to improve the accuracy of prostate cancer detection on MRI?

10.4. Challenges and Limitations in Genitourinary Imaging

Learning Outcome

1. Understand patient safety and radiation exposure
2. Focus on limitations of imaging resolution
3. Know cost implications of advanced imaging
4. Discuss accessibility of imaging services
5. Describe variability in interpretation of images
6. Explain ethical considerations in imaging
7. Know impact of patient factors on imaging outcomes
8. Understand need for standardized protocols
9. Address disparities in healthcare access

Imaging technical progress has significantly improved diagnostic precision, but genitourinary imaging nevertheless has specific challenges that detract from maximal clinical gain. Major among them is the problem of being unable to get suitable contrast and resolution to effectively separate benign and malignant tissue, particularly in very complicated anatomical locations such as adrenal glands and kidneys. Moreover, some imaging modalities can expose patients to the risk of radiation or contrast nephrotoxic media, and there exist issues of safety and repeated use. Another obstacle is the translation of new targeted imaging probes from preclinical to clinical applications, where despite promising data in early-stage studies, few actively targeted nanocarriers have progressed to regulatory approvals and widespread use in tumor imaging, precluding potential advantages in early detection and monitoring of treatment (Rosenblum *et. al.*, 2018). Additionally, conditions like congenital adrenal hyperplasia require balanced imaging approaches with both diagnostic efficiency and patient-specific factors such as safety and quality of life, further complicating imaging protocols (Speiser *et. al.*, 2018). These intricate limitations highlight the ongoing need for state-of-the-art technologies and patient-specific imaging approaches in genitourinary diagnosis (Figure 10.17).

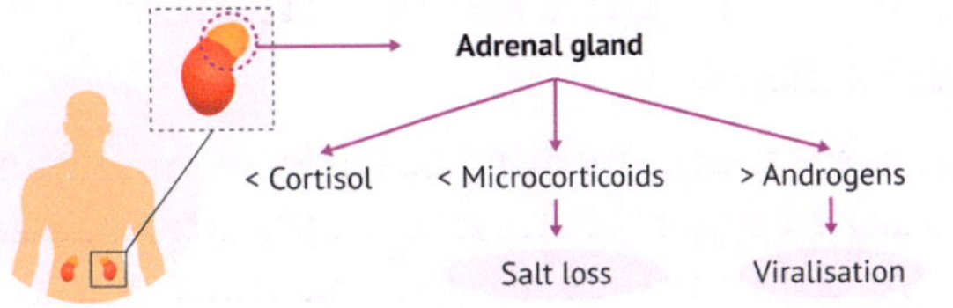

Figure 10.17. Congenital adrenal hyperplasia.

Source: https://www.invitra.com/en/wp-content/uploads/2020/07/adrenal-hyperplasia-congenita.png.

10.4.1. Patient Safety and Radiation Exposure

Safety of patients during diagnostic imaging demands strict attention to radiation exposure, particularly with genitourinary imaging where detailed visualization can be needed at greater modalities such as CT. While CT scans provide great diagnostic data, they expose patients to varying levels of ionizing radiation, which has inherent danger in the form of cancer due to radiation. Studies assessing dose variation emphasize the importance of weighing optimized scanning parameters to reduce exposure without compromising image quality, underlining the role of standard protocols and continuous monitoring in radiology departments for upholding safety standards. As an example, effective dose assessments for contrast-enhanced CT abdomen show variation based on patient demographics and scanning parameters, necessitating optimized measures to limit unnecessary radiation (Aryal *et. al.*, 2025). In the same way, research on radiation doses in the course of fluoroscopic procedures highlights the linear relationship between exposure time and lens dose, again affirming strict control measures to prevent risk (Abuş *et. al.*, 2024). By the same token, balancing diagnostic performance with radiation protection remains an essential concern in genitourinary imaging practice.

10.4.2. Limitations of Imaging Resolution

Despite tremendous advances in imaging modalities, resolution constraints continue to be a hindrance to genitourinary imaging. Resolution high imaging is required to deliver high-quality imaging of small structures such as renal calyces, ureteral walls, and prostate zones. Physical constraints inbuilt within the imaging process, such as signal-to-noise ratio and attenuation effects, however, restrict achievable spatial resolution and typically result in blurred or undetectable detail. In addition, patient movement or physiological activity can cause motion artifacts that contribute to degrading image sharpness.

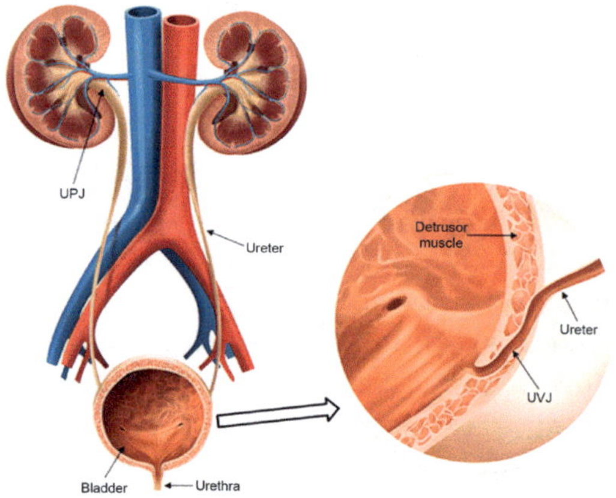

Figure 10.18. High-resolution imaging is crucial for accurately visualizing small anatomical structures such as renal calyces, ureteral walls, and prostate zones.

Source: https://pubs.rsna.org/cms/10.1148/rg.2021200078/asset/images/medium/rg.2021200078.fig1b.gif.

These limitations render precise diagnosis and treatment planning more difficult, especially in distinguishing benign from malignant lesions. Although novel approaches endeavor to obviate these challenges by utilizing more advanced software or advanced hardware, these approaches cannot reverse basic resolution limitations. Incubating novel imaging modalities with complementary diagnostic procedures remains critical to overcome these limitations in the clinic and improve outcomes in genitourinary disease (Burity *et. al.*, 2014) (Figure 10.18).

10.4.3. Cost Implications of Advanced Imaging

Incorporation of novel imaging modalities into genitourinary diagnosis has revolutionized the accuracy and comprehensiveness of clinical evaluation. These developments are accompanied by major cost effects on health care systems and patient access. High-resolution MRI, multiparametric imaging, and contrast-enhanced imaging are likely to require expensive hardware, specialized personnel, and extended operating times that increase overall costs. Such cost pressures could limit widespread use in resource-constrained settings, potentially exacerbating genitourinary care disparities. In addition, the economic cost of such imaging must be weighed against its utility in diagnosis since excessive usage can serve to fuel unneeded healthcare expense without corresponding clinical gain.

A balance between technological progress and economic sustainability is essential in light of the fact that judicious use based on indication and outcome data is most important. Even though existing literature provides some information regarding these dynamics, more research and policy discussion is needed to optimize the economic impact of advanced genitourinary imaging (Burity *et. al.*, 2014).

10.4.4. Accessibility of Imaging Services

Medical technological innovations have significantly expanded genitourinary imaging possibilities, but there are still unequalities of access within populations and geography. Geographic and socioeconomic conditions and insufficient healthcare infrastructure continue to restrict patient access to cutting-edge imaging technologies such as MRI, CT, and ultrasound. These are supplemented in rural or underserved settings where specialized machines are scarce and trained personnel are not easily accessible. Integration of innovative digital solutions has the potential to mitigate these challenges through enabling remote consultation and image sharing, streamlining diagnostic processes, and enhancing expert interpretation accessibility. The development of interrelated query systems facilitates efficient retrieval and evaluation of imaging data, guaranteeing enhanced resource organization and decision-making in genitourinary imaging (Bittencourt *et. al.*, 2018; Brinkley *et. al.*, 2012). Resolution of these access issues is critical to equal delivery of healthcare and improved outcomes for genitourinary patients (Figure 10.19).

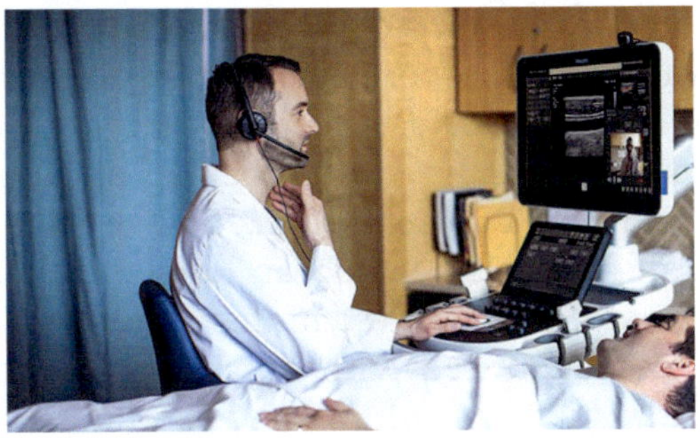

Figure 10.19. Geographic limitations, socioeconomic barriers, and insufficient healthcare infrastructure continue to restrict patient access to sophisticated imaging modalities such as MRI, CT, and ultrasound.

Source: https://www.philips.com/c-dam/corporate/innovation-and-you/global/dec-2021/teaser-blog-ultrasound.jpg.

10.4.5. Variability in Interpretation of Images

Proper interpretation of genitourinary imaging remains a challenging task due to inherent individual variability among radiologists and anatomical presentation variability. Variability can lead to inconsistencies in diagnosing conditions such as prostate cancer, where it is critical to distinguish between indolent and clinically important lesions. Experiments demonstrate that even with a well-established scoring system like PI-RADS, interobserver consensus can be low, leading to poor clinical decision-making and even affecting patient outcomes (Nather *et. al.*, 2022). ML and cluster analysis research offer promising avenues to resolve such an issue by providing a fully automated classification and measurement of anatomical structures, reducing subjectivity bias, and enhancing reproducibility in image interpretation (Kim *et. al.*, 2021). For instance, deep learning models have also shown similar or superior performance compared to experienced radiologists, indicating their potential as adjunctive tools to standardize diagnoses across clinical settings (Nather *et. al.*, 2022). Continued inclusion of such technologies might decrease variability, leading to more uniform and accurate genitourinary diagnoses.

10.4.6. Ethical Considerations in Imaging

Genitourinary imaging innovations have raised complex ethical challenges that require careful consideration to preserve patient rights and safety. Utilization of emerging technologies such as 3D scanning and printing from cadavers requires obtaining informed consent not to commodify human donors and addressing concerns regarding privacy and abuse of identifiable anatomical data (Andrew *et. al.*, 2024). Likewise, the integration of AI in imaging enhances accuracy of diagnosis but poses ethical concerns like transparency, accountability, and potential biases that can exacerbate health inequities if models are not trained on diverse datasets (Marey *et. al.*, 2024). These concerns highlight the importance of developing effective ethical standards that regulate the usage, storage, and sharing of genitourinary imaging data. Values like respect for persons, beneficence, and justice must inform ethical decision-making here, underlining the necessity for standardized procedures and regulatory monitoring in order to investigate changing technologies responsibly and equitably.

10.4.7. Impact of Patient Factors on Imaging Outcomes

Imaging findings in genitourinary diagnostics are prone to change because of underlying patient factors that can complicate exact interpretation and future treatment planning. Prostate volume, tissue density, and history of prior interventions can heavily influence the clarity and validity of imaging modalities such as MRI and ultrasound.

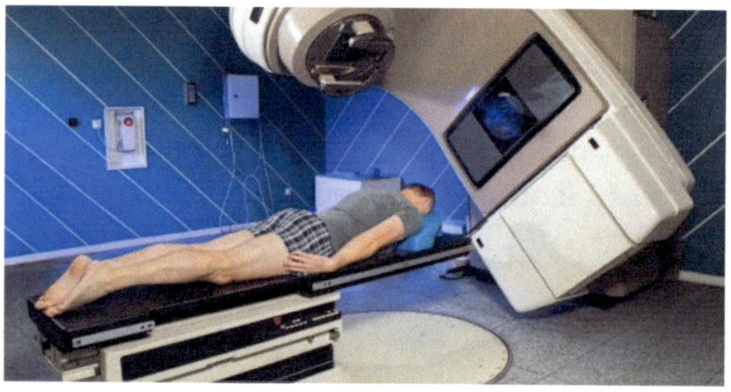

Figure 10.20. External beam radiation therapy (EBRT).

Source: https://aocancer.com/uploads/_1200x630_crop_center-center_82_none/radiation-therapy-vs-proton-therapy-for-prostate-cancer-treatment-affiliated-oncologists-chicago.jpg?mtime=1694470964

For instance, EBRT patients present unique challenges due to the post-treatment changes of tissue characteristics that may obscure tumor visualization or mimic pathological changes (Chen *et. al.*, 2019). Furthermore, the adjuvant or salvage radiation choice for post-prostatectomy patients also relies on imaging results highly influenced by patient-specific factors such as Gleason score and tumor recurrency patterns (Chen *et. al.*, 2019). These nuances call for tailored imaging protocols and specialist interpretation to ensure optimal diagnostic accuracy, thereby improving personalized therapeutic approaches in genitourinary cancer. Therefore, detection and control for patient-specific factors are critical in optimizing imaging performance in this regard (Figure 10.20).

10.4.8. Need for Standardized Protocols

Technique and interpretation variability is a frequent issue in contemporary medical imaging, detracting from the consistency and dependability of diagnostic findings. The issue is best illustrated in genitourinary imaging, where nonuniform protocols lead to variable image quality and diagnostic accuracy. Standardized protocols must be developed in order to correct reproducibility issues, regulate comparative studies, and increase the overall value of imaging modalities. For instance, standardized usability testing protocols for medical imaging software enable uniform assessment of usability and user satisfaction, finally yielding improved clinical decision-making and device optimization (Denisova *et. al.*, 2024). Similarly, in analogous areas such as lung ultrasound, use of standardized scanning protocols has been demonstrated with improved diagnostic accuracy through minimizing methodological heterogeneity (Carranza-Enríquez *et. al.*, 2023). By implementing stringent, standardized procedures in genitourinary imaging, practitioners are able to provide more precise diagnoses, improved patient care, and the facilitation of advances in imaging technology through comparable data sets and demonstrated performance measurements.

10.4.9. Addressing Disparities in Healthcare Access

Health disparities remain a significant hindrance in the best application of genitourinary imaging, particularly in disadvantaged populations. Barriers such as limited insurance, rural living, and socioeconomic factors tend to restrict patient access to state-of-the-art diagnostic equipment fundamental to the earlier diagnosis and treatment. Health insurance schemes have shown to close such gaps by improving access and affordability, but still face administrative hurdles and unequal resource distribution (Selvamuthu *et. al.*, 2025). Furthermore, the use of telemedicine to deliver genitourinary care offers promises of wider coverage but concurrently shines the light on the digital divide that disproportionately affects those with low digital literacy levels or substandard technological infrastructure (Ch *et. al.*, 2025). To face these challenges, a comprehensive approach of tailored insurance policies, community education programs, and infrastructure upgradation is needed. These steps not only make genitourinary imaging services more accessible but also improve health outcomes and early detection among the underserved populations.

Test Your Knowledge

1. What challenges are associated with the use of MRI in imaging patients with metal implants, particularly in the genitourinary system?
2. How does the low sensitivity of ultrasound limit its use in detecting small bladder or prostate cancers?

SUMMARY

In synthesizing the advances and failures shown throughout the discussion of genitourinary imaging, it is evident that the addition of novel radiographic biomarkers can be very informative for prognosis. The advancement of body composition risk scores incorporating information such as skeletal muscle index and visceral fat index has been demonstrated to provide improved predictability compared with traditional methods, such as body mass index, in patients treated with immunotherapy for urothelial carcinoma. These findings underscore the potential of imaging modalities not just to diagnose but also plan individualized treatment and predict outcomes (Martini *et. al.*, 2021). Further, the multidisciplinary focus within respective oncology imaging highlights the need for individualized patient care when optimizing complicated treatment options against conditions like pregnancy or tumor histology (Shachar *et. al.*, 2017). Lastly, continuous quality improvement and validation of the imaging biomarkers will be instrumental in establishing more precise and effective clinical management in genitourinary oncology, justifying the central position of genitourinary imaging in modern medical practice.

Technologic advances in genitourinary imaging have greatly enhanced the diagnostic precision and treatment planning of a range of urological malignancies. Tumor size, location, and depth of invasion continue to be accurately determined with direct implications for therapeutic planning and prognostic assessment. For instance, evidence shows that percutaneous thermal ablation is preferable with centrally located tumors due to fewer complications and shorter hospital stay, whereas liver resection is preferred with subcapsular tumors with the requirement of broader margins of safety (Tombesi *et. al.*, 2025). Furthermore, radiologic staging is also vital in determining the extent of disease spread by evaluating lymph node involvement and distant metastases, and these form the core of patient management algorithm planning (Rouhezamin *et. al.*, 2024). Emerging technologies such as stereotactic navigation and AI-enabled imaging software also enhance the accuracy of tumor targeting and margin assessment and may even expand the application of less invasive interventions. These developments together underscore the active role of genitourinary imaging in realizing maximal patient benefit across a broad spectrum of clinical situations.

KEY TERMS FROM THIS CHAPTER

- High-resolution visualization
- Kidney
- Prostate
- Technology
- Genitourinary tract
- Genitourinary imaging
- Bladder
- Reproductive organ diseases
- Prostate cancer
- Urologic oncology

CRITICAL THINKING QUESTIONS

1. **Which imaging modality is most commonly used for evaluating kidney stones?**
   a. MRI
   b. Ultrasound
   c. CT scan without contrast
   d. X-ray
2. **What is the best imaging modality for assessing a suspected bladder tumor?**
   a. CT urography
   b. MRI of the pelvis
   c. Intravenous pyelogram (IVP)
   d. Cystoscopy
3. **What is the primary advantage of using Doppler ultrasound in genitourinary imaging?**
   a. Provides detailed structural imaging
   b. Allows real-time evaluation of blood flow
   c. Can evaluate renal function
   d. Detects small kidney stones
4. **What imaging technique is most appropriate for staging renal cell carcinoma?**
   a. Plain X-ray
   b. MRI with contrast
   c. Ultrasound
   d. CT with contrast
5. **What is the primary advantage of using CT urography in genitourinary imaging?**
   a. It is less expensive than MRI
   b. It provides detailed images of the entire urinary tract, including the kidneys, ureters, and bladder
   c. It requires no contrast agents
   d. It is preferred for evaluating prostate cancer

Short Answer Questions

1. What imaging modality is typically used to diagnose renal stones in the emergency setting?
2. How does Doppler ultrasound aid in evaluating renal blood flow and function?
3. What role does MRI play in the assessment of prostate cancer, particularly in staging?
4. What is the preferred imaging technique for evaluating bladder cancer?
5. What are the common findings of a renal mass on contrast-enhanced CT?
6. What are the imaging characteristics of a simple renal cyst on ultrasound?
7. What are the imaging features of chronic kidney disease on radiologic studies?

Answers to Critical Thinking Questions

1. (c); 2. (b); 3.(b); 4.(d); 5.(b)

REFERENCES

1. Abuş, F., Gürçalar, A., Günay, O., Tunçman, D., Kesmezacar, F., & Demir, M. (2024). Quantification of lens radiation exposure in scopey imaging: A dose level analysis. *International Journal of Applied Sciences and Radiation Research*. https://www.semanticscholar.org/paper/834b6574556122107e9b9c22bb34a2ae6ea551d1 (accessed on 30 May 2025).
2. Agarwal, A., Majzoub, A., Baskaran, S., Panner Selvam, M. K., Cho, C. L., Henkel, R., Finelli, R., *et. al.* (2020). Sperm DNA fragmentation: A new guideline for clinicians. *The World Journal of Men's Health, 38*, 412. https://doi.org/10.5534/wjmh.200128.
3. Aguirre-Avalos, G., & Amaya-Tapia, G. (2018). Urinary tract tuberculosis. https://core.ac.uk/download/322436565.pdf (accessed on 30 May 2025).
4. Ahmed, J., & Nasir, S. (2018). A bibliometric analysis of research on Zika virus indexed in Web of Science. https://core.ac.uk/download/268082342.pdf (accessed on 30 May 2025).
5. Ali, M., Alongi, P., Benfante, V., Boldrini, L., *et. al.* (2024). Artificial intelligence and statistical models for the prediction of radiotherapy toxicity in prostate cancer: A systematic review. https://core.ac.uk/download/638998504.pdf (accessed on 30 May 2025).
6. Anand, U., Dey, A., Singh Chandel, A. K., Sanyal, R., Mishra, A., Pandey, D. K., De Falco, V., *et. al.* (2022). Cancer chemotherapy and beyond: Current status, drug candidates, associated risks and progress in targeted therapeutics. *Genes & Diseases, 10*, 1367–1401. https://doi.org/10.1016/j.gendis.2022.02.007.
7. Aryal, B., Bhat, M. R., Wani, A. A., & Islam, J. U. (2025). Assessment of radiation exposure: An in-depth analysis of dose evaluation in contrast-enhanced computed tomography abdomen imaging. *Annals of the National Academy of Medical Sciences (India)*. https://www.semanticscholar.org/paper/f0b7f1ca5fdb0fdf9af7eac1f50918f54123d5e4 (accessed on 30 May 2025).
8. Baldacchino, I., Gatt, A. S., & Saliba, I. (2016). Fetal MRI: An essential step in interpreting complex ultrasound findings. https://core.ac.uk/download/46604247.pdf (accessed on 30 May 2025).
9. Bhat, A., Goyal, S. K., & Gupta, H. (2016). Current status of nanotechnology in urology. https://core.ac.uk/download/539912362.pdf (accessed on 30 May 2025).
10. Bilican, G., Karakan, T., Eğritaş Gürkan, Ö., Sabhan, H., Hedin, C., Forss, A., Petrousis, G., *et. al.* (2025). P0376 Advancing intestinal ultrasound for IBD in Turkey: Results of a national survey. *Journal of Crohn's and Colitis*. https://www.semanticscholar.org/paper/30611e47cd0b36def50c23f1da2c6676be6ab456 (accessed on 30 May 2025).
11. Bittencourt, L. K., D'Anastasi, M., Domingues, R., Hricak, H., *et. al.* (2018). Global challenges for cancer imaging. https://core.ac.uk/download/129921504.pdf (accessed on 30 May 2025).
12. Bivalacqua, T. J., Allen, B., Brock, G., Broderick, G. A., Köhler, T., Mulhall, J. P., Oristaglio, J., *et. al.* (2021). Acute ischemic priapism: An AUA/SMSNA guideline. *The Journal of Urology, 206*, 1114–1121. https://doi.org/10.1097/ju.0000000000002236.
13. Blaszczyszyn, M., Gorzelanczyk, E. J., Kawala-Sterniuk, A., Martinek, M., *et. al.* (2020). Comparison of smoothing filters in analysis of EEG data for the medical diagnostics purposes. https://core.ac.uk/download/322825152.pdf (accessed on 30 May 2025).

14. Bresolin, A., Brioso, R. C., Crespi, L., Dei, A., *et. al.* (2024). Machine learning and lean six sigma for targeted patient-specific quality assurance of volumetric modulated arc therapy plans. https://core.ac.uk/download/638787428.pdf (accessed on 30 May 2025).

15. Brinkley, J. F., & Detwiler, L. T. (2012). A query integrator and manager for the query web. https://core.ac.uk/download/pdf/9412382.pdf (accessed on 30 May 2025).

16. Burity, J., Fonte, I. B. da, & de Melo, P. B. (2014). Radiological Society of North America (RSNA) 3D printing Special Interest Group (SIG): Guidelines for medical 3D printing and appropriateness for clinical scenarios. https://core.ac.uk/download/212867900.pdf (accessed on 30 May 2025).

17. Cahill, L. C., Rosen, S., Yoshitake, T., Wu, Y., York, L., Tsai, L., Gershman, B., *et. al.* (2021). Real-time diagnosis and Gleason grading of prostate core needle biopsies using nonlinear microscopy. *Modern Pathology, 35*, 539–548. https://www.semanticscholar.org/paper/d2c014978e1ea7ae789e304eb9b100e6253c2888 (accessed on 30 May 2025).

18. Carranza-Enríquez, F., Soto, C., Pineda, C., Rodriguez-Reyne, T. S., Ángeles-Acuña, A., Solorzano Flores, S. Y., Vazquez Ortega, A., *et. al.* (2023). POS1261 Diagnostic accuracy of lung ultrasound for detecting interstitial lung disease among patients with systemic sclerosis: A comparative study of two scanning protocols. *Annals of the Rheumatic Diseases*. https://www.semanticscholar.org/paper/be3a235c6b797b9ab440f013ca055f2c52a0a5ae (accessed on 30 May 2025).

19. Donoso Castellanos, P., Cárdenas Aguirre, C. A., Flores Bustamante, A., *et. al.* (2025). Atypical epididymis-orchitis with scrotal manifestation of Entamoeba histolytica with concurrent Morganelli morganii infection. https://core.ac.uk/download/645626183.pdf (accessed on 30 May 2025).

20. Chen, Y., Degnin, C., Hung, A. Y., McClelland, S., *et. al.* (2019). Is moderate hypofractionation accepted as a new standard of care in North America for prostate cancer patients treated with external beam radiotherapy? Survey of genitourinary expert radiation oncologists. https://core.ac.uk/download/228066084.pdf (accessed on 30 May 2025).

21. Chen, Y., Degnin, C., McClelland, S., Mitin, N., *et. al.* (2019). Adjuvant vs. salvage radiation therapy in men with high-risk features after radical prostatectomy: Survey of North American genitourinary expert radiation oncologists. https://core.ac.uk/download/228066107.pdf (accessed on 30 May 2025).

22. Cimadamore, A., Lopez-Beltran, A., Cheng, L., & Montironi, R. (2020). Molecular diagnostics in uro-oncology. https://core.ac.uk/download/589943007.pdf (accessed on 30 May 2025).

23. Daimiel Naranjo, I., Bhowmik, A., Basukala, D., Lo Gullo, R., Mazaheri, Y., Kapetas, P., Eskreis-Winkler, S., *et. al.* (2024). Assessment of hypoxia in breast cancer: Emerging functional MR imaging and spectroscopy techniques and clinical applications. *Journal of Magnetic Resonance Imaging (JMRI)*. https://www.semanticscholar.org/paper/cdda120b02a1fbc744b3dab32b2193883df094c9 (accessed on 30 May 2025).

24. Deane, A. S., & Byers, K. T. (2024). A review of the ethical considerations for the use of 3D printed materials in medical and allied health education and a proposed collective path forward. *Anatomical Sciences Education*. https://www.semanticscholar.org/paper/89ed9786b9d830939b7f34018a5cc18763c692be (accessed on 30 May 2025).

25. Denisova, E., Tiribilli, E., Luschi, A., Francia, P., Manetti, L., Bocchi, L., & Iadanza, E. (2024). Enabling reliable usability assessment and comparative analysis of medical software: A comprehensive framework for multimodal biomedical imaging platforms. *Health and Technology*. https://www.semanticscholar.org/paper/3013b1e4f20eba57894a6cf5240feac0ce60a432 (accessed on 30 May 2025).

26. Ferrero, A., Krambeck, A. E., Lieske, J. C., McCollough, C. H., *et. al.* (2019). Understanding, justifying, and optimizing radiation exposure for CT imaging in nephrourology. https://core.ac.uk/download/225126909.pdf (accessed on 30 May 2025).

27. Habib, G., Malik, I. A., Qureshi, S., Ra, I. H., Singh, S., & Sharma, S. (2025). Harnessing the power of attention for patch-based biomedical image classification. *IEEE Access, 13*, 36760–36774. https://www.semanticscholar.org/paper/cc91020efb35f685fbc6eca998f128022a169b90 (accessed on 30 May 2025).

28. Hagens, M., van Leeuwen, P. V., Wondergem, M., Boellaard, T., Sanguedolce, F., Oprea-Lager, D., Bex, A., *et. al.* (2024). A systematic review on the diagnostic value of fibroblast activation protein inhibitor PET/CT in genitourinary cancers. *The Journal of Nuclear Medicine, 65*, 888–896. https://www.semanticscholar.org/paper/ff9e9790ee4f55c391bacc3c11ca88d4c121d407 (accessed on 30 May 2025).

29. Hajiran, A., Point, D. C., & Zaslau, S. (2013). Bedside ultrasound in workup of self-inserted headset cable into the penile urethra and incidentally discovered intravesical foreign body. https://core.ac.uk/download/207770000.pdf (accessed on 30 May 2025).

30. Halpern, E. J., Kim, S., Salmanoglu, E., Thakur, S., *et. al.* (2018). A glance at imaging bladder cancer. https://core.ac.uk/download/227055407.pdf (accessed on 30 May 2025).

31. Jani, A., Schreibmann, E., Goyal, S., Halkar, R., Hershatter, B., Rossi, P., Shelton, J., *et. al.* (2021). EMPIRE-1: Randomized trial comparing conventional- vs conventional plus fluciclovine (18F) PET/CT imaging-guided post-prostatectomy radiotherapy for prostate cancer. *Social Science Research Network*. https://www.semanticscholar.org/paper/75ccd3e383b7e2c4e2c9171bcfa1314478a06fe8 (accessed on 30 May 2025).

32. Jerjes, W., Stevenson, H., Ramsay, D., & Hamdoon, Z. (2024). Enhancing oral cancer detection: A systematic review of the diagnostic accuracy and future integration of optical coherence tomography with artificial intelligence. *Journal of Clinical Medicine, 13*. https://www.semanticscholar.org/paper/3999a213b09818c64ba2f17435b118bd832cf552 (accessed on 30 May 2025).

33. Jessica, E. C. (2024). Advancements and challenges in algebraic techniques for medical imaging: A comprehensive review of MRI and CT scan applications in Nigeria. *Newport International Journal of Biological and Applied Sciences*. https://www.semanticscholar.org/paper/91654d34182d72675a759d337f27056f54aa2170 (accessed on 30 May 2025).

34. Kamagata, K., Saito, Y., Andica, C., Uchida, W., Takabayashi, K., Yoshida, S., Hagiwara, A., *et. al.* (2023). Noninvasive magnetic resonance imaging measures of glymphatic system activity. *Journal of Magnetic Resonance Imaging, 59*. https://www.semanticscholar.org/paper/0a7907971da36a770da3a760520ccb436ffdb210 (accessed on 30 May 2025).

35. Karalis, V. (2024). The integration of artificial intelligence into clinical practice. *Applied Biosciences, 3*, 14–44. https://doi.org/10.3390/applbiosci3010002.

36. Kaushik, P., & Sharma, P. (2024). Enhancing kidney disease diagnosis through advanced deep

learning techniques: A comprehensive analysis in modern medical imaging. *2024 5th IEEE Global Conference for Advancement in Technology (GCAT)*. https://www.semanticscholar.org/paper/243fcf3a3d0ce470acce4b18ba025b05851db053 (accessed on 30 May 2025).

37. Key, N. S., Khorana, A. A., Kuderer, N. M., Bohlke, K., Lee, A. Y. Y., Arcelus, J. I., Wong, S. L., *et. al.* (2019). Venous thromboembolism prophylaxis and treatment in patients with cancer: ASCO clinical practice guideline update. *Journal of Clinical Oncology, 38*, 496–520. https://doi.org/10.1200/jco.19.01461.

38. Kim, Y. H., Jeon, K., Lee, C., Choi, Y., Jung, H., & Han, S. S. (2021). Analysis of the mandibular canal course using unsupervised machine learning algorithm. *PLoS ONE, 16*. https://www.semanticscholar.org/paper/caacd3dd22c6f72e19ea05f745358cd2ad0837ac (accessed on 30 May 2025).

39. Kohan, A., Hanneman, K., Mirshahvalad, S. A., Afaq, A., Mallak, N., Metser, U., & Veit-Haibach, P. (2024). Current applications of PET/MR: Part II: Clinical applications II. *Canadian Association of Radiologists Journal = Journal Association Canadienne Des Radiologists*. https://www.semanticscholar.org/paper/506726c9a4c0fafc535571d7c38d9c719aed0426 (accessed on 30 May 2025).

40. Lowrance, W. T., Dreicer, R., Jarrard, D. F., Scarpato, K. R., Kim, S. K., Kirkby, E., Buckley, D., *et. al.* (2023). Updates to advanced prostate cancer: AUA/SUO guideline (2023). *The Journal of Urology, 209*, 1082–1090. https://doi.org/10.1097/ju.0000000000003452.

41. Mäkelä, P. (2024). MRI findings after transurethral ultrasound ablation of prostate. https://core.ac.uk/download/624259084.pdf (accessed on 30 May 2025).

42. Marey, A., Serdysnki, K. C., Killeen, B., Unberath, M., & Umair, M. (2024). Applications and implementation of generative artificial intelligence in cardiovascular imaging with a focus on ethical and legal considerations: What cardiovascular imagers need to know! *BJR|Artificial Intelligence*. https://www.semanticscholar.org/paper/0e8e3b2828235f4372d65a7e840d88b8162c62c7 (accessed on 30 May 2025).

43. Martini, D., Shabto, J., Goyal, S., Liu, Y., Olsen, T., Evans, S. T., Magod, B., *et. al.* (2021). Body composition as an independent predictive and prognostic biomarker in advanced urothelial carcinoma patients treated with immune checkpoint inhibitors. *The Oncologist*. https://www.semanticscholar.org/paper/227605825310b64d8671e8e083acf726938373fd (accessed on 30 May 2025).

44. Mastroianni, R., Ferriero, M., Tuderti, G., Anceschi, U., Bove, A. M., Brassetti, A., Misuraca, L., *et. al.* (2022). Open radical cystectomy versus robot-assisted radical cystectomy with intracorporeal urinary diversion: Early outcomes of a single-center randomized controlled trial. *The Journal of Urology, 207*, 982–992. https://doi.org/10.1097/ju.0000000000002422.

45. McCormack, B., Hampton, H. L., Speich, J., Radley, S. C., Burkett, L. S., & Klausner, A. (2024). Ultrasound urodynamics: A review of ultrasound imaging techniques for enhanced bladder functional diagnostics. *Current Bladder Dysfunction Reports, 19*, 263–271. https://www.semanticscholar.org/paper/9a3b68895b7afca5b477134804ff993ce64af17d (accessed on 30 May 2025).

46. Mikkelsen, A. F. S., Thygesen, J., & Fledelius, J. (2025). Optimizing CT imaging parameters: Implications for diagnostic accuracy in nuclear medicine. *Seminars in Nuclear Medicine*. https://www.semanticscholar.org/paper/c4f9a04d46044ff87101d0cbcc900215852c3c26 (accessed on 30 May 2025).

47. Miller, J. M., Binnicker, M. J., Campbell, S., Carroll, K. C., Chapin, K. C., Gonzalez, M. D., Harrington, A., *et. al.* (2024). Guide to utilization of the microbiology laboratory for diagnosis of infectious diseases: 2024 update by the Infectious Diseases Society of America (IDSA) and the American Society for Microbiology (ASM). *Clinical Infectious Diseases.* https://doi.org/10.1093/cid/ciae104.

48. Nagy, K., Jatsch, A., Fortner, P., Aurich, M., Seitz, S., Sommer, A., Gorich, J., *et. al.* (2024). The potential of artificial intelligence in the assessment of coronary artery stenosis in follow-up CT examinations. *European Heart Journal–Cardiovascular Imaging.* https://www.semanticscholar.org/paper/03b9debaf66776babc9e86ca7a9b07c188b691ff (accessed on 30 May 2025).

49. Nather, J., & Muglia, V. (2022). Editorial for "Performance of Artificial Intelligence-Aided Diagnosis System for Clinically Significant Prostate Cancer with MRI: A Diagnostic Comparison Study." *Journal of Magnetic Resonance Imaging, 57.* https://www.semanticscholar.org/paper/aad4335e9dfd13333f8fc8590794a03b263b209e (accessed on 30 May 2025).

50. Oudah, Q. C., Mohammed, M. Z., & Abdulkafi, A. Q. (2023). Reliability of magnetic resonance imaging in the detection of congenital anomalies of Iraqi women. *Journal of Prevention, Diagnosis and Management of Human Diseases.* https://www.semanticscholar.org/paper/5cc128acaf73666ed9eb45276952808f3376b26f (accessed on 30 May 2025).

51. Priya, P. M., & Ezhilarasan, M. (2024). A hybrid technique of diagnosing kidney disorder using deep neural network. *International Journal of Online Biomedical Engineering, 20,* 43–59. https://www.semanticscholar.org/paper/a8f1da7f4a0a20eb024b4460310d8ea89f362567 (accessed on 30 May 2025).

52. Rösch, J. (1999). Introduction. *Seminars in Interventional Radiology, 16,* 251. https://www.semanticscholar.org/paper/a41b106f0878fface557ed2d0c634d1c26939467 (accessed on 30 May 2025).

53. Rosenblum, D., Joshi, N., Tao, W., Karp, J. M., & Peer, D. (2018). Progress and challenges towards targeted delivery of cancer therapeutics. *Nature Communications, 9.* https://doi.org/10.1038/s41467-018-03705-y.

54. Rouhezamin, M. R., Lee, S. I., Harisinghani, M., & Uppot, R. N. (2024). The tipping point: Key oncologic imaging findings resulting in critical changes in the management of malignant genitourinary and gynecological tumors. *Current Problems in Diagnostic Radiology.* https://www.semanticscholar.org/paper/49819758867fb9810face1a4f2243dd7b5c0b779 (accessed on 30 May 2025).

55. Saeed, A., Pervaiz, F., Nawaz, H., Rafiq, S., Bibi, Y., Almagharbeh, W. T., Mobeen, M., *et. al.* (2025). Health equity in telemedicine: Addressing disparities in digital healthcare access—a narrative review-S. *Insights-Journal of Life and Social Sciences.* https://www.semanticscholar.org/paper/12c5c54afc3c933bf81c3be4feb47b8d31b1c9c3 (accessed on 30 May 2025).

56. Sarker, S., Sarker, P., Stone, G., Gorman, R., Tavakkoli, A., Bebis, G., & Sattarvand, J. (2024). A comprehensive overview of deep learning techniques for 3D point cloud classification and semantic segmentation. *Machine Vision and Applications, 35,* 67. https://www.semanticscholar.org/paper/f65a1ce8c49380f7e90633a9367b1efd80b90442 (accessed on 30 May 2025).

57. Selvamuthu, C. M., Lavaraju, B., & Sundaram, A. (2025). Perceptions of health insurance schemes and their role in reducing healthcare disparities across Asian populations: Insights into access, equity and policy. *Journal of Pioneering Medical Sciences.* https://www.semanticscholar.org/

paper/07933006c941fd959b639d88deb18ed8994b630e (accessed on 30 May 2025).

58. Shachar, S. S., Gallagher, K., McGuire, K., Zagar, T., Faso, A., Muss, H., Sweeting, R., *et. al.* (2017). Multidisciplinary management of breast cancer during pregnancy. *The Oncologist, 22*(3), 324–334. https://www.semanticscholar.org/paper/1db81b4031f7eeb05b9751c4a8e82727272eb4cc (accessed on 30 May 2025).

59. Soliman-Aboumarie, H., Joshi, S., Cameli, M., Michalski, B., Manka, R., Haugaa, K., Demirkıran, A., *et. al.* (2022). EACVI survey on the multi-modality imaging assessment of the right heart. *European Heart Journal. Cardiovascular Imaging*. https://www.semanticscholar.org/paper/0a1e66052bb48e8350c00a5734c91e055e4f523e (accessed on 30 May 2025).

60. Song, Y., Xu, Y., He, Y., Zhang, X., Wang, R., & Quan, W. (2024). Development of a telemedicine-based assisted system for CT imaging and gene matching. *2024 6th International Conference on Frontier Technologies of Information and Computer (ICFTIC)*. https://www.semanticscholar.org/paper/fc1052de1869422d514a029829e8673c355794c4 (accessed on 30 May 2025).

61. Speiser, P., Arlt, W., Auchus, R. J., Baskin, L. S., Conway, G. S., Merke, D. P., Meyer-Bahlburg, H. F. L., *et. al.* (2018). Congenital adrenal hyperplasia due to steroid 21-hydroxylase deficiency: An endocrine society* clinical practice guideline. *The Journal of Clinical Endocrinology & Metabolism, 103*, 4043–4088. https://doi.org/10.1210/jc.2018-01865.

62. Stöckl, A., & Diaz, D. (2025). Cultural differences in perception and engagement of AI-generated online ads. *AHFE International*. https://www.semanticscholar.org/paper/c46f0515ebf50c2a4098837f3f90efdd50cbc362 (accessed on 30 May 2025).

63. Sundar, K., Manohar, E., Vijay, K., & Ravikumar, S. (2024). Segmentation and detection of liver tumors from CT scans using TransUNet architecture in deep learning. *2024 Second International Conference on Intelligent Cyber Physical Systems and Internet of Things (ICoICI)*. https://www.semanticscholar.org/paper/f74cfadd3418871474a68c2b853ae4b765d550c4 (accessed on 30 May 2025).

64. Tombesi, P., Cutini, A., Di Vece, F., Grasso, V., Politti, U., Capatti, E., & Sartori, S. (2025). Surgery or percutaneous ablation for liver tumors? The key points are: When, where, and how large. *Cancers, 17*. https://www.semanticscholar.org/paper/214bb196b3569fd963a995208a2652d9b2a83b41 (accessed on 30 May 2025).

65. Wang, H., & Li, X. (2024). DeepBlue: Advanced convolutional neural network applications for ocean remote sensing. *IEEE Geoscience and Remote Sensing Magazine, 12*, 138–161. https://www.semanticscholar.org/paper/d2b2fc901cb85c6a12054bb1153a0e4d848e4155 (accessed on 30 May 2025).

OBSTETRIC ULTRASOUND

11

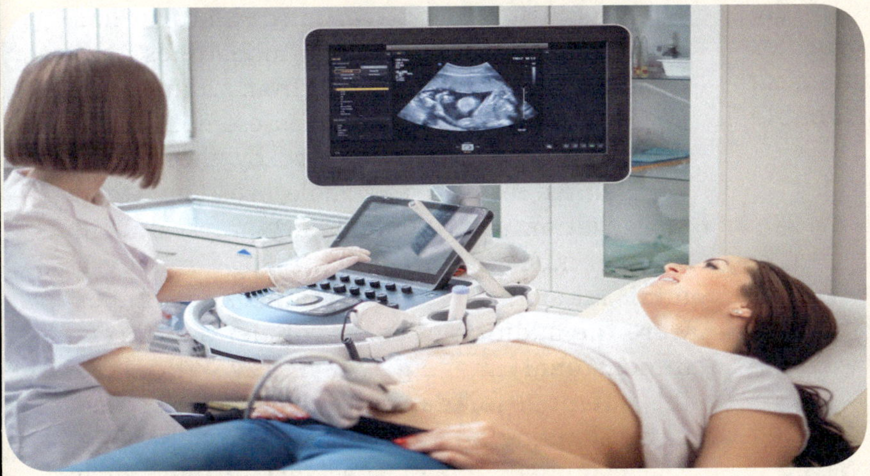

LEARNING OBJECTIVES

After studying this chapter, you will be able to:

1. Explain types of obstetric ultrasound
2. Know applications of obstetric ultrasound
3. Discuss benefits and limitations of obstetric ultrasound
4. Focus on technological advancements in obstetric ultrasound

Introduction

Medical technology has continued to advance prenatal care more and more, greatly improving with the ability to monitor fetal growth and the mother's health. Among all the advances, obstetric ultrasound has been one of the breakthrough technologies that provide real-time images with which doctors can effectively analyze a variety of fetal parameters. The recent advent of portable ultrasound machines that are mobile and can be integrated with cellular devices is one such innovation, with the ready availability and mobility beyond the confines of the traditional clinic being enabled (Plöger *et. al.*, 2024). Furthermore, obstetric ultrasound technology has been simultaneous with improvements in prenatal genetic screening, where sonographic diagnosis is complemented by molecular analysis, such as non-invasive prenatal testing (NIPT) and chromosomal microarray analysis, expanding fetal assessment scope (Tina *et. al.*, 2021). This integration reflects the growing role of obstetric ultrasound, not just as a diagnostic tool, but also as part of whole prenatal care that allows for early detection and intervention measures.

Definition of Obstetric Ultrasound

Modern medical imaging has transformed prenatal care by enabling minute visualization of the in-utero fetus and the corresponding maternal anatomy. Among the modalities, obstetric ultrasound is a non-invasive diagnostic modality employing high-frequency sound waves to produce real-time images of the placenta, uterus, and fetus. The test provides valuable information on fetal growth, anatomical development, and detection of probable abnormalities.

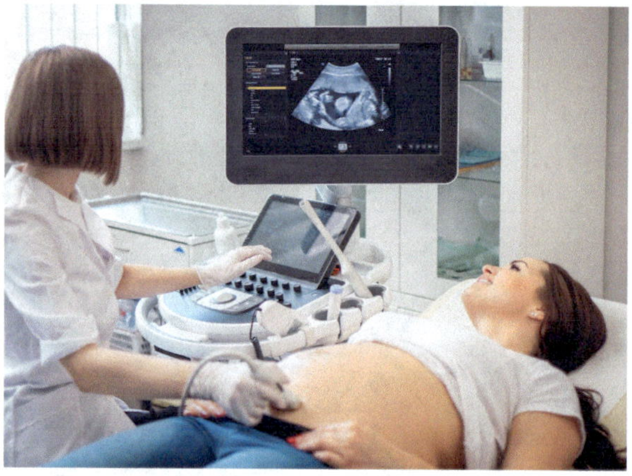

Figure 11.1. Obstetric ultrasound.

Source: https://s3.amazonaws.com/static.organiclead.com/Site-f859dd19-b65f-4524-8064-a1aa06f7055d/shutterstock_1485769484.png.

Technological improvement, such as Fusion Imaging, where ultrasonography (EUS) is fused with magnetic resonance imaging (MRI) and Computed Tomography (CT), has enhanced obstetric diagnostic accuracy beyond its traditional applications (Bellati *et. al.*, 2018). Besides, the combination of ML algorithms and obstetric ultrasound has introduced clever tools with automated detection of anomalies and functional assessment of fetoplacental and cervical health with the promise of improved prediction and control of conditions like preterm labor and fetal growth restriction (Arain *et. al.*, 2023). Thus, obstetric ultrasound remains at the core of maternal-fetal medicine, combining safety, accessibility, and evolving technology to optimize prenatal outcomes (Figure 11.1).

Historical Background of Ultrasound Technology

The evolution of ultrasound history has been marked by significant milestones that transformed obstetric practice from rudimentary imaging to sophisticated fetal assessment. Early development was spearheaded by those who, with limited resources available, broadened fetal visualization using rudimentary grayscale and Doppler modalities to pave the way for modern fetal medicine. These landmark advances were the addition of color Doppler and three-dimensional imaging, which revolutionized the potential for detecting abnormalities and understanding fetal cardiovascular physiology. The establishment of specialist forums, such as the International Society of Ultrasound in Obstetrics and Gynecology and its journal, was an international forum that accelerated research and knowledge exchange, providing a climate for collaboration essential for growth in this specialty (Chaoui, 2021). Most recently, tele-ultrasound has appeared, which has caused significant change in healthcare delivery through facilitating remote fetal imaging and consultation, particularly in resource-constrained areas, thereby increasing access and enhancing prenatal care globally (Britton *et. al.*, 2019).

Importance of Ultrasound in Prenatal Care

Medical imaging technological advancements have significantly enhanced prenatal care, and obstetric ultrasound has become a key diagnostic and monitoring tool. The non-invasive nature of ultrasound and the relative cost-effectiveness of ultrasound machines make it an economical way to check up on fetal growth and detect congenital abnormalities early, which can be crucial in managing complications during pregnancy. Evidence indicates that the majority of pregnant women enjoy ultrasound reassurance in diagnosing fetal well-being, with still unresolved questions regarding its full diagnostic potential (Alshalahi *et. al.*, 2025). Ultrasound serves not only in diagnosing normal conditions but also abnormal complications like placental tumors, whose early detection can result in proper early intervention and improve maternal-fetal outcomes (Castro-Apodaca *et. al.*, 2025). In this way, ultrasound is both a clinical requirement and a source of emotional reassurance during pregnancy, highlighting the importance that is attached to individualized education for pregnant women and continuing professional education to optimize its clinical usefulness and inform decision-making during gestation (Figure 11.2).

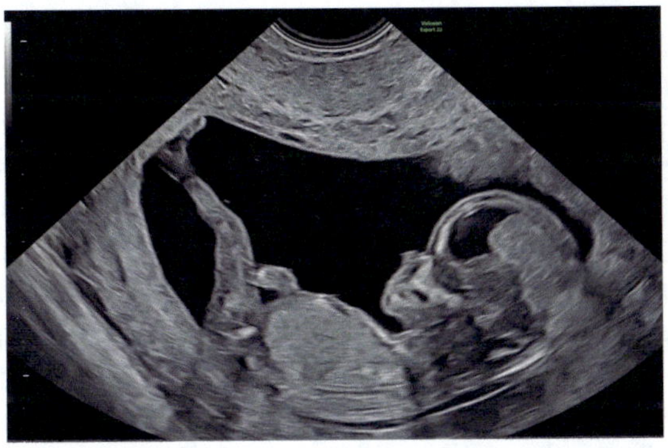

Figure 11.2. Ultrasound's non-invasive nature and relative cost-effectiveness make it an accessible option to track fetal development and detect congenital anomalies early, which can be critical in managing pregnancy risks.

Source: https://images.takeshape.io/f1ba446a-c0cf-4882-b0c9-50298f143ec2/dev/be85a2da-a08b-408a-b201-2f33170c430e/918420?auto=compress%2Cformat&crop=center.

Overview of Ultrasound Types Used in Obstetrics

Medical imaging development has also astoundingly advanced prenatal care, with numerous ultrasound techniques now employed to monitor fetal growth and maternal well-being. The standard two-dimensional (2D) ultrasound is still in most widespread use, providing the fundamental images that are needed for fetal anatomy assessment and for early detection of any abnormalities. Supplementing this, three-dimensional (3D) and four-dimensional (4D) ultrasounds provide greater visual detail and movement, enabling clinicians and parents to see fetal motion in real-time. Doppler ultrasound also plays a role by measuring blood circulation in the placenta and fetus, which is essential in determining hypertensive disorders and avoiding complications (Freeman *et. al.*, 2013). While valuable, availability and expertise to perform these ultrasounds are not consistent globally, with educational efforts to further improve practitioner competency, particularly in resource-constrained areas, as described within the context of midwifery training programs in South Africa (Gilstad *et. al.*, 2012). In combination, these disparate ultrasound modalities are a fundamental part of total obstetric care.

Significance of Advancements in Ultrasound Technology

Technological innovation in medical imaging has dramatically transformed prenatal care by allowing early and accurate diagnosis of fetal conditions. Advances in ultrasound technology have improved the quality of images and real-time monitoring, allowing for detailed assessment of fetal development and maternal well-being. These technologies not only allow clinicians to identify potential complications more precisely but also allow more informed pregnancy decision-making. But its implications extend far beyond clinical utility. As more precise in diagnosis, obstetric ultrasound also raises ethical concerns related to prenatal screening and reproductive choices, as earlier and routine application can empower as well as constrain maternal autonomy (Nakou, 2020). Moreover, the fusion of ultrasound innovation with recent monitoring technologies, e.g., heart rate variability analysis in neonatal practice, emphasizes the potential of a holistic perinatal monitoring, integrating obstetric imaging and following postnatal outcomes along with stimulating interdisciplinarity for improving infant health (Chiera *et. al.*, 2020). Hence, the significance of ultrasound innovations lies in their dual potential to create medical know-how and to escalate difficult ethical consideration (Figure 11.3).

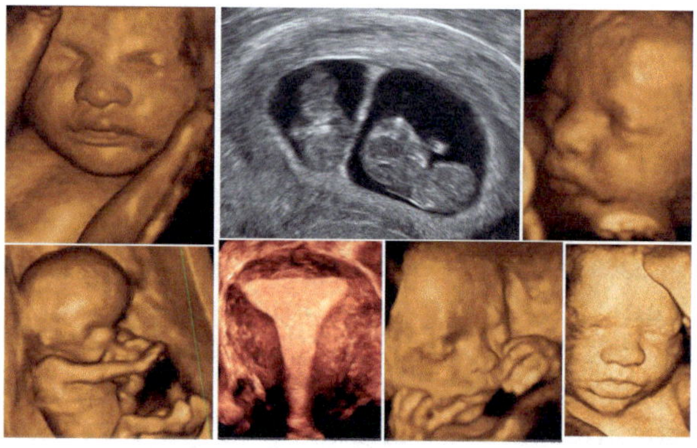

Figure 11.3. Advancements in ultrasound technology have improved image resolution and real-time monitoring capabilities, facilitating comprehensive assessments of fetal development and maternal health.

Source: https://media.vyaparify.com/vcards/blogs/114754/obstetric-colour-doppler.jpg.

Ethical Considerations in Obstetric Ultrasound

Technical advances in obstetric ultrasound have greatly enhanced prenatal care but come with complex ethical problems to be addressed with circumspection. One of the principal concerns is informed consent and how to make pregnant women fully cognizant of the purpose, benefit, and potential limitations of ultrasound scanning. Detection of anomalies, e.g., those relating to chronic hypertension, which is increasingly prevalent and impacts fetal and maternal outcomes, should be presented compassionately according to contemporary evidence in an attempt to allow decision-making and anxiety reduction. Ethical considerations are also present regarding the use of ultrasound technology for non-clinical indications, e.g., gender selection or the creation of keepsake pictures, which could detract from its clinical use. Moreover, for pandemic contexts where critical illness and conditions like COVID-19 might affect pregnancy, the health professionals are faced with the dilemma of finding a balance between required imaging and infection control, thus ensuring the safety of mother and fetus as well as ensuring fair access and ethical levels (Geoffrey *et. al.*, 2020). Careful consideration of these factors is required in order to involve ethically responsible obstetric ultrasound practice.

Future Trends in Obstetric Ultrasound

Technological innovations continue to redefine prenatal care in the promise of monumental leaps in obstetric ultrasound's prognostic and diagnostic capability. Emerging trends involve integrating machine learning (ML) algorithms for enhanced risk determination, optimized delivery planning, and better detection of fetal malformations at an early stage. These artificial intelligence tools facilitate more personalized care through processing of complex data sets, potentially anticipating complications more effectively than traditional methods (Islam *et. al.*, 2022). Additionally, ongoing research on nanomedicine and stem cell therapy directed through ultrasound imaging has the potential to revolutionize treatment of cerebral palsy, a disorder more often linked with prenatal origins recognizable by ultrasound (Paul *et. al.*, 2022). New solutions would also encompass state-of-the-art imaging techniques and clinical decision support, which will enable healthcare providers to tailor treatments efficiently and optimize neonatal care. Together, all these innovations foreshadow a future in which obstetric ultrasound is not what it currently is, but rather is an encompassing predictive instrument for prevention and therapy during pregnancy.

11.1. Types of Obstetric Ultrasound

Learning Outcome

1. Understand transabdominal and transvaginal ultrasound
2. Focus on 2D, 3D, and 4D ultrasound imaging
3. Describe Doppler ultrasound
4. Explain fetal echocardiography
5. Discuss point-of-care ultrasound
6. Give comparison of ultrasound types

Technologic advances in imaging have significantly expanded the range of obstetric ultrasound provided, enhancing the quality of prenatal care. Most commonly used, though, is still traditional two-dimensional (2D) ultrasound, providing basic anatomical details of the fetus and placenta. The three-dimensional (3D) and four-dimensional (4D) ultrasounds have added extended observation capabilities, with moving observation of fetal movement and more accurate structural assessments.

In addition, Doppler ultrasound examines fetal vessel blood flow, which is an important element for monitoring fetal health. Nowadays, fusion imaging has also been a useful tool with the integration of ultrasonography (EUS) with others like MRI in providing enhanced prenatal complex condition diagnosis as well as benign gynecopathies (Bellati *et. al.*, 2018). Not only do these developments improve diagnostic accuracy, but they also enhance multidisciplinary prenatal care to its best. Moreover, the technology is deployed in different healthcare settings, which are able to capture differences in resources and populations of patients, as have been observed in comparative studies of maternity care models (Cook *et. al.*, 2009).

11.1.1. Transabdominal Ultrasound

Prenatal care has been greatly advanced by the developments in imaging technology, making fetal evaluations more accurate and complete. Among these technologies, transabdominal ultrasound is a core non-invasive method commonly used in obstetric ultrasound to assess fetal growth and maternal well-being during pregnancy. Through the use of the transducer positioned on the abdomen, clinicians have access to real-time images that aid in monitoring fetal anatomy, placental location, and amniotic fluid levels.

This approach is very convenient according to its accessibility and adaptability in accommodating various gestational ages. Furthermore, the integration of newer point-of-care ultrasound (POCUS) machines improves the efficacy of diagnosis, enabling procedures such as neuraxial block procedures and hemodynamic assessment in complex cases (Aleshi *et. al.*, 2025). Although primarily applied in obstetrics, the basic principles of transabdominal ultrasound are identical to those applied in other organ examinations like pancreatic imaging, where intensive anatomical expertise and sequential study protocols ensure maximal diagnostic accuracy (Henker *et. al.*, 2024). The reason why transabdominal ultrasound is indispensable in prenatal diagnosis and maternal management (Figure 11.4) lies in this.

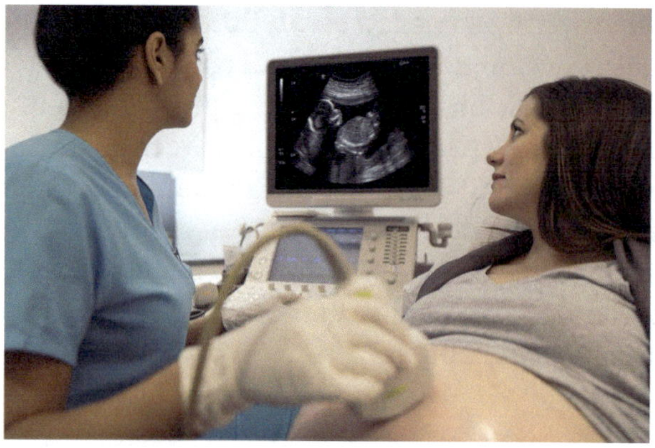

Figure 11.4. Transabdominal ultrasound.

Source: https://excelivf.com/wp-content/uploads/2023/02/What-is-the-Importance-of-Ultrasound-During-Pregnancy-Dr-Rhythm-Gupta-IVF-Doctor-Excel-IVF.jpg.

11.1.2. Transvaginal Ultrasound

Advances in imaging technology have significantly enhanced the accuracy of obstetric diagnosis, particularly with the use of transvaginal ultrasound. Transvaginal ultrasound involves the placement of an ultrasound probe within the vagina such that better images of early pregnancy structures may be obtained than with transabdominal ultrasound. It provides valuable information during the first trimester such that precise gestational age can be ascertained, ectopic pregnancy can be diagnosed, and maternal pelvic anatomy can be assessed. Also, transvaginal ultrasound offers a more comprehensive display of the cervix, which is of relevance to monitoring cervical length and preventing preterm labor. Such characteristics denote its irreplaceable role in early pregnancy management and risk stratification. The interaction with newer technology, such as fusion imaging, promises further enhancement of diagnostic accuracy with the integration of ultrasound and MRI or CT, further expanding the usage of obstetric evaluation (Bellati *et. al.*, 2018). Historically, this evolution of such ultrasound modalities owes an outstanding debt to those pioneering endeavors in the middle of the 20th century, which set the stage for modern obstetric imaging (Christie *et. al.*, 2000).

11.1.3. 2D Ultrasound Imaging

Advances in ultrasound technology have significantly enhanced prenatal care by facilitating earlier and more detailed fetal assessments. Two-dimensional ultrasound scanning plays a critical role in obstetrics, particularly the evaluation of fetal cardiac anatomy during the first trimester. Early scanning enables the identification of significant congenital heart malformations, which constitute the most common congenital abnormalities, thereby facilitating improved pregnancy management and well-informed parental decisions (Turan *et. al.*, 2020).

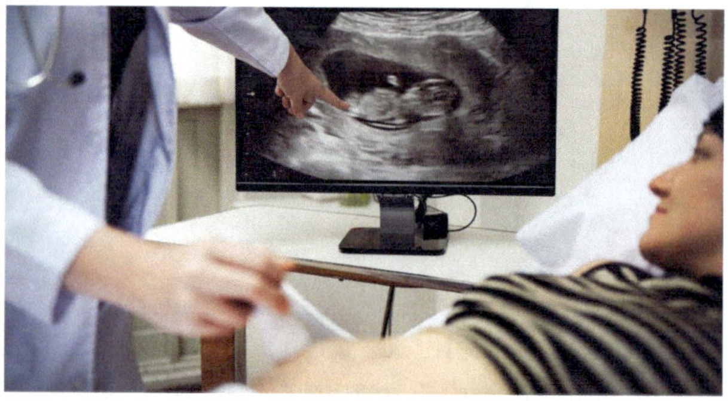

Figure 11.5. Two-dimensional ultrasound imaging plays a crucial role in obstetrics, particularly in the evaluation of fetal cardiac anatomy during the first trimester.

Source: https://www.asterhospitals.in/sites/default/files/2022-12/difference-between-anomaly-scan-and-fetal-scan.jpg.

Despite restrictions such as small fetal size and maternal body habitus, modern 2D ultrasound, especially when supplemented by color and power Doppler imaging, achieves good visualization of large cardiac structures, such as the four-chamber view and outflow tracts. Moreover, low-cost versions of 2D ultrasound have proved useful in clinical practice, being less operator dependent and finding greater use in resource-poor environments (Drews *et. al.*, 2021). Together, these developments emphasize the continuing importance of 2D ultrasound imaging as a versatile and cost-effective imaging tool in obstetric ultrasound practice (Figure 11.5).

11.1.4. 3D Ultrasound Imaging

Advances in imaging technology have revolutionized prenatal care, such that clinicians are able to access more comprehensive and accurate fetal assessment. One of the developments is 3D ultrasound imaging, where volumetric images are provided that enhance fetal anatomy visualization beyond the limitations of standard two-dimensional imaging. The technique enables detailed examination of structural deformities and spatial relationships in utero, crucial for early diagnosis and planning for congenital diseases. Furthermore, the use of cutting-edge microvascular imaging techniques, i.e., those derived from super-resolution and functional ultrasound technologies, has the possibility of contributing to improved inspection of cerebral and placental vasculature critical in fetal health monitoring and developmental disorder research (Song, 2023). In addition, advancement in ultrasound transducer technology with those employing increased bandwidth piezoelectric micromachined ultrasound transducers facilitates the provision of higher spatial resolution and image quality, allowing more precise obstetric imaging with the potential for future devices to get miniaturized and integrated (Cai *et. al.*, 2023).

11.1.5. 4D Ultrasound Imaging

Technical innovation in obstetric ultrasound has significantly enhanced prenatal diagnostic capability, and a major advance has been four-dimensional (4D) ultrasound imaging. Unlike traditional two-dimensional imaging, real-time, dynamic depiction of the fetus is provided by 4D ultrasound, encoding three-dimensional spatial and temporal alterations. With 4D ultrasound, this enables clinicians to visualize fetal motion, behavior, and anatomy with unprecedented detail, allowing earlier and more precise detection of anomalies. In addition, 4D imaging reinforces parental bonding through evocative visualizations, contributing to psychological reassurance throughout pregnancy. Nevertheless, 4D ultrasound use must be in accordance with established clinical guidelines for standardized protocols to ensure safety and diagnostic effectiveness. Operators must receive specialized training, and exams must follow documented protocols limiting informational gains while eschewing biophysical safety principles such as ALARA (As Low As Reasonably Achievable) (Caterina *et. al.*, 2023). Correct integration of 4D ultrasound into routine obstetric management demonstrates the commitment to enhancing perinatal care under the tight evidence-based practice standards (Salomon *et. al.*, 2022) (Figure 11.6).

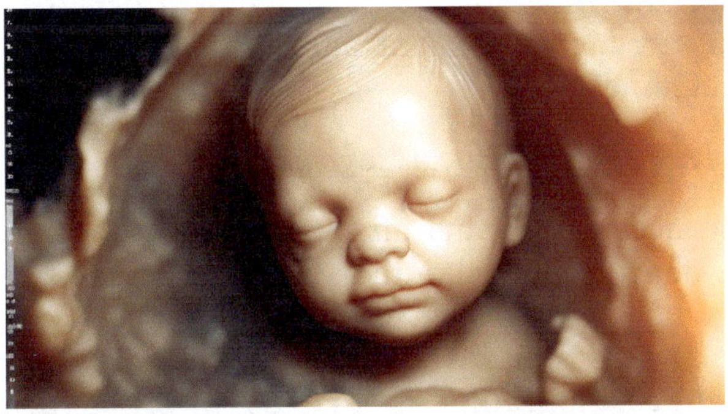

Figure 11.6. Moreover, 4D imaging offers improved parental bonding through vivid visualizations, contributing to psychological reassurance during pregnancy.

Source: https://storage.googleapis.com/msgsndr/qM4eDSgq2CZr577cFPDG/media/66485add8eb3ba7ad049785e.webp.

11.1.6. Doppler Ultrasound

Progress in obstetric imaging has transformed prenatal care, with the more accurate assessment of fetal health now being possible, a role led by Doppler ultrasound. Real-time measurement of blood flow through the umbilical artery, fetal heart, and other key vessels is possible through this technology, and it helps clinicians to assess fetal health and identify fetal growth restriction and cardiac abnormalities. Curiously, the use of Doppler ultrasound in combination with standard imaging provides complementary functional information unavailable from structural images themselves. Advances in technology, like fusion imaging, further enhance diagnostic performance by the integration of Doppler data with other modalities in order to expand vistas in obstetrically challenging cases (Bellati *et. al.*, 2018). Furthermore, careful fetal heart evaluation with Doppler imaging improved congenital heart defects in early pregnancy, despite challenges for routine screening due to variability in expertise and imaging acquisition (Tegnander *et. al.*, 2006). Consequently, Doppler ultrasound serves an important function in prenatal diagnosis to give vital information to direct management and improve perinatal outcomes.

11.1.7. Fetal Echocardiography

dvances in prenatal imaging have significantly enhanced the ability to assess fetal well-being, particularly through procedures that are not part of standard obstetric ultrasound. Fetal echocardiography is one such procedure, crucial in the early detection of congenital heart disease and in the assessment of fetal cardiac function. This modality employs high-resolution two-dimensional imaging and, more recently, advanced technology like two-dimensional speckle-tracking echocardiography (2D-STE), which enables precise quantification of global and segmental myocardial mechanics. The application of artificial intelligence (AI) in fetal echocardiography has also optimized clinical workflows by enabling less experienced operators to obtain the right functional cardiac parameters, hopefully improving diagnostic accuracy and fetal treatment outcome (Scharf *et. al.*, 2024). The increasing complexity of maternal and fetal cardiac pathology underscores the importance of standardized training routes and obstetric ultrasound critical care knowledge, underpinned by rising global demands in maternal cardiovascular care (Padilla *et. al.*, 2024). Such developments emphasize the paramount role of fetal echocardiography within overall obstetric evaluation (Figure 11.7).

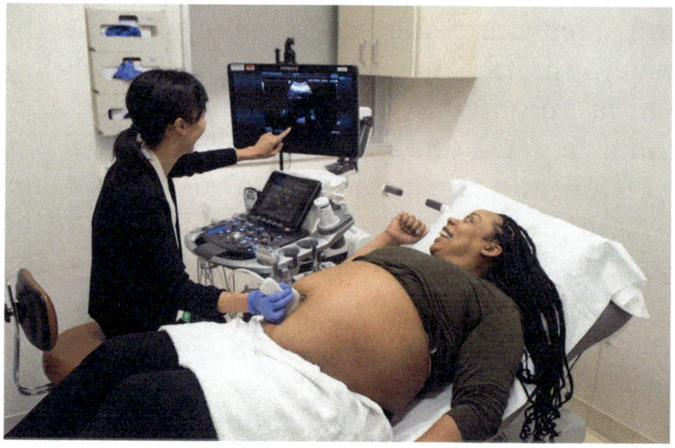

Figure 11.7. Fetal echocardiography.

Source: https://www.kidsheart.com/wp-content/uploads/2023/03/Fetal-Ad-image-scaled.jpg.

11.1.8. Point-of-care Ultrasound

The integration of POCUS into obstetric care represents a significant advance in maternal-fetal medicine, with the potential to generate bedside imaging instantly that enhances diagnostic quality and clinical decision-making. Unlike standard ultrasound techniques, which are often formalized and carried out in specialty radiology departments, POCUS allows direct, real-time visualization of fetal health and placental position at the bedside of the patient, thus allowing immediate intervention when necessary. This real-time value is particularly valuable for emergency settings and low-resource environments, optimizing outcomes through the capacity to rapidly detect complications such as fetal distress or abnormal amniotic fluid amount. The history of obstetric ultrasound is one of collaboration between clinicians and engineers, as exemplified in the pioneering work in Glasgow during the middle decades of the twentieth century, which underpinned the development of modern handheld ultrasound machines (Christie *et. al.*, 2000). In addition, advances in neonatal care have been linked directly with the evolution of diagnostic ultrasound, showing how this technological development in the specialty has keenly impacted improved perinatal outcomes.

11.1.9. Comparison of Ultrasound Types

Imaging advancements have profoundly enhanced prenatal care through diverse ultrasound techniques appropriate to individual diagnostic needs. In obstetric ultrasound, the key modalities are two-dimensional (2D), three-dimensional (3D), and Doppler ultrasound, each with its strengths and weaknesses. The traditional 2D ultrasound remains the standard for routine fetal evaluation, providing real-time images to evaluate fetal growth and anatomy. Conversely, 3D ultrasound allows precise spatial visualization of fetal anatomy, which can improve detection of congenital abnormalities and assist parental bonding by providing more realistic images. Doppler ultrasound, in turn, assesses placental and fetal circulation blood flow and is crucial in the assessment of such conditions as preterm labor, which remains a leading global health disorder (Chawanpaiboon *et. al.*, 2018). While there is a specific contribution that each modality provides to pregnancy care, collectively they enable meticulous surveillance and informed decision-making, which is consistent with the integrative approach recommended in advanced clinical guidelines such as those for polycystic ovary syndrome (Teede *et. al.*, 2018).

Test Your Knowledge

1. What is the difference between transabdominal ultrasound and transvaginal ultrasound in obstetrics?
2. When is transvaginal ultrasound typically preferred over transabdominal ultrasound in early pregnancy?

11.2. Applications of Obstetric Ultrasound

Learning Outcome

1. Perform early pregnancy assessment
2. Explain fetal growth monitoring
3. Discuss detection of fetal anomalies
4. Perform assessment of amniotic fluid levels
5. Discuss placental location and health
6. Focus on evaluation of multiple pregnancies
7. Monitor maternal health
8. Describe guidance for invasive procedures
9. Understand postnatal assessment

Medical technological innovations have hugely expanded the scope of diagnostic tools that can be utilized during prenatal care, with obstetric ultrasound having been a pivot in this advancement. It is now applied beyond mere fetal visualization, leveraging ML and AI to enhance the prediction, diagnosis, and management of complex obstetric conditions such as gestational diabetes, pre-eclampsia, and fetal growth restriction. These intelligent devices facilitate automatic detection of fetal abnormalities and provide essential information on fetoplacental and cervical function, which further promotes clinical decision-making and maternal-fetal safety during pregnancy and parturition (Arain *et. al.*, 2023). Further, ultrasound is the keystone of fetal biometry measurement, like the measurement of isolated second-trimester small head circumference, which yields prognosis and guides individualized prenatal care. Subdivision by ultrasound findings allows individualized follow-up approaches and indicates the importance of adding genetic testing and specialist referral when indicated (Diderich *et. al.*, 2024). This comprehensive use underscores obstetric ultrasound's transformative place in maternal-fetal medicine.

11.2.1. Early Pregnancy Assessment

Imaging technologies have significantly impacted prenatal care, particularly during early pregnancy when correct assessment is critical for fetal well-being. Obstetric ultrasound plays a pivotal role in early pregnancy assessment through enabling visualization of embryonic anatomy and detection of abnormalities before clinical symptoms arise. One of the more important applications is screening for chromosomal disorders such as Downs syndrome, where accurate imaging of fetal intracranial anatomy, including the Nuchal

Translucency, is critical diagnostic information. Enhancements in deep learning algorithms have made interpretation more accurate and faster from these ultrasounds, with performance on a par with human experts when trained on early risk stratification (Reshi *et. al.*, 2024). Additionally, novel techniques such as contrast-enhanced ultrasound offer promising possibilities for the investigation of placental vascularization that is key to surveillance of placental insufficiency and potential pregnancy complications. Current evidence also supports the safety of these new imaging modalities during human pregnancies, highlighting their growing role in detailed early pregnancy assessments (Dassen *et. al.*, 2024) (Figure 11.8).

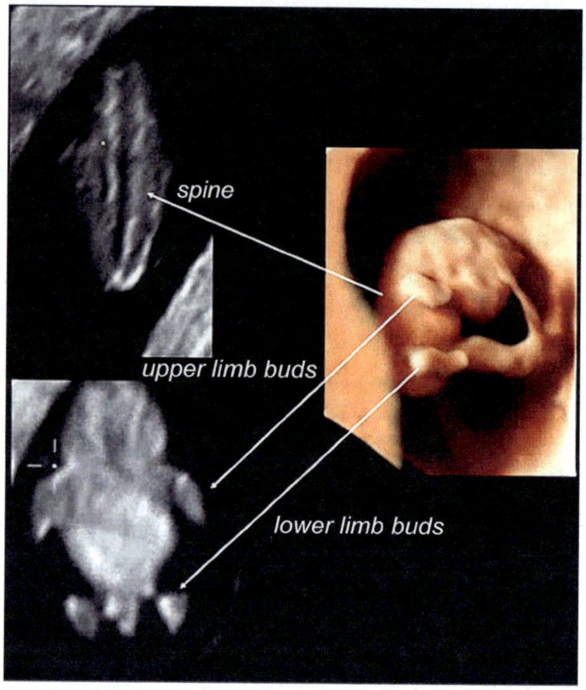

Figure 11.8. Obstetric ultrasound plays a pivotal role in early pregnancy assessment by enabling the visualization of embryonic structures and the detection of anomalies before clinical symptoms arise.

Source: https://images-glowm.cms.ama.uk.com/img/Obstetrics-V18-C02-17.jpg.

11.2.2. Fetal Growth Monitoring

Effective fetal growth surveillance is crucial in the detection of pregnancies at risk for intrauterine growth restriction (IUGR), a significant reason for perinatal mortality and morbidity. Advances in obstetric ultrasound technology have enabled the routine evaluation of fetal growth parameters, which can be useful in the early detection of aberrant growth patterns. Controversy continues to exist about the utility of routine third-trimester EUS in improving perinatal outcomes. Recent large trials, such as randomized controlled trials of routine versus indicated ultrasound, aim to determine whether systematic imaging is associated with fewer serious adverse events by permitting early clinical intervention (Bosmans *et. al.*, 2016). Despite the promise of these technologies, evidence directly demonstrating a reduction in stillbirth rates is scarce, since most methods of monitoring have unacceptably high false-positive rates without clear protocols for management in the subsequent steps (Bhutta *et. al.*, 2009). Therefore, merging fetal growth surveillance with effective clinical response systems is essential to improve its effectiveness in obstetric practice and reduce perinatal hazards.

11.2.3. Detection of Fetal Anomalies

Advances in obstetric ultrasound have far enhanced the capability for detection of fetal anomalies, making it possible to diagnose earlier and more confidently, which is crucial in prenatal diagnosis. Polyhydramnios, or the excessive accumulation of amniotic fluid, is one of the leading signs of anomaly scanning and has been very diagnostic in the detection of congenital fetal anomalies in standard scans. Research indicates that polyhydramnios is highly sensitive and specific with over 90% accuracy, thus proving to be an effective sonographic marker for further detailed evaluation (Mohsin *et. al.*, 2023).

In addition, more advanced parameters such as computerized myocardial performance index of the fetal right ventricle provide additional insight into cardiac function, differentiating between normal and affected fetuses due to maternal diabetes that may result in cardiac malformations (Ding *et. al.*, 2024). Together, these ultrasound modalities enable complete fetal evaluation, optimizing risk stratification and facilitating early intervention. The overlap of fluid assessment and cardiac functional testing demonstrates the multi-faceted contribution of obstetric ultrasound to fetal anomaly scanning (Figure 11.9).

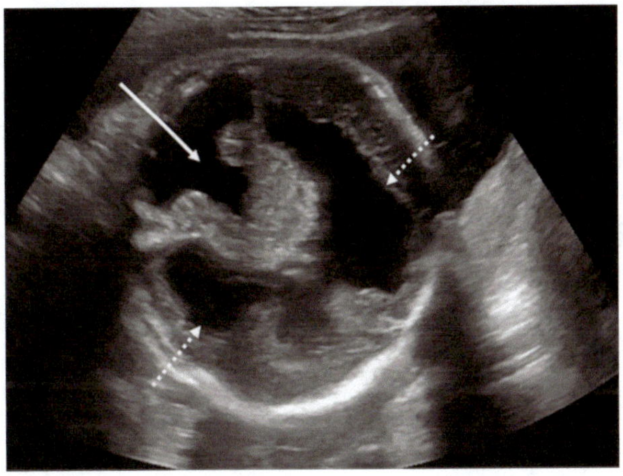

Figure 11.9. One important indicator utilized in anomaly detection is polyhydramnios, the excessive accumulation of amniotic fluid, which has demonstrated substantial diagnostic accuracy in identifying congenital fetal anomalies during routine scans.

Source: https://pubs.rsna.org/cms/10.1148/rg.220146/asset/images/medium/rg.220146.fig16.gif.

11.2.4. Assessment of Amniotic Fluid Levels

Accurate measurement of amniotic fluid volume is a critical component of prenatal care, both because it has direct implications for fetal well-being and because it guides clinical management. Obstetric ultrasound provides a safe, effective means of evaluating this volume, most frequently by using the amniotic fluid index (AFI) or single deepest pocket. These measurements enable identification of abnormal oligohydramnios or polyhydramnios that may suggest fetal or placental pathology. Current research emphasizes the importance of using locally generated reference values as traditional international nomograms may fail to express population-based variability, potentially leading to misdiagnosis and unnecessary interventions (Ignatov *et. al.*, 2024). Furthermore, POCUS advances facilitate quicker and more accessible evaluation with more real-time clinical management in maternal pathology with hemodynamic changes according to amniotic fluid volume (Aleshi *et. al.*, 2025). Therefore, amniotic fluid evaluation protocols are refined by incorporating population-derived data and embracing new ultrasound technologies, which largely enhances prenatal surveillance and outcomes.

11.2.5. Placental Location and Health

Proper placental position determination during pregnancy is important to maternal and fetal health because improper positioning can lead to placenta previa or abruption complications that are of high risk during delivery. Ultrasound of the obstetric aspect is very essential in the detection of placental positioning early to enable early interventions to prevent bad outcomes.

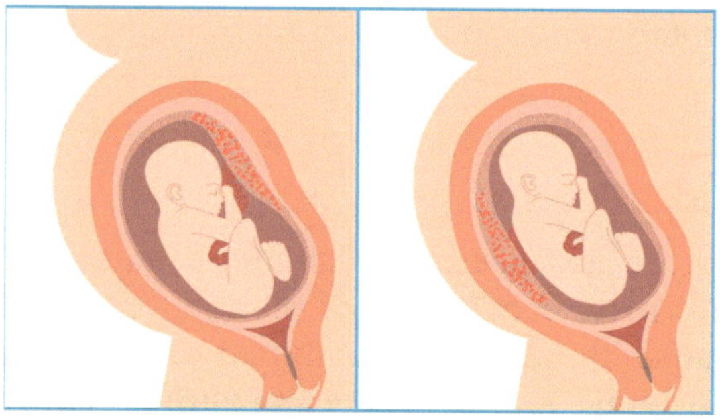

Figure 11.10. Obstetric ultrasound plays a pivotal role in identifying placental positioning early, facilitating timely interventions to mitigate adverse outcomes.

Source: https://cdn-prod.medicalnewstoday.com/content/images/articles/324/324554/anterior-placenta-illustration.jpg.

Despite its importance, the appropriate application of ultrasound in determining placental health is often undermined by inadequate training and limited facilities among clinicians, which has been attested by family medicine residents with low self-efficacy and limited practice in performing obstetric ultrasounds (Albadi *et. al.*, 2024). In addition, disparities in access to good-quality antenatal ultrasound services can affect uniformity of placental surveillance, dictating health rights and maternal outcomes in different locations (Suarayasa *et. al.*, 2024). Therefore, upgrading ultrasound training and implementing placental assessment protocols is a critical step towards improving prenatal care and safeguarding maternal-fetal health (Figure 11.10).

11.2.6. Evaluation of Multiple Pregnancies

Accurate assessment during early pregnancy is crucial to optimize outcomes, especially in multiple gestations. Determination of chorionicity and amnionicity during the early first trimester is significant for clinical management and anticipatory guidance of impending complications. EUS is the optimal modality for determining these parameters by establishment of the number of gestational sacs and presence or absence of dividing membranes, as they have direct implications on risk stratification. Furthermore, early diagnosis allows confirmation of viability and makes subsequent monitoring appropriately individualized based on the individual needs of multifetal pregnancies. Lack of proper diagnosis of chorionicity can lead to improper monitoring and increased morbidity. Systematic ultrasound evaluation through predetermined protocols, thus, ensures adequate evaluation, i.e., confirmation of number of embryos, viability, and morphological intactness, and directs future management plans. These recommendations are current expert advice and emphasize the importance of first-trimester ultrasound expertise in managing the complexities of multiple gestations (Caterina *et. al.*, 2023; Salomon *et. al.*, 2022).

11.2.7. Monitoring Maternal Health

Advanced diagnostic techniques have upgraded the maternal health surveillance during pregnancy to a high degree, significantly enhancing prenatal care. Obstetric ultrasound is one of them, a non-invasive real-time imaging technology that has played an important role in providing vital information on fetal development and maternal well-being. The intersection of AI instruments and ML with ultrasound has strengthened the capability to predict and diagnose obstetric conditions such as pre-eclampsia, gestational diabetes, and fetal growth restriction by analyzing enormous sets of data from electronic health records and imaging reports (Arain *et. al.*, 2023). These developments not only increase fetal anomaly detection sensitivity but also facilitate the assessment of fetoplacental function, essential to optimizing maternal and fetal outcome. Trends in diagnostic imaging during the past highlight sustained interest in enhancing maternal health surveillance, consistent with trends in enhancing neonatal and perinatal care. Hence, obstetric ultrasound is an important component of total surveillance of maternal welfare in modern-day obstetrics (Figure 11.11).

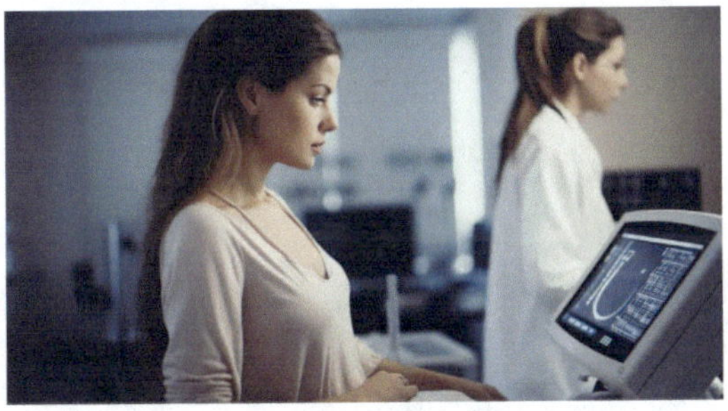

Figure 11.11. Obstetric ultrasound stands out as a non-invasive, real-time imaging modality that provides critical insights into fetal development and maternal well-being.

Source: https://ris.com.au/wp-content/uploads/2024/04/ULTRA-SOUND.webp.

11.2.8. Guidance for Invasive Procedures

The use of advanced imaging modalities has significantly enhanced the security and accuracy of invasive obstetric procedures, such as ultrasound. It delivers real-time imaging that allows doctors to guide needles into guiding amniocentesis and chorionic villus sampling more precisely, minimizing the risks to mother and fetus. Greater use of simulation workshops has also improved procedure training efficiency, as evidenced by highly rated courses providing needle guidance basics augmented with procedure-specific practice to overcome the problem of reduced clinical experience due to progressing diagnostic technologies (Codsi *et. al.*, 2022). This method of learning ensures that practitioners remain skilled, regardless of falling procedural volumes. In addition, ultrasound's capability to identify anatomical structures and detect potential complications—e.g., neurovascular injury during musculoskeletal interventions—demonstrates its use in numerous invasive environments (Paczesny *et. al.*, 2023). Consequently, ultrasound-guided injections become a versatile resource that enhances procedural success while safeguarding patient outcomes in obstetrics.

11.2.9. Postnatal Assessment

Neonatal health following delivery is a significant component of integrated obstetric care since it provides useful information about the current health of the newborn and any complications that should be intervened. Postnatal assessment, informed by experience acquired via obstetric ultrasound, facilitates earlier identification of fetal distress or hypoxia that could have persisted into the neonatal period. Doppler EUS techniques, which were used for years prenatally to assess fetal and placental blood circulation, yield valuable parameters with postnatal correlations, including the measurement of blood flow in critical vessels like the umbilical and cerebral arteries (Indira *et. al.*, 2022). The ability to image and interpret these hemodynamic markers enhances clinical decision-making and guides neonatal management. Furthermore, advancement of technology in ultrasound image quality and ML-enhanced improvement is set to enhance postnatal assessment so that precise interpretation of subtle physiological abnormalities during this critical period can be accomplished (Pegios *et. al.*, 2024) (Figure 11.12).

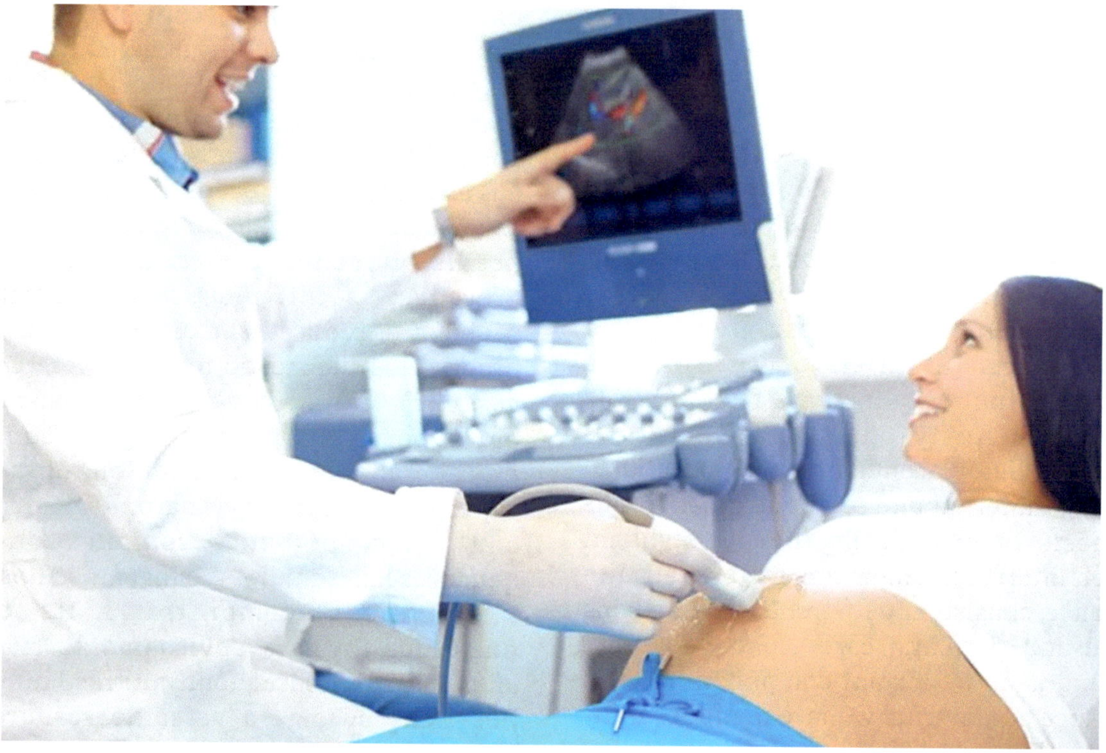

Figure 11.12. Doppler ultrasonography techniques.

Source: https://cdn.cdnparenting.com/articles/2017/11/218566381-H-768x525.webp.

Test Your Knowledge

1. What is the primary application of early pregnancy ultrasound (6–9 weeks gestation)?
2. How is obstetric ultrasound used to assess fetal viability in the first trimester?

11.3. Benefits and Limitations of Obstetric Ultrasound

Learning Outcome

1. Explain non-invasive nature of ultrasound
2. Focus on real-time imaging capabilities
3. Learn safety profile of ultrasound
4. Discuss limitations in accuracy and interpretation
5. Know potential for false positives/negatives
6. Understand accessibility and cost considerations
7. Know emotional impact on expectant parents
8. Focus on training and expertise of ultrasound technicians
9. Learn ethical concerns regarding fetal imaging

Advances in prenatal care have been greatly boosted by the use of obstetric ultrasound, which gives useful information regarding fetal anatomy, pattern of growth, and development. Obstetric ultrasound is a non-invasive technique that enables early detection of structural anomalies, assessment of fetal well-being, and estimation of gestational age, all critical for decision-making and improved perinatal outcomes (Salomon *et. al.*, 2022). Furthermore, ultrasound enables monitoring of complications like growth restriction of the fetus, a major underlying reason for stillbirth and neonatal morbidity, by using measurements like estimated fetal weight and Doppler studies to assess placental function (Melamed *et. al.*, 2021). Despite its widespread use, obstetric ultrasound has its limitations, foremost among them being variation in detection rates depending on the quality of equipment and operator experience. False positives and false negatives, especially in discriminating between growth-restricted and small for gestational age fetuses, cause diagnostic challenges. Additionally, utilizing specific reference charts and interpretative nature of the majority of findings underscore the importance of standardized algorithms and prolonged training in a bid to maximize its benefit with a minimum of potential risks (Melamed *et. al.*, 2021; Salomon *et. al.*, 2022).

11.3.1. Non-invasive Nature of Ultrasound

The evolution of methods of diagnosis in obstetrics has been concerned with patient safety and comfort, and the worth of techniques minimally risky and maximally diagnostic has been emphasized. Ultrasound embodies these values in being inherently non-invasive, giving in real-time a visual representation of fetal development without incision or exposure to ionizing radiation.

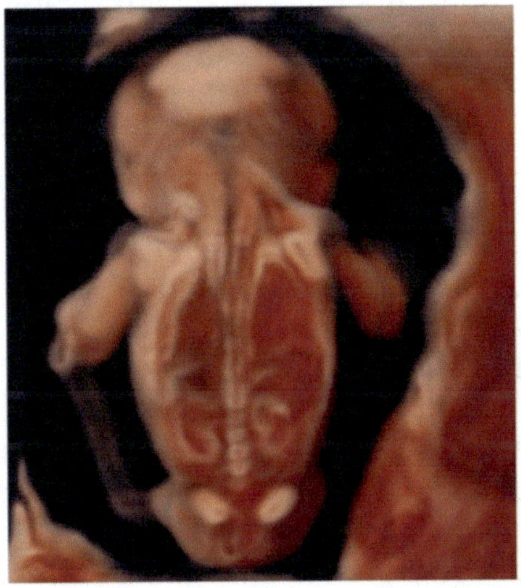

Figure 11.13. Ultrasound embodies these ideals through its inherently non-invasive nature, allowing for real-time visualization of fetal development without the need for incisions or exposure to ionizing radiation.

Source: https://ars.els-cdn.com/content/image/1-s2.0-S1084952122000623-gr3.jpg.

This feature not only reduces body harm but also alleviates psychological distress in pregnant women, making the imaging procedure more repeatable and accessible in pregnancy. Other newer technologies, such as Fusion Imaging, enhance traditional ultrasound by coupling it with modalities including MRI and CT, enhancing diagnostic accuracy without compromising non-invasiveness in obstetric evaluation (Bellati *et. al.*, 2018). These advances ensure that high-level prenatal screening and monitoring can be achieved with minimal risk, and this is a critical concern in maternal-fetal medicine (Stefanovic *et. al.*, 2020). Thus, the non-invasive nature of ultrasound remains at the center of its global use and continued progress in obstetric practice (Figure 11.13).

11.3.2. Real-time Imaging Capabilities

The evolution of obstetric ultrasound has been significantly influenced by technological advancements that allow real-time monitoring of the fetus during pregnancy. The earliest ultrasound machinery was largely static in imaging, which limited diagnosis and also led to delayed clinical decision-making. However, the introduction of real-time imaging revolutionized the assessment of the fetus by allowing real-time imaging of fetal movement, cardiac function, and blood flow, thereby enhancing diagnostic sensitivity and prenatal care. This capacity was the product of the union of clinical acumen and engineering innovation, specifically in the joint effort under Professor Ian Donald's direction in Glasgow during the mid-twentieth century, where practical demonstration of the first scanners convinced clinicians that the technology was valuable (Christie *et. al.*, 2000). Therefore, real-time imaging is a strict requirement in everyday obstetric practice, with early detection of defects and intervention, highlighting its central role in modern fetal medicine (Nicholson *et. al.*, 2003).

11.3.3. Safety Profile of Ultrasound

The employment of obstetric ultrasound has revolutionized prenatal care by providing valuable information regarding fetal development and the health of the mother. While normally safe since it is non-ionizing, there is a continuous need to review its safety profile to avoid any negative effects related to long-term or repeated exposure. The ultrasound process uses sound waves to generate images, avoiding harmful radiation used in other modalities, which significantly explains its favorable safety profile. Nevertheless, operators have to adhere to regulations for safe use, most importantly the planning of an ultrasound during pregnancy, which is emphasized in the emerging paradigm of healthcare and public health such as the COVID-19 pandemic (Bellussi *et. al.*, 2020). Moreover, accessibility and affordability issues influenced by healthcare policy, such as the Medicare Safety Net, drive the level to which services for ultrasound are utilized and monitored, indirectly influencing safety outcomes by stimulating appropriate application among diverse groups (Savage *et. al.*, 2025) (Figure 11.14).

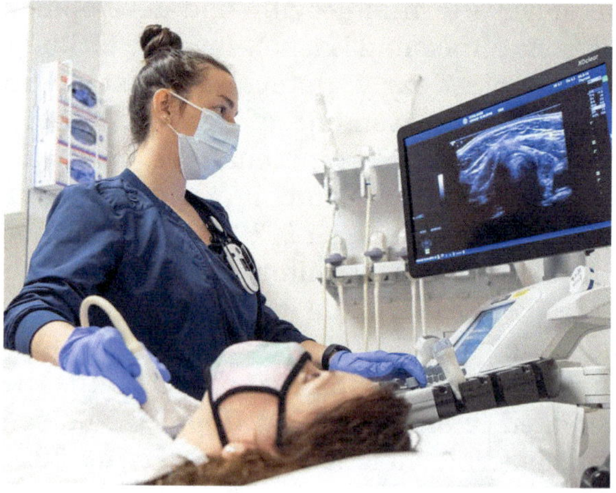

Figure 11.14. The ultrasound procedure uses sound waves to create images, avoiding the harmful radiation present in other imaging techniques, which significantly contributes to its favorable safety profile.

Source: https://my.clevelandclinic.org/-/scassets/images/org/health/articles/4995-ultrasound-imaging.

11.3.4. Limitations in Accuracy and Interpretation

In spite of great progress in obstetric ultrasound technology, inherent limitations in accuracy and interpretation continue to be a paramount issue impacting diagnostic reliability and clinical decision-making. Variability in image quality and measurement accuracy due to factors like operator expertise, fetal position, and maternal body habitus may cause inconsistencies in the detection of structural abnormalities or fetal growth monitoring (Salomon *et. al.*, 2022). Moreover, subjective judgment and interpretation bias can influence the assessment of subtle findings, leading to high risk of false positives or false negatives. Although new approaches such as deep learning present promising directions for advancing image analysis and standardizing assessments, low imaging quality issues and variability remain to keep automated and objective evaluations from being fully accepted (Liu *et. al.*, 2019). Thus, even though obstetric ultrasound is very valuable, practitioners must be mindful of its limitations and place findings in the context of overall clinical experience, employing adjunctive diagnostic modalities as necessary.

11.3.5. Potential for False Positives/Negatives

Although there has been technical advancement in imaging, obstetric ultrasound is not immune to diagnostic mistakes in the form of false positives and false negatives, which can significantly affect clinical decision-making.

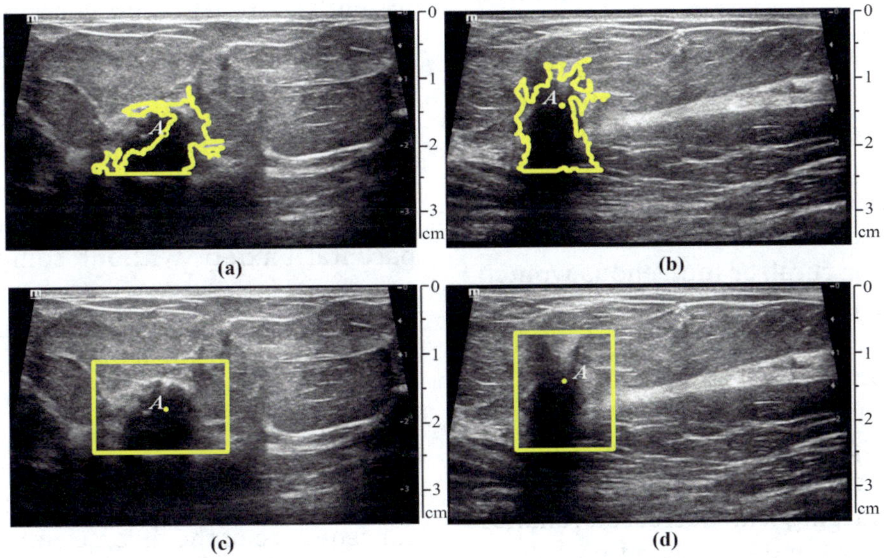

Figure 11.15. MaskFormer has shown promising reductions in false results in breast lesion segmentation.

Source: https://www.mdpi.com/sensors/sensors-25-01593/article_deploy/html/images/sensors-25-01593-g008.png.

These are facilitated by operator experience, fetal lie, and technical limitations of the apparatus and result in incorrect diagnosis or unnecessary intervention. Ultrasound application outside obstetrics has been the subject of research, and similar problems have been reported;

for instance, ultrasound's low sensitivity for detecting subtle pathologies has been noted, and staggering false-positive and false-negative rates against MRI, a more precise imaging exam (Mocanu *et. al.*, 2025). Moreover, recent work in combining AI models like MaskFormer has optimistically decreased false outcomes in breast lesion segmentation, suggesting that similar technology could improve the diagnostic capacity of obstetric ultrasound by minimizing human error and imaging interpretation (Anand *et. al.*, 2024). Elimination of the potential for false results remains central to maximizing clinical utility and obstetric ultrasound outcomes (Figure 11.15).

11.3.6. Accessibility and Cost Considerations

Health disparities usually manifest as limited access to essential diagnostic tools such as obstetric ultrasound, particularly among remote or underserved communities. Geographic remoteness and economic means usually are key determinants of profoundly limiting access to timely ultrasounds, with adverse prenatal care and health outcomes ensuing. Evidence has indicated that poor, rural, or Indigenous women have lower rates of access to second-trimester ultrasound scans, and this has identified structural barriers present in the provision of healthcare within these environments (Adams *et. al.*, 2021). Disparities may be overcome by innovations like telerobotic ultrasound, which enables remote imaging with decreased reliance on patient transport and associated cost. This approach, in addition to increasing access, reduces the economic burden on healthcare systems and patients. In addition, the availability of equipment and clinician proficiency influence the proper use of ultrasound modalities, as seen in obstetric anesthetic practice, where the restricted availability of ultrasound leads to procedural suboptimization in high-risk patients, including obese parturients (Loebig *et. al.*, 2020). All of these emphasize that overcoming cost and accessibility barriers is crucial towards enhancing quality and equity of obstetric ultrasound services.

11.3.7. Emotional Impact on Expectant Parents

The experience of undergoing an obstetric ultrasound possesses the potential to strongly influence the emotional well-being of expectant parents and is often found to form an attachment to the unborn baby. To view the baby is more frequent in order to raise parental attachment, which can have positive effects on maternal health behaviors and the parent-infant relationship following birth. But this process is not complication-free; the presentation of unforeseen or unclear results while scanning can induce immense distress. Sensing the emotional weight inherent within such situations, recent initiatives have stressed the need for sensitive and transparent communication on the part of ultrasound professionals. Recommendations include employing honest terminology in conjunction with explanations that are accessible to parents in order to alleviate parental anxiety without compromising their emotional needs. Moreover, such suggestions debar the pressure of expectant parents into making hurried decisions during the scan, in favor of a comforting environment that enables working through emotionally. In consideration of these advances, further studies are imperative to identify reliably effective interventions in consequence of the diverse emotional responses of mothers and fathers equally throughout obstetric ultrasound (Cunen *et. al.*, 2016; Harley-Roberts *et. al.*, 2020).

11.3.8. Training and Expertise of Ultrasound Technicians

The proficiency of the ultrasound technician is a critical factor in the accuracy and dependability of obstetric ultrasound imaging. The development of proficiency requires comprehensive training encompassing not only the technical operation of ultrasound equipment but also extensive study in the anatomy and development of the fetus. Extensive training enables sonographers to differentiate between normal and pathologic conditions precisely. In addition, professional education is essential due to continuous technical advancements in ultrasonics machines and clinical practices. Under resource- and formally trained personnel-limited facilities, newer methods such as unsupervised learning algorithms have the potential to aid lesser-trained sonographers by maximizing image interpretation rates, as noted in pulmonary ultrasonography assessment (Akhbardeh *et. al.*, 2023). However, the fundamental skills acquired through formal education and clinical exposure remain crucial for effective obstetric ultrasound practice, underlining the necessity of intense training for ultrasound technicians (Nicholson *et. al.*, 2003) (Figure 11.16).

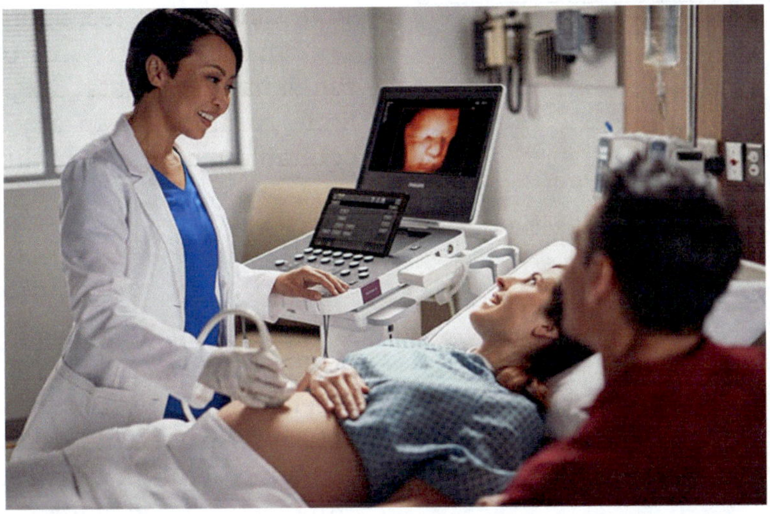

Figure 11.16. The proficiency of ultrasound technicians is a critical factor in the accuracy and reliability of obstetric ultrasound imaging.

Source: https://www.philips.com/c-dam/corporate/newscenter/global/standard/resources/healthcare/2023/isuog2023/philips-compact-5000-ob-gyn-in-use.jpg.

11.3.9. Ethical Concerns Regarding Fetal Imaging

Improved technology in obstetric ultrasound has transformed prenatal care in the form of more detailed information on fetal growth, but the advances bring abysmally difficult ethical challenges. One major challenge is how to balance respect for pregnant women's autonomy with beneficence, particularly when routine scanning can lead to overmedicalization and unwanted worry. Informed consent is complex as patients must understand not only the medical indication of imaging but also potential psychological and social impact, especially when results guide pregnancy continuation (Favaretto *et. al.*, 2024). Further, fetal imaging through AI is offering the prospect of improved diagnosis but raises issues of responsibility, data privacy, and equal access, highlighting the need for stringent regulation to prevent error or abuse (Tonni *et. al.*, 2024). These ethical considerations underscore the importance of good communication and policy-making to make technological progress in obstetric ultrasound serve both medical and social responsibilities without compromising patient autonomy.

Test Your Knowledge

1. How does obstetric ultrasound help in early detection of fetal abnormalities and birth defects?
2. What are the advantages of using ultrasound for gestational dating and determining due dates compared to other methods?

11.4. Technological Advancements in Obstetric Ultrasound

Learning Outcome

1. Understand innovations in imaging technology
2. Explain integration of artificial intelligence
3. Focus on improvements in image resolution
4. Discuss development of portable ultrasound devices
5. Learn enhanced software for analysis
6. Discuss telemedicine applications in obstetrics
7. Describe future research directions
8. Know impact of technology on prenatal care
9. Explain global disparities in access to ultrasound technology

Medical technology has significantly transformed obstetric ultrasound with new developments, both by increasing diagnostic precision and also the efficiency of clinical procedures. AI integration into ultrasound machines enables advanced analysis of images, providing enhanced fetal development and abnormality monitoring with greater accuracy. Such AI technologies aid clinicians by performing gestational age measurement and fetal malpresentation identification automatically, necessary for early treatment and improved maternal-fetal outcomes (Moses *et. al.*, 2024). Furthermore, ML algorithms allow for real-time interpretation of data, reducing the dependence on operators and increasing access to high-quality prenatal care, especially in low-resource settings. Despite these advances, ethical considerations regarding data privacy, informed consent, and transparent algorithmic decision-making remain critical to ensure responsible deployment (Karalis, 2024). With developing technological inventions, the combination of AI with obstetric ultrasound can enhance prenatal diagnostics to its utmost limit, resulting in an era of personalized and equitable maternal healthcare worldwide.

11.4.1. Innovations in Imaging Technology

Advances in medical imaging have revolutionized the power of diagnosis across numerous specialties, and obstetrics has been a significant field to have been shaped by them. The addition of high-resolution ultrasound equipment has enhanced the visualization of fetal details and accuracy, making it possible to detect fetal developmental defects earlier and more accurately. Technological advancements such as contrast-enhanced ultrasound have increased the diagnostic potential by providing detailed vascular data, which is critical in the assessment of placental well-being and fetal well-being (Shi *et. al.*, 2025).

In addition, the use of AI and ML algorithms has also improved image processing and interpretation, and hence analysis of complex data sets has become faster and accurate (Krishnarao *et. al.*, 2025). These developments complement tailored prenatal care by allowing timely intervention and more rational clinical decisions. Despite these advances, challenges in maximizing imaging sensitivity and harmoniously fusing multi-modal data remain to further enhance obstetric ultrasound's diagnostic promise, which still harbors encouraging directions for further research and clinical application (Figure 11.17).

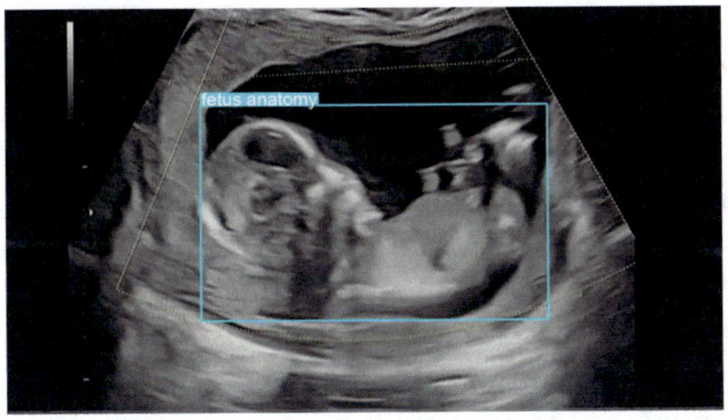

Figure 11.17. Innovations such as contrast-enhanced ultrasound have expanded the diagnostic potential by providing detailed vascular information, which is critical in assessing placental health and fetal well-being.

Source: https://miro.medium.com/v2/resize:fit:2000/1*0Pfft3-F_JzPUbHBWVtFeg.png.

11.4.2. Integration of Artificial Intelligence

The development of technology has constantly transformed clinical practices, and AI is one such very important aspect in enhancing medical diagnostics and patient treatment. In the field of obstetric ultrasound, the employment of AI offers sufficient progress by making complex image analysis automatic and facilitating more precise evaluation of fetal development, placental health, and other important parameters.

These technologies facilitate preterm identification of congenital abnormalities and enhanced prediction of adverse pregnancy outcomes required to optimize maternal-fetal management. Obstetric imaging using AI-driven equipment not only streamlines the diagnostic process but also enhances availability where resources are scarce, potentially reducing inequality in antenatal care. More importantly, the ethical implications involving confidentiality of data, consent, and disclosure must be managed with extreme care as AI solutions take larger strides. Overall, AI's incorporation into obstetric ultrasound represents a promising convergence of technology and healthcare aimed at improving clinical outcomes and decision-making processes (Horgan *et. al.*, 2023; Karalis, 2024).

11.4.3. Improvements in Image Resolution

Technical advances in obstetric ultrasound have significantly enhanced fetal anatomy visualization in clearer and more precise forms. Initial issues of image resolution had a tendency to restrict diagnostic precision, but implementation of sophisticated signal processing techniques such as tissue harmonic imaging and spatial compounding has significantly increased spatial and contrast resolution and thus enabled more reliable evaluation of fetal structures. These technological innovations allow for better quality real-time sweeps rather than two-dimensional static images, greatly enhancing normal fetal cardiac anatomy and flow dynamics detection rates. Furthermore, the shift from conventional two-dimensional imaging to three-dimensional and four-dimensional ultrasound has provided unprecedented volume rendering capability, enabling extensive examination of external malformations and vascular reconstructions. Imaging support technologies like STIC and volume contrast imaging enable improved visualization of dynamic and complex structures, transforming fetal evaluation by enhancing image quality as well as diagnostic certainty in routine prenatal care (Sammet *et. al.*, 2010; Stewart *et. al.*, 2005) (Figure 11.18).

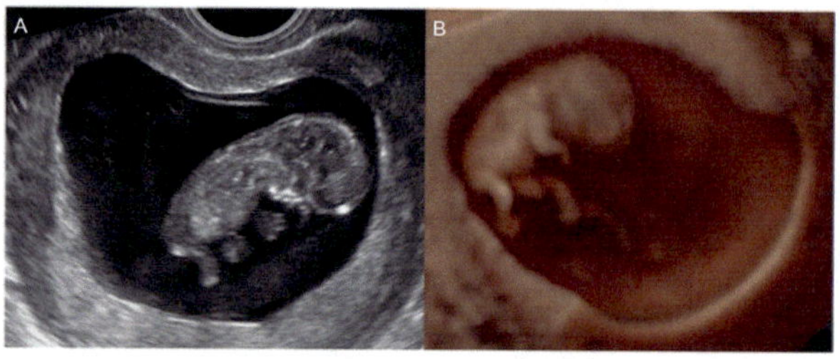

Figure 11.18. Advancements in obstetric ultrasound have profoundly enhanced the ability to visualize fetal anatomy with greater clarity and precision.

Source: https://ars.els-cdn.com/content/image/1-s2.0-S1084952122000623-gr2.jpg.

11.4.4. Development of Portable Ultrasound Devices

Advances in medical imaging have more and more transformed the practice of medicine, particularly in obstetrics, where immediate fetal assessment is of utmost importance. The development of handheld ultrasound machines has been a major achievement, bridging the gap between the large, older machines and the need for cheap, immediate diagnosis technology. Small, usually handheld units can be connected to a smartphone or tablet and deployed at the point of care in different settings outside the hospital. Current data indicate that portable ultrasound devices provide equivalence in consistency and accuracy with fixed equipment in the evaluation of significant obstetric factors such as fetal size, cardiac function, and placental location (Plöger *et. al.*, 2024). Their mobility provides additional flexibility in prenatal care, delivering exemplary benefits in both limited-resource and regular clinical settings. Besides this, application of new technologies like AI and augmented reality suggests ongoing potential for enhancing diagnostic accuracy and increasing useful applications in obstetrics as well as ancillary fields (Das *et. al.*, 2024).

11.4.5. Enhanced Software for Analysis

Enhanced technology for obstetric ultrasound in recent years has been significantly accelerated by advancements in more advanced analysis software that allows for more precise interpretation of fetal measurements and greater diagnostic potential. Advanced algorithms within ultrasound equipment enable total measurement of such critical parameters as thigh circumference, biparietal diameter, and abdominal circumference, resulting in a more precise estimation of fetal weight than previous clinical methods. This technology development not only mechanizes data analysis but also facilitates large-scale training programs that improve theoretical knowledge as well as practical skills among sonologists effectively, as seen in increased performance following formal instruction courses (Abuhamad *et. al.*, 2019).

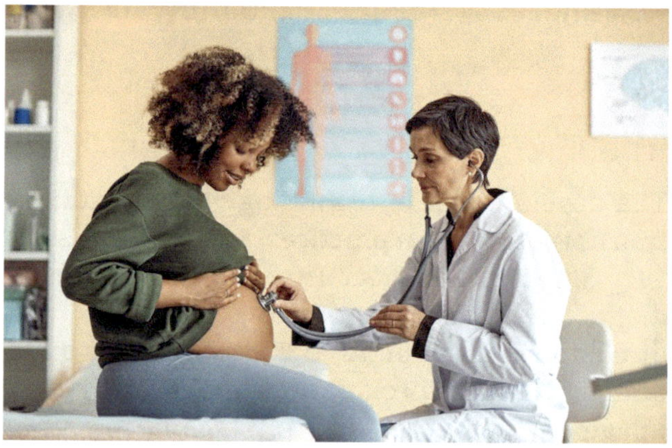

Figure 11.19. Innovative algorithms integrated into ultrasound systems enable the detailed assessment of critical parameters such as thigh circumference, biparietal diameter, and abdominal circumference, contributing to more reliable fetal weight estimations compared to traditional clinical methods.

Source: https://www.cyient.com/hubfs/shutterstock_2417854505.jpg.

In addition, newer software can merge multiple biometric inputs to produce precise predictive models, increasing the correlation between estimated and actual fetal weights and hence enabling more effective clinical decision-making (Hebbar *et. al.*, 2005). All this illustrates the pivotal function of advanced analytical tools in optimizing obstetric ultrasound findings and patient care (Figure 11.19).

11.4.6. Telemedicine Applications in Obstetrics

Advances in technology have significantly expanded the ambit of prenatal care through remote access to requisite health services, with telemedicine being most prominent among these. Telemedicine services in obstetrics have enabled monitoring and timely intervention for expectant women, especially those in underserved or distant locations. Recent studies recognize the revolutionary character of tele-obstetric platforms that not only provide educational resources tailored to the specific needs of the individual patient but also integrate real-time data from wearable technology to optimize fetal and maternal outcomes. Concurrently, the development of handheld ultrasound scanners connected to smartphones and tablets revolutionized bedside fetal evaluation by offering stable imaging that rivals conventional equipment (Plöger *et. al.*, 2024). These point-of-care technologies enhance fetal weight, cardiac activity, and placental evaluation diagnostic accuracy over logistic and geographical barriers to care. Together, telemedicine and point-of-care ultrasound systems represent a paradigm shift in obstetric ultrasound to promote equitable, accessible, and individualized prenatal care in diverse patient populations.

11.4.7. Future Research Directions

Advancements in technology continue to transform the world of obstetric ultrasound, encouraging significant exploration of potential new areas of investigation that can enhance diagnostic rates and maternal-fetal management. One such area is the application of AI to improve ultrasound imaging, enabling more accurate and early detection of conditions such as preterm labor. AI methods, including ML models and deep learning techniques, have been highly promising in interpreting complex patterns of data and providing individualized risk decisions, which can revolutionize obstetric care by allowing early intervention and better outcomes (Ahmed *et. al.*, 2024). However, future studies must address concerns of data privacy, ethics, and standardization of AI tools in the clinical process. Additionally, additional research into integrations of wearables and telemedicine with ultrasound can broaden access in disadvantaged regions. More multidisciplinary collaborations will be essential to introduce these innovations into standard clinical practice, a move that will be revolutionary in precision obstetrics (Nicholson *et. al.*, 2003).

11.4.8. Impact of Technology on Prenatal Care

Advances in technology have transformed prenatal care with enhanced diagnostic sensitivity and patient management. A classic example is the use of obstetric ultrasound in routine prenatal screening, which can diagnose fetal abnormality early on and track fetal growth in real-time. These imaging technologies, along with emerging technologies in AI, can assist clinicians in scanning large databases within a short time and improving diagnostic accuracy, thereby potentially saving poor outcomes while individualizing patient care (Karalis, 2024). In addition, these advances extend beyond diagnosis to contribute to better risk stratification as well as for interventions in some prenatal complications. Sophisticated ultrasound technologies, for example, allow for the identification of neurological diseases like cerebral palsy, and early detection and enhanced therapy techniques can be applied (Paul *et. al.*, 2022). Lastly, integration of prenatal care with technology is a move towards enhanced, personalized maternal-fetal medicine that recognizes the central place of obstetric ultrasound in this new clinical landscape (Figure 11.20).

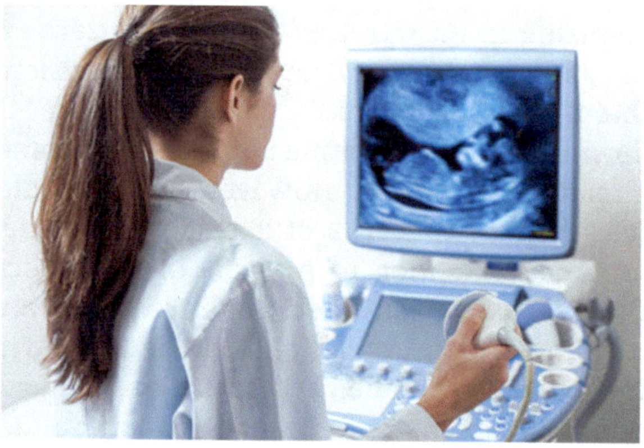

Figure 11.20. The integration of obstetric ultrasound in routine prenatal screening exemplifies this shift, allowing for early detection of fetal abnormalities and real-time monitoring of fetal development.

Source: https://www.aapc.com/codes/webroot/upload/articles_pdf/2022/oca/2022-09-15_17-47-37.webp.

11.4.9. Global Disparities in Access to Ultrasound Technology

Despite the huge leap in medical imaging, access to ultrasound technology is still disproportionately distributed at the worldwide level, and it is an enormous contribution to obstetric services in low-resource settings. The majority of the developing nations lack infrastructure backup, trained staff, and economic capital to fund the routine application of obstetric ultrasound, and hence the inhibition of early diagnosis and management of conditions such as pre-eclampsia and fetal abnormalities. Conversely, developed countries possess homogenized advice and global access to technology, maximizing fetal and maternal outcomes. Such imbalances not only preclude timely decision-making on the clinical front but also increase existing health inequalities, leading to spirals of deterioration in maternal health. Health workers ought to operate under these limitations ethically, cutting down on proximate recommendations without sacrificing quality of care, maintaining worldwide standards and local limitations (Visseren *et. al.*, 2021). Furthermore, with consideration of variability in placental states, the value of access to ultrasound is improved towards achieving early diagnosis and treatment, and therefore closing this technology gap is necessary (Graham *et. al.*, 2019).

Test Your Knowledge

1. How has the development of doppler ultrasound technology advanced the ability to assess fetal blood flow and placental function?
2. How has the integration of artificial intelligence (AI) and machine learning into ultrasound technology improved fetal anomaly detection and diagnostic accuracy?

SUMMARY

The inclusion of obstetric ultrasound in prenatal care has transformed the ability to track fetal development and detect anomalies more accurately. While providing clinical benefits, the presentation of unwanted or sensitive information during scanning calls for effective communication skills from the sonographer, making training intervention specifically addressing specific needs essential. Sonography communication training was revealed to have potential in establishing such confidence and empathetic response capability of these two professionals, thereby enhancing care humanization and patient experience overall (Kaur *et. al.*, 2024). Furthermore, the diagnostic challenges presented by rare thyroid ailments diagnosable through ultrasound also replicate the general notion that ultrasound is key in distinguishing complicated cases that require further histologic evaluation (Michell *et. al.*, 2024). Ultimately, continued advancement and uptake of obstetric ultrasound depend on achieving equilibrium between technological precision and sympathetic patient explanation, facilitated by organizational backing and pertinent research to achieve optimum success for expectant parents and clinicians alike.

Medical imaging sciences have transformed prenatal health care with valuable information regarding fetal development and maternal health. Obstetric ultrasound is a non-invasive, real-time diagnostic device that allows more precise estimation of gestational age, detects congenital anomalies, and monitors fetal health and growth. Its widespread application has improved pregnancy outcome through early intervention upon complication. But awareness of the limitations of ultrasound technology, such as operator dependence and variability of image interpretation, is required to prevent overuse of such technology. Furthermore, correlation of ultrasound findings with other diagnostic tests ensures complete evaluation of pregnancy. Patient education about the benefits and drawbacks of ultrasound also institutionalizes ethical and well-informed decision-making processes in prenatal care. In brief, obstetric ultrasound remains indispensable in modern obstetrics, yet continuous education and research must be conducted to maximize its effectiveness and safety (Barron *et. al.*, 2005; Nicholson *et. al.*, 2003).

KEY TERMS FROM THIS CHAPTER

- Obstetric ultrasound
- Non-invasive prenatal testing (NIPT)
- Fusion Imaging
- Fetal growth
- Molecular analysis
- Chromosomal microarray analysis
- Preterm labor
- Color Doppler

CRITICAL THINKING QUESTIONS

1. **At what stage of pregnancy is the first-trimester ultrasound typically performed?**
   a. 4–6 weeks
   b. 7–9 weeks
   c. 10–13 weeks
   d. 14–20 weeks
2. **What is the primary purpose of performing an ultrasound during the first trimester?**
   a. To determine fetal gender
   b. To assess fetal growth
   c. To confirm gestational age and detect any abnormalities
   d. To check for placental location
3. **Which of the following is the most reliable method for estimating the gestational age of the fetus in early pregnancy?**
   a. Crown-rump length (CRL) measurement
   b. Biparietal diameter (BPD)
   c. Femur length (FL)
   d. Placental thickness
4. **What is a common indication for a second-trimester ultrasound?**
   a. To check for fetal anomalies
   b. To confirm the fetal heartbeat
   c. To determine placental position
   d. To assess amniotic fluid volume
5. **What is the primary purpose of a third-trimester ultrasound?**
   a. To determine fetal sex
   b. To assess fetal well-being and growth
   c. To check for maternal hypertension
   d. To measure placental thickness

Short Answer Questions

1. What is the primary purpose of performing an early pregnancy ultrasound (6–9 weeks gestation)?
2. How does nuchal translucency measurement help in screening for chromosomal abnormalities during the first trimester?
3. What are the common indications for performing a second-trimester ultrasound?
4. What are the potential benefits and limitations of 3D ultrasound in obstetric imaging?
5. How does a Doppler ultrasound help in assessing fetal well-being, especially in cases of suspected fetal growth restriction?
6. What are the common findings of placental abruption on ultrasound imaging?
7. How can breech presentation of the fetus be identified on ultrasound, and why is it important?

Answers to Critical Thinking Questions

1. (c); 2.(c); 3. (a); 4.(a); 5. (b)

REFERENCES

1. Abuhamad, A., Tabor, A., Papageorghiou, A. T., Bilardo, C. M., Florescu, C. C., Hempel, D., & ISUOG. (2019). *International Society of Ultrasound in Obstetrics and Gynecology (ISUOG)–The Propagation of Knowledge in Ultrasound for the Improvement of OB/GYN Care Worldwide: Experience of Basic Ultrasound Training in Oman*. https://core.ac.uk/download/286270866.pdf (accessed on 30 May 2025).
2. Adams, S. J. (2021). *Improving Access to Ultrasound Imaging in Northern, Remote Communities*. https://core.ac.uk/download/478191195.pdf (accessed on 30 May 2025).
3. Ahmed, A. G., Elrasheed, F. E., Logman, H., Abbas, N. H., Tahir, A. S. M., Mudawi, E. M., & Ahmed, A. (2024). *Role of Artificial Intelligence in Risk Prediction of Preterm Labor: Narrative Review*. https://core.ac.uk/download/640070277.pdf (accessed on 30 May 2025).
4. Akhbardeh, A., Jacobs, M. A., & Sagreiya, H. (2023). *Automated Lung Ultrasound Pulmonary Disease Quantification Using an Unsupervised Machine Learning Technique for COVID-19*. https://core.ac.uk/download/619409492.pdf (accessed on 30 May 2025).
5. Albadi, S., & Sekhar, C. (2024). Family medicine residents' confidence in performing a basic obstetric ultrasound at primary health care centers in Qassim Province, Saudi Arabia. *Cureus, 16*. https://www.semanticscholar.org/paper/cf194df6c529d7d085b6d9f56e24e69a351be1b3 (accessed on 30 May 2025).
6. Aleshi, P., Ortner, C. M., & Butwick, A. J. (2025). Point-of-care ultrasound in obstetric anesthesia clinical practice. *Current Opinion in Anesthesiology*. https://www.semanticscholar.org/paper/8a8776d9d25105672e32a637a148c99e8f466961 (accessed on 30 May 2025).
7. Alshalahi, S., Alguizzani, N., Alqarni, D., Korkoman, S., Almassari, M., Alotayban, R., & Tehsin, F. (2025). Pregnant women's perceptions and knowledge of obstetric ultrasound in Central Region, Saudi Arabia. *International Journal of Medicine in Developing Countries*. https://www.semanticscholar.org/paper/3f7215c4897b33c290d7189e8ba097b76222f6cc (accessed on 30 May 2025).
8. Anand, A., Jung, S., & Lee, S. (2024). Breast lesion detection for ultrasound images using Mask Former. *Sensors (Basel, Switzerland), 24*. https://www.semanticscholar.org/paper/a31a8f0876e8b261c7e2440648004ff0a109cde9 (accessed on 30 May 2025).
9. Arain, Z., Chowdhury, T. T., David, A. L., & Iliodromiti, S. (2023). *Machine Learning and Disease Prediction in Obstetrics*. https://core.ac.uk/download/571216446.pdf (accessed on 30 May 2025).
10. Barnes, G. D., Burnett, A., Allen, A. L., Blumenstein, M., Clark, N. P., Cuker, A., Dager, W. E., *et. al.* (2020). Thromboembolism and anticoagulant therapy during the COVID-19 pandemic: Interim clinical guidance from the Anticoagulation Forum. *Journal of Thrombosis and Thrombolysis, 50*, 72–81. https://doi.org/10.1007/s11239-020-02138-z.
11. Barron, M. L., & Fehring, R. (2005). *Basal Body Temperature Assessment: Is It Useful to Couples Seeking Pregnancy?* https://core.ac.uk/download/213076060.pdf (accessed on 30 May 2025).
12. Bellati, F., Caserta, D., Costanzi, F., & De Marco, A. (2018). *Real-Time Virtual Sonography in Gynecology & Obstetrics: Literature's Analysis and Case Series*. https://core.ac.uk/download/195777140.pdf (accessed on 30 May 2025).

13. Bellussi, F., Berghella, V., Boelig, R. C., & Saccone, G. (2020). *MFM Guidance for COVID-19*. https://core.ac.uk/download/pdf/323187692.pdf (accessed on 30 May 2025).

14. Bhutta, Z. A., Darmstadt, G. L., Haws, R. A., & Menezes, E. V. (2009). *Reducing Stillbirths: Screening and Monitoring During Pregnancy and Labor*. https://core.ac.uk/download/pdf/8285199.pdf.

15. Bilardo, C. M., Chaoui, R., Hyett, J., Kagan, K. O., Karim, J., Papageorghiou, A. T., Poon, L. C., & ISUOG. (2023). ISUOG practice guidelines (updated): Performance of 11–14-week ultrasound scan. *Ultrasound in Obstetrics and Gynecology, 61*, 127–143. https://doi.org/10.1002/uog.26106.

16. Bockarie, M. J., Ansumana, R., Machingaidze, S., de Souza, D. K., Fatoma, P., Zumla, A., & Lee, S. S. (2024). Transformative potential of artificial intelligence on health care and research in Africa. *International Journal of Infectious Diseases, 143*, 107011. https://doi.org/10.1016/j.ijid.2024.107011.

17. Cunen Borg , N., Borg Xuereb, R., Jomeen, J., & Poat, A. (2016). *A Narrative Review of Interventions Addressing the Parental-Fetal Relationship*. https://core.ac.uk/download/151162916.pdf (accessed on 30 May 2025).

18. Bosmans, J. E., de Jonge, A., Franx, A., & Henrichs, J. (2016). *Effectiveness and Cost-Effectiveness of Routine Third Trimester Ultrasound Screening for Intrauterine Growth Restriction: Study Protocol of a Nationwide Stepped Wedge Cluster-Randomized Trial in The Netherlands (The IRIS Study)*. https://core.ac.uk/download/346483744.pdf (accessed on 30 May 2025).

19. Britton, N., Miller, M. A., Safadi, S., Siegel, A., Levine, A. R., & McCurdy, M. T. (2019). Tele-ultrasound in resource-limited settings: A systematic review. *Frontiers in Public Health, 7*. https://doi.org/10.3389/fpubh.2019.00244.

20. Burton, G. J., Redman, C. W. G., Roberts, J. M., & Moffett, A. (2019). Pre-eclampsia: Pathophysiology and clinical implications. *BMJ*. https://doi.org/10.1136/bmj.l2381.

21. Cai, J., Wang, Y., Jiang, D., Gu, Y., Lou, L., Gao, F., & Wu, T. (2023). Photoacoustic imaging based on broadened bandwidth aluminum nitride piezoelectric micromachined ultrasound transducers. *IEEE Sensors Letters, 7*, 1–4. https://www.semanticscholar.org/paper/32ac1fae74a1966f9aa7f34cb9fa4335be5b8053 (accessed on 30 May 2025).

22. Castro-Apodaca, F., Murillo-Llanes, J., Cortez-Hernández, J., Magaña-Gómez, J. A., Amézquita-López, B. A., Peña-García, G., Medina-Gutiérrez, A. R., *et. al.* (2025). Giant placental chorioangioma: Case report. *Medicine: Case Reports and Study Protocols*. https://www.semanticscholar.org/paper/b90b26bd7c4bb3db22bbc2cd4046bc2b642d64e7 (accessed on 30 May 2025).

23. Chaoui, R. (2021). Evolution of fetal cardiac imaging in 30 years of ISUOG. *Ultrasound in Obstetrics and Gynecology, 57*, 38–42. https://doi.org/10.1002/uog.23551.

24. Chawanpaiboon, S., Vogel, J. P., Moller, A.-B., Lumbiganon, P., Petzold, M., Hogan, D. R., Landoulsi, S., *et. al.* (2018). Global, regional, and national estimates of levels of preterm birth in 2014: A systematic review and modelling analysis. *The Lancet Global Health, 7*(1), e37–e46. https://doi.org/10.1016/s2214-109x(18)30451-0.

25. Chiera, M., Cerritelli, F., Casini, A., Barsotti, N., Boschiero, D., Cavigioli, F., Corti, C., *et. al.* (2020). Heart rate variability in the perinatal period: A critical and conceptual review. *Frontiers in Neuroscience, 14*. https://doi.org/10.3389/fnins.2020.561186.

26. Christie, D. A., & Tansey, E. M. (2000). *Looking at the Unborn: Historical Aspects of Obstetric Ultrasound.* https://core.ac.uk/download/30696167.pdf (accessed on 30 May 2025).

27. Codsi, E., Brost, B., & Nitsche, J. (2022). Hands-on simulation workshop for obstetric ultrasound-guided invasive procedures. *MedEdPORTAL: The Journal of Teaching and Learning Resources, 18.* https://www.semanticscholar.org/paper/983ef1f6657e89d0db76a483d8a35caa86c29cfd (accessed on 30 May 2025).

28. Cook, A., & Palmer, L. (2009). *Providing Maternity Care to The Underserved: A Comparative Case Study of Three Maternity Care Models Serving Women in Washington, D.C.* https://core.ac.uk/download/71348405.pdf (accessed on 30 May 2025).

29. Das, N. K., & Panday, S. D. (2024). Integrating radiological diagnostic tools in Shalya Tantra: Advancements and clinical applications. *International Journal for Multidisciplinary Research.* https://www.semanticscholar.org/paper/1d88e90cfb6fb61dc23f6171453f317bfab502a2 (accessed on 30 May 2025).

30. Dassen, S., Monen, L., Oei, G., Mischi, M., & van Laar, J. (2024). Safety of contrast-enhanced ultrasound using microbubbles in human pregnancy: A scoping review. *Ultra Schall in der Medizin.* https://www.semanticscholar.org/paper/54d282d56a193220a860697f9c0c0667215f856a (accessed on 30 May 2025).

31. Diderich, K. E. M., Go, A. T. J. I., Groenenberg, I. A. L., & Husen, M. (2024). *Prenatal Counseling of An Isolated Fetal Small Head Circumference During the Second Trimester Expert Ultrasound Examination.* https://core.ac.uk/download/596932849.pdf (accessed on 30 May 2025).

32. Ding, Z. J., Yue, J. Z., Zhang, Y. D., & Yin, W. (2024). Research on evaluation of fetal right ventricular function in normal and diabetic pregnant women during mid to late pregnancy using automated MPI ultrasound detection technology. *The Journal of Maternal-Fetal & Neonatal Medicine, 37*(1), 2424892. https://www.semanticscholar.org/paper/dd87bbb47d4b95cb072aec3e746591774fff0baa (accessed on 30 May 2025).

33. Drews, E., Wildman-Tobriner, B., Mathews, A., Nickenig Vissoci, J. R., Kalisz, K., Amrhein, T. J., Wiggins, W. F., *et. al.* (2021). Prospective evaluation of novice-acquired three-dimensional point-of-care ultrasound for carotid stenosis. *Academic Emergency Medicine, 28*, 1440–1443. https://doi.org/10.1111/acem.14320.

34. Favaretto, M., & Rost, M. (2024). "A picture paints a thousand words"—A systematic review of the ethical issues of prenatal ultrasound. *Journal of Bioethical Inquiry.* https://www.semanticscholar.org/paper/6c1dbdc9abed67e1ebc52dd7a1fff5e7adc58724 (accessed on 30 May 2025).

35. Findley, T. O., & Northrup, H. (2021). The current state of prenatal detection of genetic conditions in congenital heart defects. *Translational Pediatrics, 10*(8), 2157–2170. https://doi.org/10.21037/tp-20-315.

36. Freeman, D., Huda, S., Jarvie, E., McKenna, L., *et. al.* (2013). How to assess and manage hypertension during and after pregnancy. https://core.ac.uk/download/19888252.pdf.

37. Gilstad, H. (2012). Obstetric ultrasound expertise as manifest in encounters between midwives and pregnant women: A case study from KwaZulu-Natal in South Africa. https://core.ac.uk/download/636677220.pdf (accessed on 30 May 2025).

38. Harley-Roberts, A., Sims, A., McGuinness, A., Sumra, A., Hynes, C., Harrison, G., & Yaz, G. (2020).

UK Consensus Guidelines for The Delivery of Unexpected News in Obstetric Ultrasound: The ASCKS Framework. https://core.ac.uk/download/340075158.pdf (accessed on 30 May 2025).

39. Hebbar, S. N., & Varalaxmi. (2005). Role of fetal thigh circumference in estimation of birth weight by ultrasound. https://core.ac.uk/download/pdf/86659.pdf.

40. Henker, R., Blank, V., & Karlas, T. (2024). Transabdominal ultrasound for the diagnostic workup of parenchymal pancreatic diseases. *Ultraschall in der Medizin–European Journal of Ultrasound.* https://www.semanticscholar.org/paper/8f22199878ffe25dab987d5a2a1697efd5dca909 (accessed on 30 May 2025).

41. Horgan, R., Nehme, L., & Abuhamad, A. (2023). Artificial intelligence in obstetric ultrasound: A scoping review. *Prenatal Diagnosis, 43*, 1176–1219. https://doi.org/10.1002/pd.6411.

42. Ignatov, P., & Yordanova-Ignatova, T. (2024). Bulgarian Federation of Obstetrics and Gynecology (BFOG) amniotic fluid index charts. *Fetal Medicine, Obstetrics and Gynecology*. https://www.semanticscholar.org/paper/d098602882e0dedfd7c1178f77c3ea8349e9dfda (accessed on 30 May 2025).

43. Islam, M. N., Mustafina, S. N., Mahmud, T., & Khan, N. I. (2022). Machine learning to predict pregnancy outcomes: A systematic review, synthesizing framework and future research agenda. *BMC Pregnancy and Childbirth, 22*. https://doi.org/10.1186/s12884-022-04594-2.

44. Karalis, V. (2024). The integration of artificial intelligence into clinical practice. *Applied Biosciences, 3*(1), 14–44. https://doi.org/10.3390/applbiosci3010002.

45. Kaur, E., Arezina, J., Bryant, L. D., Pollak, K., Wallace, R., Harrison, G., Bender Atik, R., *et. al.* (2024). 'More like a partnership': A qualitative evaluation of communication coaching for sonographers (CCS) in obstetric ultrasound. *Ultrasound*. https://www.semanticscholar.org/paper/51ebc4f0100c6b8ff5912c8ce041f6ee7eba89ae (accessed on 30 May 2025).

46. Krishnarao, A. V., & Sharma, A. (2025). Advancements in disease detection and volume reduction: A review on medical imaging and healthcare innovations. *Journal of Information Systems Engineering and Management*. https://www.semanticscholar.org/paper/d28f2aa68fc26066d9e15b2ad3b50c3a47663c7a (accessed on 30 May 2025).

47. Liu, S., Wang, Y., Yang, X., Lei, B., Liu, L., Li, S. X., Ni, D., *et. al.* (2019). Deep learning in medical ultrasound analysis: A review. *Engineering, 5*(2), 261–275. https://doi.org/10.1016/j.eng.2018.11.020.

48. Loebig, W. F. (2020). *Nurse Anesthetists' Perceptions and Use of Ultrasound for Epidural and Spinal Needle Placement in Obese Parturient* [Doctoral dissertation, University of Michigan]. http://deepblue.lib.umich.edu/bitstream/2027.42/156390/1/Loebig2020.pdf (accessed on 30 May 2025).

49. Melamed, N., Baschat, A., Yinon, Y., Athanasiadis, A., Mecacci, F., Figueras, F., Berghella, V., *et. al.* (2021). FIGO (International Federation of Gynecology and Obstetrics) initiative on fetal growth: Best practice advice for screening, diagnosis, and management of fetal growth restriction. *International Journal of Gynecology & Obstetrics, 152*, 3–57. https://doi.org/10.1002/ijgo.13522.

50. Michell, K., Hall, S., Al Shiekh Ali, Z., Al-Hashim, M., & Howlett, D. C. (2024). Riedel's thyroiditis: A case report and review of the ultrasound findings of this rare disease entity. *Ultrasound.*

https://www.semanticscholar.org/paper/8e54e7c605206e82d06b1bef413c1dd0a13f34cd (accessed on 30 May 2025).

51. Mocanu, D., Bokwa-Dąbrowska, K., Helander, K. N., & Szaro, P. (2025). Comparative analysis of ultrasound and magnetic resonance imaging in diagnosing pain in the posterolateral region of the ankle. *Journal of Ultrasonography, 25*. https://www.semanticscholar.org/paper/82e2f34b4d5fb42fe74667fce80c157e8626cfd6 (accessed on 30 May 2025).

52. Mohsin, I., Aziz, S., Aziz, I., Azam, S., & Hamayun, P. (2023). Accuracy of polyhydramnios for detection of fetal anomalies on ultrasound. *Pakistan Armed Forces Medical Journal*. https://www.semanticscholar.org/paper/fc68b8099ef63c2861c5bd7f14bcedad7c48e1e1 (accessed on 30 May 2025).

53. Nakou, P. (2020). Is routine prenatal screening and testing fundamentally incompatible with a commitment to reproductive choice? Learning from the historical context. *Medicine, Health Care and Philosophy, 24*, 73–83. https://doi.org/10.1007/s11019-020-09985-w.

54. Nicholson, D. (2003). *Secrets of Success: The Development of Obstetric Ultrasound in Scotland, 1963–1990* [Master's thesis]. https://core.ac.uk/download/6117516.pdf (accessed on 30 May 2025).

55. Paczesny, Ł., Lorkowski, M., Pielak, T., Wójcicki, R., Huri, G., & Zabrzyński, J. (2023). The role of ultrasound guidance in mini-invasive musculoskeletal surgery—A pictorial essay. *Applied Sciences*. https://www.semanticscholar.org/paper/aa974eab5f9086f1b381ff668b594405b2206e55 (accessed on 30 May 2025).

56. Padilla, C., Ortner, C., Dennis, A., & Zieleskiewicz, L. (2024). The need for maternal critical care education, point-of-care ultrasound and critical care echocardiography in obstetric anesthesiologists training. *Obstetric Anesthesia Digest*. https://www.semanticscholar.org/paper/4df8758f751b14bf5df9808800522f0f45c5134d (accessed on 30 May 2025).

57. Paul, S., Nahar, A., Bhagawati, M., & Kunwar, A. J. (2022). A review on recent advances of cerebral palsy. *Oxidative Medicine and Cellular Longevity, 2022*, 1–20. https://doi.org/10.1155/2022/2622310.

58. Pegios, P., Lin, M., Weng, N., Svendsen, M. B. S., Bashir, Z., Bigdeli, S., Christensen, A. N., *et. al.* (2024). Diffusion-based iterative counterfactual explanations for fetal ultrasound image quality assessment. *ArXiv, abs/2403.08700*. https://www.semanticscholar.org/paper/ee9650bdc9a33431be35c4e3f44f2ee22ba2c121 (accessed on 30 May 2025).

59. Plöger, R., Behning, C., Walter, A., Jiménez Cruz, J., Gembruch, U., Strizek, B., & Recker, F. (2024). Next-generation monitoring in obstetrics: Assessing the accuracy of non-piezo portable ultrasound technology. *Acta Obstetrician et Gynecological Scandinavica, 103*, 2031–2041. https://doi.org/10.1111/aogs.14922.

60. Régia e Silva, I., Rodrigues, R. P. S., Soares da Silva, A. B., Leitão, K. R. S., de Carvalho, P. V. S., Barbosa, M. A. P. S., Sousa, F. D. C. A., *et. al.* (2022). Fetal distress during the last third of pregnancy in bitches: Evaluation by Doppler ultrasound imaging. *Acta Scientiae Veterinarian*. https://www.semanticscholar.org/paper/c13c1b200041bdef2c16d4708b18f11c157b1fce (accessed on 30 May 2025).

61. Reshi, A., Shafi, S., Qayoom, I., Wani, M., Parveen, S., & Ahmad, A. (2024). Deep learning-based architecture for Down syndrome assessment during early pregnancy using fetal ultrasound images. *International Journal of Experimental Research and Review*. https://www.

semanticscholar.org/paper/55f03f0de8626a11af7646d74bd72bf6d7a11653 (accessed on 30 May 2025).

62. Salomon, L., Alfirević, Ž., Berghella, V., Bilardo, C. M., Chalouhi, G. E., da Silva Costa, F., Hernández-Andrade, E., *et. al.* (2022). ISUOG Practice Guidelines (updated): Performance of the routine mid-trimester fetal ultrasound scan. *Ultrasound in Obstetrics and Gynecology, 59*, 840–856. https://doi.org/10.1002/uog.24888.

63. Sammet, S., & Ramos, Y. (2010). The 2008 Kenneth R. Gottesfeld Award Winners. *Journal of Diagnostic Medical Sonography, 26*(1), 1–3. https://www.semanticscholar.org/paper/f2bc129f9cf253f8780ef08b447e8fc8e7308b82 (accessed on 30 May 2025).

64. Savage, E., van Gool, K., Haas, M., Anderson, R., & Viney, R. (2025). Who's getting caught? An analysis of the Australian Medicare Safety Net. *CHERE Working Paper 2006/8*. https://core.ac.uk/download/pdf/6376798.pdf (accessed on 30 May 2025).

65. Scharf, J., Dracopoulos, C., Gembicki, M., Rody, A., Welp, A., & Weichert, J. (2024). How automated techniques ease functional assessment of the fetal heart: Applicability of two-dimensional speckle-tracking echocardiography for comprehensive analysis of global and segmental cardiac deformation using fetalHQ®. *Echocardiography, 41*. https://www.semanticscholar.org/paper/d6e44ddd4ea70894b037677b98a4ef2b183613a3 (accessed on 30 May 2025).

66. Shi, D., & Li, L. (2025). Advancements in ultrasound imaging for assessing the biological behavior of hepatocellular carcinoma. *International Journal of Biology and Life Sciences*. https://www.semanticscholar.org/paper/32138acde4044865bbb6bb26a65e8011dc2a3ddc (accessed on 30 May 2025).

67. Song, P. (2023). Small animal cerebral microvascular imaging with super-resolution ultrasound: Techniques and applications. *The Journal of the Acoustical Society of America*. https://www.semanticscholar.org/paper/426ea3a2714d1255495438e64dc5018606b56968 (accessed on 30 May 2025).

68. Stefanovic, V. (2020). Role of obstetric ultrasound in reducing maternal and neonatal mortality in developing countries: From facts to acts. https://core.ac.uk/download/335969332.pdf (accessed on 30 May 2025).

69. Stewart, E., So, M., Fennessy, F., McDannold, N., Hynynen, K., & Tempany, C. (2005). OC1.03: High-intensity focused ultrasound: The treatment of uterine fibroids and other potential applications. *Ultrasound in Obstetrics and Gynecology, 26*. https://www.semanticscholar.org/paper/1ccb8ec10ad034e5010527a6835cd93fdfc4c7df (accessed on 30 May 2025).

70. Suarayasa, K., Kasim, A., Mallawa, S. D., & Weri, A. (2024). Fulfilling the right to health of pregnant women through obstetric ultrasound examination at antenatal care (ANC) at the Palu City Health Center–Central Sulawesi, Indonesia. *International Journal of Innovative Research in Multidisciplinary Education*. https://www.semanticscholar.org/paper/395abe5f2f7160aeafd565484ddbdf15cf6964d1 (accessed on 30 May 2025).

71. Teede, H., Misso, M., Costello, M., Dokras, A., Laven, J. S. E., Moran, L., Piltonen, T., *et. al.* (2018). Recommendations from the international evidence-based guideline for the assessment and management of polycystic ovary syndrome. *Clinical Endocrinology, 89*, 251–268. https://doi.org/10.1111/cen.13795.

72. Tegnander, E. (2006). Detection of congenital heart defects in a non-selected population of 42,381 fetuses. https://core.ac.uk/download/646166949.pdf (accessed on 30 May 2025).

73. Tonni, G., Grisolia, G., Tonni, S., Lacerda, V. A., Ruano, R., & Sepulveda, W. (2024). Fetal face: Enhancing 3D ultrasound imaging by postprocessing with AI applications: Myth, reality, or legal concerns? *Journal of Clinical Ultrasound*. https://www.semanticscholar.org/paper/e21278e49cdd3b6d77c04b242d14a3458b5da189 (accessed on 30 May 2025).

74. Turan, S., & Goetzinger, K. (2020). First-trimester fetal heart evaluation: Time to move forward. *Ultrasound in Obstetrics and Gynecology, 57*(5), 677–680. https://doi.org/10.1002/uog.23572.

75. Visseren, F. L. J., Mach, F., Smulders, Y. M., Carballo, D., Koskinas, K. C., Bäck, M., Bénétos, A., *et. al.* (2021). 2021 ESC guidelines on cardiovascular disease prevention in clinical practice. *European Heart Journal, 42*, 3227–3337. https://doi.org/10.1093/eurheartj/ehab484.

GYNECOLOGICAL IMAGING

12

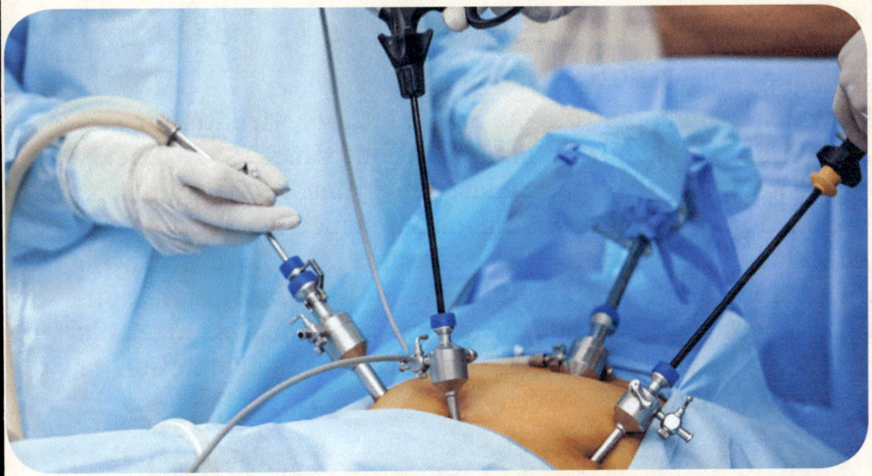

LEARNING OBJECTIVES

After studying this chapter, you will be able to:

1. Identify types of gynecological imaging
2. Describe applications of gynecological imaging
3. Know safety and risks in gynecological imaging
4. Focus on advances in gynecological imaging technology

Introduction

Medical technological advances have revolutionized diagnostic and treatment approaches throughout the specialties, significantly influencing patient outcomes. Herein, gynecologic imaging has proven to be a boon, delivering high-resolution visualization of the female reproductive system to aid in the diagnosis, management, and monitoring of a range of conditions. Their significance is brought out by the presentation of minimally invasive surgical techniques, now standard practice in gynecology, for which decreased patient morbidity and enhanced recovery periods are the highlights. Such modalities permit precise preoperative planning and postoperative evaluation, consistent with modern-day oncologic treatment protocols involving effectiveness as well as attention to patient quality of life. Moreover, ongoing developments in imaging technology offer counterparts to ongoing education in medical schools, allowing for the overall education of future gynecologic specialists (Medicine *et. al.*, 2015). This integration of imaging innovation and medical practice brings about a new age of women's health, where accurate diagnosis and personalized treatment converge.

Definition of Gynecological Imaging

Medicine technology has significantly enhanced the diagnosis and treatment of conditions in the female reproductive tract. Gynecologic imaging is referred to as the collection of diagnostic technologies employed to visualize the uterus, ovaries, fallopian tubes, and other adjacent organs. The majority of these imaging modalities include ultrasound, magnetic resonance imaging (MRI), and computed tomography (CT), which provide comprehensive anatomical and pathological information relevant to accurate diagnosis and treatment planning. For instance, imaging is employed to detect ovarian cancer, a serious disease that affects a majority of women annually and typically presents at advanced stages, complicating treatment (Blagden *et. al.*, 2015).

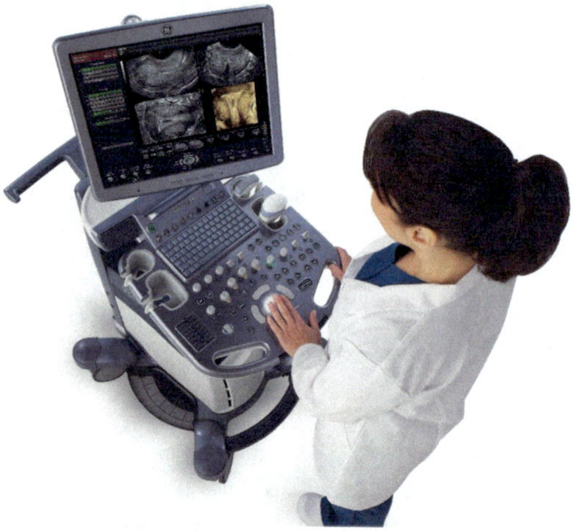

Figure 12.1. Gynecological imaging refers to the array of diagnostic techniques employed to visualize the uterus, ovaries, fallopian tubes, and other related structures.

Source: https://images.takeshape.io/f1ba446a-c0cf-4882-b0c9-50298f143ec2/dev/8456861e-be67-42e9-b962-200319f8f2d2/493786?auto=compress%2Cformat&crop=center.

Gynecological imaging also guides surgical procedures, for instance, whether patients are candidates for minimally invasive hysterectomy or open abdominal surgery, thereby affecting patient outcomes and healthcare equality (Haji-Noor *et. al.*, 2023). With the union of precision and non-invasiveness, gynecologic imaging is now at the forefront of today's women's health care, enabling early treatment and improved prognosis (Figure 12.1).

Importance of Imaging in Women's Health

Proper diagnosis and timely treatment are crucial to maximize outcomes in women's health, particularly in gynecologic conditions where symptoms are nonspecific or reversible with other illnesses. Imaging plays a central role in this by providing high-resolution, non-invasive imaging of internal structures to enable early detection and precise determination of disease severity.

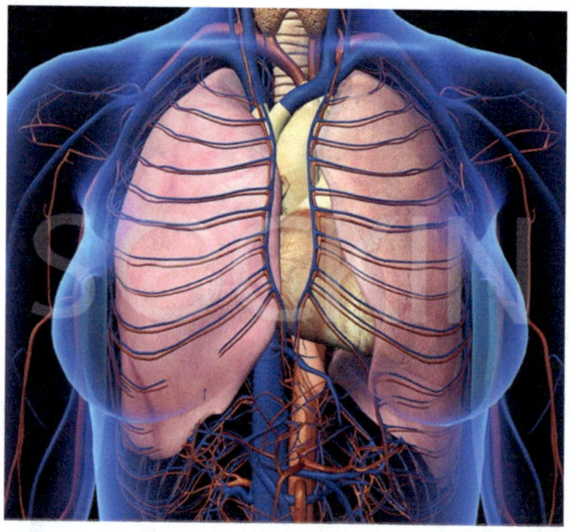

Figure 12.2. Thoracic endometriosis.

Source: https://drseckin.com/wp-content/uploads/2022/04/thoracic-cavity.jpg.

For instance, advanced modalities like high-resolution CT and MRI have enabled diagnosis of complex disorders like thoracic endometriosis, a rare but incapacitating disease most often not diagnosed due to presenting with non-specific respiratory symptoms (Bałoniak *et. al.*, 2025). Similarly, transvaginal ultrasound is extremely useful for myometrial invasion assessment in endometrial cancer, whereby specialist reporting after adequate training significantly increases diagnostic utility (Alcázar *et. al.*, 2023). These capabilities not only facilitate on-time treatment options but also alleviate the burden of chronic conditions, highlighting the manner in which imaging innovation impacts better management and better quality of life in women's medicine (Figure 12.2).

Historical Context of Gynecological Imaging

Medical imaging, over the years, has had a major impact on diagnostic and therapeutic strategies across specialties, even gynecology. The earliest imaging methods were crude, and the focus remained largely on physical examination and basic visualization techniques, which prevented precise diagnosis and treatment planning. The introduction of technologies like CT and MRI offered a critical turn in the history of imaging, permitting precise visualization of gynecological anatomy and pathology to an unmatched degree. These developments made more precise surgical interventions and improved patient outcomes through customized treatment regimens. Moreover, emerging technologies like three-dimensional printing, which are a byproduct of CT and MRI scans, also augmented the surgical management of gynecological pathologies by offering customized preoperative planning and intraoperative navigation (José *et. al.*, 2022). Alongside technological developments, the use of artificial intelligence (AI) for image analysis has also contributed to greater diagnostic accuracy and efficiency, depicting the ongoing change in gynecologic imaging against a broader clinical backdrop (Karalis, 2024).

Current Trends in Gynecological Imaging

Technological advancements have significantly impacted diagnostic capabilities in gynecology, facilitating the advancement of new imaging technologies that enhance precision and patient outcomes. Current trends aim at the integration of digital platforms that offer distant access to images such that experts can research and diagnose more accurately irrespective of geographical variations. Web-based applications with Extensible Markup Language (XML) have been essential in managing huge amounts of medical data, including imaging and patient records, thus facilitating interoperability and effective communication among healthcare systems (Lalande *et. al.*, 2017). In addition, more use of high-resolution ultrasound and MRI offers improved visualization of soft tissues, facilitating early detection and improved characterization of gynecologic pathologies. These advances are followed by protocols for safe data transfer that maintain patient confidentiality while facilitating multidisciplinary care. Advances such as these are contributing to a bigger shift towards gynecological imaging digitization, which allows for greater accuracy and accessibility in diagnosis.

Target Audience for Gynecological Imaging

Understanding the characteristics and needs of the target audience plays a pivotal role in optimizing gynecological imaging protocols and screening programs. Primarily, women of varied age groups who are at risk for cervical cancer or other gynecological conditions constitute the main recipients of these imaging services. Awareness levels regarding cervical cancer and associated preventive measures, such as Pap tests and HPV vaccination, directly influence participation rates in screening initiatives. Data suggest significant gaps in knowledge, with over 30% of women unaware of curability aspects or protective measures tied to HPV vaccination, highlighting the need for tailored educational interventions to enhance screening uptake (Chantziantoniou *et. al.*, 2019). Furthermore, symptomatic women presenting at later disease stages underscore the urgency of early diagnostic imaging and population-based screenings to improve outcomes. Healthcare providers must therefore focus on reaching asymptomatic yet at-risk women through organized calls to screening and reallocating resources for comprehensive imaging availability. Visual tools and educational materials, as represented in clinical summaries (The University of Texas MD Anderson Cancer Center, 2023), can further aid in clarifying the importance of timely gynecological imaging (Figure 12.3).

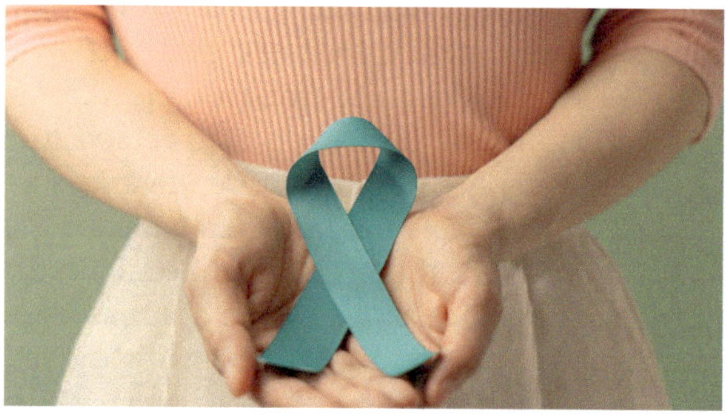

Figure 12.3. Awareness levels regarding cervical cancer and associated preventive measures, such as Pap tests and HPV vaccination, directly influence participation rates in screening initiatives.

Source: https://static.toiimg.com/thumb/msid-112175853,width-1280,height-720,resizemode-4/112175853.jpg.

Challenges in Gynecological Imaging

In spite of tremendous progress in imaging technology, various challenges still exist in gynecologic imaging that hinder precise diagnosis and successful planning of treatment. The intricacy of the female reproductive system, along with the frequently subtle and overlapping presentation of gynecologic pathologies, necessitates extremely sensitive and specific imaging methods. Moreover, identification and discrimination of malignant and benign lesions remain problematic with overlapping imaging characteristics, possibly leading to misdiagnosis or delayed diagnosis. The integration of serum tumor biomarkers with imaging holds promise for enhancing diagnostic accuracy, but standardized protocol and interpreting criteria are yet to be formulated (Anastasi *et. al.*, 2018). In addition, enabling early diagnosis through prompt screening is hindered by disparities in access to health care and variability in patient compliance with recommended screenings (Nilufar *et. al.*, 2023). Addressing these obstacles is essential for improving outcomes in gynecologic cancer detection and treatment, serving to justify ongoing study and interdisciplinarity.

Future Directions

Technological innovations continue to advance in the field of medical imaging, with future potential to further improve gynecologic diagnosis. Emerging modalities based on AI and ML algorithms are promising for optimizing accuracy and efficiency in image interpretation, reducing diagnostic errors, and facilitating personalized treatment plans. Additionally, the development of low-energy, portable imaging tools can revolutionize access to care, especially in settings with scarce resources where even coverage with uniform power supply is not a straightforward matter, as pointed out in energy storage technology across various industries (Sadavar *et. al.*, 2024). The transition to the convergence of imaging technology with real-time data monitoring, consistent with other health devices such as insulin pumps (Rimon *et. al.*, 2024), is indicative of an age where fluid integration defines patient outcome enhancement. Such advancements not only allow for earlier diagnosis of gynecological pathologies, but may also enable minimally invasive intervention, which changes patient management radically through precision imaging.

12.1. Types of Gynecological Imaging

Learning Outcome

1. Explain ultrasound imaging
2. Discuss magnetic resonance imaging (MRI)
3. Focus on computed tomography (CT)
4. Learn X-ray imaging
5. Define hysterosalpingography (HSG)
6. Describe sonohysterography and laparoscopy
7. Understand endovaginal ultrasound
8. Identify 3D imaging techniques

Imaging advances have enabled detection and monitoring of gynecologic disorders with increased precision. Among the various imaging modalities, ultrasound is a leader due to its accessibility and effectiveness in evaluating ovarian masses, often complemented by risk assessment models such as the ADNEX model that classifies tumors as benign and several malignant subtypes to allow more reliable clinical management (Anthoulakis *et. al.*, 2015).

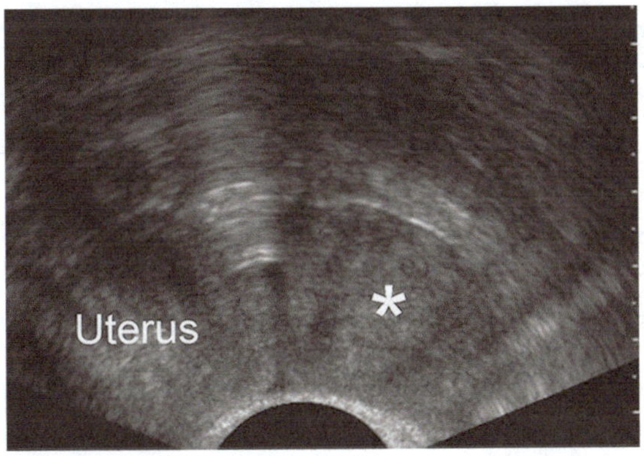

Figure 12.4. ADNEX method.

Source: https://ajronline.org/cms/10.2214/AJR.05.0905/asset/images/05_0905_05a.jpeg.

Furthermore, MRI and CT provide accurate anatomical and functional data, which is critical to staging cancers and planning treatment. Integration of these modalities with biomarker evaluation is a multimodal approach that optimizes tumor detection and follow-up. Such combined strategies are imperative in the context of the rising incidence of gynecological cancers because they improve diagnostic efficacy and therapeutic outcomes by facilitating early management and patient-centered care (Anastasi *et. al.*, 2018) (Figure 12.4).

12.1.1. Ultrasound Imaging

Growth in imaging modalities has significantly contributed to the evaluation of gynecological conditions by facilitating real-time non-invasive visualization of pelvic anatomy and pathology. Of the various modalities, ultrasound imaging stands out in that it is safe, readily available, and extremely versatile and therefore has become a first-line diagnostic modality in gynecology. This modality takes advantage of sound wave conduction and reflection principles such that clinicians can see soft tissue structures in real time, and this is of utmost value in assessing conditions like uterine disease and ovarian masses.

Developments like Doppler imaging and elastography further augmented diagnostic insight by assessing tissue vascularity and stiffness to identify pathological changes with greater accuracy with enhanced precision (Ammar *et. al.*, 2024). Particularly, Morphological Uterus Sonographic Assessment (MUSA) standardizes sonographic evaluation of abnormal uterine bleeding (AUB), effectively separating serious conditions from one another like adenomyosis and fibroids based on meticulous sonographic criteria and optimizing diagnostic precision and informing treatment options (Khaladkar *et. al.*, 2024). As a result, sonography continues to be an essential part of total gynecological assessment and patient management.

12.1.2. Magnetic Resonance Imaging (MRI)

Technological advancements in imaging have greatly enhanced diagnostic accuracy for such a complex gynecologic condition, with MRI having a major contribution. MRI offers high soft tissue contrast resolution, enabling high-resolution imaging of pelvic anatomy, which is invaluable when disease conditions like peritoneal carcinomatosis and endometriosis are being evaluated.

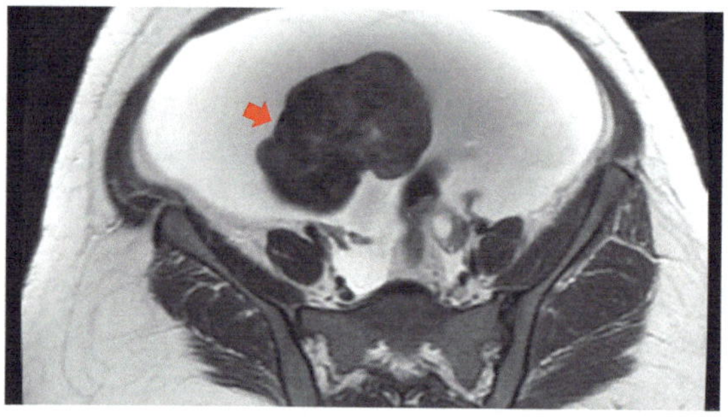

Figure 12.5. MRI has shown utility in detecting peritoneal spread from ovarian and endometrial malignancies.

Source: https://www.clinicalradiologyonline.net/cms/10.1016/j.crad.2024.07.004/asset/544601c6-8fe2-41e6-b6a7-b7a6d2c2cbda/main.assets/gr18_lrg.jpg.

MRI is a non-invasive technique with the added benefit of multiplanar imaging, thereby facilitating precise anatomical definition, enabling early diagnosis and planning of treatment. In particular, MRI has been particularly helpful in the diagnosis of peritoneal dissemination of endometrial and ovarian cancer, complementing the other imaging techniques like CT and PET scans, although the degree of accuracy in detection varies depending on technical and patient conditions (Meucci *et. al.*, 2024). In addition, advances have been made to enhance MRI-based detection of deep pelvic abnormalities, including pouch of Douglas obliteration in endometriosis, using novel techniques like distillation algorithms that exploit the complementary information from transvaginal ultrasound data, while increasing sensitivity and specificity (Zhang *et. al.*, 2023). All these advances highlight the critical role of MRI in gynecologic imaging (Figure 12.5).

12.1.3. Computed Tomography (CT)

Technologic advances in imaging have markedly enhanced the diagnostic capability in numerous fields of medicine, including gynecology. CT, which was long overshadowed by ultrasound and MRI in gynecologic imaging, provides valuable cross-sectional details that complement the assessment of complicated pelvic disease. Its extremely high spatial resolution allows accurate definition of pelvic anatomy and is useful in the detection of malignancies, abscesses, or complications of disease such as hemorrhage and fistulas. Apart from this, CT's rapid acquisition time and overall accessibility make it a suitable option in a case of emergency or when MRI is not feasible. New developments in image processing and automated detection technologies, as discussed in the case of tumors and lesions in other organs, reveal opportunities for applying similar segmentation and classification methods to gynecological CT imaging, enhancing diagnostic precision and workflow efficiency (Abdullah *et. al.*, 2024; Tasnim *et. al.*, 2024). Thus, the blending of CT and advanced computational algorithms may strengthen the detection and characterization of gynecological illness.

12.1.4. X-Ray Imaging

Advances in diagnostic technologies have significantly enhanced the consistency of gynecologic examinations, with X-ray imaging being the focal point even in the presence of other modalities. Specifically, radiographic tests such as hysterosalpingography (HSG) provide useful visualization of the uterine cavity and tubal patency, which are useful for infertility workup and structural abnormality detection. The relative availability and accuracy of X-ray imaging make it appropriate for initial investigations where non-invasive modality is preferred.

In spite of that, its application is specifically warranted due to radiation exposure problems and lower contrast between soft tissues compared to ultrasound or MRI. Enhanced image resolution and dose-reduction technology over recent years have mitigated some risks without loss of diagnostic usefulness, permitting more accurate definition of anatomy needed for successful treatment planning in gynecologic health. Thus, X-ray imaging continues as an adjunct but useful part of gynecologic imaging protocols.

12.1.5. Hysterosalpingography (HSG)

In evaluation for female infertility, it is necessary to test the patency and morphology of the fallopian tubes as these are powerful predictors of reproductive potential. HSG is an important radiologic modality used to characterize the uterine cavity and evaluate the functioning of the uterus and fallopian tubes by the instillation of a contrast medium and followed by X-ray imaging. This method has a less invasive alternative to laparoscopy with subsequent diagnostic data essential to tubal obstruction or uterine disease leading to subfertility. While laparoscopy remains the optimum method of comprehensive pelvic assessment, HSG is an outpatient investigation as a first option since it is accessible and of lower risk. Its utility in defining tubal status is aligned with the need for effective fertility workups, especially in the presence of high levels of subfertility by the World Health Organization's definition (Bhattacharya *et. al.*, 2019). HSG integration into diagnostic workups enhances patient management by allowing early intervention (Khouri *et. al.*, 2004) (Figure 12.6).

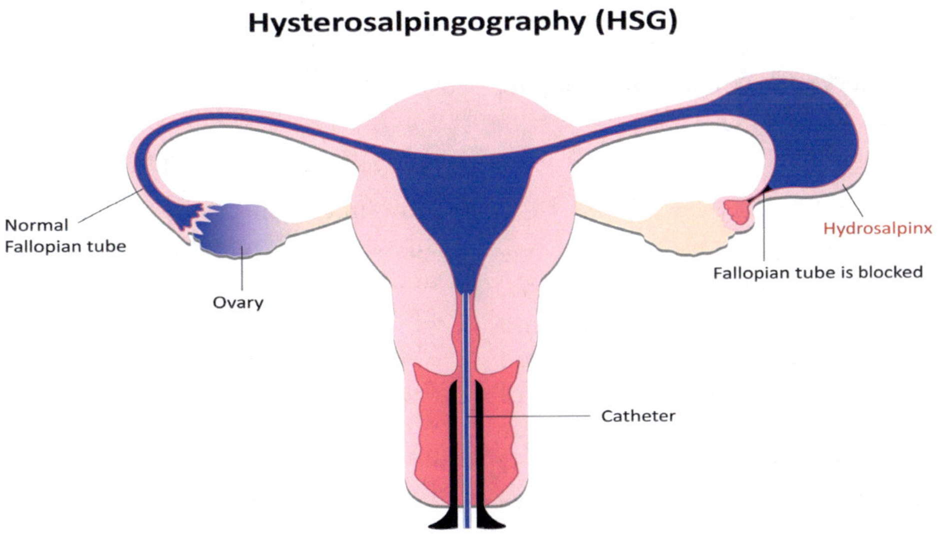

Figure 12.6. Hysterosalpingography.

Source: https://vitaalteraivf.com/wp-content/uploads/2025/01/Hysterosalpingography.jpeg.

12.1.6. Sonohysterography

Technological progress in imaging the gynecological apparatus has significantly improved diagnostic accuracy in different uterine diseases, particularly in diagnosing AUB and infertility. Among these techniques, sonohysterography has proven to be a helpful modality due to enhanced visualization of the endometrial cavity by distending the uterus with saline infusion, which provides clearer images than the standard transvaginal sonography. Comparative studies demonstrate that sonohysterography is superior in sensitivity and specificity in diagnosing submucosal myomas and other uterine pathology and has much greater diagnostic accuracy than transvaginal sonography (Goyal *et. al.*, 2017). The technique is specifically valuable in assessment of patients with a history of recurrent pregnancy loss and suspected congenital uterine anomaly, where precise characterization of uterine morphology is essential for therapy planning. In such environments, sonohysterography with additional high-technology modalities like three-dimensional ultrasound and MRI has a significant role in improving reproductive outcomes after an appropriate intervention Calç, G., Calagna, G., Cucinella, G., *et. al.* (2014).

12.1.7. Laparoscopy

Sophisticated diagnostic techniques are important in the management of multifactorial gynecological conditions such as infertility and endometriosis. Of these, laparoscopy has emerged as a watershed technology with the benefit of immediate visual inspection of pelvic organs over the sensitivity of non-surgical imaging tests. It allows for precise identification of abnormalities such as tubal obstruction, adhesions, and endometriotic lesions that are most frequently implicated in infertility and chronic pelvic pain. Research has established laparoscopy not only to deliver accurate diagnosis but also enable targeted surgical intervention towards improved patient outcomes. In the case of infertility, for example, laparoscopy has established a high prevalence of polycystic ovaries, tubal disease, and uterine abnormalities and consequently guided appropriate treatment modalities (Shruti *et. al.*, 2019). Moreover, despite the success of less invasive imaging technology in the diagnosis of endometriosis, laparoscopy remains the "gold standard" for both diagnosis and treatment as it has the capability to directly assess and treat disease progression (Domino *et. al.*, 2025) (Figure 12.7).

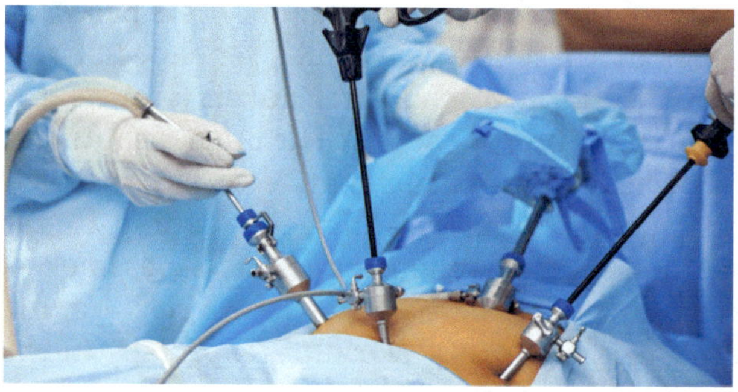

Figure 12.7. Laparoscopy.

Source: https://www.nufertility.com/blog/wp-content/uploads/2024/01/Shutterstock_525787207-compressed-1140x600.png.

12.1.8. Endovaginal Ultrasound

Advances in imaging technologies have significantly improved gynecologic diagnostic abilities, particularly in the evaluation of the pelvic anatomy. Of these, endovaginal ultrasound stands out because it is capable of creating high-resolution images of the uterus, ovaries, and surrounding tissues, with early detection and characterization of pathology. It allows for thorough assessment of the morphology and vascularity of tissue, necessary to differentiate benign from malignant lesions. Also, imaging methods such as three-dimensional shear wave elastography complement endovaginal ultrasound with the measurement of tissue stiffness, improving lymph node evaluation in gynecologic cancers and potentially reducing invasive procedures (Shen *et. al.*, 2025). Moreover, inclusion of artificial intelligence (AI) in pelvic ultrasound imaging will maximize diagnostic accuracy and streamline workflow, though the technologies require additional multi-center validation to minimize bias and meet regulatory sign-off (Cai *et. al.*, 2024). Endovaginal ultrasound, supplemented with elastography and AI, forms a cornerstone of modern gynecological imaging practice.

12.1.9. 3D Imaging Techniques

Advances in medical imaging have revolutionized the diagnostic process, particularly in gynecology, where precise visualization of anatomical structure is at the heart of effective treatment planning. Three-dimensional imaging techniques such as MRI, PET, and CT scans have rich images that surpass conventional two-dimensional routines with fine detailed evaluations of uterine and tumor morphology. These modalities support better segmentation accuracy, isolating a single tissue or pathology, increasing diagnostic accuracy and assisting in tailored therapeutic interventions. In fact, deep learning-based automatic segmentation algorithms have been highly promising, particularly with MRI scans with high Dice coefficients indicating the utility in delineating uterine and tumor margins. Accuracy in segmentation remains inferior for PET and CT scans, however. HameshingHarnessing hybrid CNN-transformer models has the potential to go beyond limitations of the past, with improved performance in 3D imaging applications which are crucial in gynecological oncology (Aggarwal *et. al.*, 2025; Desai *et. al.*, 2024) (Figure 12.8).

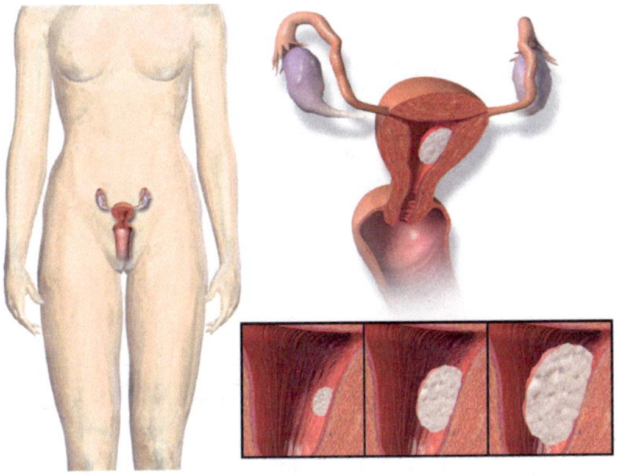

Figure 12.8. Assessments of uterine and tumor morphology.

Source: https://upload.wikimedia.org/wikipedia/commons/9/9b/Blausen_0348_EndometrialCancer.png.

Test Your Knowledge

1. Which imaging modality is commonly used for the assessment of ovarian cysts and ovarian tumors in gynecology?
2. What role does 3D ultrasound play in the assessment of uterine fibroids, endometrial polyps, and congenital uterine abnormalities?

12.2. Applications of Gynecological Imaging

Learning Outcome

1. Understand diagnosis of ovarian cysts
2. Perform evaluation of uterine abnormalities
3. Learn assessment of pelvic inflammatory disease
4. Monitor pregnancy complications
5. Detect gynecological cancers
6. Discuss guidance for biopsies and interventions
7. Explain evaluation of infertility issues
8. Focus on preoperative planning for gynecological surgeries
9. Describe postoperative assessment

Technological advancements in gynecologic imaging have significantly enhanced diagnostic accuracy of different conditions of the female reproductive system. For instance, ultrasonography (EUS) is now the imaging modality of choice to differentiate between benign and malignant adnexal masses using pattern recognition and gray-scale imaging to identify tumor characteristics with high accuracy. Synergistic application of color Doppler imaging provides additional information on blood flow patterns, though its clinical application remains controversial. Future clinical applications are perceived in developments such as three-dimensional vascular indices and computer-aided diagnosis algorithms, the potential for which is for earlier diagnosis and enhanced decision-making for treatment (Piras *et. al.*, 2015). In addition, polarimetric imaging technologies like Mueller matrix imaging have a non-invasive tool for cervical tissue structure examination, with the potential to enhance early diagnosis of cervical cancer and other pathological processes (Gonzalez *et. al.*, 2022). These technologies are especially useful in poor communities, where portable, simplified devices can facilitate mass screening and alleviate the global burden of cervical cancer.

12.2.1. Diagnosis of Ovarian Cysts

Advances in imaging have significantly enhanced the diagnostic yield of many gynecologic conditions, including ovarian cysts. Accurate characterization and identification of ovarian cysts are extremely crucial in determining the optimal management plan and separating benign from possibly malignant lesions. EUS remains the imaging modality of first choice owing to its widespread availability, cost-effectiveness, and high-fidelity visualization of cyst morphology. However, indeterminate or complex cases may be supported by further imaging modalities such as MRI or CT, since these will provide further anatomic and tissue-specific detail. The combination of fusion imaging technology, which unites EUS with MRI or CT, has been very promising in increasing diagnostic sensitivity and specificity, thus enabling accurate cyst assessment and well-informed clinical decision-making (Bellati *et. al.*, 2018).

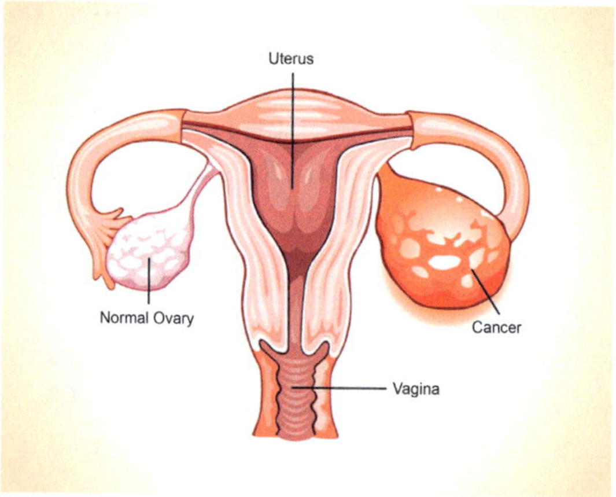

Figure 12.9. Accurate identification and characterization of ovarian cysts are crucial for determining the appropriate management strategy and differentiating benign from potentially malignant lesions.

Source: https://journals.sagepub.com/cms/10.1177/1533034614547445/asset/a4742972-68ee-492e-8a32-7433dd46d8d1/assets/images/large/10.1177_1533034614547445-fig1.jpg.

In addition, combined evaluation of serum tumor markers with imaging findings represents an efficient multimodal approach to ovarian cyst and related gynecological tumor diagnosis and follow-up monitoring (Anastasi *et. al.*, 2018) (Figure 12.9).

12.2.2. Evaluation of Uterine Abnormalities

Technical advancements in imaging equipment have significantly enhanced diagnostic accuracy for most gynecologic conditions, with the greatest progress seen in uterine pathology. Traditionally, ultrasound and MRI have been utilized; nevertheless, uterine pathology diagnosis is more commonly augmented nowadays by fusion imaging techniques which blend EUS with other imaging modalities such as MRI or CT, which permits better visualization of complex uterine anatomy and lesions. This enables more precise detection of congenital anomalies, fibroids, and adenomyosis. By overlaying real-time ultrasound images over high-resolution cross-sectional images, fusion imaging lessens diagnostic doubt and enhances preoperative planning. However, although promising early results have demonstrated its potential to enhance uterine assessment, more clinical trials must be undertaken to establish standard protocols and demonstrate its efficacy in diverse patient groups (Bellati *et. al.*, 2018). Advanced imaging methods, including image fusion advancements, highlight the changing scenario of uterine abnormality assessment in gynecological imaging.

12.2.3. Assessment of Pelvic Inflammatory Disease

Diagnosis of pelvic inflammatory disease (PID) is essential since, if left untreated, it can potentially lead to severe reproductive morbidity. Imaging is a valuable part of the evaluation of suspected PID and contributes to clinical findings and laboratory tests. Ultrasound is most commonly the first imaging modality since it is minimally invasive, widely available, and can produce very good visualization of the pelvic organs, thereby allowing complications such as tubo-ovarian abscess or hydrosalpinx to be identified. Transvaginal ultrasound's ability to produce real-time images further enhances diagnostic accuracy, facilitating differentiation between non-gynecological and gynecological pelvic pathology (Ajossa *et. al.*, 2022). However, for instances where ultrasounds' findings are indefinite or further assessment is needed, MRI may be considered since it offers superior soft tissue contrast without the use of ionizing radiation. The selection of imaging modality should balance diagnostic yield with patient safety, based on recommendations now for women of reproductive age with pelvic pain (Cantisani *et. al.*, 2022) (Figure 12.10).

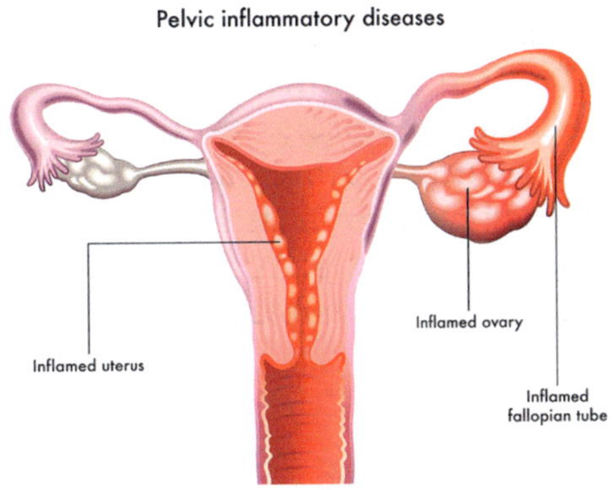

Figure 12.10. Accurately diagnosing pelvic inflammatory disease (PID) is essential due to its potential to cause significant reproductive morbidity if left untreated.

Source: https://media.healthdirect.org.au/images/inline/original/t5ff2c_8af49ae9-73f8-48af-995c-9dcc6af6d41f-ee154f.jpg.

12.2.4. Monitoring of Pregnancy Complications

The optimal management of pregnancy complications relies on early and precise monitoring, which in turn relies heavily on advanced gynecological imaging modalities. Ophthalmic abnormalities such as Mullerian duct anomalies (MDA), which are leading causes of infertility and pregnancy complications, should be identified early to offer the best possible outcomes to patients. MRI is the modality of choice for visualization with high resolution of these abnormalities, allowing exact characterization and aiding in clinical decision-making without rigidly confining findings into known categories (Dixit *et. al.*, 2025). In addition, ultrasound, including three-dimensional transvaginal sonography, complements MRI by offering low-cost and dynamic assessments during pregnancy. Along with structural evaluations, meticulous imaging plays an important role in minimizing risk of surgery in relation to gynecologic procedures during pregnancy because the choice of operative strategy can have direct implications for maternal and fetal safety (Chimenea *et. al.*, 2025). Through the integration of state-of-the-art imaging protocols into prenatal health, early intervention programs are simplified, and pregnancy complication monitoring is improved, ultimately elevating maternal-fetal health outcomes in complex clinical scenarios.

12.2.5. Detection of Gynecological Cancers

Advances in technology, with imaging devices have revolutionized the ability to detect and characterize gynecologic malignancies, improving patient prognosis through earlier and more precise diagnosis. Although traditional CT scanning and ultrasound remain useful, they often fail to accurately distinguish between malignant and benign lymph node disease, a crucial parameter in staging and treatment planning. New approaches, such as three-dimensional shear wave elastography (3D-SWE), provide quantitative assessment of lymph node stiffness with higher diagnostic performance, especially when the comparison of elasticity levels from different planes is taken into account to minimize dependence on invasive biopsy (Shen *et. al.*, 2025). Positron emission tomography and computed tomography (18F-FDG PET/CT) have also been very helpful for the detection of small peritoneal metastatic implants in ovarian cancer patients that are commonly missed using conventional imaging modalities. Such sensitivity augments loco-regional recurrence and distant metastases detection and thereby the therapeutic approach and management outcome (El-Din *et. al.*, 2024). As a group, the imaging modalities are important early and accurate detecting tools in gynecological malignancies (Figure 12.11).

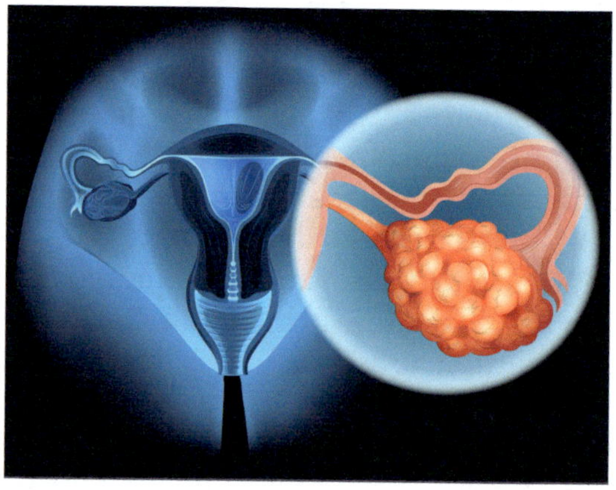

Figure 12.11. Gynecological cancers.

Source: https://www.openaccessgovernment.org/wp-content/uploads/2015/11/dreamstime_s_59495028.jpg.

12.2.6. Guidance for Biopsies and Interventions

Proper diagnosis and effective planning of treatment for gynecologic cancers rely heavily on precise biopsy procedures and duly aimed interventions. Imaging techniques play an important role in the guidance of biopsies so that tissue samples are adequately obtained from the best available sites to enhance diagnostic reproducibility. Literature on tru-cut biopsies demonstrates that, in the hands of skilled clinicians, such interventions are able to realize high adequacy and accuracy with no significant chances of complications, supporting the rationale for technical expertise in taking biopsies. Furthermore, intraoperative frozen section evaluation provides real-time diagnostic feedback required for maximizing surgical planning, particularly in ovarian cancer where discriminating malignancy grade impacts therapeutic management (Kraemer *et. al.*, 2008). Integration of preoperative CT assessment with biopsy results facilitates global evaluation of tumor dimension and guides selection of candidates for primary debulking operation, eventually improving prognostic outcomes. These multidisciplinary activities highlight that central management and imaging-guided specialty intervention significantly improve diagnostic accuracy and therapeutic efficacy in gynecologic oncology (Kraemer *et. al.*, 2008).

12.2.7. Evaluation of Infertility Issues

Improvements in gynecologic imaging have significantly enhanced infertility evaluation by enabling more precise anatomical and functional assessment of the female reproductive tract. For instance, three-dimensional transvaginal ultrasonography has been extremely useful in diagnosing uterine anomalies such as septate uterus, a common etiology of recurrent miscarriage and infertility. A recent study indicated that 3D ultrasound-guided diode laser hysteroscopic metroplasty not only successfully corrected the septum but also increased endometrial volume, a positive prognostic indicator of reproductive outcomes (Angioni *et. al.*, 2021). Furthermore, merging various imaging modalities like MRI with new ultrasound technologies enables comprehensive evaluation of conditions like endometriosis, adenomyosis, and ovarian masses that are often implicated in infertility (Gilbert *et. al.*, 2021). These imaging technologies provide valuable information to aid diagnosis and therapeutic planning, increasing the success of conception and pregnancy maintenance. Lastly, imaging of gynecology is the foundation of the treatment of infertility under a multidisciplinary framework (Figure 12.12).

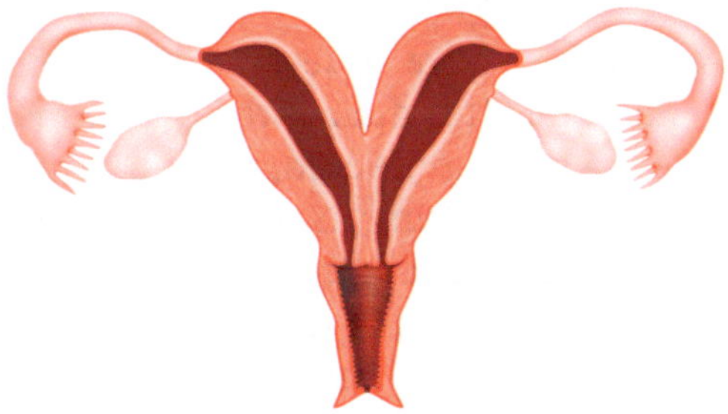

Figure 12.12. Congenital uterine abnormalities.

Source: https://www.melakafertility.com/wp-content/uploads/2020/09/Figure-11.2-Uterine-didelphus-1024x731.png.

12.2.8. Preoperative Planning for Gynecological Surgeries

Effective surgical outcomes in gynecology typically rely on meticulous preoperative planning, increasingly from cutting-edge imaging modalities. Multidimensional visualization of pelvic anatomy ensures precise surgical planning, limiting intraoperative complexity and optimizing operative efficiency. For instance, image-guided platforms enable surgeons to view specific anatomical variations and optimize device placements before intervention, optimizing procedure accuracy (Egger *et. al.*, 2013). Furthermore, intensive preoperative imaging fosters the standardization of procedure for minimally invasive techniques, as revealed by improvements in laparoscopic surgery training that align operative strategies with patient-specific anatomy (Rabischong *et. al.*, 2023). Not only does such planning reduce operative time and intraoperative bleeding, but it also provides similar postoperative outcomes for various clinical practices. Therefore, the integration of advanced imaging modalities into preoperative routines becomes obligatory for optimizing the conduct of surgery, improving patient safety, and enhancing the quality of gynecologic treatment.

12.2.9. Postoperative Assessment

Precise postoperative assessment is a critical factor in order to guarantee good patient outcomes after gynecological operations, particularly if imaging is obligatory for the evaluation of anatomical restoration and functional restoration. It is an integral process whereby imaging findings are integrated with clinical considerations in order to detect early complications such as infections, hematomas, or anatomical distortions. As with postoperative care in all specialties, it emphasizes both functional and cosmetic outcomes, objectively quantifiable using validated patient self-reports, focusing on the importance of patient satisfaction as well as on clinical success (Cordray *et. al.*, 2025). Monitoring recovery with noninvasive imaging modalities also aids in tracking tissue healing and identifying deviations that can jeopardize rehabilitation. Additionally, postoperative assessments extend beyond imaging into the arena of physiological assessments, e.g., studies comparing airway management approaches' impact on recovery in the postoperative period, highlighting the fact that best perioperative care contributes significantly towards patient overall health (Mahaseth *et. al.*, 2025). Thus, careful postoperative assessment in gynecological imaging is the pillar to advancing personalized treatment and raising surgical success rates.

Test Your Knowledge

1. What are uterine abnormalities?
2. Write some infertility issues.

12.3. Safety and Risks in Gynecological Imaging

Learning Outcome

1. Know radiation exposure concerns
2. Explain contrast agent reactions
3. Know psychological impact of imaging procedures
4. Identify risks associated with invasive procedures
5. Focus on guidelines for safe imaging practices
6. Understand patient education on imaging risks
7. Give comparison of risks across imaging modalities
8. Know importance of informed consent
9. Define regulatory standards in imaging safety

Technological development in gynecological imaging has significantly improved diagnostic accuracy, as well as therapeutic planning, but safety concerns and inbuilt risks always come first. Imaging modalities, particularly fluoroscopy when using interventional radiology, necessitate careful evaluation of patient stability and procedure timing to prevent complications. For instance, the requirement for timely decision-making using embolization, in which laparotomy is advisable when patient status renders waiting impossible (Abutaima *et. al.*, 2018). In addition, challenging situations such as large retroperitoneal masses mimicking gynecological tumors illustrate the challenges in preoperative imaging interpretation and the necessity of proper surgical planning to avoid unintentional injury. The intricacy of pelvic anatomy necessitates a multidisciplinary exercise with special focus on surgeon expertise and the tailored, deployment of imaging techniques to avoid operative risks and enhance outcomes (Abis *et. al.*, 2024). Thus, weighing the benefits of high-level imaging against potential procedural risk remains at the heart of ensuring optimum patient safety in gynecological practice (Figure 12.13).

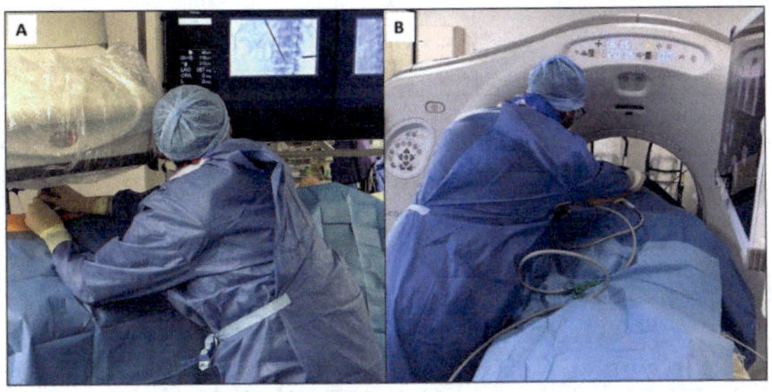

Figure 12.13. Imaging techniques, particularly when involving interventional radiology, demand careful evaluation of patient stability and the timing of procedures to minimize complications.

Source: https://pub.mdpi-res.com/medicina/medicina-57-00500/article_deploy/html/images/medicina-57-00500-g001.png?1621305084.

12.3.1. Radiation Exposure Concerns

In the complex management of gynecological pathology, particularly in pregnancy, diagnostic imaging needs a balanced trade-off between the clinician's risks and benefits. The use of ionizing radiation is a prevalent issue considering its teratogenic and carcinogenic effects in an evolving fetus. It thus demands strict precautions in the avoidance of ionizing radiation whenever possible. Nonionizing imaging technologies, such as ultrasound and MRI, are used to reduce fetal risk; nevertheless, prudent use of ionizing technologies may become inevitable to ensure appropriate diagnosis and effective planning for treatment in certain cases. Multidisciplinary coordination is needed to modify imaging protocols for optimal maternal well-being and fetal protection. This approach is especially apt in cancers like cervical cancer, where timely and precise imaging influences therapy but not fetal outcome (Gökçü *et. al.*, 2016). Lastly, continued research and guideline refinement are important to maximize risk stratification and provide safer gynecologic imaging in pregnancy.

12.3.2. Contrast Agent Reactions

In gynecologic imaging, intravenous contrast agent administration is of pivotal importance in maximizing diagnostic accuracy but demands utmost vigilance regarding potential adverse effects. While frequent utilization of contrast media has excellent safety profiles, hypersensitivity and nephrotoxicity are inherently significant concerns. Reactions range from self-limiting complaints such as rash and nausea to marked anaphylactic reactions with an urgent need for clinical intervention.

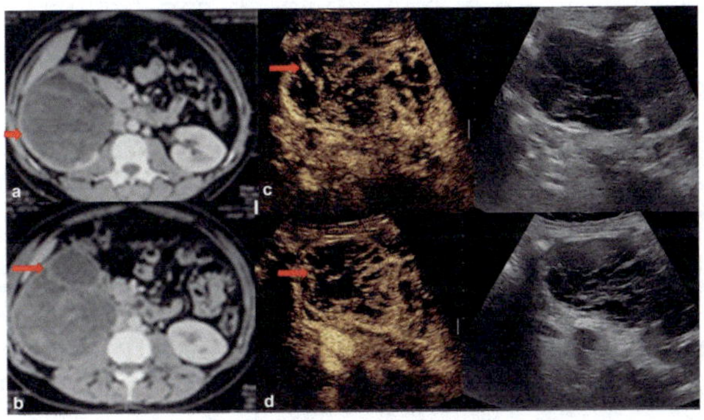

Figure 12.14. While commonly used contrast agents generally exhibit a favorable safety profile, hypersensitivity and nephrotoxicity remain significant concerns.

Source: https://media.springernature.com/lw1200/springer-static/image/art%3A10.1007%2Fs00261-022-03438-z/MediaObjects/261_2022_3438_Fig4_HTML.jpg.

Patient-specific factors and the choice of contrast agent define the risk profile importantly. Pioneering contrast-enhanced ultrasound agents, like Sonazoid, initially intended for hepatic applications, demonstrate special features on diagnostic sensitivity and specificity, which indirectly defines their paradigms of safety use (Cao *et. al.*, 2024; Liu *et. al.*, 2024). An appreciation of these insidious reactions in a range of imaging circumstances underscores the merit of specialized protocols to avoid dangers, thus ensuring patient safety whilst maximizing imaging efficacy in gynecologic evaluations (Figure 12.14).

12.3.3. Psychological Impact of Imaging Procedures

The experience of having gynecological condition imaging tests rarely ends in bodily pain, significantly affecting a patient's mental well-being. Anxiety is most often generated by concerns over radiation exposure, potential diagnoses, and the invasiveness of procedures, especially in periods of utmost need such as pregnancy. Emotional distress can become a part of a patient's quality of life and willingness to adhere to ensuing treatment or imaging protocols. It is therefore critical that psychological treatment be included in multidisciplinary team treatment to offset these impacts and optimize patient outcomes. In addition, psychological distress may be potentially amplified where imaging results generate complex treatment options, like in chemotherapy treatment with adverse effects of nausea further reducing quality of life (Atthobari *et. al.*, 2011). Treatment of these interrelated physical and psychological burdens is essential to finish gynecological care, emphasizing the need for improved communication, informed consent, and supportive interventions throughout the imaging continuum.

12.3.4. Risks Associated with Invasive Procedures

Gynecological treatment continues to put increasingly more emphasis on minimally invasive procedures in an effort to reduce patient morbidity, yet the risks of invasive procedures also require commensurate prudence. For instance, real-time three-dimensional trans-esophageal echocardiography, although instrumental in guiding minimally invasive procedures, has been associated with the risk of thermal esophageal mucosal injury as a result of probe-induced heat, leading to the development of cooling equipment to obviate such risks without compromising image quality (Parrotta *et. al.*, 2025). Similarly, uterine artery embolization, while offering an alternative minimally invasive procedure to traditional surgery for fibroid management, carries complications like ischemic complications and possibly untested long-term reproductive effects that require keen patient counseling and patient selection (Balamurugan *et. al.*, 2025). Such complications reflect the fine balance in gynecologic imaging and intervention between therapeutic gain and procedural safety. Even with improvements in surgical methods, every attempt is made to limit collateral injury and preserve fertility, highlighting the need for continuing research and development of techniques to reduce and counteract the complications of invasive gynecologic surgery (Figure 12.15).

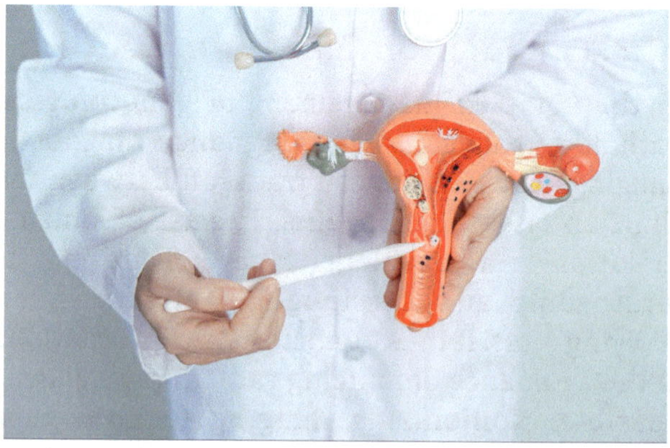

Figure 12.15. Uterine artery embolization.

Source: https://blog-revamp.s3.ap-south-1.amazonaws.com/wp-content/uploads/2023/09/12224700/image2-13-1-1.jpg.

12.3.5. Guidelines for Safe Imaging Practices

Technologic advances in imaging have tremendously improved diagnostic capacity in gynecology but also require stringent adherence to safety standards so that patients are not exposed to excess risk. Safe imaging is all about meticulous choice of appropriate modalities, optimization of radiation dose rates, and careful use of contrast agents so as not to provoke unwanted reactions. Present guidelines emphasize the importance of thorough patient assessment, including contraindication screening for conditions such as allergy or renal impairment, particularly with the application of contrast media. The employment of standard questionnaires also enhances patient safety by substantiating risk factors before the application of imaging methods. Guidelines further propose continuous monitoring of contrast agents and dosage patterns in accordance with recently released evidence-based guidelines to prevent side effects and drug interactions. Such open guidelines, approved by governing bodies like the American College of Radiologists and the European Society of Urogenital Radiology, create a robust platform for implementing secure image practices in gynecological practice (Kim *et. al.*, 2024; Sinitsyn *et. al.*, 2024).

12.3.6. Patient Education on Imaging Risks

Effective communication between health practitioners and patients is central to informed decision-making, particularly in gynecologic imaging where ionizing radiation or contrast media exposure may pose potential harm. Instructing the patient on the risks in relation to the benefits of diagnosis enhances empowerment to become an active participant in their own management and alleviates anxiety due to lack of knowledge. Physicians have to provide clear, specific answers to each patient's needs, employing visual aids and simple language to ensure optimal comprehension. Additionally, interoperable electronic health records facilitate universal risk disclosure and continuity of care through integration of relevant patient information by means of standardized ontologies to maternal well-being (Almeida *et. al.*, 2016). While imagery supports accurate diagnosis, visual aids in the form of annotated images can similarly improve explanation of risk information so patients are cognizant of its contextual applicability. Not only is this an ethical practice, it also leads to trust, thereby optimizing patient-centered outcomes in gynecologic imaging (Figure 12.16).

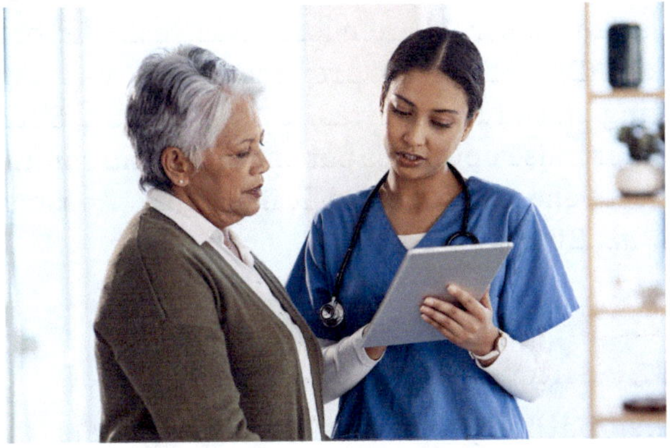

Figure 12.16. Clinicians should provide clear explanations tailored to individual patient needs, incorporating visual aids and accessible language to enhance understanding.

Source: https://www.acpdecisions.org/wp-content/uploads/2019/07/GettyImages-1169325038-1.jpg.

12.3.7. Comparison of Risks Across Imaging Modalities

Technological advances in imaging modalities have transformed diagnosis and treatment for gynecologic illness, but the risk they pose varies greatly across modalities. Ultrasound, generally the initial imaging modality of choice, is uniformly recognized for its risk profile of being free of ionizing radiation and, as such, is extremely suitable for follow-up scans and surveillance. Conversely, CT and PET, including PET/CT and PET/MRI, offer greater diagnostic precision at the cost of exposure to ionizing radiation, with the risk of cumulative doses of radiation being a concern, especially in younger patients or in patients who require sequential scans.

MRI does not expose patients to radiation but involves intravenous contrast agents that are associated with allergic reactions or nephrotoxicity. Selection of imaging modalities thus demands an educated compromise of these risks against the diagnostic benefit. Such compromises are crucial in the treatment of ovarian cancer, wherein less invasive modalities like FDG PET/MRI are promising without being harmful (Anastasi *et. al.*, 2015). Such compromise optimizes patient safety and clinical effectiveness in gynecological imaging (Anastasi *et. al.*, 2015).

12.3.8. Importance of Informed Consent

The pathway to accurate diagnosis in gynecologic imaging is typically complicated procedures with built-in risks or nuisances, and thus patient understanding is critical to ethical and good practice. One important point of departure here is informed consent, which guarantees patients the knowledge about the reason, advantages, limitations, and potential complications of imaging modalities such as transvaginal ultrasound or high-technology MRI scans. Such openness is based on trust and allows patients to participate actively in their care choices, particularly when diagnosing diseases like thoracic endometriosis or assessing myometrial infiltration in endometrial cancer.

Further, the nuance of interpretation required—highlighted by the steep learning curve even for echogenic confrontation among clinicians evaluating myometrial infiltration—again underscores the importance of informing patients regarding the diagnostic difficulties and assumptions of imaging appearances (Alcázar *et. al.*, 2023). Ethical consent processes thus uphold both patient autonomy and enhance clinical results by aligning expectations with the realities of gynecologic imaging (Bałoniak *et. al.*, 2025) (Figure 12.17).

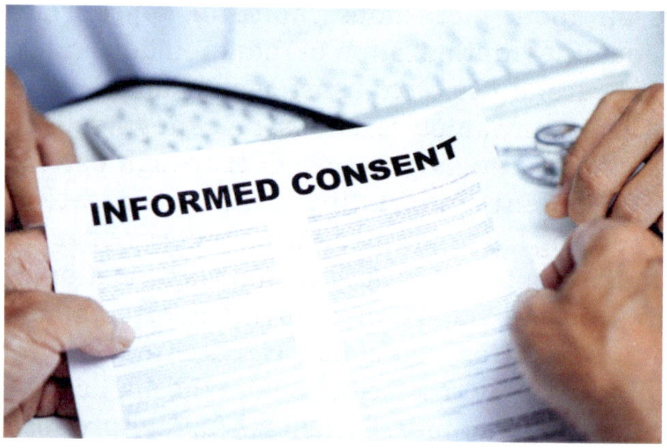

Figure 12.17. Informed consent.

Source: https://depts.washington.edu/bhdept/sites/default/files/InformedConsent.png.

12.3.9. Regulatory Standards in Imaging Safety

The progress of gynecological imaging has been powerfully directed by rigorous regulatory requirements for patient safety and maximum achievement of diagnostic performance. The control requirement covers not only the performance of the imaging equipment but also emphasizes strong validation, testing, and clearance procedures that are essential before any clinical release. These paradigms minimize risks from radiation exposure, machine failure, and user errors to protect patient health. The challenges associated with attaining such standards tend to hold back the availability of new imaging technology, demanding tangible proof of safety and efficacy in order to provide a match for regulatory demands. The lessons from surgical robotics caution against the necessity of systematic checking and ongoing assessment in filling gaps for clinical application, as an example of a good investment for imaging technology used within gynecology (Haidegger *et. al.*, 2015). Also, continuing professional education and adherence to evolving guidelines foster responsibility and safety culture in medical imaging practice (Copeland *et. al.*, 2019). This syncretic method of regulatory control is required to enhance gynecological imaging without compromising patient health.

Test Your Knowledge

1. What are the potential risks of using X-ray and CT scans in gynecological imaging, particularly in pregnant women?
2. What are the safety concerns associated with radiation exposure during CT imaging of the pelvis, especially for reproductive-aged women and young patients?

12.4. Advances in Gynecological Imaging Technology

Learning Outcome

1. Understand innovations in ultrasound technology
2. Explain development of high-resolution MRI
3. Learn integration of artificial intelligence in imaging
4. Focus on enhanced imaging software and analysis tools
5. Define telemedicine and remote imaging consultations
6. Describe 3D printing applications in gynecological imaging
7. Explain use of contrast-enhanced imaging techniques
8. Discuss future potential of molecular imaging
9. Know impact of technology on patient outcomes

The inclusion of new diagnostic technology has significantly enhanced the accuracy and efficiency of gynecologic cancer detection in the last few years. The advancements are relevant since early diagnosis and correct monitoring have major implications on the outcome of treatment and patient prognosis. The effect of new imaging technologies, with the addition of serum tumor biomarkers, includes a complete multimodal approach which improves tumor presence, extent, and recurrence assessment. This collaboration facilitates more individualized treatment strategies and more precise response evaluation, a concrete improvement over the traditional method. Above all, non-invasive imaging innovations make better visualization of tumors of the gynecologic system possible with less requirement for exploratory surgery and earlier treatment. These advances further suggest more targeted, patient-specific care in gynecology as it speaks to the necessity of integrating molecular biology results and advanced imaging modalities (Anastasi *et. al.*, 2018). Graphic depiction of these innovations also helps standardize diagnostic procedures, a gynecological imaging technology breakthrough.

12.4.1. Innovations in Ultrasound Technology

Recent imaging developments have had a crucial effect on diagnostic precision in the majority of specialties, including gynecology. Among them, ultrasound technology has been the foremost example of noninvasive technology with real-time imaging. Present ultrasound machines employ high-frequency transducers and advanced Doppler techniques, which allow for improved delineation of intricate pelvic anatomy and blood flow patterns, essential in the assessment of uterine and ovarian function. Three-dimensional and four-dimensional ultrasound imaging have also improved diagnostic precision further by providing comprehensive volumetric imaging that facilitates better evaluation of challenging anatomical variations and pathologies. Additionally, the incorporation of contrast-enhanced ultrasound improves lesion characterization without ionizing radiation exposure. These developments have not only raised detection precision of abnormalities such as fibroids, cysts, and endometrial lesions but also enhanced guided interventional procedures. These developments represent a significant step forward in imaging in gynecology, optimizing patient outcomes through more precise and dynamic assessments (Figure 12.18).

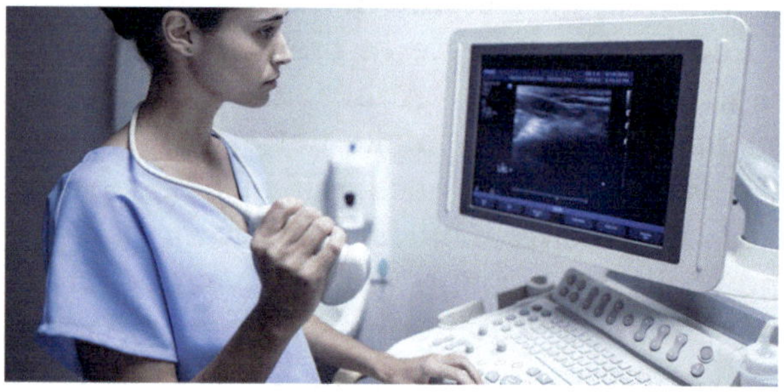

Figure 12.18. Advanced doppler techniques.

Source: https://artemiscardiac.com/speciality/65a8f929e54fdColor%20Doppler%20-%20Header%20Image.webp.

12.4.2. Development of High-resolution MRI

Technical advancement in imaging has significantly enhanced the diagnosis and treatment of gynecological disorders with improved patient outcomes. Among such developments, the improvement of high-resolution MRI has been particularly groundbreaking, with its unparalleled soft tissue contrast and high anatomical resolution. This enables clinicians to accurately classify gynecological tumors, assess extent of disease, and quantify response to treatment with greater precision (Anastasi *et. al.*, 2018). Moreover, high-resolution MRI has also been promising in the diagnosis of challenging cases such as thoracic endometriosis, where standard imaging is insufficient due to non-specific symptoms and anatomical nuances (Bałoniak *et. al.*, 2025). The capacity to combine and enhance the imaging quality with novel biomarkers facilitates early detection and individually crafted treatment procedures, further corroborating the role of this technology in contemporary gynecological imaging. Thus, high-resolution MRI is a significant method in maximizing patient care and enhancing diagnostic accuracy in the discipline.

12.4.3. Integration of Artificial Intelligence in Imaging

Technological innovations have steadily revolutionized diagnostic medical methods, and AI is currently a major driving force in improving imaging methods in gynecology. Through the capability to employ ML algorithms and pattern recognition, AI provides more precise analysis of complex imaging information, thereby assisting in overcoming challenges like early gynecological malignancy diagnosis. Particularly with ovarian cancer, conventional diagnostic methods are short on effective biomarkers. The application of AI in imaging not only improves diagnostic performance but also supports prognostic assessment and individualized treatment planning, culminating in benefit to the patient. Moreover, AI aids clinicians by rendering the decision-making process more cost-effective in obstetrics and gynecology, domains that are often afflicted by fetal physiology complexities and cancer management. With this technology's advancement, there is a need for ongoing research to further develop AI applications and implement them effectively in clinical practice, eventually revolutionizing gynecologic imaging modalities and improving healthcare provision (Bacalbasa *et. al.*, 2024; Sinha *et. al.*, 2023) (Figure 12.19).

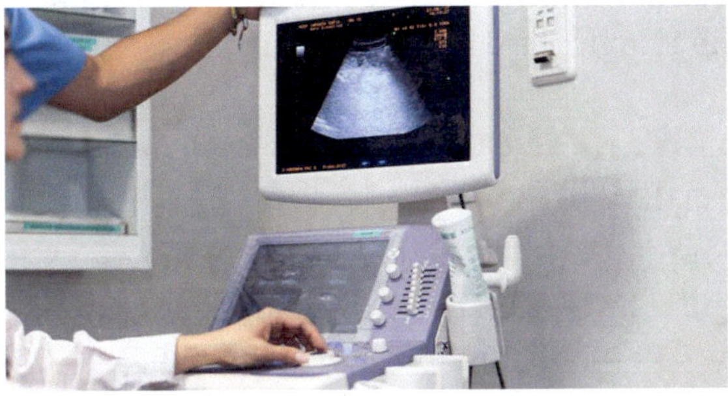

Figure 12.19. Advancements in technology have consistently transformed medical diagnostics, with artificial intelligence emerging as a pivotal tool in enhancing imaging techniques within gynecology.

Source: https://medicalbuyer.co.in/wp-content/uploads/2025/01/Ultrasound-%E2%80%93-Leading-the-future-of-diagnostics-imaging.jpg.

12.4.4. Enhanced Imaging Software and Analysis Tools

Trailblazers of diagnostic techniques have significantly transformed the landscape of gynecological imaging, facilitating more precise identification and treatment of malignancies. The impetus behind this revolution is latest imaging software and analysis tools which integrate advanced algorithms for facilitating better visualization and interpretation of complex anatomical structures. These tools enable high-resolution image reconstruction, quantitative imaging, and functional imaging, thus empowering clinicians with comprehensive information beyond existing imaging limits. For example, positron emission tomography in combination with computed tomography or magnetic resonance imaging (FDG PET/CT and FDG PET/MRI) applies advanced analytical software to increase sensitivity and specificity for the identification of gynecologic cancers like ovarian and endometrial cancers, as thoroughly reviewed in recent articles (Alkatout *et. al.*, 2023). Also, such advanced tools enable the evaluation of biochemical markers and their compatibility with the imaging findings, offering multi-dimensional diagnosis and monitoring of treatment (Anastasi *et. al.*, 2015). Consequently, such developments not only enhance diagnostics but also optimize personalized patient management approaches.

12.4.5. Telemedicine and Remote Imaging Consultations

The evolution of health care technologies has compelled health care providers to innovate with strategies in patient care, particularly under the constraints of global health crises. The COVID-19 pandemic qualitatively evolved telemedicine uptake by addressing the two-pronged challenge of persistent management of patients and preventing physical contacts in clinical settings (Eva *et. al.*, 2020). Remote imaging consultation and telemedicine in gynecologic imaging are very helpful in that they enable specialists to remotely evaluate diagnostic images and provide timely specialist input without requiring patients to travel to health centers.

This is especially helpful in infertility management, in which the initial interviews, review of test results, planning of treatment, and supervision of medication can be efficiently conducted through virtual interfaces, enhancing patient compliance and accessibility (Palagiano *et. al.*, 2023). Moreover, telemedicine facilitates ongoing emotional support and guidance, which is needed in cases with psychological complications related to reproductive health. Consequently, integrating telemedicine in gynecologic imaging ensures the optimum delivery of care with safety and continuity despite dynamic healthcare needs.

12.4.6. 3D Printing Applications in Gynecological Imaging

Advances in medicine through technology have increasingly enhanced accuracy in treatment planning and patient individualized treatment, particularly through such developments as three-dimensional (3D) printing. In gynecological imaging, 3D printing has contributed importantly to the creation of personalized applicators, improving the precision and effectiveness of treatments like brachytherapy. With patient-specific anatomical details derived from imaging modalities, physicians can quickly create biocompatible, sterilizable devices that are uniquely tailored to individual anatomical variations, leading to enhanced dose delivery and lowered tissue toxicity.

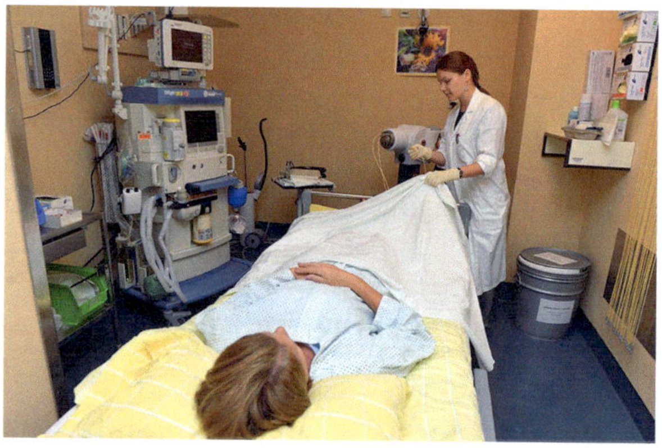

Figure 12.20. Brachytherapy.

Source: https://www.iaea.org/sites/default/files/brachytherapy_1.jpg.

As an example, patient-specific vaginal applicators in patients with complex anatomical demands have shown superior treatment outcomes without severe side effects, demonstrating the clinical effectiveness of this technology (Cunha *et. al.*, 2016). Although extensive application in gynecology is at present restricted compared to other specialties, growing evidence suggests that the integration of 3D-printed tools with imaging information has vast promise for enhancing personalized treatment planning in gynecologic oncology (Mäkitie *et. al.*, 2019). This intersection of additive manufacturing and imaging is a groundbreaking advancement in personalized gynecologic care (Figure 12.20).

12.4.7. Use of Contrast-enhanced Imaging Techniques

Advances in imaging technology have significantly improved the diagnostic accuracy and treatment planning of gynecology. Among these, contrast-enhanced imaging modalities have gained prominence because of their ability to provide precise vascular and tissue characterization, which is essential for the evaluation of pelvic pathologies. Contrast agents, typically stabilized microbubbles within a biocompatible shell, improve ultrasound imaging by more clearly delineating blood circulation and tissue perfusion, which is the key to differentiating between benign and malignant lesions. More recent developments in contrast agents, such as nanobubbles, offer further promise with their smaller size and higher concentration, allowing for better tissue penetration and novel diagnostic applications. These developments align with broader clinical trends in contrast-enhanced ultrasound, which have proven to be invaluable in other fields for lesion detection and treatment monitoring (Wegierak *et. al.*, 2024). Technical expertise is required to maximize benefits and minimize deficits in terms of operator reliance and image disturbance, as has been the case in other organ systems (Ying *et. al.*, 2025).

12.4.8. Future Potential of Molecular Imaging

Growth in imaging technology promises to revolutionize the field of gynecological diagnostics, particularly by synergistically integrating molecular imaging techniques. They can potentially enhance detection at an early stage and accurate characterization of malignant and pre-malignant conditions, which so far remain challenging with conventional imaging.

For instance, molecular imaging could dramatically increase the preoperative discrimination of leiomyosarcoma of the uterus from leiomyoma by establishing definite cellular or molecular markers of malignancy and permitting timely and targeted interventions (Adishesh *et. al.*, 2020). Similarly, handheld vital microscopy demonstrates the potential of real-time visualization of microvascular changes to facilitate instant clinical decision-making in cervical intraepithelial neoplasia and cervical cancer, emphasizing the utility of molecular-scale imaging for real-world communities (Berg *et. al.*, 2024). As molecular imaging evolves, its ability to provide accurate functional and metabolic information alongside anatomical information has the potential to revolutionize patient-specific treatment planning, reduce unnecessary surgical procedures, and ultimately improve outcomes for gynecologic cancer patients.

12.4.9. Impact of Technology on Patient Outcomes

Advances in technology have changed gynecological imaging tremendously to a large extent, greatly affecting patient outcomes with improved diagnostic accuracy and personalized therapy. Integration of AI in imaging enables the detection of extremely subtle abnormalities that can be omitted with standard approaches, thereby enabling earlier treatment and improved prognoses. AI-based algorithms review complex imaging and patient history information to tailor diagnosis and treatment plans specific to each patient's pathology and risk profile. This transition toward precision medicine not only enhances treatment efficacy but also lowers the side effects of treatment, optimizing patient compliance and satisfaction. Furthermore, AI advancements reduce the number of hospital admissions via remote care and electronic consultations, thereby improving continuity and access to care . There remain challenges in ethical use and data integration, but ongoing improvement emphasizes the transformative potential of technology in enhancing the extent of gynecological treatment and patient survival (Ananya *et. al.*, 2024; Forkuo *et. al.*, 2024).

Test Your Knowledge

1. How has the integration of AI and machine learning enhanced diagnostic accuracy in gynecological ultrasound imaging?
2. What technological improvements have been made in contrast-enhanced ultrasound (CEUS) for characterizing adnexal masses and vascular structures?

SUMMARY

Technical advancement in imaging modalities has significantly enhanced the diagnosis and treatment of gynecologic conditions, with earlier detection and improved patient outcomes. Technologies such as high-resolution MRI and PET/CT allow for greater insights than before into function and anatomy, enabling tailored treatment planning to maximize therapeutic targeting and minimize invasive procedures (Bałoniak *et. al.*, 2025; Carsrud *et. al.*, 2024). Moreover, the use of novel biomarkers in combination with imaging techniques is promising for non-invasive diagnostics with the potential to transform disease stratification and monitoring protocols (Bałoniak *et. al.*, 2025). Despite some of the limitations, including resolution problems and the need for standard methods, research continues to advance these tools to fill the gaps further. The effect of these innovations combined puts into perspective the irreplaceable role of comprehensive gynecological imaging in practice, augmenting diagnostic confidence and therapeutic precision. To sum up, the intersection of imaging innovation and biomarker research is a revolution towards more efficient, patient-centered gynecological treatment (Bałoniak *et. al.*, 2025; Carsrud *et. al.*, 2024).

Gynecologic imaging advances have enhanced diagnostic sensitivity and patient management by visualizing in detail reproductive anatomy and disease. Imaging techniques such as EUS, MRI, and CT yield overlapping information about conditions ranging from benign cysts to malignancy, thereby influencing treatment and prognostic evaluation. Integration of accurate imaging with clinical assessment allows early detection of abnormalities, such as those defined by systemic conditions such as obesity, presenting additional barriers to imaging interpretation and management of the patient (Fionnuala *et. al.*, 2020). Furthermore, awareness of the biochemical context, such as elements such as matrix metalloproteinases and their inhibitors, contributes to imaging interpretation regarding remodeling of tissue and progression of disease (Griselda *et. al.*, 2020). Collectively, the key points emphasize the requirement for a multidisciplinary team and adherence to evolving guidelines to ensure imaging modalities are maximally utilized to maximize outcomes in women's health through evidence-based, individualized treatment.

KEY TERMS FROM THIS CHAPTER

- Gynecology
- Personalized treatment
- Open abdominal surgery
- Diagnostic accuracy
- Morbidity
- Minimally invasive hysterectomy
- Artificial intelligence

CRITICAL THINKING QUESTIONS

1. **What is the primary imaging modality used for routine gynecological examinations?**
   a. X-ray
   b. Ultrasound
   c. CT scan
   d. MRI
2. **Which of the following imaging techniques is most commonly used to assess ovarian cysts?**
   a. CT scan
   b. MRI
   c. Transvaginal ultrasound
   d. Mammography
3. **In gynecological imaging, which imaging modality is considered the gold standard for the evaluation of endometriosis?**
   a. CT scan
   b. Ultrasound
   c. MRI
   d. Hysterosalpingography (HSG)
4. **Which imaging modality is most commonly used to assess the uterine anatomy and detect abnormalities such as fibroids or polyps?**
   a. Ultrasound
   b. MRI
   c. Hysterosalpingography (HSG)
   d. CT scan
5. **In the diagnosis of uterine cancer, which imaging modality is typically used to evaluate the extent of the disease?**
   a. Ultrasound
   b. MRI
   c. CT scan
   d. PET scan

Short Answer Questions

1. What is the most common imaging technique used for the evaluation of uterine fibroids?
2. How does transvaginal ultrasound differ from transabdominal ultrasound in the assessment of gynecological conditions?
3. What is the role of MRI in the evaluation of endometriosis?
4. How does 3D ultrasound improve the assessment of uterine anomalies compared to traditional 2D ultrasound?
5. What are the indications for using MRI in the assessment of pelvic masses or ovarian tumors?
6. How does Doppler ultrasound help in evaluating uterine blood flow and diagnosing conditions such as uterine artery abnormalities?
7. What is the primary imaging modality for diagnosing ectopic pregnancy, and why is it preferred over others?

Answers to Critical Thinking Questions

1. (b); 2. (c); 3. (c); 4. (a); 5. (b)

REFERENCES

1. Abdullah, M. F., Sulaiman, S. N., Osman, M. K., Karim, N., Ani, A. I. C., & Ahmad, N. (2024). Identification of lung lesions in computed tomography scan images using machine learning techniques. In *2024 IEEE 14th International Conference on Control System, Computing and Engineering (ICCSCE)*. https://www.semanticscholar.org/paper/f69516500d9c72af8ef9ebe5686b4b76c80eb66f (accessed on 30 May 2025).
2. Abis, P., D'Angelo, N., Maccio, A., Madeddu, C., *et. al.* (2024). A giant pelvic infiltrating schwannoma misdiagnosed as an ovarian neoplasm that was resected using a laparoscopic approach: A case report. https://core.ac.uk/download/621427776.pdf (accessed on 30 May 2025).
3. Abutaima, A. J. A., Al-Nagri, A. M., Alsaleh, S. A. S., Dehbash, F., *et. al.* (2018). Gynecological disorders and the management of interventional radiology. https://core.ac.uk/download/234692393.pdf (accessed on 30 May 2025).
4. Adishesh, M., DeCruze, S. B., Hapangama, D. K., Lane, G., *et. al.* (2020). Developing a preoperative algorithm for the diagnosis of uterine leiomyosarcoma. https://core.ac.uk/download/334602144.pdf (accessed on 30 May 2025).
5. Aggarwal, K., Singhal, A., Singh, S., & Naqvi, N. (2025). Advancements in automated segmentation techniques for endometrial cancer: A comprehensive review. In *2025 10th International Conference on Signal Processing and Communication (ICSC)*. https://www.semanticscholar.org/paper/87a1448483614e16cca30e56118bc7d07ddcd109 (accessed on 30 May 2025).
6. Ajossa, S., Alcázar, J. L., Browne, J. L., Graupera, B., *et. al.* (2022). Extra-gynecological pelvic pathology: A challenge in the differential diagnosis of the female pelvis. https://core.ac.uk/download/558773528.pdf (accessed on 30 May 2025).
7. Alcázar, J. L., Chacón, E., Guerriero, S., Laza, R., *et. al.* (2023). Learning curve for ultrasound assessment of myometrial infiltration in endometrial cancer visualizing videoclips: Potential implications for training. https://core.ac.uk/download/558773519.pdf (accessed on 30 May 2025).
8. Alkatout, I., Allahqoli, L., Fallahi, A., Ghiasvand, F., *et. al.* (2023). 18F-FDG PET/MRI and 18F-FDG PET/CT for the management of gynecological malignancies: A comprehensive review of the literature. https://core.ac.uk/download/599096231.pdf (accessed on 30 May 2025).
9. Almeida, M., Elkin, P., Farinelli, F., Smith, B., *et. al.* (2016). OntONeo: The obstetric and neonatal ontology. https://core.ac.uk/download/131214730.pdf (accessed on 30 May 2025).
10. Alnawafleh, T. M., Radzi, Y., Alshipli, M., Oglat, A., & Alflahat, A. (2024). A comprehensive review of the recent advancements in imaging segmentation and registration techniques for glioblastoma and focusing on the utilization of magnetic resonance imaging (MRI) and computed tomography (CT) scans. *Current Medical Imaging, 20*(1), e15734056309829. https://www.semanticscholar.org/paper/ae87c4cf6856748d0b441675af777db7633b96a8 (accessed on 30 May 2025).
11. Ananya, S., Suresh, N., & Pullela, P. K. (2024). Revolutionizing healthcare: The impact of artificial intelligence on precision diagnoses and patient outcomes. *2024 Fourth International Conference on Multimedia Processing, Communication & Information Technology (MPCIT)*. https://www.semanticscholar.org/paper/607826beafe78c939b68834bc7b9e00498235705 (accessed on 30 May 2025).

12. Anastasi, E., Angeloni, A., Ballesio, L., Gigli, G., *et. al.* (2018). The complementary role of imaging and tumor biomarkers in gynecological cancers: An update of the literature. https://core.ac.uk/download/153370712.pdf (accessed on 30 May 2025).

13. Anastasi, E., Angeloni, A., Granato, T., Manganaro, L., *et. al.* (2015). Low 25-OH vitamin D levels at time of diagnosis and recurrence of ovarian cancer. https://core.ac.uk/download/54521407.pdf (accessed on 30 May 2025).

14. Angioni, S., Bollino, M., De Feo, V., Falagario, T., *et. al.* (2021). The use of hysteroscopic metroplasty with diode laser to increase endometrial volume in women with septate uterus: Preliminary results. https://core.ac.uk/download/541245238.pdf (accessed on 30 May 2025).

15. Anthoulakis, C., Bourne, T., Froyman, W., Kaijser, J., *et. al.* (2015). Practical guidance for applying the ADNEX model from the IOTA group to discriminate between different subtypes of adnexal tumors. https://core.ac.uk/download/77000315.pdf (accessed on 30 May 2025).

16. Asp, M. (2022). Advanced ovarian cancer: A multimodal diagnostic approach to predict outcome. https://core.ac.uk/download/543787062.pdf (accessed on 30 May 2025).

17. Atthobari, J., Dwiprahasto, I., Gelderblom, H., Guchelaar, H. J., *et. al.* (2011). Impact of chemotherapy-induced nausea and vomiting on quality of life in Indonesian patients with gynecologic cancer. https://core.ac.uk/download/11820685.pdf (accessed on 30 May 2025).

18. Bacalbașa, N., Balalau, C., Bălescu, I., *et. al.* (2024). *Artificial Intelligence in Ovarian Cancers—from Diagnosis to Treatment: A Literature Review.* https://core.ac.uk/download/624145776.pdf (accessed on 30 May 2025).

19. Balamurugan, S., Shah, R., Panganiban, K., Lehrack, M., & Agrawal, D. K. (2025). Uterine artery embolization: A growing pillar of gynecological intervention. *Journal of Radiology and Clinical Imaging, 8*(1), 1–17. https://www.semanticscholar.org/paper/8f90e21d8323ced2b698a2e5d899ed1b6ec848d3 (accessed on 30 May 2025).

20. Bałoniak, J., Bałoniak, Z., Doligalska, M., *et. al.* (2025). *Diagnostic Challenges and Innovations in Thoracic Endometriosis (TE): Exploring the Role of Imaging and Biomarkers. A Narrative Review.* https://core.ac.uk/download/636385653.pdf (accessed on 30 May 2025).

21. Bellati, F., Caserta, D., Costanzi, F., *et. al.* (2018). *Real-Time Virtual Sonography in Gynecology & Obstetrics: Literature's Analysis and Case Series.* https://core.ac.uk/download/195777140.pdf (accessed on 30 May 2025).

22. Berg, A. V. V., Ince, C., Kastelein, A. W., *et. al.* (2024). *Handheld Vital Microscopy for The Identification of Microcirculatory Alterations in Cervical Intraepithelial Neoplasia and Cervical Cancer.* https://core.ac.uk/download/591475272.pdf (accessed on 30 May 2025).

23. Bhattacharya, S., Boivin, J., Farquhar, C. M., *et. al.* (2019). *Female Subfertility.* https://core.ac.uk/download/162930981.pdf.

24. Blagden, S., Fotopoulou, C., Gabra, H., *et. al.* (2015). *The Next Steps in Improving the Outcomes of Advanced Ovarian Cancer.* https://core.ac.uk/download/77021701.pdf (accessed on 30 May 2025).

25. Bouwsma, E. V. A., Jones, B. P., Lees, C., Stalder, C., Barcroft, J., Ben Nagi, J., Yazbek, J., *et. al.* (2020). *Implications for the Future of Obstetrics and Gynecology Following the COVID-19 Pandemic: A Commentary.* https://core.ac.uk/download/328757402.pdf (accessed on 30 May 2025).

26. Cabral-Pacheco, G. A., Garza-Veloz, I., Castruita-De la Rosa, C., Ramirez-Acuña, J. M., Perez-Romero, B. A., Guerrero-Rodriguez, J. F., Martínez-Avila, N., *et. al.* (2020). The roles of matrix metalloproteinases and their inhibitors in human diseases. *International Journal of Molecular Sciences, 21*(24), 9739. https://doi.org/10.3390/ijms21249739.

27. Cai, L., & Pfob, A. (2024). Artificial intelligence in abdominal and pelvic ultrasound imaging: Current applications. *Abdominal Radiology, 50*, 1775–1789. https://www.semanticscholar.org/paper/55314a35acef6c9e235b37b28972c8abfbcc0089 (accessed on 30 May 2025).

28. Calç, G., Calagna, G., Cucinella, G., *et. al.* (2014). *Septate Uterus: Nosographic Overview and Endoscopic Treatment.* https://core.ac.uk/download/53293073.pdf (accessed on 30 May 2025).

29. Cantisani, V., Caruso, M., Dell'Aversano Orabona, G., *et. al.* (2022). *Pelvic Pain in Reproductive Age: US Findings.* https://core.ac.uk/download/566522949.pdf (accessed on 30 May 2025).

30. Cao, J., Wang, H., Ruan, X., Yang, J., Ren, Y., & Ling, W. (2024). The American College of Radiology contrast-enhanced ultrasound Liver Imaging Reporting and Data System and its modified version in diagnosing hepatocellular carcinoma via Sonazoid: A meta-analysis. *Quantitative Imaging in Medicine and Surgery, 14*, 4555–4566. https://www.semanticscholar.org/paper/daeda5a0759741ad0accc541ff139ba123b23dfd (accessed on 30 May 2025).

31. Carsrud, N. D. V., Flores, J. V., Holets, H. M., *et. al.* (2024). *Transformative Precision: Investigative Summary of Pet/Ct-Guided Radiation Therapy Simulation in Comprehensive Cancer Management.* https://core.ac.uk/download/603903713.pdf (accessed on 30 May 2025).

32. Chantziantoniou, N. (2019). *Impediments to the Historical Development of The Clinical Pap Test in the United States: Their Relevance in Optimizing Cervical Cancer Screening in the State of Qatar.* https://core.ac.uk/download/268253145.pdf (accessed on 30 May 2025).

33. Chimenea, Á., & Calderón, A. M. (2025). Enhancing safety in gynecologic surgery: Innovative access and lymphadenectomy techniques to reduce complications. *Complications.* https://www.semanticscholar.org/paper/31e4d49f0d365a527043b8dcdbd4d0f72774b5d7 (accessed on 30 May 2025).

34. College of Medicine. (2015). *University of South Alabama College of Medicine annual report for 2015–2016.* https://core.ac.uk/download/568546361.pdf (accessed on 30 May 2025).

35. Copeland, L. I. B. T., Duinkerken, M. S. I., Gordon, K., *et. al.* (2019). *Jefferson Digital Commons Quarterly Report: October–December 2019.* https://core.ac.uk/download/286097805.pdf (accessed on 30 May 2025).

36. Cordray, H., Shah, A. S., Buttrick, E., Chang, B., Little, K. J., Al-Muhtaseb, T., & Mendenhall, S. D. (2025). Postoperative and long-term patient-reported outcomes of Type A ulnar polydactyly. *Plastic and Reconstructive Surgery.* https://www.semanticscholar.org/paper/874c0e5ad8fc28282d63b2177d7cbc56a9f11955 (accessed on 30 May 2025).

37. Cornejo, J., Cornejo, J., Vargas, M., Helguero, C. G., Andrade, R. M., Torres, S., Asensio-Salazar, J., *et. al.* (2022). Anatomical engineering and 3D printing for surgery and medical devices: International review and future exponential innovations. *BioMed Research International, 2022*, 1–28. https://doi.org/10.1155/2022/6797745.

38. Cunha, A., Diederich, C., Hsu, I. C., *et. al.* (2016). *Clinical Applications of Custom-Made Vaginal Cylinders Constructed Using Three-Dimensional Printing Technology.* https://core.ac.uk/download/323074295.pdf.

39. Desai, M. B., Pandey, S., & Kumar, Y. (2024). Advancements in artificial intelligence techniques for diagnosis and detection in 3D medical images. In *2024 International Conference on Intelligent Systems for Cybersecurity (ISCS)*. https://www.semanticscholar.org/paper/d5818850e85ded7e8754c2bc0d05a3b25aaf4d78 (accessed on 30 May 2025).

40. Dixit, R., Duggireddy, C. S., & Pradhan, G. S. (2025). Mullerian anomalies: Revisiting imaging and classification. *Insights into Imaging, 16*. https://www.semanticscholar.org/paper/d941d5228e1aacafd378ccb5d42cf322197d9db9 (accessed on 30 May 2025).

41. Domino, W., Śnieżna, J., Florczak, W., Dzwonnik, K., Zelik, U., Włodyka, J., Trestka, G., *et. al.* (2025). Innovative diagnostic approaches and treatment strategies for endometriosis: Current trends and future direction–Review. *Quality in Sport*. https://www.semanticscholar.org/paper/14ef6ac1b1b836fdfad05d55b97b4e22e6948bc6 (accessed on 30 May 2025).

42. Egger, J. (2013). *Image-Guided Therapy System for Interstitial Gynecologic Brachytherapy in A Multimodality Operating Suite*. https://core.ac.uk/download/pdf/81056936.pdf (accessed on 30 May 2025).

43. El-Din, O., Amin, M., & Abdelsatar, S. A. E. (2024). Evolving role of whole-body 18F-FDG PET/CT in post therapeutic evaluation of ovarian malignancy. *Benha Medical Journal*. https://www.semanticscholar.org/paper/1e73b1099e9eebca9f26e723a989da9195e1e042 (accessed on 30 May 2025).

44. Forkuo, A. Y., Ikhalea, N., Chianumba, E. C., & Mustapha, A. Y. (2024). Reviewing the impact of AI in improving patient outcomes through precision medicine. *International Journal of Advanced Multidisciplinary Research and Studies*. https://www.semanticscholar.org/paper/0b0962e87408dc4a1aeb920f4b4681fbdff32f39 (accessed on 30 May 2025).

45. Gilbert, S. (2021). *Imaging in Women's Health*. https://core.ac.uk/download/520100775.pdf (accessed on 30 May 2025).

46. Gökçü, M., Güngördük, K., Köse, M. F., *et. al.* (2016). *Management of Cervical Cancer During Pregnancy*. https://core.ac.uk/download/288333035.pdf (accessed on 30 May 2025).

47. Gonzalez, M. (2022). *Polarimetric Imaging of the Uterine Cervix*. https://core.ac.uk/download/572717141.pdf (accessed on 30 May 2025).

48. Goyal, A. S., Chaudhari, J., Sejal, Shrivastava, A. R., *et. al.* (2017). *Comparison of Transvaginal Sonography and Saline Infusion Sono Hysterography for the Diagnosis of Causes of Abnormal Uterine Bleeding: A Diagnostic Accuracy Study*. https://core.ac.uk/download/539902244.pdf (accessed on 30 May 2025).

49. Haidegger, T., & Rudas, I. J. (2015). *From Concept to Market: Surgical Robot Development*. https://core.ac.uk/download/42938958.pdf (accessed on 30 May 2025).

50. Haji-Noor, Z. M. (2023). *Classifying Eligibility for Minimally Invasive Hysterectomy in the Carolina Hysterectomy Cohort, 2014–2017*. https://core.ac.uk/download/596785709.pdf (accessed on 30 May 2025).

51. Rimon Islam , M. T., Hasan, M. W., Hassan, M., & Cesmeci, S. (2024). Advancements in insulin pumps: A comprehensive exploration of insulin pump systems, technologies, and future directions. *Pharmaceutics, 16*. https://www.semanticscholar.org/paper/2bd8813d206cff837eb62ca6aa3f53cdd8b3768b (accessed on 30 May 2025).

52. Karalis, V. (2024). The integration of artificial intelligence into clinical practice. *Applied Biosciences, 3*, 14–44. https://doi.org/10.3390/applbiosci3010002.

53. Khaladkar, S., Dhande, A., Shah, R. N., & KirdatPatil, P. P. (2024). Application of the morphological uterine scoring assessment in ultrasound for abnormal uterine bleeding. *Cureus, 16*. https://www.semanticscholar.org/paper/662019ce6dcecedde96c8787cde69fb40c9c9e18 (accessed on 30 May 2025).

54. Khouri, A. (2004). *Evaluation of Diagnostic Culdoscopy in Women with Infertility*. https://core.ac.uk/download/326710925.pdf (accessed on 30 May 2025).

55. Kim, Y. R., & Jeong, S. (2024). Evaluating the interaction between orthodontic appliances and magnetic resonance imaging: Establishing clinical guidelines for safe imaging practices. *Clinical Journal of Korean Association of Orthodontists*. https://www.semanticscholar.org/paper/0339fe5f46fd931ef4bc129abf004d2261ec6183 (accessed on 30 May 2025).

56. Kraemer, B., Cox, D., Wallwiener, D., Baez, E., Hoffmann, G., Schulz, K. D., Freidel, K., *et. al.* (2008). *Vacuum-Assisted Breast Biopsy: A Comparison of 11-Gauge And 8-Gauge Needles in Benign Breast Disease*. https://core.ac.uk/download/pdf/8072063.pdf.

57. Lalande, A., Bonmatí, J. M., Miquel, C. M., Malagelada, O., *et. al.* (2017). On the use of XML in medical imaging web-based applications. https://core.ac.uk/download/81581709.pdf (accessed on 30 May 2025).

58. Liu, Q., Liu, T., Liu, X., Zhang, F., Yang, J., Cheng, Y., & Yang, Q. (2024). The efficacy of modified contrast-enhanced ultrasound Liver Imaging Reporting and Data System (CEUS LI-RADS) using Sonazoid in diagnosis of hepatocellular carcinoma: A systematic review and meta-analysis. *Quantitative Imaging in Medicine and Surgery, 14*, 2927–2937. https://www.semanticscholar.org/paper/89a750c8d101b5d4e428481d1a773fdff8041ec8 (accessed on 30 May 2025).

59. Mahaseth, R., Gupta, B., Jain, G., Bahadur, A., Singla, D., & Tripathy, D. (2025). Proseal laryngeal mask airway and endotracheal intubation in lower abdominal gynecological surgeries for perioperative gastric volume assessment and assessing postoperative recovery of gastrointestinal functions: A randomized controlled trial. *Saudi Journal of Anesthesia, 19*, 27–33. https://www.semanticscholar.org/paper/d52b22276d62f66397b4857e1bdc123265bce412 (accessed on 30 May 2025).

60. Mäkitie, A. A., Pettersson, A. B. V., Salmi, M., & Serlo, W. (2019). Main clinical use of additive manufacturing (three-dimensional printing) in Finland restricted to the head and neck area in 2016–2017. https://core.ac.uk/download/479166410.pdf (accessed on 30 May 2025).

61. McAuliffe, F. M., Killeen, S. L., Jacob, C. M., Hanson, M. A., Hadar, E., McIntyre, D., Kapur, A., *et. al.* (2020). Management of prepregnancy, pregnancy, and postpartum obesity from the FIGO Pregnancy and Non-Communicable Diseases Committee: A FIGO (International Federation of Gynecology and Obstetrics) guideline. *International Journal of Gynecology & Obstetrics, 151*, 16–36. https://doi.org/10.1002/ijgo.13334.

62. Meucci, R., Prosperi, D., Lauri, C., Campagna, G., Nayak, P., Garaci, F., & Signore, A. (2024). Peritoneal carcinomatosis of malignant gynecological origin: A systematic review of imaging assessment. *Journal of Clinical Medicine, 13*. https://www.semanticscholar.org/paper/c9dc71c2796ba3e636eaba36e4794d260fcafdb0 (accessed on 30 May 2025).

63. Oglat, A. A., & Abukhalil, T. (2024). Ultrasound elastography: Methods, clinical applications,

and limitations: A review article. *Applied Sciences*. https://www.semanticscholar.org/paper/0bc80b40eaf5c4e7484d0c0537133c7ebebe57e9 (accessed on 30 May 2025).

64. Palagiano, A., Bulletti, C., Bulletti, F. M., Berrettini, M., Guido, M., & Sciorio, R. (2023). Telemedicine in IVF programs. https://core.ac.uk/download/620489861.pdf (accessed on 30 May 2025).

65. Parrotta, F., Faoro, G., Tognarelli, S., Menciassi, A., & Giannoni, A. (2025). A miniaturized cooling system for trans-esophageal echocardiographic probes may improve patients' safety in minimally invasive cardiac surgery or trans-catheter percutaneous interventions. *European Heart Journal–Cardiovascular Imaging*. https://www.semanticscholar.org/paper/5e12a6f2494f07d987389a13de54d4fa51fa232d (accessed on 30 May 2025).

66. Piras, A., Peddes, C., Pilla, F., Sedda, F., Melis, G. B., Alcázar, J. L., Saba, L., *et. al.* (2015). Past, present and future ultrasonographic techniques for analyzing ovarian masses. https://core.ac.uk/download/572833132.pdf.

67. Rabischong, B., Spadoto-Dias, D., Bueloni-Dias, F. N., França, M. L. M., Canis, M., Bourdel, N., Chauvet, P., *et. al.* (2023). *The Impact of Laparoscopic Gynecological Surgery Training on The Technicity Index of a Developing Country Center*. https://core.ac.uk/download/579829818.pdf (accessed on 30 May 2025).

68. Rasulova, N., Teshabaeva, K., Ozodova, M., & Rakhmatullaeva, N. (2023). *Early Diagnosis and Prevention of Gynecological Diseases*. https://core.ac.uk/download/586551571.pdf (accessed on 30 May 2025).

69. Sadavar, S., Lee, S., & Park, S.-J. (2024). Advancements in asymmetric supercapacitors: From historical milestones to challenges and future directions. *Advanced Science, 11*. https://www.semanticscholar.org/paper/6293f91c0a7141c721b0dac7f55c8cedf9a273f8 (accessed on 30 May 2025).

70. Shen, Y., Dai, J., Li, J., & Lu, M. (2025). The application of three-dimensional shear wave elastography in the detection of inguinal lymph node metastasis in gynecological malignancies. *Clinical and Experimental Obstetrics & Gynecology*. https://www.semanticscholar.org/paper/c755e5f12f1cf8e5771904048c0db6744487c9b3 (accessed on 30 May 2025).

71. Shruti, & Sen, S. (2019). The prospective study of laparoscopic finding in infertility cases. *International Journal of Reproduction, Contraception, Obstetrics and Gynecology*. https://www.semanticscholar.org/paper/3770b15154c6c1d297be77753cfff883c91de2bc (accessed on 30 May 2025).

72. Sinha, V. (2023). *A Systemic Review on The Future of Obstetrics and Gynecology: Harnessing Artificial Intelligence*. https://core.ac.uk/download/595722139.pdf (accessed on 30 May 2025).

73. Sinitsyn, V., Tyurin, I., Shimanovskiy, N. L., Karmazanovskiy, G. G., Bychenko, V., Rubtsova, N., & Filatova, D. (2024). Safe use of contrast media in radiology (clinical guidelines). *Journal of Radiology and Nuclear Medicine*. https://www.semanticscholar.org/paper/7c5dd4e5d1a892ec058bcfbf12b68282ef268d36 (accessed on 30 May 2025).

74. The University of Texas MD Anderson Cancer Center. (2023). *2023 Summer Experience Program Abstracts*. https://core.ac.uk/download/578908493.pdf

75. Wegierak, D., Nittayacharn, P., Cooley, M. B., Berg, F., Kosmides, T., Durig, D., Kolios, M., *et. al.*

(2024). Nanobubble contrast enhanced ultrasound imaging: A review. *Wiley Interdisciplinary Reviews: Nanomedicine and Nanobiotechnology, 16*. https://www.semanticscholar.org/paper/448565e59d59d5bfe2cdb4d10ca731f9af3f46d4 (accessed on 30 May 2025).

76. Ying, X., Dong, S., Zhao, Y., Chen, Z., Jiang, J., & Shi, H. (2025). Research progress on contrast-enhanced ultrasound (CEUS) assisted diagnosis and treatment in liver-related diseases. *International Journal of Medical Sciences, 22*, 1092–1108. https://www.semanticscholar.org/paper/36455cb54dbad49b95ce8ca257accbed7cc950a6 (accessed on 30 May 2025).

77. Zhang, Y., Wang, H., Butler, D., To, M. S., Avery, J., Hull, M. L., & Carneiro, G. (2023). Distilling missing modality knowledge from ultrasound for endometriosis diagnosis with magnetic resonance images. In *2023 IEEE 20th International Symposium on Biomedical Imaging (ISBI)*. https://www.semanticscholar.org/paper/4ce5198b2d4bf7b7eeed621d19effee64045cec8 (accessed on 30 May 2025).

BREAST IMAGING

13

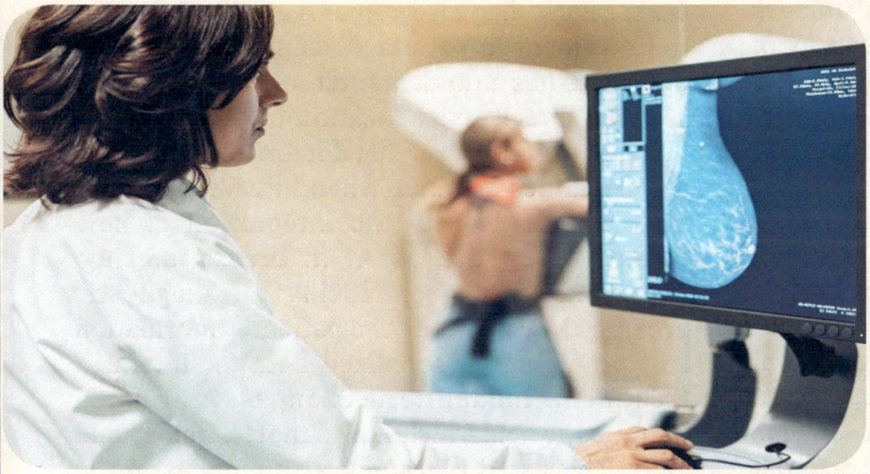

LEARNING OBJECTIVES

After studying this chapter, you will be able to:

1. Identify types of breast imaging techniques
2. Describe indications for breast imaging
3. Know benefits and limitations of breast imaging
4. Focus on future directions in breast imaging

Introduction

Medical technology breakthroughs have significantly impacted the early detection and diagnosis of illnesses, particularly in cancer. Of these breakthroughs, breast imaging has turned out to be a critical application in the detection of breast cancer in stages where rates of cure are ideal. Breast imaging encompasses numerous modalities with their forte and limitations that define performance in diagnosis, tolerance of patients, and healthcare expenditure. New advancements, like photoacoustic imaging, offer promising options by way of cost-saving and non-invasive, promising to replace traditional methods like X-ray mammography and EUS at the near diagnosis phase (Hilgerink *et. al.*, 2011). This is coupled with the application of deep learning algorithms in medical image analysis that has enhanced the accuracy and efficiency of breast imaging interpretation, rendering previously time-consuming and operator-dependent tasks such as classification and segmentation feasible (Bejnordi *et. al.*, 2017). All these concepts combined demonstrate the evolving face of breast imaging and highlight the essence of future investigations to streamline diagnostic methods.

Definition of Breast Imaging

Medical technology has significantly expanded the number of methods that can be employed to image breast tissue, enabling early detection and improved diagnosis of breast pathology. Breast imaging encompasses different modalities that are used to acquire extensive internal images of the breast, which aid in the detection of abnormalities such as tumors, cysts, or calcifications. Conventional methods, like X-ray mammography and EUS, remain in vogue, but newer modalities like photoacoustic imaging and ultrasound tomography offer promising advances. Photoacoustic imaging, for example, is the combination of optical and ultrasound technologies to provide low-cost and non-invasive diagnostic options that might rival existing imaging standards in the detection of initial breast cancer (Hilgerink *et. al.*, 2011). Similarly, three-dimensional ultrasound tomography reconstructs accurate sound speed maps in the breast tissue, which results in improved diagnostic accuracy and removal of artifacts typical of conventional imaging (Cox *et. al.*, 2020).

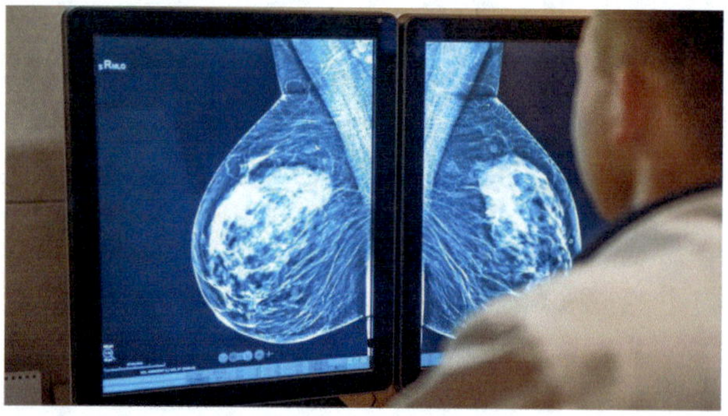

Figure 13.1. Breast imaging.

Source: https://www.dinw.com/wp-content/uploads/2021/10/Breast-Imaging-820x460.jpg.

In total, these modalities reflect the evolving concept of breast imaging as a multidisciplinary specialty where various technologies come together to improve patient care (Figure 13.1).

Importance of Breast Imaging in Healthcare

Technological changes have transformed the healthcare setting, particularly in the detection and management of diseases such as breast cancer. Early diagnosis remains a major factor for improvement in patient outcome, and imaging of breasts has a fundamental role in this aspect. Through precise visualization of breast tissue, imaging procedures assist doctors in identifying abnormalities at times when interventions are most effective. Also, the integration of new technologies, such as AI in breast imaging, will contribute to enhancing the diagnostic accuracy by combining the patient's information and providing personalized data for intended treatment modalities. Changes in related therapeutic fields, including nanotechnology and electric-assisted therapies, also emphasize the importance of precise imaging in managing the treatment process and evaluating response. As the progress in healthcare continues through such interdisciplinarity, the worth of breast imaging as a basis for integrated breast cancer care increasingly becomes apparent (Fadlil *et. al.*, 2024; Marano *et. al.*, 2024).

Overview of Breast Imaging Techniques

Technological advances have revolutionized the world of breast imaging, enhancing detection and planning of treatment. Traditional methods such as mammography remain the cornerstone, providing essential screening function, with ultrasound and magnetic resonance imaging (MRI) giving added information, particularly in dense breasts or high-risk individuals. Additionally, image-guided localizing techniques for wire positioning and novel magnetic seed localizing methods have refined the accuracy of preoperative interventions, balancing oncological safety and aesthetic outcomes (Franceschini *et. al.*, 2021). Artificial intelligence (AI) also aids these imaging technologies by reducing diagnostic errors and enhancing workflow, though data quality problems and ethical restraints persist (Goyal, 2021). Collectively, these approaches provide an integrated model for the diagnosis and treatment of breast cancer, emphasizing the importance of individual evaluation to maximize clinical wisdom (Figure 13.2).

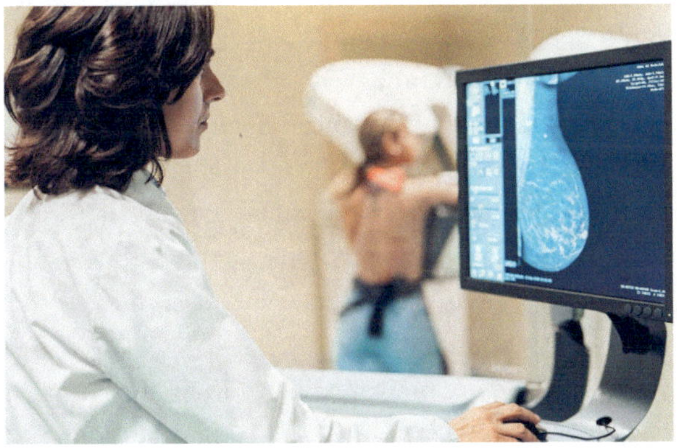

Figure 13.2. As technology evolves, multidisciplinary collaboration remains critical to leveraging these tools effectively for improved patient care.

Source: https://www.yashodahealthcare.com/blogs/wp-content/uploads/2021/08/mammography-test-cost-in-delhi-ncr.jpeg.

Historical Context of Breast Imaging

Breast imaging development follows overall progress in medical technology and diagnostic modalities, following a trend from rudimentary modalities to highly sophisticated, AI-based ones. Early breast imaging was extensively based on palpation and basic radiography, with no great sensitivity and specificity. The introduction of mammography represented a breakthrough, enabling the detection of breast pathology at an earlier stage and reducing mortality by increasing the screening level. With the advancement of technology, three-dimensional tomosynthesis and digital imaging became increasingly precise in their diagnosis. Even more recently, the addition of AI transformed breast imaging through the ability to recognize patterns and make predictions more effectively, thereby increasing the precision and speed of diagnosis. All these innovations address problems such as minimizing human errors and ensuring maximum personalized care, in line with broader healthcare digitization and AI adoption trends. An appreciation of this historical evolution outlines the manner in which this fusion of technological and clinical advances has all convergently impacted contemporary breast imaging practice, reinforcing the imperative of continued interdisciplinarity (Iqbal, 2022; Shuroug *et. al.*, 2023).

Current Trends in Breast Imaging

Technological innovation in the field of medicine has had a significant influence on the subspecialty of breast imaging, promoting improvements towards more targeted and less invasive diagnostic techniques. The trend today includes the use of newer imaging technologies such as spectral imaging that offer more ability to quantitate multiple molecular and cellular parameters simultaneously, offering richer prognostic and diagnostic information than conventional methods (Beechem *et. al.*, 2012). In addition, technological progress in imaging has been accompanied by technological progress in breast surgery and reconstructive surgery, facilitating enhanced preoperative planning and postoperative monitoring. Instrumentation and implant developments used in breast surgery reflect a larger trend toward personalized image-guided therapy, allowing for better results and patient safety (Darzi *et. al.*, 2016). These trends manifest a growing interest in combining quantitative imaging data with advances in surgery to make breast cancer detection and treatment more optimal. This interdisciplinary collaboration holds out a rosy future for breast imaging, characterized by greater specificity and individualized care.

Target Audience

Effective breast imaging practice must be modified to meet the requirements of special populations, and interventions in screening and diagnosis must be well-suited to patient characteristics. The target population is primarily composed of women at average or greater than average risk for breast cancer, highly heterogeneous in age, genetic risk, and general health status. These are crucial considerations because treatments and recommendations are more applicable based on varying individual clinical presentations. For instance, application of sexual health and quality of life in cancer patients through timely counseling and targeted medical interventions is crucial in a general care plan, highlighting the need for individualized strategies based on patient demographics and side effects of treatments (Carter *et. al.*, 2017).

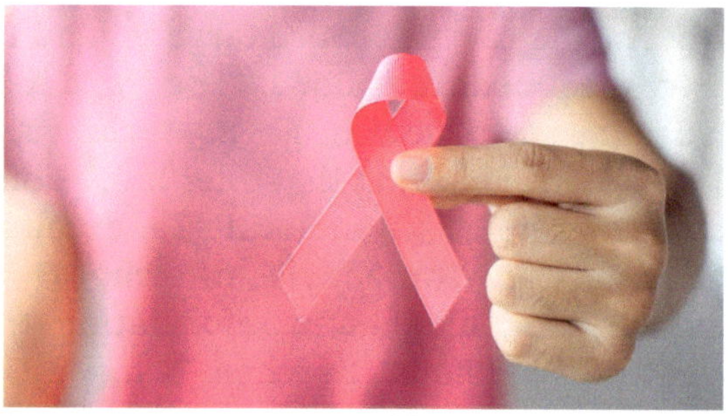

Figure 13.3. The target audience primarily includes women at average or elevated risk for breast cancer, who vary widely in age, genetic predisposition, and overall health status.

Source: https://d35oenyzp35321.cloudfront.net/introduction_to_cancer_1_37fa93bd5f.jpg.

Moreover, there are simultaneous observations that can be made regarding pediatric obesity guidelines with the necessity of individualized screening strategies and care plans intended for controlling comorbidities and risk factors in a high-risk population effectively (Dennis *et. al.*, 2017). Thus, it defines the target audience for breast imaging such that patient-specific care becomes more targeted, maximizing outcomes while improving timely intervention (Figure 13.3).

13.1. Types of Breast Imaging Techniques

Learning Outcome

1. Understand mammography
2. Focus on ultrasound
3. Know magnetic resonance imaging (MRI)
4. Define tomosynthesis (3D mammography)
5. Explain breast-specific gamma imaging (BSGI)
6. Describe contrast-enhanced mammography
7. Explain digital breast tomosynthesis
8. Understand elastography
9. Identify emerging technologies in breast imaging

As medical technology advances, the range of breast imaging modalities increases, raising the level of diagnostic accuracy and outcome in patients. Mammography remains the first-line screening procedure since it can detect early malignancies through X-ray imaging, but is handicapped by dense breasts. In comparison to this limitation, ultrasound imaging is another method that employs sound waves to distinguish cystic from solid masses without the application of radiation. MRI provides high-resolution, three-dimensional images that are useful in high-risk populations and complex cases, leveraging contrast agents that highlight vascular activity commonly present in tumors. Emerging technologies, such as circulating tumor cell (CTC) detection using microfluidic platforms, suggest future integration of non-invasive cellular biomarkers to accompany imaging and improve prognosis determination

(Che *et. al.*, 2016). However, the exact estimation of their impact on these innovations is still difficult, owing to economic as well as social factors that will determine their integration into standard breast imaging practices (Fortina *et. al.*, 2015). This multi-dimensional approach mirrors the dynamic trend in the identification of breast cancer.

13.1.1. Mammography

Advances in breast cancer diagnosis have led to a focus on imaging devices that maximize diagnostic yield and patient comfort and safety. Among these, mammography remains a cornerstone in the early detection of breast cancer due to its ease of access and demonstrated efficacy. Yet, newer technologies such as photoacoustic imaging hold promising prospects that could overcome some of the shortcomings of traditional mammography, specifically in minimizing invasiveness and ionizing radiation exposure without compromising diagnostic performance.

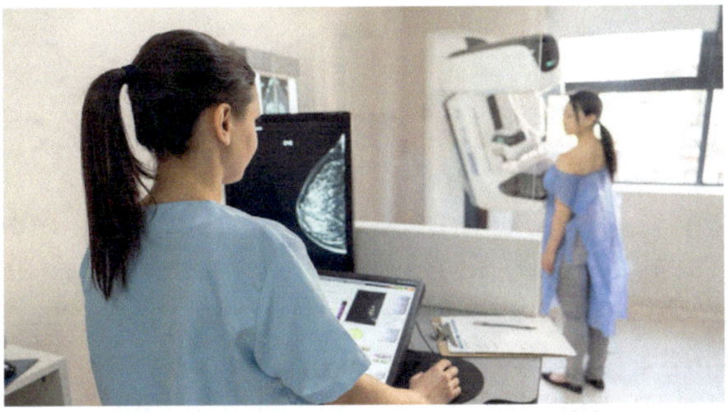

Figure 13.4. Mammography test.

Source: https://srivastavamriandimagingcentre.com/images/content/slider/Mammography.jpg.

Expert opinion suggests that enhancement of features such as detector sensitivity and reconstruction algorithms can render these novel modalities much more efficient, making them good substitutes for the traditional x-ray mammography and EUS combination in early detection programs (Hilgerink *et. al.*, 2011). Microwave imaging systems also present new avenues using specialized antenna design for maximum signal coupling and resolution within tissue in the breast (Busawon *et. al.*, 2010). These ongoing developments show an ever-changing field where mammography's role is reassessed in light of emerging techniques, in pursuit of more effective and patient-focused breast imaging modalities (Figure 13.4).

13.1.2. Ultrasound

Advances in imaging technology have significantly enhanced the use of ultrasound in breast imaging with enhanced diagnostic precision and lesion characterization. Advanced ultrasound techniques, particularly when combined with state-of-the-art computational models such as EfficientNet-B7, enable highly precise classification of breast lesions as benign, malignant, or normal. By using several image enrichment methods like Random Horizontal Flip, Rotation, and Color Jitter, these models reduce data imbalances and increase generalizability to achieve classification grades of 99% accuracy, precision, recall, and F1-score, which are critical in reducing diagnostic errors in medical practice. In addition, more recent breakthroughs in Doppler imaging, i.e., Angio-PLUS, facilitate noncontrast observation of microvasculature through subtle examination of tissue motion, overcoming the previous shortcomings of loss of low-flow signals in small vessels. This heightened sensitivity to vascularity allows better estimation of the aggressiveness and possible malignancy of lesions, giving radiologists valuable information for accurate diagnosis without contrast agents (Mohindra *et. al.*, 2024).

13.1.3. Magnetic Resonance Imaging (MRI)

Advances in imaging technology have significantly enabled the early detection and treatment of breast cancer, particularly through the use of MRI. Compared with routine mammography, MRI is much more sensitive in tumor detection, particularly in dense breasts where mammograms are less effective. This increased sensitivity renders MRI a valuable tool in screening at-risk populations as well as in pre-treatment planning, allowing the clinician to more precisely measure tumor size and extent. Beyond detection, MRI also plays a central role in planning breast biopsy when lesions are detected only on this modality. MRI-guided biopsies, with drawbacks including contraindications from implants and relatively high benign yields, remain the modality of choice since they can sample regions inaccessible to other imaging modalities (Preste *et. al.*, 2024). Ongoing technological innovations, including the integration of robotic assistance in image-guided biopsies, will further augment the specificity and efficiency of breast MRI, establishing it even more firmly in breast imaging protocols (Preste *et. al.*, 2024) (Figure 13.5).

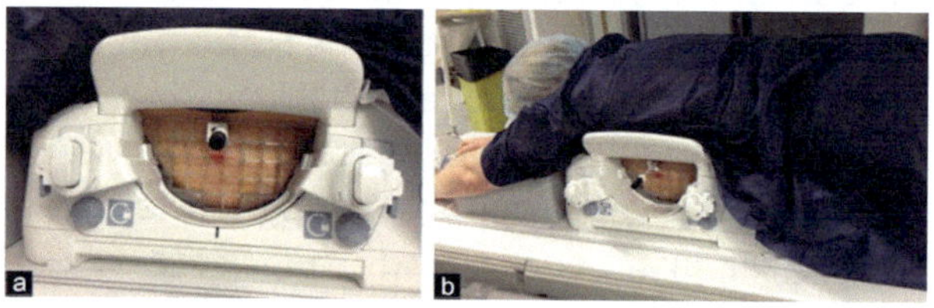

Figure 13.5. MRI-guided biopsies, despite challenges such as contraindications from implants and a relatively high rate of benign findings, remain the preferred method due to their ability to target areas inaccessible by other imaging techniques.

Source: https://ars.els-cdn.com/content/image/1-s2.0-S2211568413004312-gr3.jpg.

13.1.4. Tomosynthesis (3D Mammography)

Advances in technology of breast imaging have significantly enhanced detection and description of breast lesions, reducing some of the built-in disadvantages of traditional mammography. Among such advances is tomosynthesis, also known as 3D mammography, where a pseudo-3D image of the breast is reconstructed, thus circumventing the issue of tissue overlap that is common with traditional 2D imaging. This facilitates improved visualization of normal fibroglandular tissue and pathological lesions, allowing for more accurate detection of potential malignancies. Furthermore, modern-day algorithms integrate image registration and reconstruction steps, offering better image fidelity and enhanced spatial correspondence between time sequences, which are critical to following changes over time (Arridge *et. al.*, 2013). Despite such innovation, challenges persist, such as low contrast at X-ray frequencies between tumors and normal tissue, in some cases leading to false positives or false negatives. To do this, new multimodal methods combining tomosynthesis with other imaging modalities, like near-field radar imaging, are also being created in a bid to leverage the strengths of both methodologies, potentially enhancing diagnostic accuracy and patient outcomes (Dagheyan *et. al.*, 2017).

13.1.5. Breast-specific Gamma Imaging (BSGI)

Breast imaging has evolved, focusing more on improving diagnostic performance and minimizing invasive tests. Among more recent techniques, BSGI is a valuable alternative to standard mammography and EUS in inconclusive cases. Studies have indicated that BSGI can achieve a remarkable negative predictive value of 98.4% and maintain sensitivity of about 90%, being quite effective in preventing unnecessary biopsies and associated healthcare costs (Ko *et. al.*, 2024). In addition, the incorporation of BSGI with mammography or EUS has been shown to enhance diagnostic performance, especially for BI-RADS category 0 and 4a, by increasing specificity and positive predictive values, enhancing patient management (Ryu *et. al.*, 2022). Though beneficial, tumor growth rates can influence the accuracy of BSGI, which emphasizes the need for prudent interpretation within a multidisciplinary context. Finally, BSGI is a thrilling imaging modality that complements existing techniques, enabling differential diagnosis and optimizing therapeutic decisions (Figure 13.6).

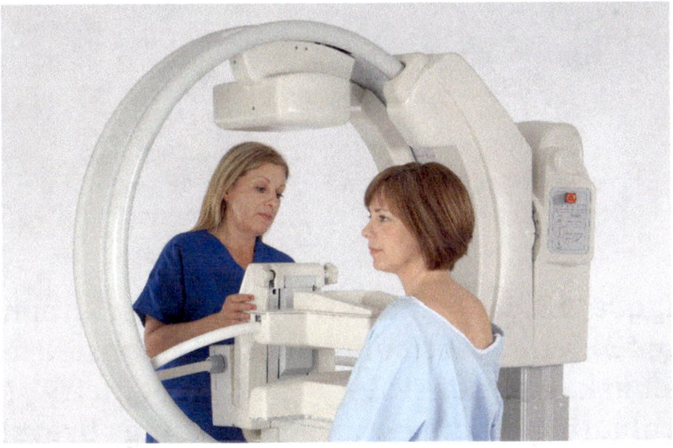

Figure 13.6. Breast-specific gamma imaging (BSGI).

Source: https://www.itnonline.com/sites/default/files/field/image/X0000_Gamma%20Medica_LumaGEM%204_0.jpg.

13.1.6. Contrast-enhanced Mammography

Technological advancements in breast imaging have increasingly emphasized techniques that maximize the early detection and accurate diagnosis of cancer. Among these, Contrast-Enhanced Mammography (CEM) has been an optimistic modality, employing contrast agents to maximize the visualization of tumors over standard mammography. In comparison to the norm set by breast MRI, CEM has similar sensitivity and specificity in detecting suspicious breast lesions, based on pooled data indicating sensitivities of 96% for CEM and 97% for MRI, and both modalities having a specificity of 77% (Neeter *et. al.*, 2023). While MRI has a slightly higher diagnostic odds ratio overall, the potential for CEM is to image faster with fewer contraindications and better accessibility. Furthermore, new techniques using deep learning to assess CEM images claim to directly predict histological tumor characteristics, which may decrease delay to diagnosis and enhance treatment planning (Popello *et. al.*, 2024). These developments mean that CEM is well placed to take an increasingly major part in breast imaging protocols.

13.1.7. Digital Breast Tomosynthesis (DBT)

Innovations in breast imaging have been directed in greater degrees toward surpassing the limitations of standard mammography, in particular the issue of tissue overlap, which obscures lesions. DBT addresses this issue by reconstructing pseudo-three-dimensional images from a series of low-dose X-ray projections and thus enhancing visualization of fibroglandular architecture and underlying pathology. One of the key developments in DBT technology is image registration techniques built into it, which improve temporal change detection through image registration of images taken at different times to track disease progression. Conventional methods are typically hampered by artifacts produced by limited-angle data acquisition but have been surpassed by newer techniques employing simultaneous reconstruction and registration, where greater accuracy was demonstrated through joint estimation of image intensities and transformations. These methods, like non-rigid B-spline models, allow for more accurate deformation recovery without image fidelity loss, enhancing diagnostic assurance and potential early cancer detection further (Arridge *et. al.*, 2013). These advances underscore the clinical value of DBT for breast imaging (Figure 13.7).

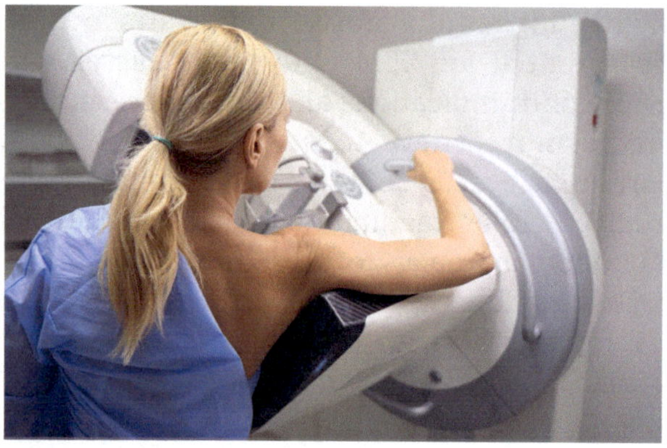

Figure 13.7. Digital breast tomosynthesis (DBT).

Source: https://www.insideprecisionmedicine.com/wp-content/uploads/2024/09/Tomosynthesis-1799926176.jpg.

13.1.8. Elastography

Imaging modalities have turned more and more to measuring tissue mechanical properties in a bid to improve diagnostic yield. Among these more recent approaches, elastography involves the use of tissue elasticity to more accurately distinguish between malignant and benign masses than standard imaging. Particularly, quantitative micro-elastography (QME) has proved to be highly sensitive and specific in the evaluation of tumor margins of breast-conserving surgery, offering intraoperative guidance that can reduce the frequency of reoperation for suboptimal margins. Unlike traditional optical coherence tomography, QME provides three-dimensional images of microscale tissue stiffness, making it possible to differentiate tumor cells within 1 mm from the surgical margin accurately. This increased accuracy not only enables better surgical outcomes but can be made to automate in real-time diagnosis (Kelsey *et. al.*, 2020). In addition, recent imaging technologies including photoacoustic techniques also have the ability to augment elastography by providing high-resolution imaging which is non-ionizing with contrast abilities varied, potentially bettering breast cancer treatment planning and screening (Steinberg *et. al.*, 2019) (Figure 13.8).

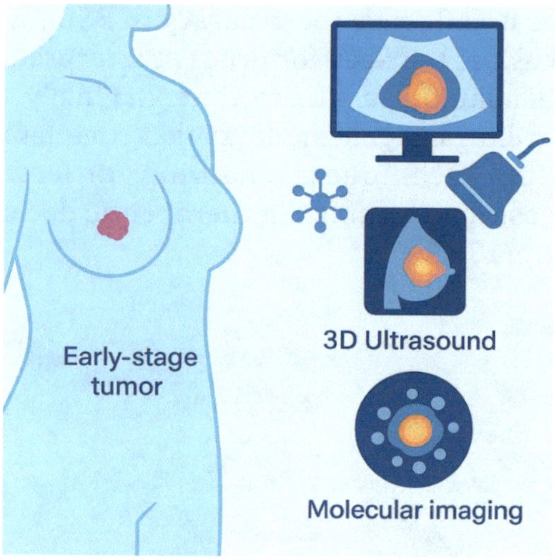

Figure 13.8. Quantitative micro-elastography (QME), in particular, has demonstrated remarkable sensitivity and specificity in evaluating tumor margins during breast-conserving surgery.

Source: https://publinestorage.blob.core.windows.net/066823f7-a05a-4a02-bd5b-0be3408adb30/csp-2024-00032-ga.jpg.

13.1.9. Emerging Technologies in Breast Imaging

Recent advances in medical imaging have revolutionized diagnostic capability, particularly in breast imaging, by integrating emerging technologies such as AI, multimodal data analysis, and novel imaging modalities. The introduction of AI-based technologies such as generative AI and explainable AI has significantly improved image interpretation accuracy and reduced diagnostic errors, enabling the early detection of breast lesions and enhanced personalized therapy. In addition, technologies like digital twins and augmented reality provide clinicians with high-fidelity 3D models for preoperative planning and more precise interventions. These technological advancements are supported by developments in data infrastructure, regulation, and interprofessional collaboration, enabling smooth incorporation into clinical workflows.

The future of breast imaging also holds the promise of using blockchain and quantum imaging to further secure data and to enhance the resolution of images, respectively. These revolutionizing developments emphasize the central role that transformational technologies contribute to improving patient outcome and operational efficiency in breast imaging (Gwendolyn *et. al.*, 2024). Concurrent development of surgical application, such as microsurgical intervention aided by enhanced imaging, likewise portrays this convergence (Ayala *et. al.*, 2024).

Test Your Knowledge

1. What are the primary imaging techniques used for breast cancer screening?
2. When is breast ultrasound typically used, and what types of lesions is it best suited to evaluate?

13.2. Indications for Breast Imaging

Learning Outcome

1. Perform screening for breast cancer
2. Learn diagnostic evaluation of breast abnormalities
3. Monitor treatment response
3. Assess breast density
4. Evaluate high-risk patients
5. Investigate breast pain
6. Discuss follow-up after breast surgery
7. Describe research and clinical trials
8. Focus on patient education and awareness

Accurate diagnosis and management of breast pathology largely rely on appropriate imaging modalities in response to individual clinical circumstances. Imaging of the breast is not merely indicated for screening but also when routine work-up results are indeterminate, e.g., evaluation of ambiguous lesions or determination of estrogen receptor status in metastatic breast carcinoma. For example, 18F-FES PET scans are particularly helpful in clarifying uncertain cases by establishing estrogen receptor status in metastatic disease, especially in the bone, thereby raising diagnostic confidence and informing therapy (van *et. al.*, 2012). However, its sensitivity varies by site, and liver metastases are less reliably detected. In addition, tools, like automated 3D breast ultrasound and digital breast tomosynthesis, have expanded the use of breast imaging, offering greater mass, microcalcification, and multifocal disease visualization, as well as supplementing traditional mammography and ultrasound for diagnostic and screening applications (European Society for Gastrointestinal and Abdominal Radiology, 2012). These tools underscore the significance of personalized imaging strategies to provide best-in-class patient outcomes.

13.2.1. Screening for Breast Cancer

Medical imaging technologies have played a major role in the early diagnosis of breast cancer, an important determinant of survival improvement. Mammography is the gold standard for breast cancer screening and is highly effective in older women but may be less sensitive in younger women because of dense breasts, making image interpretation more difficult. As a result, adjunct modalities like ultrasound and MRI are now used more frequently to improve detection. Ultrasound is particularly valuable in the evaluation of indeterminate findings but not as a standalone screening test in asymptomatic women. MRI, more costly and less available, is more sensitive to be applied in high-risk populations and provides an accurate assessment of tumor size. Emerging technologies like digital infrared thermal imaging offer the possibility of detection of subtle early vascular changes prior to mammographic change. Furthermore, the incorporation of AI is revolutionizing breast imaging with improved lesion detection, classification, and risk estimation, ultimately contributing to optimizing the effectiveness of screening and patient outcomes (Ahmed *et. al.*, 2024) (Figure 13.9).

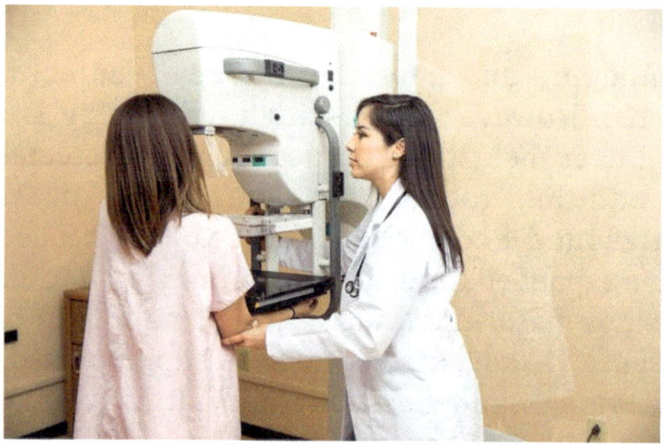

Figure 13.9. Screening for breast cancer.

Source: https://axisimagingnews.com/wp-content/uploads/2018/01/dreamstime_s_82298992.jpg.

13.2.2. Diagnostic Evaluation of Breast Abnormalities

Technical innovations in imaging modalities significantly enhanced the diagnostic evaluation of breast pathology by promoting detection and characterization of lesions. Traditional methods, like color Doppler ultrasound, are mostly restricted in sensitivity, particularly for identifying low-flow signals in small vessels, which are of paramount significance in differentiating benign and malignant lesions. These older ultrasound-based microvascular imaging techniques are surpassed by the newer ones, which provide improved visualization of the vascularity of tumors without contrast agents, enabling more accurate diagnosis and treatment planning (Mohindra *et. al.*, 2024). Additionally, AI-supported modalities such as Thermalytix, a thermal imaging device, also hold promise as adjunct diagnostic tools. Research confirms that Thermalytix offers good sensitivity and specificity, particularly in the dense breast tissue cases of women, when conventional mammography might be non-diagnostic (Bansal *et. al.*, 2023). Adding these newer techniques adds confidence to diagnosis, optimizes patient management, and reduces the risk of breast cancer missed or delayed detection in breast imaging protocols.

13.2.3. Monitoring Treatment Response

Breast cancer treatment has tried to increasingly put its focus on the contribution of dynamic assessment techniques to measure the outcome of intervention methods. Traditional imaging devices, while very important for initial diagnosis, are not sensitive in the measurement of response to treatment and identification of residual disease on a continuous basis. Liquid biopsies, which assess CTCs and circulating tumor DNA (ctDNA), are a promising complement to standard breast imaging by offering real-time insight into the dynamics of the tumor and clonal evolution during treatment (Gabriel *et. al.*, 2020). In particular, both the number and description of the clusters of CTCs, which possess significantly enhanced metastatic potential compared to solitary CTCs, have demonstrated strong prognostic value in monitoring disease recurrence and treatment responses (Emma *et. al.*, 2021). Combining these molecular biomarkers with existing imaging modalities can further enable personalized therapeutic approaches, permitting the earlier identification of resistance mechanisms and metastasis and, therefore, improved patient outcome via timely intervention adjustment (Figure 13.10).

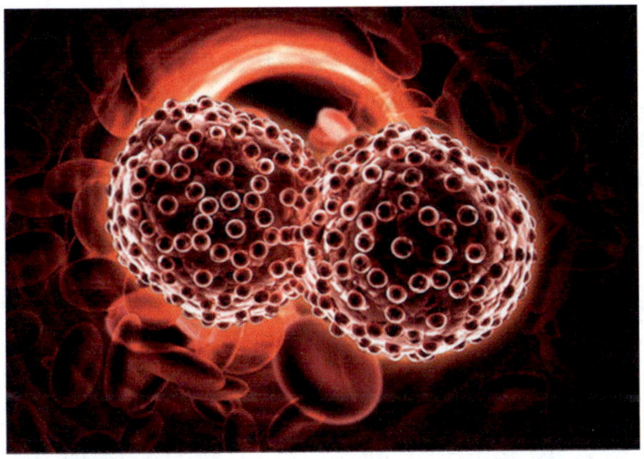

Figure 13.10. Circulating tumor cells (CTCs).

Source: https://actorius.co/wp-content/uploads/2019/08/3.jpg.

13.2.4. Assessing Breast Density

Recent technological progress in breast imaging has kept the spotlight on the central role of breast density estimation in cancer risk stratification and diagnostic performance. Breast density, as seen on mammograms, is a powerful independent predictor of breast cancer and affects screening effectiveness and patient treatment. A number of risk estimation models, such as Tyrer–Cuzick and BOADICEA, integrate mammographic density with genetic data to enhance risk estimation accuracy, although with challenges in appropriately individualizing risk assessment (Evans *et. al.*, 2016). Significantly, research emphasizes the heterogeneity of density measurement techniques, where visual inspection is often better than automated versions despite inherent variability, and prompting the use of standardized measures. In addition, emerging imaging technologies to assess microvascular density in breast cancer, such as AngioPLUS Doppler technology, hold out promise for new avenues to correlate vascular morphology with tumor biology with a potential increase in diagnostic specificity (Kim *et. al.*, 2018). These technologies all collectively draw attention to the evolving face of breast density measurement as part of whole breast imaging.

13.2.5. Evaluating High-Risk Patients

Accurate diagnosis and personalized management are critical considerations in optimizing results for patients considered to be at high risk for breast cancer. These individuals will generally require more extensive imaging studies beyond the standard mammogram due to the complexity and subtlety of potential malignant presentation. The addition of cutting-edge modalities such as breast MRI improves sensitivity, especially for the diagnosis of pathologic nipple discharge-associated abnormalities, a symptom that is frequently complained of and associated with malignancy in a high percentage of cases (Panzironi *et. al.*, 2019). Moreover, fusion imaging technology, which integrates EUS with MRI or CT, holds promising potential for maximizing anatomical visualization and guiding targeted interventions, though its application in breast imaging is nascent and requires further research (Bellati *et. al.*, 2018).

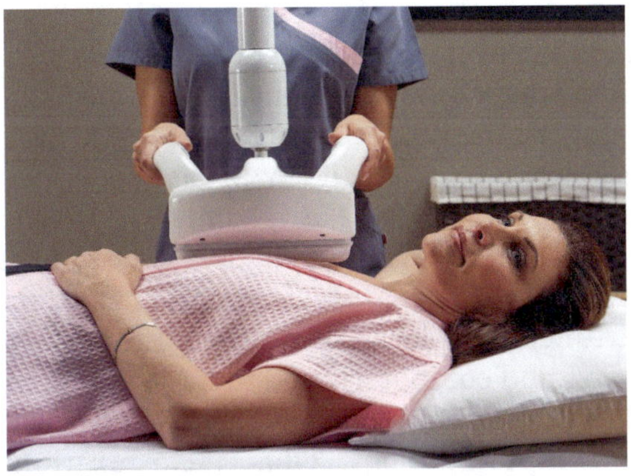

Figure 13.11. Accurate diagnosis and personalized management are crucial components in optimizing outcomes for patients considered at high risk for breast cancer.

Source: https://images-cdn.welcomesoftware.com/ Zz05MGRlMTFhMG IwNGYxMWVjODBm OGQ2OWI0Nz NiNzUzZA= =/GE%20and%20Intel%20Article% 20Banner%20Image%20.jpeg.

By tailoring imaging protocols to the individual patient's risk profile and symptoms, clinicians can maximize early detection rates, facilitate minimally invasive diagnosis, and reduce unnecessary surgery. This integrated approach underlines the usefulness of innovative imaging techniques in the subtle evaluation of high-risk breast patients (Figure 13.11).

13.2.6. Investigating Breast Pain

Effective evaluation of breast pain requires an aggressive approach that integrates clinical examination with advanced imaging techniques to resolve benign etiology from possibly severe pathology. Even though breast pain is generally associated with hormonal fluctuations or benign processes such as cysts or mastitis, persistent or atypical symptoms require further assessment with directed imaging modalities. Fusion imaging, being the union of EUS and more high-resolution imaging like MRI, is a cutting-edge diagnostic technology that best illustrates the enhanced visualization of breast tissue and enhanced discrimination of lesions, thereby aiding clinical decision-making (Bellati *et. al.*, 2018). The technology, although used more extensively in breast imaging in other departments, has promising potential to enhance assessment algorithms in breast imaging by offering precise anatomical details and functional data. Also, altering radiological reports and computerized databases are helpful points of reference to correlate imaging findings and symptomatology. Thus, incorporation of advanced imaging modalities in the diagnostic algorithm of breast pain is essential in order to provide correct diagnosis and proper management.

13.2.7. Follow-Up After Breast Surgery

Effective follow-up care after breast cancer treatment in patients is crucial to optimize long-term outcomes and detect recurrences early. In patients treated with breast-conserving surgery, studies have demonstrated that adhering to a follow-up regimen with diagnostic mammogram every six months for the first two years significantly enhances the detection rate of ipsilateral breast tumor recurrence, with nearly one-third of recurrent events detected by this approach (Miah *et. al.*, 2024). This pro-active surveillance regimen rounds off physical assessment and ancillary modalities in addressing the daunting requirement for earlier intervention for invasive recurrences. Moreover, new axillary management strategies after breast surgery, such as tailored axillary surgery with or without irradiation, are being explored to reduce morbidity with adequate disease control (Weber *et. al.*, 2024). These advances highlight the importance of individualized follow-up imaging regimens that navigate between intensive surveillance and avoiding excessive invasive procedures and ultimately enhance patient quality of care and survival advantage in breast cancer treatment (Figure 13.12).

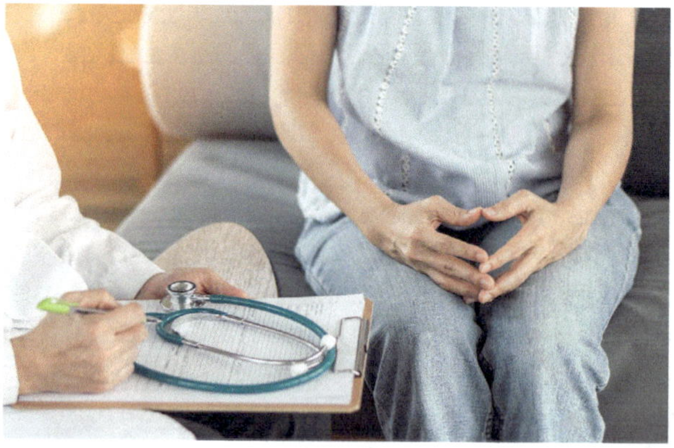

Figure 13.12. Effective post-surgical management in breast cancer patients is essential to optimize long-term outcomes and detect recurrences early.

Source: https://www.verywellhealth.com/thmb/qjwJoyUn87I_gHj1eKS6xvTkc3o=/1500x0/filters:no_upscale():max_bytes(150000):strip_icc()/iStock-989387872-a87c953e4a4c44c488d5aeb446bfd5ca.jpg.

13.2.8. Research and Clinical Trials

Technologic advancements in breast imaging have increasingly become reliant on the use of AI and deep learning (DL) to enhance diagnostic accuracy and treatment follow-up. Research continues to examine how AI potentially would identify, segment, and classify tumor lesions on its own, minimizing the workload of radiologists and enhancing consistency across clinical sites (Zheng *et. al.*, 2023). Encouraging initial results are reported, especially in mammography and digital breast tomosynthesis, but extensive randomized clinical trials are needed, keeping broad clinical application out of reach. Additionally, DL algorithms have performed as well as or even better than radiologists in image interpretation tasks, but in-depth validation through large trials must be achieved to establish their clinical utility in full (Balkenende *et. al.*, 2022). Moreover, the applications of DL in modalities such as ultrasound, MRI, and nuclear medicine are yet to come, and additional research must be done to evaluate their effectiveness and ethics. Hence, ongoing clinical trials are critical in evaluating these technologies on a systemic level and validating them as worthy prior to utilization in routine breast cancer practice.

13.2.9. Patient Education and Awareness

Effective breast imaging and early detection of cancer largely rely on education and awareness among patients, which allows patients to get timely screening and understand implications of mammographic results. Despite rapid advancements in imaging technologies, disparity exists in outcomes of breast cancer, particularly among the uninsured or underinsured, who have more advanced disease and mortality. Programs like Indiana's Breast and Cervical Cancer Program, that are dedicated to maximizing access and recognition, demonstrate the importance of targeted education alongside expanded coverage under insurance to eradicate these inequalities and improve prognosis (Fisher *et. al.*, 2018). Visual aids and readily accessible information resources also help with comprehension, so patients become proactively engaged in their healthcare decisions and adhere to recommended screening protocols. Ultimately, encouraging patient awareness lies at the center of taking full advantage of breast imaging technologies and better overall health outcomes through early detection and knowledge-based participation in care.

Test Your Knowledge

1. What are the primary indications for performing screening mammography in women over age 40?
2. In which clinical scenarios is diagnostic mammography preferred over screening mammography?

13.3. Benefits and Limitations of Breast Imaging

Learning Outcome

1. Focus on early detection of breast cancer
2. Explain reduction in mortality rates
3. Know non-invasive nature of imaging techniques
4. Identify limitations of mammography
5. Understand false positives and negatives
6. Describe cost-effectiveness of imaging
7. Focus on patient anxiety and psychological impact
8. Focus on accessibility and availability of services
9. Explain technological advancements and their implications

Advances in breast imaging have revolutionized the identification and diagnosis of breast lesions at an early stage, enhancing the outcome of patients through timely and accurate interventions. Techniques such as elastography complement traditional EUS and mammography by offering non-invasive assessment of tissue elasticity, enabling the differentiation between benign and malignant tumors with greater accuracy, hence reducing unnecessary biopsies and anxiety associated with them (Michał *et. al.*, 2025). However, they are offset by limitations like operator dependence and homogeneity between various imaging machinery, which are known to affect diagnostic consistency and reliability. Moreover, although modalities like MRI are accurate volumetric and complication assessments, their costliness and restricted accessibility make them difficult to apply on a large scale (Bogdan *et. al.*, 2024). EUS, though precise and non-invasive, may lack the fine detail of more advanced methods and underscores the need to integrate multiple imaging modalities. This tension between technical potential and practical constraint characterizes recent investigation and clinical application in breast imaging.

13.3.1. Early Detection of Breast Cancer

Advances in imaging technology have significantly enhanced the detection of early breast cancer, the cornerstone for improved patient outcomes. The traditional X-ray mammography, ultrasound, and MRI remain the foundation; however, their limitations have led to explorations of still more sensitive and less costly approaches. Deep learning-based models applied to mammogram analysis in recent years have performed very well, with classification accuracy rates of nearly 99% through ensemble methods that aggregate various convolutional neural networks for improved diagnostic accuracy (Chakravarthy *et. al.*, 2024). At the same time, microwave imaging was suggested as a likely alternative founded upon its being non-invasive, non-ionizing, and cost-effective. Together with sophisticated machine learning (ML) algorithms, microwave sensing enhances the rapid and accurate identification of breast tumors and holds the potential to break the limitations of conventional imaging (Wang, 2023). All these developments emphasize cumulatively the value of cutting-edge breast imaging technologies in facilitating early detection, which is critical in preventing mortality from breast cancer (Figure 13.13).

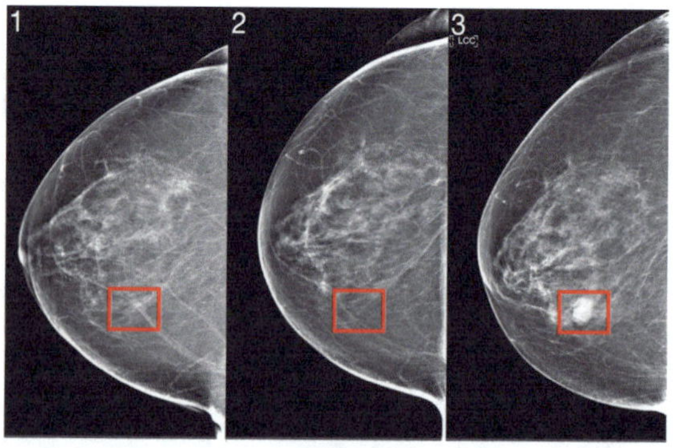

Figure 13.13. Deep learning models applied to mammogram analysis have demonstrated remarkable effectiveness.

Source: https://news.mit.edu/sites/default/files/images/202101/MIT-Mirai_0.jpg.

13.3.2. Reduction in Mortality Rates

The advances in breast imaging technology have been instrumental in the reduction of breast cancer mortality, which remains a leading cause of cancer mortality in women globally (Bray *et. al.*, 2018). Early detection using mammography, ultrasound, and MRI enables the identification of tumors at curable stages, significantly improving prognosis in patients. The application of periodic screening programs has contributed to timely intervention, reducing the advanced-stage diagnoses that are otherwise linked with poorer outcomes. In addition, enhanced imaging accuracy also assists in more precise surgical planning and focal treatments, restricting morbidity related to treatment. This two-way approach also facilitates monitoring of disease progression and response, thereby optimizing clinical management. With the advancement of systemic therapies, these imaging modalities have contributed to declining breast cancer mortality trends, reinforcing the central role of breast imaging in comprehensive cancer control strategies (Vogel *et. al.*, 2018). Continued innovation and equitable access to optimal imaging are crucial to sustaining and expanding these gains.

13.3.3. Non-Invasive Nature of Imaging Techniques

Breast imaging technology advances have, in addition, highlighted non-invasive approaches with reduced physical discomfort and procedural hazards, in contrast to invasive procedures such as galactography, which require ductal discharge and can cause pain. New technologies like ultrasound and MRI, with high accuracy rates for precise visualization, represent an even less intrusive approach to breast tissue compared to mammography. Ultrasound, being highly sensitive, is a useful ancillary to mammography, especially in cases of pathologic nipple discharge, permitting good detection with minimal discomfort. MRI further enhances this non-invasive method by enabling complete assessment of tumor size and spread, both for screening high-risk individuals and pre-treatment staging, despite the need for intravenous contrast injection. This shift towards non-invasive technology not only increases patient compliance but also optimizes the early detection of cancer, reflecting the evolving face of breast imaging modalities (Panzironi *et. al.*, 2019) (Figure 13.14).

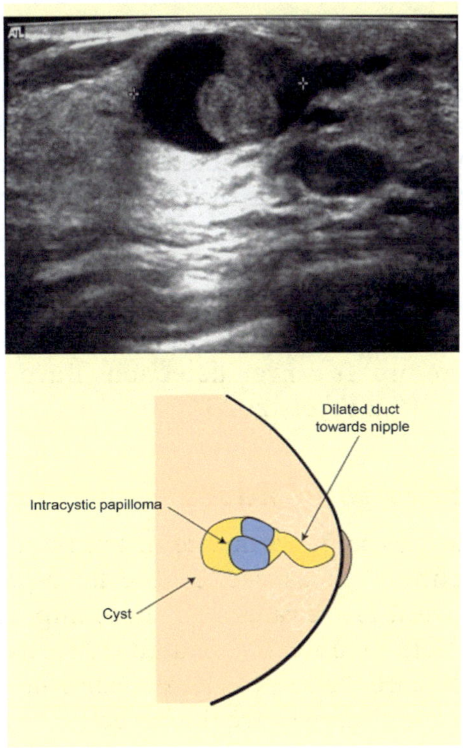

Figure 13.14. Ultrasound, with its high sensitivity, serves as an essential adjunct to mammography, especially in cases of pathologic nipple discharge, facilitating effective detection with minimal discomfort.

Source: https://ars.els-cdn.com/content/image/1-s2.0-S026393191200227X-gr4.jpg.

13.3.4. Limitations of Mammography

While the traditional gold standard method for breast cancer screening, mammography, is not without significant limitations that impair its overall performance. It decreases its sensitivity, particularly in populations with dense breast tissue, leading to false-negative findings that devalue efforts at early screening. The procedure also contains high levels of false positives that not only create unnecessary anxiety but also result in unwarranted diagnostic tests and health costs. These constraints highlight the imperative need for adjunctive imaging technologies and new modalities. Inroads developed in recent years, such as contrast-enhanced mammography and AI, have the potential to reduce some of these constraints by improving diagnostic precision and reducing false positives. Algorithmic bias and variability in performance with heterogeneous patient populations are issues that must be addressed with care to deliver fair benefits. Combined, while mammography is the cornerstone, its limitations necessitate ongoing innovation and the use of supplementary techniques to optimize breast cancer detection (Dave *et. al.*, 2025; Hafeez *et. al.*, 2025).

13.3.5. False Positives and Negatives

The diagnostic performance of breast imaging is essentially measured by the false-positive and false-negative rates, and these importantly affect patient outcome and the effectiveness of healthcare. False positives occur when non-malignant findings are incorrectly reported as malignancies, resulting in unwarranted worry, additional tests, and potentially invasive procedures. False negatives also result in cancer misses, and the treatment is delayed and prognosis is compromised. The dilemma of balance between sensitivity and specificity echoes through all interpretations, even those of qualified radiographers who conduct mammogram screening and have achieved sensitivity comparable to radiologists but with much higher false-positive findings, highlighting the risk of overdiagnosis (Mohar *et. al.*, 2015). On top of that, advances in ML and deep neural networks aim to reduce such diagnostic errors by improving pattern recognition and image examination, and ultimately lower false-negative and false-positive rates. These developments are a promising direction towards more precise, reliable breast cancer screening and diagnosis (Ayub *et. al.*, 2019) (Figure 13.15).

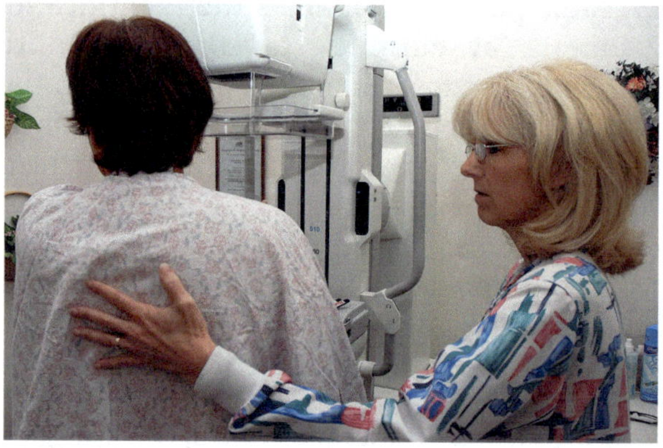

Figure 13.15. False positives occur when benign findings are incorrectly identified as malignancies, leading to unnecessary anxiety, additional testing, and invasive procedures.

Source: https://upload.wikimedia.org/wikipedia/commons/thumb/2/26/US_Navy_080922-N-2688M-004_Lead_Mammography_Technologist_Carmen_Waters_assists_a_patient.jpg/1200px-US_Navy_080922-N-2688M-004_Lead_Mammography_Technologist_Carmen_Waters_assists_a_patient.jpg.

13.3.6. Cost-Effectiveness of Imaging

Effective screening for breast cancer requires not merely clinical accuracy but also cautious consumption of healthcare resources. Cost-effectiveness analysis (CEA) is an important tool in evaluating imaging technologies by a comparison of health outcomes and cost, generally presented in terms of life years gained rather than money. Studies have shown that mammography and MRI are still the modalities of choice for breast cancer detection, although newer methods such as contrast-enhanced mammography and digital breast tomosynthesis can provide better cost-effectiveness in certain clinical contexts. Additionally, tailored screening approaches according to genetic predisposing factors have proven to be cost-effective; for example, the use of mammography in combination with MRI is effective cost-wise for BRCA1 mutation carriers, particularly in the middle-aged population, while for BRCA2 mutation carriers, mammography is sufficient cost-wise (Li *et. al.*, 2022; Waller *et. al.*, 2022). While helpful, CEAs may overlook certain qualitative findings and are not always certain when determining whether benefits exceed costs, and therefore, there is a necessity to add different economic evaluation methods to guide breast imaging guidelines appropriately.

13.3.7. Patient Anxiety and Psychological Impact

Breast imaging is not just an important instrument in the detection and diagnosis of breast cancer but also an active agent moulding patients' psychological journeys down the healthcare path. The fear aroused by imaging procedures and resulting diagnostic uncertainty is enough to take a heavy toll on mental health, augmented by breast cancer stigma in society. This internalized and enacted stigma is likely to exacerbate patients' body image and increase heightened psychological distress through stress, anxiety, and depression. Evidence shows a mediating effect of body image between stigma and psychological distress, suggesting that distorted self-perception worsens emotional suffering among infected women (Amini *et. al.*, 2021). Additionally, examinations in breast cancer patients undergoing treatment reveal widespread anxiety-depressive syndromes and sleep disorders related to unsatisfaction with the body image and also to the treatments (Kherchi *et. al.*, 2021). These findings emphasize the relevance of adding psychological support to breast imaging protocols to decrease anxiety and generally enhance well-being, optimizing both diagnostic performance and patient quality of life (Figure 13.16).

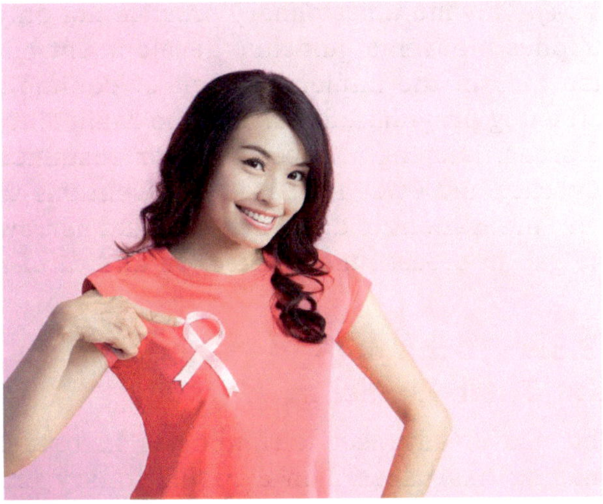

Figure 13.16. Breast imaging plays a pivotal role not only in the detection and diagnosis of breast cancer but also in shaping patients psychological experiences throughout their healthcare journey.

Source: https://www.asvinshospitals.com/wp-content/uploads/2023/08/breast-cancer-treatment.jpg.

13.3.8. Accessibility and Availability of Services

Breast imaging innovation has played a large role in early discovery and personalized treatment planning; however, disparities in accessibility and availability of these services are prevalent globally. While high-income countries enjoy extensive genetic testing and advanced imaging modalities, many low- and middle-income nations have limited access, particularly to genetically tailored diagnostics that are paramount for risk stratification and preventive care (Antone *et. al.*, 2025). Moreover, payment policy and organization of the healthcare system have a direct influence on services availability, as they influence the outcomes of patients. Health services research serves as the key solution to these problems by analyzing patterns of care for delivery, cost, and policy guidelines that govern the availability of breast imaging (Randy *et. al.*,

2024). This multidisciplinary practice not only supplies input into guideline development but also aids in the implementation of equitable screening programs. Enhancing the availability of breast imaging services calls for sustained advocacy and evidence-based interventions to drive innovations to diverse groups and narrow the gap in breast cancer detection and care.

13.3.9. Technological Advancements and Their Implications

The use of advanced technologies in breast imaging has ushered in a revolutionary era with greater precision and improved patient outcomes. Technologies such as electromagnetic tracking, initially designed for radiation therapy, have a tremendous potential to improve imaging accuracy with real-time localization with no additional radiation exposure, thus permitting more accurate targeting of the treatment with less collateral damage (Kupelian *et. al.*, 2011). Furthermore, the emergence of imaging technologies like CT and MRI in the clinical setting is itself a paradigmatic instance of the intricate relationship between technological innovation and organizational learning. Installation of these technologies is not an issue of unproblematic uptake but involves dynamic processes by which clinical practice, interdisciplinarity, and evolving institutional routines shape and are shaped by technological know-how (Sinozic *et. al.*, 2014). These developments broaden out diagnostic choices, making earlier diagnosis and individualized breast cancer therapy possible, but also come with costs, training, and integration problems attached, necessitating ongoing assessment of both the technological and social consequences.

Test Your Knowledge

1. How does breast ultrasound complement mammography, and in which scenarios is it most useful?
2. What are the limitations of mammography in women with dense breast tissue?

13.4. Future Directions in Breast Imaging

Learning Outcome

1. Learn innovations in imaging technology
2. Focus on artificial intelligence in breast imaging
3. Define personalized imaging approaches
4. Focus on integration of imaging with other diagnostic tools
5. Explain research on imaging biomarkers
6. Describe global disparities in breast imaging access
7. Understand education and training for radiologists
8. Know policy implications for breast imaging
9. Explain future research priorities

Advances in technology also have beendriving unprecedented progress in the application of breast imaging, leading to improved diagnosis and personalized treatment planning. New techniques like electromagnetic tracking, initially pioneered for radiation therapy, hold the promise of enhancing the localization of tumors without additional exposure to radiation, thus making management of breast cancer more accurate (Kupelian *et. al.*, 2011).

Moreover, the integration of AI through concepts like the Bionic Radiologist offers a revolutionary solution in the form of the marriage between computer imaging analysis and human expertise. The integration improves science-driven decision-making, standardization of image interpretation between environments, and seamless correlation of imaging findings with treatment recommendations (Dewey *et. al.*, 2019). Shattering barriers such as faith in computerized systems and offering continuous educational advancement for radiologists will be the key to making these advancements unlock their complete potential. Ultimately, future breast imaging will likely focus on precision, productivity, and patient-focused care, reducing gaps while being able to detect breast abnormalities sooner and more consistently.

13.4.1. Innovations in Imaging Technology

The application of novel computational techniques in medical diagnosis has changed the face of breast cancer identification, promising future improvements in accuracy and efficiency. Traditional imaging technology is satisfactory but susceptible to human error and radiologists' workload. New research with AI and ML algorithms has demonstrated significant promise to overcome these limitations.

For instance, computer-assisted mammography screening revealed comparable cancer detection rates to standard double-reading by radiologists but at much reduced screen-reading workload, and this is a viable solution for resource optimization for high-burden healthcare systems (Nasr *et. al.*, 2025). Complementary, ML algorithms like K-Nearest Neighbor (KNN) have achieved near-perfect classification accuracy in distinguishing between benign and malignant breast lesions, which signals the potential for accurate automated histological image analysis (Aisha *et. al.*, 2025). These developments are a paradigm shift in breast imaging technology, facilitating early diagnosis and improved patient outcomes with more reliable and scalable procedures for diagnosis (Figure 13.17).

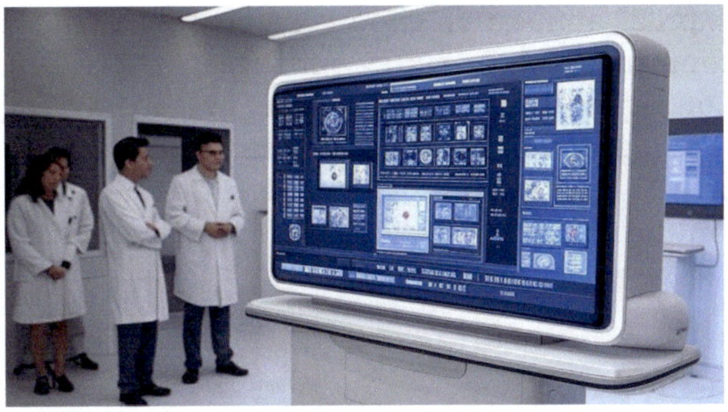

Figure 13.17. The integration of advanced computational techniques in medical diagnostics has transformed the landscape of breast cancer detection, offering promising improvements in accuracy and efficiency.

Source: https://media.licdn.com/dms/image/v2/D5612AQEAST8cHRy-jA/article-cover_image-shrink_720_1280/B56ZXFCp9PHoAI-/0/1742767562998?e=2147483647&v=beta&t=3Zz602d4pGRxPVFi18xwCPr9Qc_zfdJGBKFs4UnCd2M.

13.4.2. Artificial Intelligence in Breast Imaging

Medical imaging technologies have progressively relied on AI to enhance diagnostic efficiency and accuracy. In breast imaging, AI algorithms have been developed to process ultrasound and dynamic contrast-enhanced magnetic resonance imaging (DCE-MRI) data, breaking the hurdles of heterogeneity in image interpretation and time-consuming manual analyses. By employing ML techniques, artificial intelligence models can identify subtle patterns in breast tissue, improving early diagnosis of benign and malignant tumors, reducing radiologist fatigue and diagnostic inaccuracies (Yao *et. al.*, 2023). Additionally, AI-assisted tumor segmentation in multi-phase DCE-MRI enables defining the tumor boundaries with accuracy, supporting clinical decision-making and treatment planning. These algorithms for computer vision demonstrate strength across numerous imaging protocols and significantly accelerate workflows, cutting manual annotation time considerably without compromising accuracy (Zhang *et. al.*, 2023). Consequently, the use of AI in breast imaging is a huge breakthrough with the power to make screening and diagnosis processes more efficient and ultimately improve patients' outcomes.

13.4.3. Personalized Imaging Approaches

Advances in technology have significantly impacted the practice of breast imaging to be able to offer more tailored diagnostic approaches with the potential to improve patient-specific treatment. These personalized imaging techniques leverage cutting-edge technologies, such as AI and deep learning algorithms, to improve detection sensitivity and reduce false positives.

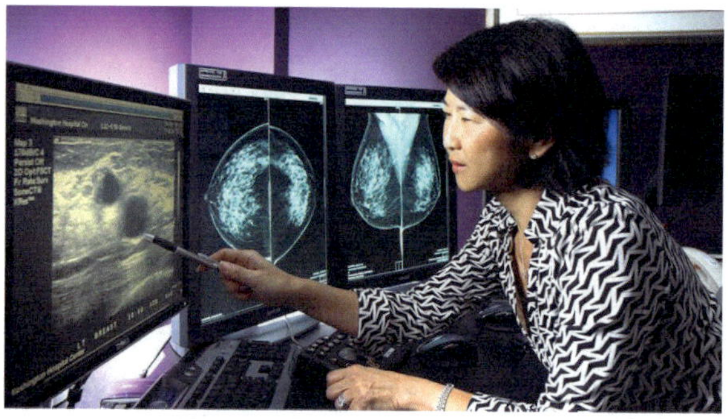

Figure 13.18. Personalized imaging approaches in breast imaging.

Source: https://medstarhealth-delivery.sitecorecontenthub.cloud/api/public/content/CHOI_Anna_breast_scans.

As an example, the addition of novel Convolutional Neural Network models has been promising with over 95% accuracy in cancerous and non-cancerous breast tissue differentiation, and enabling earlier and more precise diagnosis (Mahesh *et. al.*, 2024). Moreover, shift from traditional mammography, towards more sophisticated methods, like contrast-enhanced mammography is a nod towards personalized assessment, based on heterogeneous risk profiles of patients and breast tissue characteristics (Nicosia *et. al.*, 2023). These technologies seek to optimize diagnostic precision with fewer avoidable interventions, ultimately improving clinical decision-making and reducing breast cancer fatalities through personalized imaging strategies that adapt based on the unique features of each patient's condition (Figure 13.18).

13.4.4. Integration of Imaging with Other Diagnostic Tools

Breast cancer diagnosis has increasingly relied on the combination of imaging modalities with complementary diagnostics to enhance precision and reduce diagnostic error. For instance, use of AI in mammography has registered significant enhancements in sensitivity and specificity through use of ML algorithms that can handle complex imaging data along with clinical data to assist radiologists in making improved decisions (Dave *et. al.*, 2025). Moreover, combining cutting-edge image processing such as Wiener filtering with state-of-the-art AI models, such as vision transformers and U-KAN, recovers image quality and diagnostic performance on various datasets, improving lesion segmentation and classification outcomes (Zhu *et. al.*, 2024). Such multimodal imaging not only improves visual interpretation but also combines patient history, genetic markers, and pathology results, leading to a more comprehensive assessment of breast abnormalities. Lastly, imaging integration with other diagnostic methods facilitates earlier diagnosis and treatment strategies for individual patients, transcending the constraints of single-disease diagnostic methods and elevating the quality of breast cancer care.

13.4.5. Research on Imaging Biomarkers

Technological progress in breast imaging has increasingly emphasized the role of imaging biomarkers for enhancing diagnostic accuracy and treatment follow-up. Existing research highlights how biomarkers in respect of modalities such as cardiac magnetic resonance imaging (CMR) can provide crucial insights into systemic effects of breast cancer therapy, particularly in respect of vascular risk to health in specific subsets of patients. For instance, studies show that premenopausal women and triple-negative breast cancer patients exhibit remarkable increases in vascular stiffness, which can be quantified using imaging biomarkers like aortic pulse wave velocity and aortic distensibility, with corresponding biochemical markers like renin, cholesterol, and interleukin-6, accentuating underlying treatment complications of the cardiovascular system (Lorraine *et. al.*, 2025). Concurrently, the merge of ML and AI in deciphering complex imaging data facilitates the identification and detection of diagnostic biomarkers, improving tumor detection accuracy and prediction of response to neoadjuvant chemotherapy. All these collectively provide more personalized treatment for breast cancer by improving prognostic assessment and therapeutic decision-making (Saleh *et. al.*, 2023) (Figure 13.19).

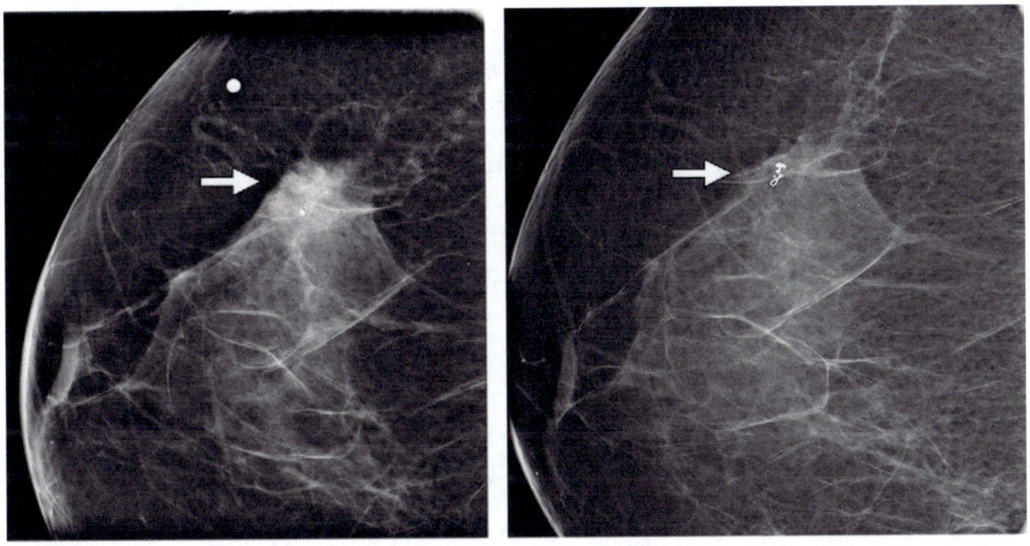

a. b.

Figure 13.19. Advancements in breast imaging have increasingly emphasized the role of imaging biomarkers in enhancing diagnostic accuracy and treatment monitoring.

Source: https://www.researchgate.net/publication/320769162/figure/fig5/AS:1110691368968201@1641820866320/mages-of-a-65-year-old-woman-with-a-palpable-mass-in-the-right-breast-a-Spot.ppm.

13.4.6. Global Disparities in Breast Imaging Access

Despite advances in breast imaging modalities, significant worldwide disparities in access to these important diagnostic resources persist. Within the majority of low- and middle-income countries, shortages of healthcare infrastructure and trained radiologists cause delays in breast cancer detection, resulting in increased morbidity and mortality rates compared to high-income environments. Attempts at unifying digital radiology and artificial intelligence, such as the concept of the Bionic Radiologist envisions, have the promise to bring more uniformity and accessibility of breast imaging services worldwide, potentially reducing such disparities by allowing remote image assessment and decision-making assistance (Dewey *et. al.*, 2019). For such technologies to be adopted, however, systemic hurdles such as resource organization and workforce training need to be conquered. In addition, sensitivity to the diverse needs of all populations, including vulnerable ones such as transgender women, is necessary for equitable provision of breast imaging (Defreyne *et. al.*, 2019). Without effective strategies, inequities in access to breast imaging will persist in threatening the global efforts toward control of cancer.

13.4.7. Education and Training for Radiologists

Advances in breast imaging technologies have necessitated complementary advances in the education and training of radiologists for proper diagnosis and best outcomes. Current professional development courses are needed for radiologists to be proficient with new modalities such as digital breast tomosynthesis and AI-based diagnostics. Such training programs increasingly include interdisciplinary collaboration, cultural sensitivity, and awareness to tackle disparities in breast cancer screening and improve patient communication, as seen in efforts to reduce healthcare inequalities and foster diversity among radiologists (Pesapane *et. al.*, 2023). Moreover, incorporating AI into practice requires radiologists to learn new skill sets that entail interpreting data produced by AI and being sensitive to its pitfalls to avoid bias and uphold ethical levels (Shuroug *et. al.*, 2023). Robust education programs encompassing hands-on imaging skills, technology trends, and patient care are critical to enabling radiologists with the skills required to manage the sophisticated requirements of contemporary breast imaging effectively (Figure 13.20).

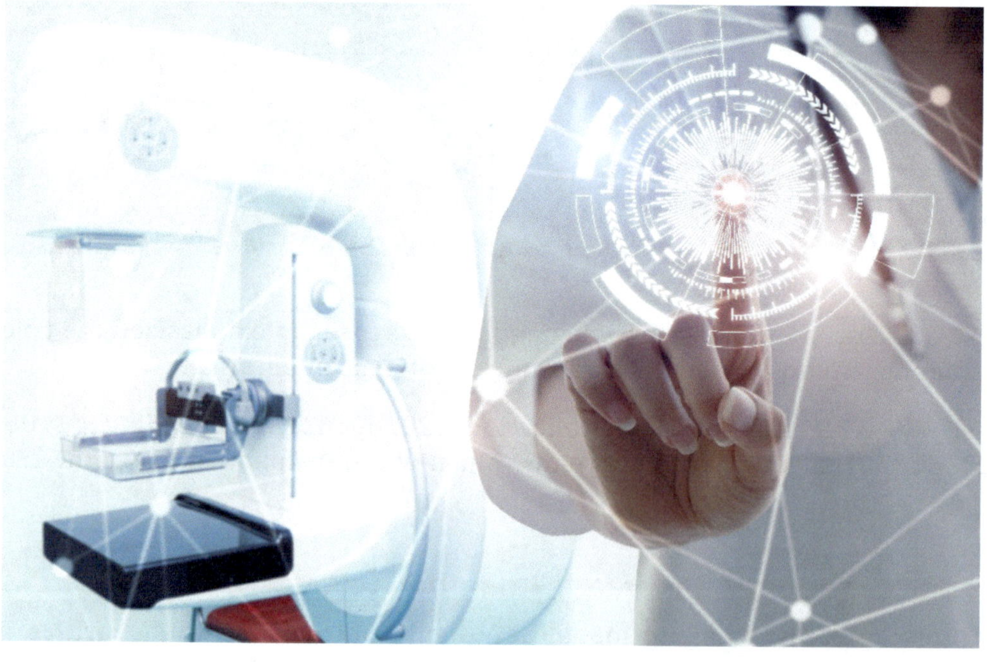

Figure 13.20. Continuous professional development programs are essential for radiologists to remain proficient with emerging modalities such as digital breast tomosynthesis and AI-assisted diagnostics.

Source: https://www.itnonline.com/sites/default/files/field/image/GettyImages-1127307436.jpg.

13.4.8. Policy Implications for Breast Imaging

A background of breast imaging is inextricably tied with ongoing evolving health policy that seeks to optimize both clinical outcomes and resource utilization. Recent advances in health services research have illustrated the value of evidence-based guidelines to specify appropriate use of imaging, particularly with regard to screening and diagnostic algorithms. Through an evaluation of cost-effectiveness and accessibility, policymakers can optimize reimbursement plans that balance patient demand against system sustainability, ultimately improving care delivery (Randy *et. al.*, 2024). In addition, identification of unusual and underdiagnosed breast imaging conditions such as breast amyloidoma enhances the necessity for protocol-based diagnostic and management guidelines to prevent misdiagnosis and standardize care (Michael *et. al.*, 2025). Therefore, these problems bring into focus the critical role of policy in controlling technology adoption, impacting clinical practice, and ensuring equitable access to advanced breast imaging technologies, thereby enhancing patient outcomes as well as healthcare efficiency.

13.4.9. Future Research Priorities

Technological advancement has transformed the field of breast imaging, but there remain colossal opportunities to make it more effective and accurate. New research needs include using AI to boost breast cancer risk prediction and screening protocols. Specifically, the implementation of AI-driven models with computational mammographic phenotypes can enable more individualized and accurate risk prediction, thereby optimizing screening protocols to reduce harm and maximize early detection (Gastounioti *et. al.*, 2022). Meanwhile, systematic clinical testing of AI applications beyond preliminary multireader studies should be conducted to confirm that they are valid in routine practice and in different populations (Leslie *et. al.*, 2022). Workflow integration, ethics, and governance must also be assessed in future research to realize successful implementation of AI in clinical practice (Leslie *et. al.*, 2022). Through focus on these areas of research, breast imaging research can advance towards more individualized patient care and improved clinical outcomes, eventually enhancing the precision medicine paradigm for the detection and treatment of breast cancer.

Test Your Knowledge

1. How is artificial intelligence (AI) expected to improve breast cancer detection and reduce false positives in mammography?
2. What potential does contrast-enhanced mammography hold as a more accessible alternative to breast MRI?

SUMMARY

Breast imaging technology and scientific research breakthroughs have significantly improved early detection accuracy and effectiveness of breast cancer. Technological innovation, like the integration of electromagnetic and ultrasonic imaging, enhanced with sophisticated ML algorithms like the Bayesian Neural Network, promises higher image resolution and diagnostic capability, particularly in dense breast tissue scenarios (No Vël *et. al.*, 2025). Parallel to this, corresponding health services research endeavors emphasize the practical and policy-making fronts of breast imaging, driving value-based care through evidence-based practice, cost assessment, and improved access to imaging (Randy *et. al.*, 2024). Collectively, these structural and technological innovations accentuate a breast imaging strategy that is not only optimized for clinical outcomes but also educational in nature for healthcare provision and policy. Lastly, the union of sophisticated imaging modalities and integrative health services research offers the foundation for ongoing progress in breast cancer screening, diagnosis, and patient care.

Advancements in breast imaging have significantly enhanced the detection of benign versus malignant lesions, improving diagnostic performance and patient outcomes. New techniques like ultrafast UF-DCE MRI offer high temporal resolution that allows accurate kinetic analysis, with over 77% sensitivity and specificity rates, without a significant difference between the most significant parameters such as maximum slope and time to enhancement (Amitai *et. al.*, 2024). Concurrently, computerized clinical decision support systems implemented in electronic health records have been shown to optimize imaging appropriateness and reduce unnecessary tests and their healthcare costs. These types of systems, particularly those with real-time decision support with enforcement like hard stops, result in less wasteful use of advanced imaging modalities without risking potential overuse and patient harm (Goldzweig *et. al.*, 2015). These advances collectively represent a two-fold focus on clinical decision support and technological progress toward maximizing the effectiveness and use of breast imaging.

KEY TERMS FROM THIS CHAPTER

- Photoacoustic imaging
- Tumors
- Calcifications
- Pathology
- X-ray mammography
- Cysts
- Radiography

CRITICAL THINKING QUESTIONS

1. **Which of the following is the most commonly used screening tool for breast cancer in women over 40 years?**
   a. Ultrasound
   b. MRI
   c. Mammography
   d. PET scan
2. **What is the main advantage of digital breast tomosynthesis (3D mammography) over conventional 2D mammography?**
   a. Lower radiation dose
   b. Better detection of microcalcifications
   c. Reduced false positives due to overlapping tissue
   d. More comfortable for the patient
3. **Which imaging modality is most sensitive for detecting breast cancer in women with dense breast tissue?**
   a. Ultrasound
   b. Digital Mammography
   c. Breast MRI
   d. CT scan
4. **In what clinical situation is breast ultrasound most commonly used?**
   a. Routine screening in women over 50
   b. Evaluation of palpable breast masses
   c. Detection of microcalcifications
   d. Screening in men
5. **Which feature on mammography is most suspicious for malignancy?**
   a. Round, well-circumscribed mass
   b. Clustered microcalcifications
   c. Fat-containing lesion
   d. Simple cyst

Short Answer Questions

1. What are the main imaging modalities used in breast imaging, and how do they differ in clinical application?
2. When is mammography recommended as a screening tool, and what age guidelines are generally followed?
3. How does breast density affect the sensitivity of mammography in detecting abnormalities?
4. What role does ultrasound play in evaluating a palpable breast mass?
5. How is breast MRI used in the detection and staging of breast cancer?
6. What are the BI-RADS categories, and how do they guide patient management?
7. How is stereotactic-guided biopsy performed, and when is it indicated?
8. What are the advantages and limitations of 3D mammography (digital breast tomosynthesis) over conventional 2D mammography?
9. What imaging findings are suggestive of a benign lesion versus a suspicious or malignant one?

Answers to Critical Thinking Questions

1. (c); 2. (c); 3. (c); 4. (b); 5. (b)

REFERENCES

1. Ahmed, M. H., Ajam, T., Al-Karawi, D., *et. al.* (2024). A review of artificial intelligence in breast imaging. https://core.ac.uk/download/613174187.pdf (accessed on 30 May 2025).
2. Alowais, S. A., Alghamdi, S. S., Alsuhebany, N., Alqahtani, T., Alshaya, A., Almohareb, S. N., Aldairem, A., *et. al.* (2023). Revolutionizing healthcare: The role of artificial intelligence in clinical practice. *BMC Medical Education, 23*. https://doi.org/10.1186/s12909-023-04698-z.
3. Amini-Tehrani, M., Zamanian, H., Daryaafzoon, M., Andikolaei, S., Mohebbi, M., Imani, A., Tahmasbi, B., *et. al.* (2021). Body image, internalized stigma and enacted stigma predict psychological distress in women with breast cancer: A serial mediation model. *Journal of Advanced Nursing, 77*, 3412–3423. https://doi.org/10.1111/jan.14881.
4. Amitai, Y., Freitas, V., Golan, O., Kessner, R., Shalmon, T., Neeman, R., Mauda-Havakuk, M., *et. al.* (2024). The diagnostic performance of ultrafast MRI to differentiate benign from malignant breast lesions: A systematic review and meta-analysis. *European Radiology, 34*, 6285–6295. https://www.semanticscholar.org/paper/b563628865ca5118ef6194fee797845582a197ed (accessed on 30 May 2025).
5. Antone, N., Pintican, R., Manole, S., Fodor, L., Lucaciu, C., Roman, A., Trifa, A., *et. al.* (2025). Predicting pathogenic variants of breast cancer using ultrasound-derived machine learning models. *Cancers, 17*. https://www.semanticscholar.org/paper/ee73fb260bf29c53f6cddf83447aebcf3bf5e856 (accessed on 30 May 2025).
6. Arridge, S., Hawkes, D., Hipwell, J., *et. al.* (2013). Numerical methods for coupled reconstruction and registration in digital breast tomosynthesis. https://core.ac.uk/download/77002591.pdf (accessed on 30 May 2025).
7. Ayala, R. M., Bustos, J. A. R., Jativa, M. A. G., *et. al.* (2024). Advances in the use of microvascular flaps for postoperative defect repair in complex abdominal surgery: Innovative approaches to recovery and functionality. https://core.ac.uk/download/620836747.pdf (accessed on 30 May 2025).
8. Ayub, A., Elahi, H., Frezza, F., *et. al.* (2019). Cancer diagnosis using deep learning: A bibliographic review. https://core.ac.uk/download/231746843.pdf (accessed on 30 May 2025).
9. Bailey, G., Farinha, J., Mochan, A., Polvora, A., Rodriguez, L., & Zanca, F. (2024). Imaging the future–Horizon scanning for emerging technologies and breakthrough innovations in the field of medical imaging and AI. https://core.ac.uk/download/642862319.pdf (accessed on 30 May 2025).
10. Balkenende, L., Teuwen, J., & Mann, R. M. (2022). Application of deep learning in breast cancer imaging. *Seminars in Nuclear Medicine, 52*(6), 584–596. https://doi.org/10.1053/j.semnuclmed.2022.02.003.
11. Bansal, R., Collison, S., Krishnan, L., Aggarwal, B., Vidyasagar, M., Kakileti, S., & Manjunath, G. (2023). A prospective evaluation of breast thermography enhanced by a novel machine learning technique for screening breast abnormalities in a general population of women presenting to a secondary care hospital. *Frontiers in Artificial Intelligence, 5*. https://www.semanticscholar.org/paper/a1bc2cce5e448c18f0c13e8ad11ce6aeba849aef (accessed on 30 May 2025).

12. Beechem, J., Levenson, R., & McNamara, G. (2012). Spectral imaging in preclinical research and clinical pathology. https://core.ac.uk/download/323068082.pdf.

13. Bejnordi, B. E., Ciompi, F., Ghafoorian, M., *et. al.* (2017). A survey on deep learning in medical image analysis. http://arxiv.org/abs/1702.05747 (accessed on 30 May 2025).

14. Bellati, F., Caserta, D., Costanzi, F., *et. al.* (2018). Real-time virtual sonography in gynecology & obstetrics: Literature's analysis and case series. https://core.ac.uk/download/195777140.pdf (accessed on 30 May 2025).

15. Bogdan, R. G., Helgiu, A., Cimpean, A. M., Ichim, C., Todor, S. B., Iliescu-Glaja, M., Bodea, I. C., *et. al.* (2024). Assessing fat grafting in breast surgery: A narrative review of evaluation techniques. *Journal of Clinical Medicine, 13*. https://www.semanticscholar.org/paper/3f77ab3ad13797297867da1571621274103f3519 (accessed on 30 May 2025).

16. Bray, F., Ferlay, J., Soerjomataram, I., Siegel, R. L., Torre, L. A., & Jemal, A. (2018). Global cancer statistics 2018: GLOBOCAN estimates of incidence and mortality worldwide for 36 cancers in 185 countries. *CA: A Cancer Journal for Clinicians, 68*, 394–424. https://doi.org/10.3322/caac.21492.

17. Busawon, K., Elsdon, M., Fernando, M., *et. al.* (2010). Fundamental issues in antenna design for microwave medical imaging applications. https://core.ac.uk/download/4148450.pdf (accessed on 30 May 2025).

18. Carter, J., Lacchetti, C., Andersen, B. L., Barton, D. L., Bolte, S., Damast, S., Diefenbach, M. A., *et. al.* (2017). Interventions to address sexual problems in people with cancer: American Society of Clinical Oncology clinical practice guideline adaptation of Cancer Care Ontario guideline. *Journal of Clinical Oncology, 36*(5), 492–511. https://doi.org/10.1200/jco.2017.75.8995.

19. Chakravarthy, S., Bharanidharan, N., Kumar, V. V., Mahesh, T., Alqahtani, M. S., & Guluwadi, S. (2024). Deep transfer learning with fuzzy ensemble approach for the early detection of breast cancer. *BMC Medical Imaging, 24*. https://www.semanticscholar.org/paper/e0a3c4ffc28e87992dd8413046c0ab3062da4270 (accessed on 30 May 2025).

20. Chan, M. F., & Hoyt, T. L. (2025). Imaging characteristics and diagnostic implications of breast amyloidoma. *Case Reports in Radiology*. https://www.semanticscholar.org/paper/859483e6063a639ba8b06d2eeedfe80e8c221d33 (accessed on 30 May 2025).

21. Che, J., Dhar, M., Di Carlo, D., *et. al.* (2016). Classification of large circulating tumor cells isolated with ultra-high throughput microfluidic vortex technology. https://core.ac.uk/download/323080454.pdf.

22. Cox, B., Javaherian, A., & Lucka, F. (2020). Refraction-corrected ray-based inversion for three-dimensional ultrasound tomography of the breast. https://core.ac.uk/download/385866374.pdf (accessed on 30 May 2025).

23. Dagheyan, A. G., Lorenzo, J. M., Martinez, A. K., *et. al.* (2017). Near-field radar microwave imaging as an add-on modality to mammography. https://core.ac.uk/download/322432094.pdf (accessed on 30 May 2025).

24. Darzi, A., Hettiaratchy, S., Hughes-Hallett, K., Kwasnicki, M., *et. al.* (2016). Fifty years of innovation in plastic surgery. https://core.ac.uk/download/77010125.pdf (accessed on 30 May 2025).

25. Dave, D., Akhunzada, A., Ivković, N., Gyawali, S., Cengiz, K., Ahmed, A., & Al-Shamayleh, A. S.

(2025). Diagnostic test accuracy of AI-assisted mammography for breast imaging: A narrative review. *PeerJ Computer Science, 11*. https://www.semanticscholar.org/paper/1ce00c0b564871b0c3c034bfa23dfa92a1f219fc (accessed on 30 May 2025).

26. Defreyne, J., Iwamoto, S. J., Motmans, J., *et. al.* (2019). Health considerations for transgender women and remaining unknowns: A narrative review. https://core.ac.uk/download/237010802.pdf (accessed on 30 May 2025).

27. Dewey, M., & Wilkens, U. (2019). The bionic radiologist: Avoiding blurry pictures and providing greater insights. https://core.ac.uk/download/228064788.pdf (accessed on 30 May 2025).

28. El Kherchi, O., Aquil, A., El Khoudri, N., Mouallif, M., Daghi, M., Guerroumi, M., Saad, E., *et. al.* (2021). Anxiety and depression comorbidities in Moroccan patients with breast cancer. *Frontiers in Psychiatry, 11*. https://doi.org/10.3389/fpsyt.2020.584907.

29. European Society for Gastrointestinal and Abdominal Radiology. (2012). ECR 2012 book of abstracts–D–Satellite symposia. *Insights into Imaging, 3*, 367–374. https://www.semanticscholar.org/paper/a99aba2f5ebf9e07093507cb57b7ae7fc1dbdcd7 (accessed on 30 May 2025).

30. Evans, D. G., Astley, S., Stavrinos, P., Harkness, E. F., Donnelly, L. S., Dawe, S., Jacob, I., *et. al.* (2016). Improvement in risk prediction, early detection and prevention of breast cancer in the NHS Breast Screening Programmed and family history clinics: A dual cohort study. *Programmed Grants for Applied Research, 4*, 1–210. https://doi.org/10.3310/pgfar04110.

31. Fadlil, F., Handayani, L., Satrian, P., Hendril, W., *et. al.* (2024). Electricity-assisted cancer therapies: Nanotechnology, electrochemotherapy, and machine learning. https://core.ac.uk/download/616887103.pdf (accessed on 30 May 2025).

32. Fisher, C. S., Haggstrom, D. A., Ludwig, K. K., *et. al.* (2018). The implications of insurance status on presentation, surgical management and mortality among non-metastatic breast cancer patients in Indiana. https://core.ac.uk/download/187423863.pdf (accessed on 30 May 2025).

33. Fortina, P., Kricka, L. J., Park, J. Y., & Polsky, T. G. (2015). The future of laboratory medicine – A 2014 perspective. https://core.ac.uk/download/54509579.pdf (accessed on 30 May 2025).

34. Franceschini, G., Mason, E. J., Grippo, C., D'Archi, S., D'Angelo, A., Scardina, L., Sánchez, A. M., *et. al.* (2021). Image-guided localization techniques for surgical excision of non-palpable breast lesions: An overview of current literature and our experience with preoperative skin tattoo. *Journal of Personalized Medicine, 11*, 99. https://doi.org/10.3390/jpm11020099.

35. Gastounioti, A., Desai, S., Ahluwalia, V. S., Conant, E. F., & Kontos, D. (2022). Artificial intelligence in mammographic phenotyping of breast cancer risk: A narrative review. *Breast Cancer Research, 24*. https://doi.org/10.1186/s13058-022-01509-z.

36. Goldzweig, C., Orshansky, G., Paige, N. M., Miake-Lye, I. M., Beroes, J. M., Ewing, B. A., & Shekelle, P. (2015). Electronic health record-based interventions for improving appropriate diagnostic imaging. *Annals of Internal Medicine, 162*, 557–565. https://www.semanticscholar.org/paper/49901c59a983e94e78ba71f659ba50add7c6e57f (accessed on 30 May 2025).

37. Goyal, S. (2021). An overview of current trends, techniques, prospects, and pitfalls of artificial intelligence in breast imaging. *Reports in Medical Imaging, 14*, 15–25. https://doi.org/10.2147/rmi.s295205.

38. Hafeez, S. A. M. R. (2025). Risk-adapted breast cancer screening: Combining DOT and ultrasound with AI to overcome mammography limitations. *2025 International Conference on Machine*

Learning and Autonomous Systems (ICMLAS). https://www.semanticscholar.org/paper/5fe88c29b6dc536986a8b266ca12ba1286f8450f (accessed on 30 May 2025).

39. Hilgerink, M. P., Hummel, J. M., IJzerman, M. J., *et. al.* (2011). Assessment of the added value of the Twente photoacoustic mammoscope in breast cancer diagnosis. https://core.ac.uk/download/pdf/11481011.pdf.

40. Kennedy, K. M., Zilkens, R., Allen, W. M., Foo, K. Y., Fang, Q., Chin, L., Sanderson, R. W., *et. al.* (2020). Diagnostic accuracy of quantitative micro-elastography for margin assessment in breast-conserving surgery. *Cancer Research, 80*(8), 1773–1783. https://doi.org/10.1158/0008-5472.can-19-1240.

41. Kim, S., Lee, H. J., Ko, K. H., Park, A. Y., Koh, J., & Jung, H. K. (2018). New Doppler imaging technique for assessing angiogenesis in breast tumors: Correlation with immunohistochemically analyzed micro vessels density. *Acta Radiological, 59*, 1414–1421. https://doi.org/10.1177/0284185118769690.

42. Ko, A., Vo, A. M., Miller, N., Liang, A., Baumbach, M., Argue, J. R., Manche, N., *et. al.* (2024). The use of breast-specific gamma imaging as a low-cost problem-solving strategy for avoiding biopsies in patients with inconclusive imaging findings on mammography and ultrasonography. *Journal of Breast Imaging*. https://www.semanticscholar.org/paper/6b566201852e9cbb096e08c6300f7bd35ab7311a (accessed on 30 May 2025).

43. Kupelian, P. A., Meeks, S. L., Shah, A. P., & Willoughby, T. R. (2011). Expanding the use of real-time electromagnetic tracking in radiation oncology. https://core.ac.uk/download/323076551.pdf.

44. Lamb, L. R., Lehman, C. D., Gastounioti, A., Conant, E. F., & Bahl, M. (2022). Artificial intelligence (AI) for screening mammography, from the *AJR* special series on AI applications. *American Journal of Roentgenology, 219*(2), 369–380. https://doi.org/10.2214/ajr.21.27071.

45. Li, J., Jia, Z., Zhang, M., Liu, G., Xing, Z., Wang, X., Huang, X., *et. al.* (2022). Cost-effectiveness analysis of imaging modalities for breast cancer surveillance among BRCA1/2 mutation carriers: A systematic review. *Frontiers in Oncology, 11*. https://doi.org/10.3389/fonc.2021.763161.

46. Mahesh, T. R. (2024). Enhancing diagnostic accuracy in breast ultrasound imaging through deep learning and image augmentation techniques. *2024 International Conference on Emerging Research in Computational Science (ICERCS)*. https://www.semanticscholar.org/paper/423439701360c41bc17085e01de27ccaf8f5845b (accessed on 30 May 2025).

47. Mahesh, T. R., Thakur, A., Gupta, M., Sinha, D. K., Mishra, K. K., Venkatesan, V. K., & Guluwadi, S. (2024). Transformative breast cancer diagnosis using CNNs with optimized ReduceLROnPlateau and early stopping enhancements. *International Journal of Computational Intelligence Systems, 17*. https://doi.org/10.1007/s44196-023-00397-1.

48. Marano, L., Polom, K., Skokowski, J., & Zydowicz, W. M. (2024). Navigating the metaverse: A new virtual tool with promising real benefits for breast cancer patients. https://core.ac.uk/download/622822691.pdf (accessed on 30 May 2025).

49. Miah, P., Fiedler, L., Baez, A., Sevdalis, A., Marmer, A., DiMaggio, C., Pak, L., *et. al.* (2024). Abstract PO5-23-05: The impact of bi-annual diagnostic imaging on detecting ipsilateral breast recurrence in patients undergoing breast conserving surgery for breast cancer. *Cancer Research*. https://www.semanticscholar.org/paper/7b2d3b2d15020a33c2663caaffc7482297bb5314 (accessed on 30 May 2025).

50. Miles, R. C., Chou, S. H. S., Lamb, L. R., Narayan, A. K., Tran, N. T., & Lee, J. M. (2024). Framework for successful integration of health services research into a breast imaging career. *Journal of Breast Imaging*. https://www.semanticscholar.org/paper/60b44a3fa62f203e1ddb4437273a08f213dd6fcc (accessed on 30 May 2025).

51. Mohar, A., Chapman, A. H., Dowdy, A. H., Bogart, A., Angeles-Llerenas, A., Mucci, B., Hillman, B. J., *et. al.* (2015). Radiographers supporting radiologists in the interpretation of screening mammography: A viable strategy to meet the shortage in the number of radiologists. https://core.ac.uk/download/323073234.pdf.

52. Mohindra, N., & Soni, N. (2024). Ultrasound-based noncontract microvascular imaging for evaluation of breast lesions: Imaging techniques and review of diagnostic criteria. *The Indian Journal of Radiology & Imaging, 34*, 702–713. https://www.semanticscholar.org/paper/fe11165c5d10a433a72a28bbc41ede3e5d0620fe (accessed on 30 May 2025).

53. Nasr, M. U., & Saleem, M. K. (2025). Embracing innovations to fight breast cancer: A letter to the editor. *JPMA. The Journal of the Pakistan Medical Association, 75*(4), 682. https://www.semanticscholar.org/paper/bc89808ae00d7be18b40c311096bee87834a3716 (accessed on 30 May 2025).

54. Neeter, L., Robbe, M. M. Q., van Nijnatten, T. V., Jochelson, M., Raat, H., Wildberger, J., Smidt, M., *et. al.* (2023). Comparing the diagnostic performance of contrast-enhanced mammography and breast MRI: A systematic review and meta-analysis. *Journal of Cancer, 14*, 174–182. https://www.semanticscholar.org/paper/4a34d3a38cd48c067a9274200be71544c35d77a8 (accessed on 30 May 2025).

55. Nicosia, L., Gnocchi, G., Gorini, I., Venturini, M., Fontana, F., Pesapane, F., Abiuso, I., *et. al.* (2023). History of mammography: Analysis of breast imaging diagnostic achievements over the last century. *Healthcare, 11*(11), 1596. https://doi.org/10.3390/healthcare11111596.

56. Noël, V., Rodet, T., & Lesselier, D. (2025). Transfer learning for data fusion for electromagnetic and ultrasound breast imaging. *IEEE Transactions on Computational Imaging, 11*, 546–555. https://www.semanticscholar.org/paper/b3e264453efc59c82ad4831cecdded76108ba9ce (accessed on 30 May 2025).

57. Panzironi, G., Pediconi, F., & Sardanelli, F. (2019). Nipple discharge: The state of the art. https://core.ac.uk/download/188829787.pdf (accessed on 30 May 2025).

58. Pesapane, F., Tantrige, P., Rotili, A., Nicosia, L., Penco, S., Bozzini, A. C., Raimondi, S., *et. al.* (2023). Disparities in breast cancer diagnostics: How radiologists can level the inequalities. *Cancers, 16*, 130. https://doi.org/10.3390/cancers16010130.

59. Popello, V., Zucco, C., Conti, G., Alessio, C., & Cannataro, M. (2024). A software pipeline for multimodal and network-based analysis of breast cancer data. *2024 Fourth International Conference on Digital Data Processing (DDP)*. https://www.semanticscholar.org/paper/117cf08ab067a203353a87c79594d5b6d6a56b16 (accessed on 30 May 2025).

60. Preste, M. (2024). MRI-guided breast biopsy. https://core.ac.uk/download/616695397.pdf (accessed on 30 May 2025).

61. Ryu, R. R., Kim, Y. J., Seo, J. Y., Kim, K., & Kim, J. S. (2022). Breast-specific gamma imaging (BSGI) as a complementary imaging tool for BI-RADS 0 and 4a lesions on mammography or ultrasonography. *Iranian Journal of Radiology*. https://www.semanticscholar.org/paper/821617842b309d44a9bef61ac8e7f4428b8e5a67 (accessed on 30 May 2025).

62. Saadoun, A. W., Mishaal, D. A., Nadhim, A. N., Abdul Wahab, R., Matti, M. S., Hamdon, Z. T., Ghaleeb, R. R., *et. al.* (2025). Breast cancer detection through histological imaging: A machine learning approach. *International Research Journal of Innovations in Engineering and Technology*. https://www.semanticscholar.org/paper/e1d07401ab05f76b1f264cd3b2c136699bd6d6a1 (accessed on 30 May 2025).

63. Saleh, G., Batouty, N., Gamal, A., Elnakib, A., Hamdy, O., Sharafeldeen, A., Mahmoud, A. M., *et. al.* (2023). Impact of imaging biomarkers and AI on breast cancer management: A brief review. *Cancers, 15.* https://www.semanticscholar.org/paper/d4e17e5011995549e425cbaceb06a99435045567 (accessed on 30 May 2025).

64. Sarker, I. H. (2022). AI-based modeling: Techniques, applications and research issues towards automation, intelligent and smart systems. *SN Computer Science, 3.* https://doi.org/10.1007/s42979-022-01043-x.

65. Schuster, E. J., Taftaf, R., Reduzzi, C., Albert, M. K., Romero-Calvo, I., & Liu, H. (2021). Better together: Circulating tumor cell clustering in metastatic cancer. *Trends in Cancer, 7*, 1020–1032. https://doi.org/10.1016/j.trecan.2021.07.001.

66. Sinozic, T. (2014). Learning in clinical practice: Findings from CT, MRI and PACS. https://core.ac.uk/download/30608478.pdf.

67. Steinberg, I., Huland, D. M., Vermesh, O., Frostig, H., Tummers, W. S., & Gambhir, S. S. (2019). Photoacoustic clinical imaging. *Photoacoustic, 14*, 77–98. https://doi.org/10.1016/j.pacs.2019.05.001.

68. Styne, D. M., Arslanian, S., Connor, E. L., Farooqi, I. S., Murad, M. H., Silverstein, J., & Yanovski, J. A. (2017). Pediatric obesity—Assessment, treatment, and prevention: An endocrine society clinical practice guideline. *The Journal of Clinical Endocrinology & Metabolism, 102*(3), 709–757. https://doi.org/10.1210/jc.2016-2573.

69. Gabriel Tellez , M., Knutsen, E., & Perander, M. (2020). Current status of circulating tumor cells, circulating tumor DNA, and exosomes in breast cancer liquid biopsies. *International Journal of Molecular Sciences, 21*(24), 9457. https://doi.org/10.3390/ijms21249457.

70. van Kruchten, M., Glaudemans, A., de Vries, E. D., Beets-Tan, R., Schröder, C., Dierckx, R., de Vries, E., *et. al.* (2012). PET imaging of estrogen receptors as a diagnostic tool for breast cancer patients presenting with a clinical dilemma. *The Journal of Nuclear Medicine, 53*(2), 182–190. https://www.semanticscholar.org/paper/150504d74c44551fe36a14f70c19e4c15eb1a513 (accessed on 30 May 2025).

71. Vélez-Torres, L. N., Thomas, A., Hatcher, S., D'Agostino, R. B., O'Conell, N. S., Park, C. J., Hundley, W., *et. al.* (2025). Abstract 791: Increased aortic stiffening in premenopausal women and triple negative breast cancer patients: Impact of biomarkers and breast cancer therapy–Findings from the PREVENT Trial (WF-98213). *Cancer Research.* https://www.semanticscholar.org/paper/d6c123aac71b2089572137642caa116bbf14b3e8 (accessed on 30 May 2025).

72. Vogel, A., Cervantes, A., Chau, I., Daniele, B., Llovet, J. M., Meyer, T., Nault, J. C., *et. al.* (2018). Hepatocellular carcinoma: ESMO clinical practice guidelines for diagnosis, treatment and follow-up. *Annals of Oncology, 29*, iv238–iv255. https://doi.org/10.1093/annonc/mdy308.

73. Waller, J., DeStefano, K., Dempsey, J., Leckron, J., Tucker, A., & Umair, M. (2022). A primer to cost-effectiveness analysis in breast cancer imaging: A review of the literature. *Cureus.* https://doi.org/10.7759/cureus.28356.

74. Wang, L. (2023). Microwave imaging and sensing techniques for breast cancer detection. *Micromachines, 14*. https://www.semanticscholar.org/paper/3009fe7917ed36605741616edb2616902d3df9db (accessed on 30 May 2025).

75. Weber, W., Mátrai, Z., Hayoz, S., Tausch, C., Henke, G., Zimmermann, F., Montagna, G., *et. al.* (2024). Tailored axillary surgery with or without axillary lymph node dissection followed by radiotherapy in patients with clinically node-positive breast cancer (OPBC-03/SAKK 23/16/IBCSG 57-18/ABCSG-53/GBG-101-TAXIS). *Journal of Clinical Oncology*. https://www.semanticscholar.org/paper/3e6584ff519dc490a270ca1119efc9fa477fd7bc (accessed on 30 May 2025).

76. Wijata, M., Wijata, A., Dutkiewicz, J., Przybyłek-Stępień, Z., Bartosiński, R., Szustak, J., Mączyńska, W., *et. al.* (2025). The role of elastography in differentiating benign and malignant breast lesions. *Journal of Education, Health and Sport*. https://www.semanticscholar.org/paper/c305a18b84bc33b7396ac7157223655f40958e24 (accessed on 30 May 2025).

77. Yao, J., Zou, Y., Du, S., Wu, H., & Yuan, B. (2023). Progress in the application of artificial intelligence in ultrasound diagnosis of breast cancer. *Frontiers in Computing and Intelligent Systems, 6*(1), 56–59. https://doi.org/10.54097/fcis.v6i1.11.

78. Zhang, J., Cui, Z., Shi, Z., Jiang, Y., Zhang, Z., Dai, X., Yang, Z., *et. al.* (2023). A robust and efficient AI assistant for breast tumor segmentation from DCE-MRI via a spatial-temporal framework. *Patterns, 4*, 100826. https://doi.org/10.1016/j.patter.2023.100826.

79. Zheng, D., He, X., & Jing, J. (2023). Overview of artificial intelligence in breast cancer medical imaging. *Journal of Clinical Medicine, 12*, 419. https://doi.org/10.3390/jcm12020419.

80. Zhu, Z., Sun, Y., & Honarvar Shakibaei Asli, B. (2024). Early breast cancer detection using artificial intelligence techniques based on advanced image processing tools. *Electronics*. https://www.semanticscholar.org/paper/df0faa8d4dc23e29958b42e5be7872759f003e6f (accessed on 30 May 2025).

INDEX

U

V

W

X

Z